Spinal Trauma: Imaging, Diagnosis, and Management

Spinal Trauma: Imaging, Diagnosis, and Management

ERIC D. SCHWARTZ, MD

Associate Professor of Radiology
Department of Radiology
University of Pittsburgh Medical Center
Pittsburgh, Pennsylvania

ADAM E. FLANDERS, MD

Professor of Radiology and Rehabilitation Medicine
Department of Radiology, Thomas Jefferson University
Co-director, Division of Neuroradiology/ENT
Thomas Jefferson University Hospital
Philadelphia, Pennsylvania

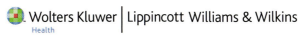

Philadelphia • Baltimore • New York • London
Buenos Aires • Hong Kong • Sydney • Tokyo

Acquisitions Editor: Lisa McAllister
Managing Editor: Kerry Barrett
Project Manager: Nicole Walz
Manufacturing Coordinator: Kathy Brown
Marketing Manager: Angela Panetta
Creative Director: Doug Smock
Cover Designer: Shawn Girsberger
Production Services: TechBooks
Printer: Walsworth Publishing Company

Library of Congress Cataloging-in-Publication Data

Spinal trauma / edited by Eric D. Schwartz, Adam E. Flanders.
   p. ; cm.
  Includes bibliographical references and index.
  ISBN-13: 978-0-7817-6248-9
  ISBN-10: 0-7817-6248-0 (case : alk. paper)
  1. Spinal cord—Wounds and injuries. I. Schwartz, Eric D.
II. Flanders, Adam E.
  [DNLM: 1. Spinal Cord Injuries–diagnosis. 2. Diagnostic Imaging
—methods. 3. Spinal Cord Injuries–therapy.   WL 400 S767 2007]
RD594.3.S695 2007
617.4'82044—dc22

                                                        2006026934

10 9 8 7 6 5 4 3 2 1

To my wonderful wife, Heidi.
(EDS)

For D & d–you make everything worthwhile!
(AEF)

CONTENTS

CONTRIBUTORS

C. Craig Blackmore, MD, MPH
Professor of Radiology and Adjunct Professor of Health
  Services
Department of Radiology
University of Washington
Associate Director of Radiology
Department of Radiology
Harborview Medical Center
Seattle, Washington

Anthony S. Burns, MD
Assistant Professor
Department of Rehabilitation Medicine
Thomas Jefferson University
Assistant Director
Regional SCI Center of the Delaware Valley
Thomas Jefferson University Hospital
Philadelphia, Pennsylvania

Hana Choe, MD
Resident
Department of Neurosurgery
Thomas Jefferson University Hospital
Philadelphia, Pennsylvania

Daniel R. Fassett, MD
Spine Fellow
Department of Neurosurgery
Thomas Jefferson University Hospital
Philadelphia, Pennsylvania

Steven Falcone, MD
Associate Professor
Department of Radiology, Neurosurgery, and
  Ophthalmology
University of Miami
Medical Director of Radiology Services
Department of Radiology
University of Miami Hospitals and Clinics
Miami, Florida

Adam E. Flanders, MD
Professor of Radiology and Rehabilitation Medicine
Department of Radiology
Thomas Jefferson University
Co-director
Division of Neuroradiology/ENT
Thomas Jefferson University Hospital
Philadelphia, Pennsylvania

James Harrop, MD
Department of Neurosurgery
Jefferson Medical Center
Philadelphia, Pennsylvania

Stephen M. Henesch, DO
Former Pediatric Radiology Fellow
Department of Radiology
The Children's Hospital of Philadelphia
Philadelphia, Pennsylvania
Director of Pediatric Radiology, Radiology Consulting of
  Long Island
Department of Radiology
Good Samaritan Hospital Medical Center
West Islip, New York

B. Timothy Himes, PhD
Research Instructor
Department of Neurobiology and Anatomy
Drexel University College of Medicine
Microbiologist
Department of Medical Research
Philadelphia VA Medical Center
Philadelphia, Pennsylvania

George Koulouris, MBBS, MMED (Radiology), FRANZCR
Musculoskeletal Radiologist
Department of Radiology
Alfred Hospital
Commercial Rd
Prahran, Victoria
Australia

Ken F. Linnau, MD, MS
Senior Fellow
Department of Radiology
University of Washington
Resident
Department of Radiology
Harborview Medical Center
Seattle, Washington

Ralph J. Marino, MD, MSCE
Associate Professor
Department of Rehabilitation Medicine
Thomas Jefferson College
Thomas Jefferson University
Clinical Director
Spinal Cord Injury Center
Department of Rehabilitation Medicine
Thomas Jefferson University Hospital
Philadelphia, Pennsylvania

William B. Morrison, MD
Associate Professor
Department of Radiology
Thomas Jefferson University
Division of Musculoskeletal and General
   Diagnostic Imaging
Department of Radiology
Thomas Jefferson University Hospital
Philadelphia, Pennsylvania

Marion Murray, PhD
Professor
Department of Neurobiology and Anatomy
Drexel University College of Medicine
Philadelphia, Pennsylvania

Diego B. Núñez, Jr., MD, MPH
Clinical Professor
Department of Radiology
Yale University School of Medicine
Chairman
Department of Radiology
Hospital of St. Raphael
New Haven, Connecticut

Avrum N. Pollock, MD, FRCPC
Assistant Professor of Radiology
Department of Radiology
University of Pennsylvania
Director of Pediatric Radiology Fellowship
   and Residency
Department of Radiology/Division of
   Neuroradiology
The Children's Hospital of Philadelphia
Philadelphia, Pennsylvania

Alejandro Zuluaga Santamaria, MD
Professor
Department of Radiology
Instituto de Ciencias de la Salud, CES
Radiologist
Department of Radiology
Cedimed
Medellin, Antioquia
Columbia

Eric D. Schwartz, MD
Associate Professor of Radiology
Department of Radiology
University of Pittsburgh Medical Center
Pittsburgh, Pennsylvania

Ashwini D. Sharan, MD
Assistant Professor of Neurosurgery and Neurology
Department of Neurosurgery
Thomas Jefferson University
Philadelphia, Pennsylvania

Laura Snyder, BS
Department of Neurosurgery
Thomas Jefferson University
Department of Neurosurgery
Thomas Jefferson University Hospital
Philadelphia, Pennsylvania

Amy Y. I. Ting, MBBS
Resident
Department of Radiology
The Alfred Hospital
Prahran, Victoria
Australia

PREFACE

Thou shouldst say concerning him: *One having a crushed vertebra in his neck; he is unconscious of his two arms [and] his two legs, [and] he is speechless. An ailment not to be treated.*

Edwin Smith Papyrus, ~1700 BCE (1)

And Hector with his sharp spear struck Eioneus on the neck below the well-made helmet of bronze, and loosed his limbs.

Homer, *The Iliad*, 600-800 BCE (2)

During ancient times, spinal trauma and paralysis was untreatable and fatal. Even in 1805, Admiral Nelson recognized the severity of his spinal injury and his imminent death after he was shot in the back and paralyzed during the Battle of Trafalgar (3). Thankfully, major advances over the past 50 to 60 years in the medical, surgical, and rehabilitation fields now allow spinal cord injury (SCI) patients to lead long and productive lives.

Despite vast improvements in conventional therapies and increased public safety awareness programs, SCI remains a significant cause of disability in the United States. This tragedy is compounded by the fact that SCI frequently afflicts the younger segment of the population—individuals who still have most of their lives to live and the greatest capacity for productivity in society. The emotional, social, and financial costs to these patients and their families are enormous. In many instances, technology provides some compensation for the functionality that is lost. The disabled patient has greater opportunities for mobility and independent living today through mechanized assist devices, portable ventilators, retrofitted automobiles, and improved public access to buildings than ever before. Adaptive computer input devices have given many SCI patients greater access to communications and control of their environments as well as opportunities for employment. Today, paralysis is no longer considered an obstacle to conceiving, bearing, or raising children.

Regaining lost function, however, remains an elusive goal. Basic scientists have identified treatments that protect and regenerate axons, and success has been achieved in animal models. Clinical application of these treatments moves slowly, and the late Christopher Reeve was known to say "Oh, to be a rat" (4). What is it going to take to move these advances from the bench to the bedside in a timely manner? While this answer is not straightforward, there are a number of promising discoveries on the horizon that may translate into effective therapies in the near future. This text promises to provide the reader with a glimpse into the future of these new therapies and diagnostic imaging methodologies in addition to a comprehensive discussion of current therapies for SCI.

Although there are a number of individual texts that touch on the various medical, surgical, and imaging aspects of spinal trauma and SCI, there is no single comprehensive text that encompasses all of the clinical, basic scientific, and therapeutic issues involved with spinal injury and treatment. This richly illustrated text focuses on using state–of-the-art imaging to diagnose and treat SCIs, and it also contains excellent reviews of the medical and surgical aspects of this disease that supplement treatises on the neuropathology, neurophysiology, and potential novel therapies. We have enlisted the help of recognized experts in their respective fields to provide content covering a wide range of topics in order to appeal to a broad audience. Additionally, we have included chapters on experimental imaging modalities and treatments with the desire of spurring discussion as to the best use of these techniques. By bringing a broad and varied subject base to this text, it is our hope that all professionals who are working to provide care and to find cures for spinal trauma (radiologists, spine surgeons, neurologists, physiatrists, physical therapists, occupational therapists and neuroscientists) will find this new material of great interest.

EDS & AEF

REFERENCES

1. Goodrich JT. History of spine surgery in the ancient and medieval worlds. *Neurosurg Focus*. 2004;16(1):E2.
2. Sahlas DJ. Functional neuroanatomy in the pre-Hippocratic era: observations from the Iliad of Homer. *Neurosurgery*. 2001;48(6):1352–1357.
3. Hanigan WC, C Sloffer. Nelson's wound: treatment of spinal cord injury in 19th and early 20th century military conflicts. *Neurosurg Focus*. 2004;16(1):E4.
4. Christopher Reeve Foundation, 2005. http://www.christopher-reeve.org/site/apps/nl/content2.asp?c=geIMLPOpGjF&b=1029401&ct=1495035.

ACKNOWLEDGMENTS

When presented with the opportunity to edit a book on spinal trauma imaging, my first thought was to ask Adam Flanders for help. We had been part of a symposium on spinal trauma imaging in 2002, and I knew his experience and knowledge of the clinical aspects of spinal cord injury would be crucial in creating this book. I also guessed correctly that his sense of humor would make this project more fun, and I am looking forward to many more cups of coffee with him.

I would like to thank my mentors (and friends) over the past decade who led me into the rewarding field of neuroradiology and spinal cord injury. I am thankful to have trained and published at the University of Miami with Robert Quencer, MD; Pradip Pattany, PhD; and Steven Falcone, MD, MBA. As a fellow, and then a staff member, at the University of Pennsylvania, I have been fortunate to have been mentored by David Hackney, MD and Elias Melhem, MD, PhD, and I am grateful to have worked with the most talented and hardworking staff I have known: Linda Bagley, MD; Ed Herskovits, MD, PhD; Bob Hurst, MD; Frank Lexa, MD; Laurie Loevner, MD; Gul Moonis, MD; John Weigele, MD, PhD; Ron Wolf, MD, PhD; John Woo, MD; and Lisa Desiderio, RT.

When I first arrived in Philadelphia, I began collaborating and studying under leading spinal cord injury neuroscientists at the Drexel University College of Medicine, including Marion Murray, PhD and Alan Tessler, MD. Working with them has been a highlight of my professional career, and their dedication to developing a cure for spinal cord injury is inspirational. I am happy to continue my association with them and other talented members of this group, including Jonathan Nissanov, PhD; Jed Shumsky, PhD; Tim Himes, PhD; and Theresa Connors.

Our LWW editors, Kerry Barrett and Lisa McAllister, have been fantastic and unbelievably patient. They are probably still wondering if Adam and I understand the definition of *deadline*. Adam and I were lucky to recruit contributors who are a veritable *who's who* in the field of spinal cord injury and imaging. Every chapter is fantastic and editing this volume has been a tremendous learning experience for me.

Most importantly, I have been blessed with a loving family. My mother and father, Nancy and David, have always been there for me from my childhood to the present, and their love of education and reading is one I hope to instill in my own children.

My children, Noah and Rebecca, are looking forward to the publication of the book. Noah continues to show interest in learning about the human body, especially with radiological images, and Rebecca loves books with lots of pictures.

I have saved the final paragraph for my beautiful wife Heidi. I would be lost without her, both professionally and personally. She is a terrific mother and role model for our children. By the time the book is published, we will have celebrated our tenth wedding anniversary, and I see only more happy years in our future.

EDS

The creation of a textbook usually involves a lot more effort *behind the scenes* than just the contribution of the authors and editors. There are a number of people who helped nurture this book to fruition to whom I would like to express my appreciation. I would like to acknowledge Anthony Burns, MD who first encouraged Eric Schwartz and I to meet and collaborate on projects of mutual interest. I am grateful to Eric for being the driving force behind this project, for working around my hectic schedule, for doing *more* than his share of the work, for keeping us as close to schedule as humanly possible, and for making the entire process fun and enjoyable.

I want to express my gratitude to Barbara L. Malamut, PhD and Laurence S. Shtasel, JD for providing their expert advice and helping us get this project off the ground.

My 19-year collaboration with the staff of The Regional Spinal Cord Injury Center of the Delaware Valley (RSCICDV) fostered my interest in spinal cord injury research and this experience has been both unique and unbelievably gratifying. The RSCICDV is one of the few model systems centers for spinal cord injury. Being a part of their team has been extremely rewarding professionally. Weekly participation in multidisciplinary clinical spinal cord injury conferences for the RSCICDV was primarily responsible for nurturing my interest in spinal injury and has provided me with a tremendous sense of appreciation of how multiple clinical services can work together for a common goal. Over the years, I have had the privilege of working closely with and learning from several exceptional spine surgeons who specialized in spinal trauma at Thomas Jefferson University Hospital: Jerome M. Cotler, MD; Bruce E. Northrup, MD; Jewell L. Osterholm, MD; and Dale M. Schaefer, MD; and currently: James S. Harrop, MD; Ashwini D. Sharon, MD; and Alexander R. Vaccaro, MD. I have been particularly fortunate to have been mentored by one of the most respected leaders of the American Spinal Injury Association (ASIA) and the current Project Director of the RSCICDV, John F. Ditunno, MD. Doctor Ditunno was visionary in his support of advanced imaging as an adjunct to the clinical examination. He has been instrumental in the incorporation of advanced imaging into RSCICDV clinical protocols, and he has been an evangelist for imaging in clinical research trials. Another highlight of my early collaboration with the RSCICDV was having the privilege to work and learn from Gerald J. Herbison, MD—a man who is not only a model clinician, teacher, and researcher, but also has a heart of gold. I am eternally grateful to the RSCICDV staff, in particular Mary Patrick, RN and Belinda Siegfried, for their amazing level of support and assistance in all of our cooperative projects.

I would also like to acknowledge my colleagues in the division of Neuroradiology/ENT at Thomas Jefferson University Hospital: Scott Enochs, MD, PhD; Steven Finden, MD; David P. Friedman, MD; Richard J.T. Gorniak, MD; Vijay M. Rao, MD; Dinesh K. Sharma, MD; Lisa M. Tartaglino, MD; Pamela Van Tassel, MD; and Michael J. Wolf, MD for their encouragement and for promoting an atmosphere conducive to academic pursuits.

I am also indebted to my parents: Norman, who instilled in me the sense to make good thoughtful decisions in life, and Eileen, who encouraged me to question everything (especially when it doesn't make sense). To my older brother (*Brot*) Sam, I am grateful that you paved the way to make my life easier.

Lastly, I owe a huge debt of gratitude and love to my wife, Deborah, and my daughter, Danielle, for enduring many weekday evenings alone while Eric and I hunkered down at the local Borders to work on our book. This project never would have happened without your understanding and encouragement!

AEF

FOREWORD

Since the 1980s, there have been significant advances in the evaluation and assessment of the spine-injured patient, particularly in the imaging of such injuries. With the evolution of magnetic resonance imaging (MRI), which can show fine soft tissue details, and with the widespread use of multidetector computed tomography (CT) yielding astonishingly high-quality bony detail in primary and reformatted (including three-dimensional) planes, the treating physician now has a clearer picture of the nature of the injury and how to best formulate a treatment strategy. In many cases, imaging has modified the clinical and surgical approach to these patients, and it has altered our understanding of the nature of these injuries. From acute spine column and spinal cord injuries, through the evolving pathophysiologic changes of neural tissue over time, to the more chronic stages of injury, imaging now gives us the opportunity to closely monitor and potentially treat new and/or evolving neurologic symptoms. Therefore, it is noteworthy that Dr Eric Schwartz, Associate Professor of Radiology at the University of Pittsburgh, and Dr Adam Flanders, Professor of Radiology at Thomas Jefferson University, have compiled the latest information on spine trauma under one cover, *Spinal Trauma*. Not only are both of these neuroradiologists well known for their publications in imaging literature, but they have received contributions from authors who have extensive experience in the evaluation of spine trauma. Because of the co-authorship across multiple disciplines, this book speaks with authority.

The book has been wisely divided into three sections, starting the reader first with the basic pathophysiology, neurology, and surgery of spine and spinal cord injury, which leads to the largest section of the book, imaging, and then to a final experimental section. A wealth of knowledge lays at the reader's doorstep, and one quickly realizes the ongoing biochemical and functional changes in neural and perineural tissues and the critical intersection of image interpretation and clinical care. For instance, the long-held but now discredited theory of the static nature of the chronically or previously injured spinal cord is dealt with not only on the basis of imaging but with critical surgical

correlations. This type of correlation is prominent throughout the book and makes the material presented applicable to the daily care of spine injured patients. In addition, from a practical standpoint, the proper sequencing of imaging studies (plain films, CT, MRI), and the protocols most useful in CT and MRI, incrementally adds to the book's value. This material, therefore, primarily serves to integrate the imaging and treatment of patients

It is of particular interest that the book does not confine itself to the imaging and clinical aspects of spine injury, but rather that it ends with a chapter on experimental therapies of spinal cord injury. Here again, the reader will begin to appreciate the possibilities for the intersection of novel therapies and advanced imaging. MRI will presumably lead the way in monitoring many of the issues mentioned, such as cellular transplantation and neural related growth factors, the effects of such interventions on the structural integrity of the cord determined with diffusion imaging and tractography, and the physiologic improvement or deterioration of such patients with MR-based neural activation studies (fMR). When a second edition of this book is published, one would expect an increasing correlation between experimental work and clinical interventions. This first edition affords a springboard to that future.

To those seeking a basic understanding of the mechanisms and neurologic sequela of spinal cord injury and the basics of the medical and surgical management of various types of spine injury, to those wanting an in-depth explanation of the imaging of all phases of spine injury, and to those engaged in basic cord injury research who wish to know what is important clinically, this book should have great appeal. Drs Flanders and Schwartz and the multiple contributing authors are to be congratulated on producing a book, which will be of great use to both the radiologist and treating clinician.

Robert M. Quencer, MD
Chairman, Department of Radiology
The Robert Shapiro, MD Professor of Radiology
University of Miami Miller School of Medicine
Miami, Florida

SECTION I

Clinical

Chapter 1

Pathophysiology of Spinal Cord Injury

B. Timothy Himes

Spinal cord injury is not one event, but a sequence of interrelated processes that can ultimately lead to destruction of neural tissue and, as a consequence, a dramatic loss of locomotor and sensory function. Understanding these processes and their chronology starting immediately after trauma and continuing for the weeks, months, and even years afterward is vital to the development of a comprehensive repair strategy for spinal cord injury (SCI). Unlike the peripheral nervous system (PNS), where injured axons can regenerate their damaged axons and reestablish functional connections with peripheral targets, regeneration in the central nervous system (CNS) and spinal cord is extremely limited. Neurons that die as a result of SCI are not replaced by proliferation from stem cells, and the severed axons of surviving neurons cannot reconstruct damaged axonal pathways. However, most human spinal cord injuries, even those that are physiologically complete, are anatomically incomplete and spare both intraspinal and peripheral pathways. Limited but substantial reorganization of unlesioned circuits has been proposed to contribute to the spontaneous recovery of sensory and motor function often seen following SCI. Injured spinal cord neurons do have the capacity to regenerate, however, and for almost 50 years it has been known that injured axons can send out regenerative sprouts in the acute phase following injury (1) and that axonal growth can be extensive if injured axons are provided with a permissive environment (2). Unfortunately the regenerative response collapses before functional benefits are realized. Successful spinal cord repair will ultimately involve several factors, not only restoration of neural cells and circuits lost as a direct consequence of SCI, but also management of factors within the CNS that inhibit successful regeneration.

EMBRYOLOGY, ANATOMY, HISTOLOGY, AND FUNCTION OF NORMAL SPINAL CORD

Embryology

The spinal cord is a roughly cylindrical structure located in the spinal canal of the vertebral column. In humans the spinal cord is about 42 to 45 cm long and 1 cm in diameter. This bilaterally symmetrical structure extends from the medulla caudally, ending, on average, at the level of the disc between the first and second lumbar vertebrae (Fig. 1-1). The spinal cord is conical in shape at its caudal end, a region known as the *conus medullaris*. From this tapered cone a thin filament, the *filum terminale*, continues caudally. At approximately the second sacral segment the filum terminale alone becomes ensheathed in dura and continues as the coccygeal ligament to attach to the

dorsum of the coccyx. Until the third month of fetal development the spinal cord extends the entire length of the spinal canal. After the third fetal month the lengthening rate of the spinal column is greater than the spinal cord such that in the adult the spinal cord occupies only the rostral two thirds of the spinal canal. It is therefore necessary for the lumbar and sacral nerve roots to descend within the spinal canal a considerable distance in order to exit from the appropriate intervertebral foramina. The filum terminale, surrounded by these lumbosacral nerve roots, comprises a structure known as the *cauda equina*, which extends in the spinal canal from the second lumbar to the second sacral vertebral segment. This region is also known as the *lumbar cistern* since there is sufficient subarachnoid space for the accumulation of cerebrospinal fluid (CSF). The withdrawal of a CSF sample by lumbar puncture between the third and fourth lumbar vertebrae can be accomplished in the lumbar cistern with minimal risk of damage to neural tissue, due to the absence of the spinal cord in this region. Covering the spinal cord are the same layers of meninges (pia mater, arachnoid, and dura mater) as those that cover the brain. The spinal cord is suspended in CSF within the subarachnoid space and held in place by a series of *denticulate ligaments*. The denticulate (dentate) ligaments are extensions of the pia mater that connect the spinal cord to the dura mater laterally. They are located midway between the dorsal and ventral roots and extend from the foramen magnum to below the exit of the first lumbar spinal nerve (Fig. 1-2).

Although the spinal cord grossly appears uniform and symmetrical on the exterior, it is anatomically arranged in segments with paired spinal nerves exiting into the body at each of 31 levels (8 cervical [C], 12 thoracic [T], 5 lumbar [L], 5 sacral [S], and 1 coccygeal) via the intervertebral foramina (Fig. 1-1). In the cervical spinal cord the nerves exit through the intervertebral foramina just rostral to the vertebra of the same name, but since there are eight cervical nerve roots and only seven cervical vertebrae, the eighth cervical spinal nerve exits through the intervertebral foramina just rostral to the first thoracic vertebra. The thoracic, lumbar, and sacral spinal nerves exit through the intervertebral foramina just caudal to the vertebra of the same name. The spinal nerve is composed of a dorsal root of afferent fibers and a ventral root containing efferent fibers. The dorsal and ventral roots are within the dural sheath of the spinal cord until they reach the intervertebral foramina where the dorsal root ganglion is located. An anatomical variation seen in humans is that the C1 dorsal root ganglia and root are missing in almost 50% of the cases with only a C1 ventral root being present. Each spinal nerve is related to a specific somite during development such that in the adult spinal cord segments form a systematic sensory relationship to areas of skin, muscle, and bone. This unit is known as a dermatome, and the understanding of the segmental

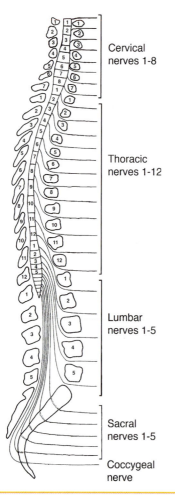

Cervical nerves 1-8

Thoracic nerves 1-12

Lumbar nerves 1-5

Sacral nerves 1-5

Coccygeal nerve

FIGURE 1-1. Illustrates the anatomical relationship between the spinal cord and the segmentally arranged spinal nerves of the vertebral column. The dorsal surface is to the left. Note that there are eight cervical spinal cord segments but only seven cervical vertebrae.

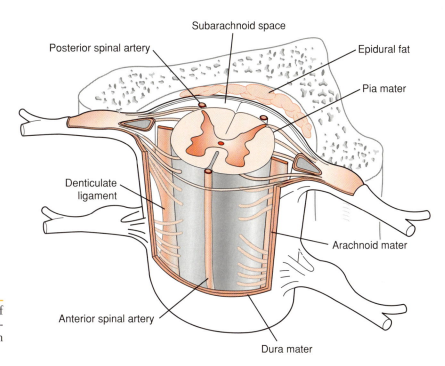

Subarachnoid space

Posterior spinal artery

Epidural fat

Pia mater

Denticulate ligament

Arachnoid mater

Anterior spinal artery

Dura mater

FIGURE 1-2. Illustrates the relationship of the denticulate ligaments to the other structures that surround the spinal cord within the spinal canal.

innervation of muscles and cutaneous regions is an important clinical tool for diagnosing the site of damage to the spinal cord (Fig. 1-3). Axons outside the spinal cord, in either the dorsal or ventral roots, are no longer associated with processes of CNS glia (astrocytes, oligodendrocytes), but are now nurtured, supported, and myelinated by the Schwann cells of the PNS.

Gray Matter and Neuronal Pathways

A cross section through the spinal cord shows its organization generally to be opposite that of the brain; with a butterfly-shaped gray matter core of neurons and glia surrounded by myelinated axon fiber bundles and tracts in the outer white matter (Fig. 1-4). Rexed (3,4) first described the cytoarchitectural organization of the spinal cord gray matter in the cat spinal cord. The gray matter was subdivided into ten layers or laminae (Fig. 1-4C). This organizational map has been applied to the spinal cord of other mammals, including humans. The histological differences seen in the gray matter correspond to functional differences (Table 1-1). Laminae I through V are found in the dorsal horn, laminae VI and VII comprise the intermediate zone gray matter, laminae VIII and IX make up most of the ventral horn, and lamina X surrounds the central canal.

Many of the neurons within the spinal cord are spinal interneurons, neurons whose synaptic connections are completely within the spinal cord. Projection neurons are neurons whose cell bodies are located in the spinal cord and that send their axons out of the spinal cord rostrally

into the brainstem and cerebellum. Spinal motor neurons are neurons in the ventral spinal cord that send their axons via the ventral root directly to muscles in the periphery. In lamina IX of the spinal cord there are two types of spinal motor neurons. The larger alpha (α) motor neurons innervate the extrafusal fibers of striated skeletal muscles. The smaller and less numerous gamma (γ) motor neurons innervate intrafusal muscle fibers of the neuromuscular spindles. Information from the brain ultimately reaches motor neurons in the ventral (anterior) horn gray matter and leaves the spinal cord via the ventral roots to innervate appropriate muscles. Preganglionic sympathetic neurons supplying the entire body lie in a column of cells known as the intermediolateral cell column located in spinal segments T1 through L3. Their axons exit the spinal cord via the ventral roots (Fig. 1-5). Cells in a similar location in S2 to S4 make up the sacral parasympathetic nuclei, and their axons leave the spinal cord in the ventral roots to synapse on postganglionic parasympathetic neurons in the pelvic viscera.

Afferent information from the body is transmitted to the spinal cord via the dorsal root ganglia and dorsal roots into the dorsal (posterior) horn for processing and relay to higher brain levels. The dorsal root at each spinal cord segment consists of six to eight rootlets. The axons in each rootlet are divided into two divisions. The lateral division contains mostly unmyelinated (group C) and many finely myelinated (small group A) axons that convey sensory information related to pain and temperature. These axons enter the dorsolateral (Lissauer) tract and send ascending and descending branches that give off

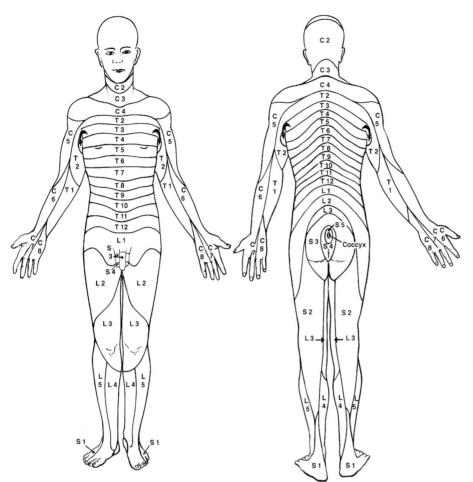

FIGURE 1-3. Dermatomes represent the cutaneous distribution of territories innervated by spinal nerves. For example, the T5 dorsal nerve root supplies sensory function to a band of skin at the nipple line, whereas the L2 dorsal nerve root provides sensory function to the skin of the anterior thigh.

collateral axons as they enter the dorsal horn of the spinal cord. The majority of these collateral axons terminate in the spinal cord segment in which they enter, but the branching can extend many segments rostral and caudal to their level of entry. These small diameter afferents terminate mainly in laminae I, II, and V of the gray matter. The medial division of the dorsal root consists of larger caliber faster conducting axons (large group A) carrying sensory information related to discriminative touch and conscious proprioception. As these axons enter the spinal cord they send collateral axons into the gray matter of the segment where they enter the spinal cord and also send branches rostral and caudal to the segment of entry. Locally these axons terminate in the deeper layers of the dorsal horn (laminae III and IV), and some branches terminate on motor neurons in the ventral horn (lamina IX) and are part of the stretch reflex.

Spinal Cord White Matter Tracts

The white matter is composed of longitudinally arranged myelinated and unmyelinated axons and subdivided into three regions: the dorsal (or posterior), lateral, and ventral

(or anterior) funiculi. Within the funiculi long tract axons can ascend or descend the length of the spinal cord, connecting the brain and spinal cord. The funiculi also contain propriospinal axons connecting spinal cord segments that are close together or far apart (Fig. 1-4).

The dorsal funiculus contains mostly ascending axons from first-order neurons of the dorsal root ganglia (the dorsal column pathway). The afferents from segments T6 and rostral ascend more laterally in the fasciculus cuneatus, while afferents from segments caudal to T6 ascend medially in the fasciculus gracilis. The fasciculi gracilis and cuneatus are also referred to as the dorsal (posterior) columns. Between the dorsal and lateral funiculus, at the lateral edge of the dorsal horn, is the Lissauer tract (fasciculus dorsolateralis), a region of white matter that contains finely myelinated and unmyelinated primary afferent axons entering lamina II (substantia gelatinosa). The lateral and ventral funiculi contain both ascending and descending tracts. The positions of these tracts have been determined from clinical and pathological studies and from comparison with experiments conducted in animals (Fig. 1-4). Of the described pathways, the dorsal column, spinothalamic,

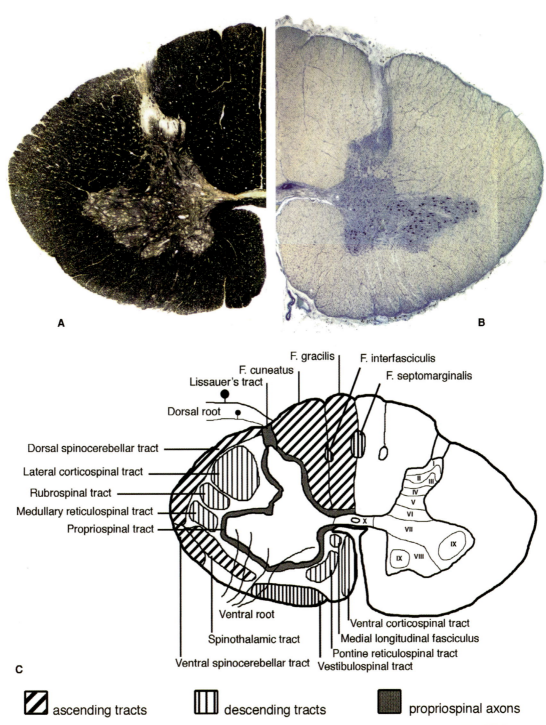

FIGURE 1-4. The structure of the human spinal cord represented in cross section at the level of the eighth cervical segment (C8). By convention, the ventral surface of the spinal cord is oriented inferiorly. **A:** The left half of the spinal cord is shown stained for myelin. Heavily myelinated axons in the white matter stain darkly for myelin while the butterfly-shaped gray matter in stained less strongly. The superficial dorsal (posterior) horn and the gray matter around the central canal contain very little myelin. **B:** The right half of the spinal cord shown after staining for Nissl substance. The density of cell bodies in the gray matter is much higher than in the white matter. The cell bodies of large motor neurons can be seen in the ventral (anterior) horn. **C:** A drawing of the major anatomical features present in the spinal cord. Many of the major axon tracts are represented on the left side of the drawing. The right side shows the lamination of the spinal cord gray matter as described by Rexed (3,4) and detailed in Table 1-1.

▶ **TABLE 1-1** **Laminar Organization of the Spinal Cord Gray Matter**

La	Structures	Input(s)	Output
Mina			
I	Marginal zone cells	Nociceptors, thermoreceptors	Spinothalamic tract
II	Substantia gelatinosa	Nociceptors	Local propriospinal
III–IV	Nucleus proprius	Low threshold mechanoreceptors, substantia gelatinosa	Spinothalamic, postsynaptic dorsal column
V		Low threshold mechanoreceptors, corticospinal and rubrospinal tracts	Spinothalamic tract
VI	Present in cervical and lumbar segments	Muscle spindle and joint afferents, corticospinal and rubrospinal tracts	Spinothalamic, spinoreticular, spinomesencephalic
VII	Clarke nucleus (T1–L2), intermediolateral cell column (T1–L2), sacral parasympathetic nuclei (S2–S4)	Muscle and tendon afferents	Dorsal spinocerebellar tract, preganglionic axons of autonomic system
VIII	Motor interneurons and long propriospinal neurons	Muscle, skin, and joint afferents, vestibulospinal and reticulospinal tracts	Motor neurons, other interneurons
IX	Motor neurons	Ia afferents, interneurons	Muscle
X	Gray matter around central canal	Nociceptors, visceral afferents	Spinoreticular, propriospinal

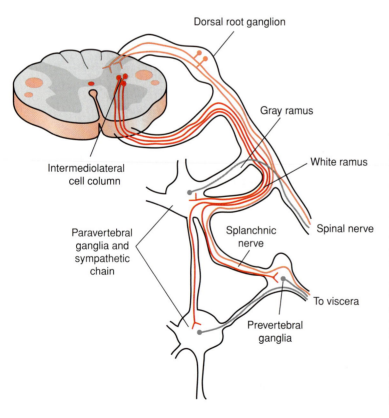

Dorsal root ganglion

Gray ramus

White ramus

Intermediolateral
cell column

Spinal nerve

Paravertebral
ganglia and
sympathetic
chain

Splanchnic
nerve

To viscera

Prevertebral
ganglia

FIGURE 1-5. The sympathetic nervous system and its relationship to the central nervous system. Sympathetic preganglionic neurons (red) are located in the intermediolateral cell column of the thoracic spinal cord. Their axons leave the spinal cord via the ventral root and enter paravertebral and sympathetic chain ganglia on the ipsilateral side of the body through the white communicating ramus. Some fibers synapse within ganglia at the same segmental level, others travel up and down the sympathetic chain to other ganglia. Postganglionic sympathetic fibers arising from cells in the paravertebral or sympathetic chain ganglia (green) join a spinal nerve by passing through a gray communicating ramus. These supply smooth muscle and glands of the body wall. Other postganglionic fibers travel through a splanchnic nerve to innervate viscera of the body cavities. Axons from sensory (pain) neurons (blue) supplying an internal organ may pass through autonomic ganglia, but they originate from neurons in the dorsal root ganglia.

spinocerebellar, corticospinal, reticulospinal, rubrospinal, and vestibulospinal pathways are somatotopically arranged.

Dorsal Funiculus

The majority of axons in the dorsal funiculus originate from dorsal root ganglia. There is also a component arising from neurons within the dorsal horn. As the tracts ascend the spinal cord axons from each spinal cord segment are added to the lateral side of the funiculus. As a result, in the upper cervical spinal cord the lowest levels of segmental innervation are located in the most medial part of the funiculus. Many of these axons convey sensory information about discriminative touch sensations and the ability to detect changes in the positions of tactile stimuli to the skin. This information is conveyed directly to nuclei in the caudal brainstem—the cuneate nucleus receives information from the body above T6 via the *fasciculus cuneatus*; the gracilis nucleus receives information from the body below T6 via the *fasciculus gracilis*. Conscious awareness of joint movement and position sense of a limb (proprioception) is conveyed from muscle spindles and, to a lesser degree, Golgi tendon organs. This information from the upper limb is carried ipsilaterally to the external or lateral cuneate nucleus in the brainstem. Similar information from the lower limb is sent to the ipsilateral nucleus dorsalis of Clarke within the thoracic spinal cord, and second order axons from these cells ascend the spinal cord ipsilaterally as the dorsal spinocerebellar tract in the lateral funiculus.

Within the dorsal funiculus there are also axons that descend the spinal cord. These axons arise from three sources: neurons in the gracile and cuneate nuclei, spinal cord gray matter, and dorsal root ganglia. The descending axons from the dorsal column nuclei form connections throughout the spinal cord, allowing the modification of sensory information sent from the spinal cord to the brain. Spinal to spinal axons can run almost the entire length of the spinal cord in both directions and could be involved in reflex coordination between the upper and lower limbs. Descending branches of primary afferents provide a means of communication between adjacent segmental levels of the body and may be part of a system that allows the regulation of signals to eventually be transmitted to the brain through long ascending tracts. Some of the long descending primary afferent axons of the dorsal funiculi are organized in distinct bundles: the *fasciculus septomarginalis*, adjacent to the dorsal septum, and the *fasciculus interfascicularis*, between the gracile and cuneate fasciculi.

Lateral Funiculus

The *lateral corticospinal tract* is located in the dorsal portion of the lateral funiculus and is comprised of axons

from neurons in the contralateral frontal and parietal lobes of the cerebral cortex (Fig. 1-6). The axons of this tract arise from layer 5 cells of the precentral cortical area (area 4), the premotor and supplementary motor areas (area 6), and the postcentral gyrus (areas 3, 1, and 2). Approximately 90% of these axons decussate at the medullary pyramid before entering the lateral funiculus. There is also a very small component (2%) of corticospinal axons that do not cross at the medullary pyramid

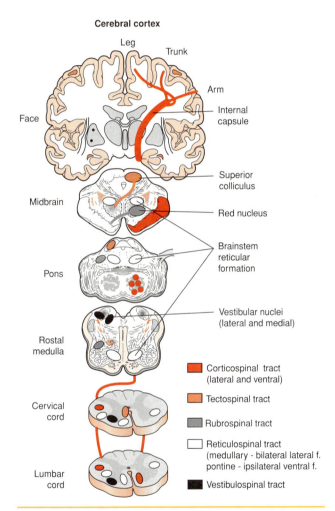

FIGURE 1-6. A diagrammatic representation of the main descending motor pathways connecting the brain to the spinal cord for one side of the body. Approximately 90% of the corticospinal axons cross at the spinomedullary junction and comprise the lateral corticospinal tract. The remaining 10% form the ipsilateral ventral corticospinal tract. Axons from cells in the contralateral superior colliculus pass through the brainstem and enter cervical levels of the spinal cord in the tectospinal tract. The red nucleus sends axons to the contralateral spinal cord in the rubrospinal tract. Neurons from many levels and both sides of the reticular formation form the reticulospinal tract. The medial and lateral vestibular nuclei send axons to the spinal cord in the vestibulospinal tract. This is mainly and ipsilaterally projecting pathway.

and synapse on ipsilateral neurons throughout the spinal cord. The tract is known as the *uncrossed lateral corticospinal tract*. Corticospinal fibers from the frontal cortex synapse mainly in the intermediate gray matter and the ventral horn. Fibers from parietal cortex end in the dorsal horn. The lateral corticospinal tract is somatotopically organized so that fibers directed for the most caudal levels of the spinal cord are located most laterally in the tract. This tract controls voluntary movement of the contralateral limbs.

Axons of the *raphespinal tract* originate from the nucleus raphe magnus in the reticular formation of the medulla and terminate in laminae I, II, and III of the spinal cord. This tract of unmyelinated axons is located in the most dorsal part of the lateral funiculus. Many of these axons contain serotonin, which may be used as a neurotransmitter in this system. The raphespinal tract acts to modify transmission from the dorsal horn of impulses initiated by noxious or painful stimuli.

The *rubrospinal tract* arises from the red nucleus in the rostral midbrain tegmentum. The axons from this nucleus cross in the ventral midbrain (the ventral tegmental decussation) and descend to the contralateral spinal cord. Rubrospinal tract axons are somatotopically arranged such that cervical spinal cord segments receive fibers for the dorsal part of the red nucleus, which receives input from the upper limb region of the sensorimotor cortex. Similarly, lumbosacral spinal cord segments are contacted by axons from the ventral half of the red nucleus, which receives input from the leg region of sensorimotor cortex. Rubrospinal axons synapse on interneurons in spinal cord layers V through VII. These neurons in turn project to motor neurons in the ventral horn. Many of the projections and functions of the rubrospinal tract have been defined from rodent studies. This tract may in fact not be of clinical significance since it has not been shown to project past the most rostral cervical spinal cord segments in primates and humans (5).

The major descending tract in the ventral portion of the lateral funiculus is the *medullary (lateral) reticulospinal tract*. It is derived mainly from the gigantocellulare reticular nucleus of the medulla. Most of the fibers are uncrossed but a small proportion cross the midline in the medulla. Whereas the corticospinal tract controls skilled voluntary movements, the reticulospinal tracts control activities that do not require constant conscious control. It is also responsible for the suppression of extensor spinal reflex activity.

Axons of neurons located in the Clarke nucleus ascend ipsilaterally forming the *dorsal (posterior) spinocerebellar tract* and reach the cerebellum via the inferior cerebellar peduncle. The tract is seen most caudally at L2 and increases in size until it reaches C8. Afferent fibers in segment caudal to L2 ascend in the fasciculus gracilis and synapse in the Clarke nucleus at L2. The dorsal spinocere-

bellar tract transmits information about muscle spindle and tendon afferents from the ipsilateral lower limb and provides the cerebellum with information about the status of individual as well as groups of muscles, thus enabling the control of movement of lower limb muscles and posture.

The *ventral (anterior) spinocerebellar tract* is located in the superficial ventrolateral funiculus. It originates from neurons at the base of the dorsal horn and the spinal border cells that are located along the lateral edge of the ventral horn in the lumbosacral spinal cord. Most of the axons cross the spinal cord at the level of origin and ascend contralaterally. The tract ascends as far as the midbrain and then the axons cross the midline for a second time to enter the cerebellum through the superior cerebellar peduncle. Both spinocerebellar tracts therefore transmit sensory information from one side of the body to the same side of the cerebellum.

The *spinothalamic tract* forms in the ventral portion of the lateral funiculus from ascending axons of neurons located in the gray matter of the opposite side of the spinal cord (Fig. 1-7). The cells of origin are in the nucleus proprius (laminae IV to VI) as well a smaller contribution from cells in laminae I, VII, VIII, and X. The axons grow across the midline in the ventral white commissure near the central canal and through the contralateral ventral horn to enter the ventrolateral and ventral funiculi. The spinothalamic tract carries information regarding tactile, thermal, and painful sensations. Its fibers are somatotopically arranged with those for the lower limb lying most dorsolaterally and those for the upper limb are more ventromedial. The main pathway in the spinothalamic tract connects second order neurons of the spinal cord gray matter with the ventral posterolateral nucleus of the thalamus (Fig. 1-8). Other axons running within the

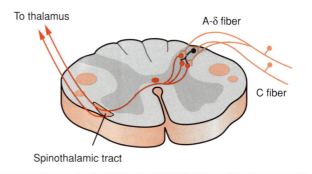

FIGURE 1-7. Primary afferents carrying pain synapse on neurons in the spinal cord dorsal horn. A-δ afferents enter laminae I and V and synapse on a second order projection neurons that transmit the information directly to the thalamus. C fibers enter the spinal cord and synapse on interneurons primarily in lamina II that then synapse on other neurons in lamina I or V. The axons of these neurons then enter either the spinothalamic or other (spinoreticular, spinomesencephalic) pathways.

spinothalamic tract form multisynaptic connections with several locations in the brain including midline and intralaminar thalamic nuclei, reticular formation, hypothalamus and limbic system and are involved in the activation of pain-inhibiting mechanisms (Fig. 1-8, Table 1-2).

There are two other small tracts that ascend the spinal cord in the ventral portion of the lateral funiculus. The *spinotectal* or *spinomesencephalic tract* originates from cells in laminae IV to VIII. Their axons cross the midline and then project rostrally to the periaqueductal gray matter, superior colliculus, and several nuclei in the reticular formation of the midbrain. The *spinoreticular tract* also

▶ **TABLE 1-2** Direct and Indirect Pathways of Pain Transmission from the Body

Tract	Spinothalamic	Spinoreticular
Body representation	Contralateral	Bilateral
Minimum number of synapses between primary afferent neuron and thalamus	One	Two or more
Final targets other than cortex	None	Hypothalamus, limbic system, autonomic nuclei
Thalamic nuclei in pathway	Ventral posterio-lateral (VPL)	Intralaminar nuclei
Cortical termination	Parietal lobe (SI)	Cingulate gyrus
Function	Discriminative pain (type, intensity, location)	Affective and arousal components of pain

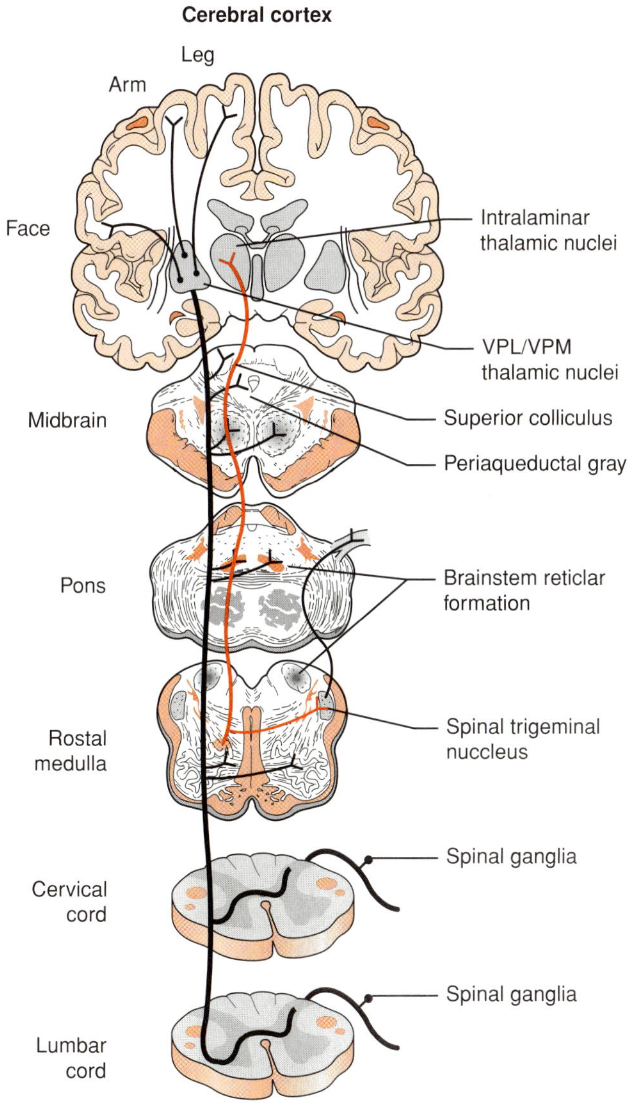

FIGURE 1-8. The transmission of pain from the body to the brain occurs in the anterolateral system, also called the spinothalamic tract. Axons of the anterolateral system terminate in the several regions including the reticular formation throughout the brainstem, superior colliculus, periaqueductal gray, and several thalamic nuclei.

originates in laminae IV to VIII and includes crossed fibers that terminate in the pontine reticular formation and uncrossed fibers that terminate in the medullary reticular formation. Many of these axons are thought to be collateral branches of spinothalamic axons. They are part of the ascending reticular activating system and may be involved in the perception of pain and of various sensations that originate in internal organs (Fig. 1-8, Table 1-2).

Ventral Funiculus

The *vestibulospinal tract* is an uncrossed pathway originating from neurons of the lateral vestibular (Deiters) nucleus in the medulla. These axons leave the tract and enter the spinal cord at all levels and synapse on neurons in laminae VII and VIII and also terminate directly on motor neurons at the cervical and lumbar levels. It is the principal route by which the vestibular system brings about postural changes to compensate for tilts and movements of the body.

Within the medial aspect of the pontine reticular formation are two groups of neurons: the nucleus reticularis pontis caudalis (caudal pontine reticular nucleus) and nucleus reticularis pontis oralis (oral pontine reticular nucleus), which give rise to the *pontine (medial) reticulospinal tract*. These neurons project ipsilaterally along the entire spinal cord with their principal function being the facilitation of extensor spinal reflexes.

Another important nucleus located in the brainstem that projects to the spinal cord is the *locus coeruleus (ceruleus)*. This nucleus is located dorsolateral to the oral pontine reticular nucleus. Neurons of the locus coeruleus contain the neurotransmitter norepinephrine (noradrenaline). The axons of these neurons branch widely and project to virtually all regions of the CNS, including the cerebral cortex, diencephalons, brainstem, cerebellum, and spinal cord. Axons projecting to the spinal cord are diffusely scattered in the ventral and lateral funiculus.

The ipsilateral and contralateral medial vestibulospinal nucleus projects to the cervical spinal cord as part of the *medial longitudinal fasciculus* (MLF). Descending axons of the MLF are located in the dorsal part of the ventral funiculus and project mainly to upper cervical spinal cord segments. These axons monosynaptically inhibit motor neurons located in the upper cervical spinal cord. It is responsible for stabilizing the head position during movement. In the brainstem, many secondary vestibular fibers project directly through the MLF to the motor neurons of the oculomotor, trochlear, and abducens nuclei, forming the basis of the vestibulo-ocular reflex. A small group of descending axons entering the spinal cord and, running in the superficial ventromedial portion of the ventral funiculus, come from neurons in the superior colliculus and form the *tectospinal tract*. These axons terminate in laminae VI, VII, and VIII in rostral segments of the cervical spinal cord and are involved with directing head movements in response to visual and auditory stimuli.

Another component of corticospinal fibers, the *ventral (anterior) corticospinal tract*, is located in the most medial portion of the ventral funiculus and is compose of 8% of corticospinal axons that did not cross at the medullary pyramid. These axons descend the spinal cord and eventually cross the midline of the spinal cord at different segmental levels to synapse on cells in the contralateral ventral horn.

Propriospinal Tract

In all three funiculi, the white matter immediately adjacent to gray matter contains the majority of propriospinal axons, both ascending and descending within the spinal cord. Shorter axons are found closer to the gray matter than longer fibers. Some of these axons can cross the midline of the spinal cord, while others remain ipsilateral. They connect different segments of the spinal cord and mediate intrinsic reflex mechanisms of the spinal cord including the coordination of upper and lower limb movements.

HISTOLOGY AND PATHOPHYSIOLOGY OF ACUTE SPINAL CORD INJURY

Experimental Models of Spinal Cord Injury

Cases of SCI that involve gunshot or stab injuries (sharp trauma) may result in complete severing of the spinal cord, but in most cases patients present with an anatomically incomplete lesion of the spinal cord. Compression or contusion injury (blunt trauma) is more frequent, occurring as a result of fracture or subluxation of the vertebrae. These types of injury can cause contusion and laceration of the spinal cord. Animal models have been developed to better study the events following SCI. These have been very important in understanding the cause, effect, and sequence of events, especially in the acute phase of injury (6–8). Many different animal species have been used to model SCI, with the majority of the studies carried out in rodents. A wide range of surgical approaches have also been developed to investigate SCI, most involve exposing the spinal cord with a laminectomy and then either surgically transecting specific tracts or regions of the spinal cord or creating a contusion injury using one of several types of weight drop devices (Fig. 1-9) (6). Other models have created SCI within the closed vertebral column by inserting and inflating a balloon (9–11) or the intravascular injection of a photosensitive dye, which is then activated in the vessels of the spinal cord, causing local vascular damage and subsequent injury (12,13). Care must be taken in interpreting any animal model of SCI; not only in using the results to better understand human injury but also in recognizing that the animal species and strain chosen for an experiment can influence the outcomes (14).

Hemorrhage and Edema

SCI has been described as developing in three phases: acute, secondary, and chronic (15–18). The direct mechanical trauma to the spinal cord is quickly followed by local ischemia and hemorrhage, resulting in edema. These events cause neural cells in the immediate vicinity to die, resulting in the loss of local synaptic contact and blockage of signal transmission through the injury site. Multiple hemorrhage points appear within minutes of the insult and increase over the next several hours (15,19,20). The physical breakdown of the microvasculature leads to a loss of the blood-brain barrier and leakage of fluid into the spinal cord. Edema is seen for the first few days following injury. The increased fluid resulting from edema can further compress the spinal cord, causing more edema and thus additional damage. Several treatments to reduce edema have been tried experimentally, leading to some improvement (21–24).

Spinal Shock

The term *spinal shock* was introduced to describe a patient's condition following acute SCI; muscle paralysis, flaccid muscle tone, and loss of tendon reflexes below the level of the lesion (25). Spinal shock worsens in degree and duration with increasing severity of the injury (26), and, if untreated, it can last for up to 6 weeks. During this

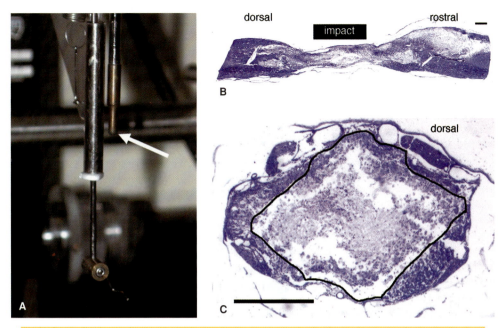

FIGURE 1-9. Examples of a severe contusion injury in the adult rat spinal cord. The injury is in the midthoracic region of the spinal cord and was created using the MASCIS impactor (141). This device is designed to deliver reproducible weight drop contusion injuries using a 10 gram weight that is dropped from a specified distance onto the exposed thoracic rat spinal cord at T9-10 level. Standard distances for the weight drop include 12.5, 25.0, or 50.0 mm, resulting in mild, moderate, or severe spinal cord contusion injury. Other parameters can be measured such as the impact velocity, cord compression distance, cord compression time, and cord compression rate. **A:** White arrow points to the 10-g impactor head of the MASCIS device which is 2.0 mm in diameter. **B:** Sagittal section through a contusion site 2 weeks after severe injury. The large bar indicates the impactor head size and the injury epicenter. In this Nissl/myelin stained section it can be seen that the injury extends both rostral and caudal to the area of impact. **C:** A cross section through the spinal cord at the epicenter of the injury, 1 week after contusion. Only a rim of white matter remains at the outer edge of the spinal cord. The dark line shows an approximate boundary between surviving host white matter and the severely damaged core of the spinal cord. Virtually no gray matter remains. The bars in A and B equal 500 μm.

time the brain and rostral spinal cord cannot communicate with the spinal cord below the level of damage. This will make the loss of function below the injury appear complete, and it is only once the swelling associated with the injury subsides that the true extent of the damage can be determined. During the months after SCI, spasticity develops with exaggerated tendon reflexes, increased muscle tone, and muscle spasms. A hypothesis has been developed to explain this dramatic change in symptoms. A change from hypoexcitability of α-motor neurons during spinal shock to hyperexcitability during spasticity is presumed (27). According to this theory, the α-motor neuron hypoexcitability in spinal shock is due to an acute loss of supraspinal excitatory input, resulting in a hyperpolarized α-motor neuron (28). Hyperpolarization of spinal motor neurons has been observed in spinal cords of transected (spinalized) cats (29). H reflexes, which are elicited with electrical stimulation of the nerve as opposed to the tendon reflex, which is secondary to mechanical stretch, have been described in humans early after SCI (25,30);

this finding argues against the theory of α-motor neuron depression as the single reason for the loss of tendon reflexes during spinal shock. This led to the idea of coincident γ-motor neuron depression since even though a physical tap does not elicit a tendon tap reflex, electrical stimulation of group I afferent nerve fibers leads to an H-reflex response (25). The interruption of descending noradrenergic (locus coeruleus) and serotonergic (raphe nucleus) pathways from the brainstem could also be involved (31–33).

Vascular Damage and Hypoxia

Along with factors such as posttraumatic hypotension and loss of autoregulation below the level of the injury, direct vascular damage causes reduced local blood flow and consequent abnormally low oxygen levels. Most vascular damage following a compression or contusion injury appears to effect capillaries in the center of the spinal cord, while the larger blood vessels around the perimeter of the spinal cord remain intact. Perhaps related to this is that damage in the spinal cord appears to spread from the gray matter outward into the white matter. Postmortem studies from human tissue show that damage to the anterior sulcal arteries following SCI causes vascular perfusion to be less efficient in gray matter than in white matter (34). Because of their high metabolic activity, neurons are particularly susceptible to death by hypoxia. An experimental 5-minute occlusion of the descending aorta leads to significant cell death in the lumbar spinal cord (35). Depending on the severity of the injury, apoptotic and necrotic neurons and glia can be seen within minutes to hours following spinal cord injury (35,36).

Ionic Imbalance

Dramatic ionic changes occur in the injury zone after SCI. Immediately after SCI, intracellular sodium concentration $[Na^+]$ and extracellular potassium concentration $[K^+]$ increases, causing cell depolarization and leading to conduction block. Damage to cell membranes at the injury eventually leads to a decrease in local extracellular $[K^+]$ (37). Intra-axonal calcium ion concentration $[Ca^{2+}]$ increases to toxic levels within minutes following SCI and remains elevated for at least a week (38,39). This influx may be from many sources: voltage-dependent calcium channels or the *N*-methyl D-aspartate (NMDA) receptor channels, release of stores from the smooth endoplasmic reticulum, or the breakdown of the Ca^{2+}-ATPase exchange pump. Increased $[Ca^{2+}]$ activates calcium-dependent phospholipase C and A_2, resulting in the breakdown of cellular membranes and the release of arachidonic acid (40). Metabolism of arachidonic acid produces prostaglandins, thromboxanes, leukotrienes, and free radicals, all known factors in causing tissue damage and inflammation through their damage to the microvasculature (41,42). Prostaglandin E_2 and thromboxanes B_2 are synthesized at the injury site starting immediately following injury, with a peak 4 hours after injury and continuing production at elevated levels for at least 72 hours (43). Blocking the increase in the levels of these factors could prevent the resultant decrease in perfusion rate of the spinal cord following SCI and reduce the amount of secondary injury (44). The iron in hemoglobin released from spinal cord hemorrhage catalyzes formation of oxygen free radicals and lipid peroxidation, resulting in damage to cell membranes (45). Under normal conditions the toxicity of oxygen free radicals is minimized by intrinsic cellular protection mechanisms, including superoxide dismutase, catalase, peroxidases, and endogenous antioxidants (46), but in cases of severe injury, the amount of oxygen free radical release overwhelms intrinsic protection mechanisms. Pharmacological agents used in the acute treatment of SCI, such as

GM1 ganglioside and methylprednisolone, act by preventing lipid peroxidation, thereby preserving the integrity of cell membranes. Following the initial ischemia caused by SCI, the injured spinal cord is reperfused with oxygenated blood, causing another increase in oxygen-derived free radicals that can lead to increased secondary injury (47,48).

Effects of Axotomy

The most severe immediate consequence of SCI is the mechanical disruption of projection axons passing through the injury. Usually, however, a rim of white matter is spared. Minimal motor function has been seen with approximately 7% of the normal axon number spared below the level of injury (20,49,50). Animal experiments suggest that some function is preserved with sparing of 1.4% to 12% of the normal complement of axons passing through the injury (51–53). Injured axons almost immediately show signs of swelling and formation of spaces between the axons and their surrounding myelin sheaths. Much of this swelling is due to edema, but vacuoles also develop as the increase in fluid volume causes disruption of the layers within the myelin sheath (54–56). Within 4 hours after SCI, white matter at the center of an injury develops a spongy appearance. Swollen axons also contain organelles, such as mitochondria, lysosomes, and smooth endoplasmic reticulum (54,57), that are usually found mainly in the cell body, suggesting a breakdown of the cytoskeletal elements that maintain the organelles in the cell body. In cases of blunt force trauma, which make up the majority of SCI cases, early intervention could preserve axons that were not severed as a direct consequence of the injury but are at risk because of the hostile environment that develops following SCI.

SECONDARY INJURY

The initial injury is just the beginning of degenerative and repair processes that occur after SCI. The consequences of secondary injury events can lead ultimately to an expansion of the lesion and the loss of additional neurons and axons that had connections in, or passed through, the injury. Hemorrhage at the injury site means that the blood-brain barrier that normally regulates substances entering or leaving the CNS is no longer intact. Blood-borne cells such as neutrophils and macrophages can now enter the parenchyma of the spinal cord in response to factors released from necrotic cells and initiate an inflammatory response. Microglia intrinsic to the CNS are also activated. Axon dieback, the retraction of the remaining proximal axon away from the injury site, and demyelination continue to hamper signal conduction across the injury. Scarring begins to wall off the damaged CNS tissue from healthy regions of the spinal cord. Neurons that have been isolated from their normal targets begin the process of apoptotic cell death. Most therapies currently employed to treat SCI attempt to minimize the problems that develop during the secondary injury phase, as it is critical to preserve as much remaining spinal cord tissue as possible and thereby maintain established circuits in the spinal cord.

Inflammatory Response

The inflammatory response following SCI removes debris from the injury and also initiates the repair process. Macrophages, neutrophils, and T cells enter the injury site from the vasculature of the compromised blood-brain barrier. Microglia, immune cells that are resident within the CNS, are also activated. These cells secrete a variety of factors, including cytokines, metabolites of arachidonic acid, and complement (20) factors that not only mediate the inflammatory response but also contribute to additional damage to the spinal cord (58,59). One of the cytokines released by many types of cells in the injury is tumor necrosis factor (TNF-α) (60). TNF-α causes additional damage in the injury site (61,62), but it also may have beneficial properties necessary for CNS repair and be neuroprotective (63). Other cytokines, such as IL-10, have anti-inflammatory properties (64). IL-10 has also been demonstrated to be neuroprotective and has been hypothesized to turn on anti-apoptotic genes (61,65). Many other factors released after SCI also have functions both destructive and beneficial (20,66), suggesting that treatments developed to repair SCI will necessarily need to take all functions of a factor into account.

The Failure to Regenerate

Neurons that have had their axons severed initially show changes in gene expression that suggest an initial attempt at regeneration. Genes normally associated with developing neurons are turned on following injury, stress, or other abnormal activity. Immediate early genes (IEGs) are activated soon after injury (67,68) and may initiate the process of adaptive change following a stimulus. The activation of IEGs such as c-Jun and c-Fos genes can depend on the type of neuron, stimulus, and distance from the injury (69). The cytoskeletal growth-associated protein, GAP-43, is important in neurons during development and is re-expressed following damage to the axon. It is re-expressed in many different types of neurons but is expressed at higher levels following injury in the PNS. It is also seen at higher levels in axons in the PNS than in the CNS (15). In the vast majority of circumstances following CNS injury and the re-expression growth promoting genes, regeneration is unsuccessful and is aborted (70,71). Intervention with treatment of neurotrophic factors or cellular transplants supports prolonged expression of these regeneration associated genes (72–74), but the longer the treatment is delayed the less likely it is to be successful (75). Axon dieback has been proposed as one reason for the diminishing response to treatment, perhaps because the active tip of the injured axon is too far from the site of treatment or the forming glial scar prevents access. A thoracic transection in adult rats caused corticospinal tract axon degeneration as far away as 2.5 mm by 8 weeks following injury (76). More recent reports suggest that axon retraction is not so severe in other systems and that terminal end bulbs of many axons remain within 500 μm of the injury (77,78).

The Role of Myelin

Myelin and molecules derived from CNS myelin have been shown to be inhibitory to axonal growth or regeneration. The expression of GAP-43 appears to be suppressed by CNS myelin (79,80). Three different myelin-derived inhibitors, NogoA, myelin-associated protein (MAG), and oligodendrocyte myelin glycoprotein (OMgp), all act through a common receptor—Nogo receptor NgR— reviewed in (81). NgR transmits its inhibitory signals via the low affinity neurotrophin receptor p75 (82,83). This pathway activates the GTPase RhoA; activation of RhoA activates Rho kinase, initiating changes in the cytoskeleton that inhibit regeneration by causing growth cone collapse. The Rho family of guanosine triphosphateases (GTPases) includes RhoA, Rac1, and Cdc42. They are important in the regulation of actin dynamics in the growth cone. Many pathways converge and act through the Rho pathway, and therapeutic intervention at this level can counteract inhibition of axonal growth at several levels (84).

Axons that are not severed following SCI may be unable to conduct action potentials because they have lost the surrounding myelin sheath. If oligodendrocytes associated with an axon die due to the injury, the myelin sheath will degenerate (85). Loss of the myelin sheath results in the exposure of internodal voltage-gated potassium channels, drastically altering the conduction properties of the demyelinated axons, leading to conduction block and the functional loss of the pathway (86).

Isolation of the Injury from Healthy Spinal Cord

Resident astrocytes and microglia in the spinal cord rapidly respond to injury (87). This process of reactive gliosis, or glial scarring, is thought to be an attempt by host astrocytes to isolate the area of injury and protect adjacent healthy spinal cord. Astrocytes also migrate to the injury site from healthy undamaged spinal cord. By 3 to 5 days after injury, astrocytes have begun to wall off the injury. A dense barrier of astrocytes develops with tightly interdigitating processes. The glial scar that is formed by this process is thought to be one of the major physical and biochemical inhibitors of successful regeneration within the CNS (88,89). In vivo experiments have also shown that reactive astrocytes can establish a barrier to regeneration (90,91). Molecules that inhibit axonal growth, such as chondroitin sulfate proteoglycans, semaphorins and tenascins, are found in the scar. Chondroitin sulfate proteoglycans, and tenascins are produced by astrocytes (92), and tenascins and semaphorin 3A by fibroblasts (93). This suggests many cell types besides astrocytes are involved in the initiation of the scar and repair processes. Following the initiation of the inflammatory response, leptomeningeal cells and fibroblasts migrate into the injury site and participate in the formation of new basal lamina (94). Fibroblasts produce basic fibroblast growth factor, a powerful angiogenic factor (95,96) that may participate in revascularization of the injury site (97). Schwann cells can also migrate into the injury from the PNS and may participate in the remyelination of sprouting or regenerating axons (66,98,99). There is proliferation of ependymal cells from the central canal in the injury (99), and these progenitor cells have been shown to express nestin and vimentin, suggesting that these progenitor cells have been stimulated to differentiate into astrocytes (100).

Neuronal Cell Death

Considerable neural cell death or atrophy occurs in the hours, days, and weeks following SCI. There are two morphologic types of cell death after SCI. Necrosis results from the direct physical and chemical attack upon cells. Necrotic neurons and glia can no longer produce ATP, often swell, and show disruption of organelle membranes. Ultimately, the cell membrane ruptures, releasing the intracellular contents into extracellular space, which then leads to a local inflammatory response.

Much of the cell death after SCI, however, is attributed to apoptotic mechanisms. Apoptosis is a mechanism used during development to eliminate excess cells in a tissue and results from the activation of an intrinsic cell suicide program. It is characterized by condensation of the nucleus and cytoplasm, intact organelles, intranucleosomal cleavage, and rapid removal of the stricken cell by resident phagocytes or adjacent cells without initiating an inflammatory response. Apoptosis requires the activation of a "cell death" program and the synthesis of new proteins by the cell that then initiate a cascade of intracellular pathways (101). This leads to the activation of a family of enzymes known as caspases. These target cytoskeletal and nuclear proteins cause the cell to stop functioning and die. Mature cells have in place antiapoptotic mechanisms to prevent cell death, but in times of stress or injury these mechanisms can be overwhelmed and result in the loss of the cell.

The particular characteristics of cell death in response to trauma, ischemia or axotomy, are likely to be influenced by a number of variables, including the severity of injury (35), type of neuron (77,102–105), the proximity to the injury (106), and what type of free radical response occurs (107). The importance of the accumulation of large concentrations of excitatory amino acids, especially glutamate, has received increasing attention as a crucial contributor to cell death after various insults (108–110). In those cases in which it has been examined, retrograde neuron death in response to axotomy has shown the morphological and biochemical features of apoptosis (111–113). Exogenous administration of neurotrophic factors, particularly the specific ligands of receptors expressed by the injured neurons, has been demonstrated to rescue axotomized neurons. Whether the success of this treatment means that the survival of adult neurons, like that of immature neurons, depends on a supply of target-derived neurotrophic factors, or whether the neurotrophic factor acts pharmacologically, is unknown. It has become clear that additional sources of trophic support are available to neurons besides those that originate in the target, including support from glia, extracellular matrix, afferent neurons, and the neurons themselves (114). Since there are so many potential sources of trophic support available to mature neurons, it has been difficult to determine whether the survival of mature neurons continues to depend on neurotrophic support and, if so, to identify the sources of this support. Exogenously administered neurotrophic factors may therefore rescue axotomized neurons by supplementing survival-promoting factors available to the neuron through its collateral axons, the axons afferent to it, and those available by an autocrine mechanism (115).

CHRONIC INJURY

Long-term Consequences

Within a few weeks of SCI a cystic cavity forms that is surrounded by an astrocytic scar. Over months and years this develops into a multilobular cystic structure bounded by astrocytes (116). If the initial injury resulted in violation of the dura, the scarring is increased by acellular, collagenous tissue produced by cells from the meninges (117). Few if any axons can grow through the chemical and physical barrier created by the glial scar at the injury. However, even where the injury site is stabilized, there are still changes occurring in the CNS as a result of the injury. The degeneration of an axon distal to an injury was first described by Waller (118) and is known as Wallerian degeneration. It is the process of breakdown and degradation of the myelin sheath and distal axon that has been severed from its neuronal cell body. In the PNS these breakdown products are removed rapidly and the environment is favorable for axonal regeneration. In the CNS, however, the debris persists months or years following injury (85).

In the chronic phase of SCI most patients have stable neurological deficits. However, some patients continue to show a progressive loss of neurologic function. The two most common causes of this continuing deterioration are progressive spinal deformity at the original site and posttraumatic syringomyelia (119,120).

Tethering

During flexion movements in the normal individual the spinal cord slides freely up and down within the vertebral column. Following SCI arachnoiditis or meningeal scarring may tether the spinal cord and prevent rostrocaudal movements. This results in pulling or stretching of the spinal cord and can cause neurological damage as the tightness increases, and can even cause ischemia in the spinal cord. Symptoms of posttraumatic cord tethering include weakness, sensory loss, and increasing pain (121), and can develop over an extended time course (122). Spinal cord tethering can also cause delayed myelopathy in patients with traumatic cord injury. Surgical release of the tethered cord is considered even when a posttraumatic syrinx is not found. Examination of the patient using magnetic resonance imaging (MRI) may show that the spinal cord is attached to the wall of the spinal canal at the site of the original injury and the spinal cord may appear misshapen. The subarachnoid space may appear to contain septa or even be absent around the injury. If no treatment is undertaken the neurologic decline will continue.

Myelomalacia and Syringomyelia

Myelomalacia can be the result of the concussive effects of a trauma. The disease process can begin within the first months and proceed for years after injury, causing a progressive increase in the size of the injury and therefore an increase in the loss of neurons and axons. Myelomalacia is a combination of ischemic and hemorrhagic infarction of the spinal cord, resulting in diffuse softening, hemorrhagic infiltration, demyelination, and polymorphonuclear infiltration of the spinal cord. Rostral and caudal extension of necrotic tissue occurs at the base of the dorsal funiculus. Cystic myelomalacia may be a precursor of posttraumatic syringomyelia. A syrinx may develop months to years after the injury. The cause of posttraumatic syrinxes is unknown, but inflammation, arachnoiditis, or myelomalacia interacting with spinal canal stenosis and kyphotic deformities is thought to play a role (120,123). A cavity forms at the site of the original SCI, in the central gray matter, which is a relatively avascular zone between the dorsal and ventral arterial supply (124). This can lead to increased tension on the spinal cord and a decrease in the circulation of CSF. Tension on the spinal cord can open cystic spaces or cause ischemia-related myelomalacia, also leading to syrinx formation. Changes in the flow of CSF have also been implicated in advancing syringomyelia (120). The syrinx may begin to enlarge over time, extending rostrally or caudally through the intermediate gray matter, in some case unilaterally. Posttraumatic syringomyelia is very difficult to manage and even with aggressive treatment only about 80% of cases have stabilized when the patients are examined 5 to 10 years after treatment (120).

Chronic Pain and Spasticity

Following SCI, chronic pain and spasticity may develop. Within the first several months to years, the majority of patients develop chronic central pain (CCP) syndrome. Two thirds of patients with SCI report pain, and, for one third of these patients, the pain is severe and debilitating (125). SCI pain is often difficult to treat and is a major cause of discomfort and disability among patients with SCI. There are two general categories of chronic pain that result from SCI. At-level neuropathic pain is located in the dermatomes near the injury and is present from the time of injury or soon after the injury. Below-level neuropathic pain has a gradual onset after SCI and is localized to dermatomes related to spinal cord segments below the level of injury (126). The causes of CCP have not been clearly determined, but both animal models and human studies provide evidence that neuronal hyperexcitability in the spinal cord central gray matter rostral to the injury and loss of the ascending spinothalamic pathway are contributors to the syndromes (126,127). Other experiments have shown hypersensitivity to painful stimuli is greater in experimental lesions restricted to the gray matter of central cord and dorsal horn than in complete injuries (128). This is consistent with clinical findings of increased allodynia/hyperalgesia after central cord injuries as compared to complete lesions of the spinal cord (129). Another component that may contribute to CCP involves excitatory amino acids and their receptor-mediated development of hyperexcitability in dorsal horn neurons (130,131). This may instigate changes in the activation state of excitatory and inhibitory receptors and their transporters (132,133).

Spasticity is often seen in patients with SCI. Patients with posttraumatic spasticity are very likely to have problems such as flexion contractures, decubitus ulcers, and poor perineal hygiene because of adductor spasms (125). Animal experiments suggest that spasticity, like CCP, is a combination of events that result from damage to long tract pathways and abnormal activity in the central gray matter of the spinal cord (134). The loss of descending corticospinal fibers probably results in decreased activity of inhibitory interneurons. Inhibitory interneurons activated from tendon organs (Ib afferents) may be one of the populations with reduced activity. This would mean that the normal inhibition of α-motor neurons from tendon organs, when muscle tension increases, could be missing in patients with SCI. The consequence of these events is a strong facilitation of the monosynaptic reflex pathway from Ia sensory neurons to α-motor neurons (125).

Peripheral Nervous System Regeneration

Unlike injuries in the CNS, injuries in the PNS are very likely to show spontaneous improvement if the endoneurial tubes remain intact. Injured neurons increase their expression of growth-associated factors, initiating a regenerative response. Schwann cells, macrophages, and fibroblasts enter the injury site, rapidly removing myelin debris, producing neurotrophic factors and substrate molecules. These features create an environment in the distal nerve stump that is conducive to axon regrowth. This environment also causes a proliferation of Schwann cells in the endoneurial tubes that act as guides, directing regenerating axons back to their denervated targets (135). However, if the distal nerve segment and peripheral target are denervated for a prolonged period of time, then there is much less recovery of function. If the delay is more than 6 months between injury and surgical repair, the likelihood of effective functional recovery is very poor (136). There are at least two elements contributing to the decline in regenerative capability of neurons projecting into the PNS. Experimental evidence suggests that chronically injured motor neurons attempt a regenerative response after a delayed second surgery, but the regenerative response is not maintained long enough to permit regeneration (137,138). The environment for regeneration also becomes less favorable over time because of the decline in the number of Schwann cells in the injury. This leads to a loss of the endoneurial tubes and basement membrane and a loss of the neurotrophic factors released by Schwann cells (139,140).

SUMMARY: DIFFICULTIES IN CENTRAL NERVOUS SYSTEM REPAIR

SCI is a dynamic process in the days, weeks, and months following initial injury. The many issues discussed regarding the pathology of SCI are important not only for the treatment and stabilization of patients after injury but also for the eventual development of a cure of SCI. The major categories for interventions can be summarized into one or more of the following: (a) *neuroprotection*, preventing the death of neurons and supporting cells threatened by the injury; (b) *initiating successful regenerative response*, involving both stimulation of a successful regenerative response from host neurons and engineering an environment within the CNS that guides and encourages axonal growth rather than inhibits; (c) *bridging the gap*, providing a graft of tissue or artificial substrate to replace lost or damaged host tissue and encourage axonal regeneration across the injury with continuation into the host spinal cord; (d) *restoration of axonal transmission*, successful remyelination of demyelinated host axons so that conduction block can be reversed, and (e) *physical therapy*, to stimulate function within spared circuits and encourage recovery via regeneration of lost plasticity in forming new functional circuits.

Within each of these elements there are the additional issues of when and where treatment should be initiated and for how long. If a cell graft is used as part of the therapy, when is the appropriate time to introduce the graft? If the graft is introduced too early, will the host inflammatory response still be so strong as to prevent good integration with the host? If the graft is delayed for too long, host neurons may have already died or aborted gene expression that could lead to a successful regenerative response, and a glial scar could have formed that would inhibit connections between the graft and host tissue. Strategies combining several types of therapies would also need to be coordinated in order to optimize the benefits of treatment; if neurotrophic factors are used to support neurons and initiate a regenerative response, when should physical therapy be started to encourage strengthening of functional circuits? After answers are found to questions like these, the final set of problems may well be how to guide regenerating axons to their correct target(s) to replace the functional circuits lost following SCI. These are some examples of the current challenges in treating SCI, and the solutions to these challenges will bring us closer to the cure for SCI.

ACKNOWLEDGMENTS

I would like to thank my colleagues Dr. Marion Murray, Dr. Alan Tessler, and Mrs. Theresa Connors for their helpful comments on the manuscript.

REFERENCES

1. Liu CN, Chambers WW. Intraspinal sprouting of dorsal root axons. *Arch Neurol Psychiatry*. 1958;79:46–61.
2. Richardson PM, McGuiness UM, Aguayo AJ. Axons from CNS neurones regenerate into PNS grafts. *Nature*. 1980; 284:264–265.
3. Rexed B. The cytoarchitectonic organization of the spinal cord in the cat. *J Comp Neurol*. 1952;96(3):414–495.
4. Rexed B. A cytoarchitectonic atlas of the spinal cord in the cat. *J Comp Neurol*. 1954;100:297–379.

5. Nathan PW, Smith MC. The rubrospinal and central tegmental tracts in man. *Brain*. 1982;105(Pt 2):223–269.

6. Rosenzweig ES, McDonald JW. Rodent models for treatment of spinal cord injury: research trends and progress toward useful repair. *Curr Opin Neurol*. 2004;17(2):121–131.

7. Stokes BT, Jakeman LB. Experimental modeling of human spinal cord injury: a model that crosses the species barrier and mimics the spectrum of human cytopathology. *Spinal Cord*. 2002;40(3):101–109.

8. Kwon BK, Oxland TR, Tetzlaff W. Animal models used in spinal cord regeneration research. *Spine*. 2002;27(14):1504–1510.

9. Tarlov IM, Klinger H. Spinal cord compression studies. II. Time limits for recovery after acute compression in dogs. *AMA Arch Neurol Psychiatry*. 1954;71(3):271–290.

10. Tarlov IM. Spinal cord compression studies. III. Time limits for recovery after gradual compression in dogs. *AMA Arch Neurol Psychiatry*. 1954;71(5):588–597.

11. Purdy PD, Replogle RE, Pride GL Jr, et al. Percutaneous intraspinal navigation: feasibility study of a new and minimally invasive approach to the spinal cord and brain in cadavers. *AJNR Am J Neuroradiol*. 2003;24(3):361–365.

12. Bunge MB, Holets VR, Bates ML, et al. Characterization of photochemically induced spinal cord injury in the rat by light and electron microscopy. *Exp Neurol*. 1994;127:76–93.

13. Watson BD, Prado R, Dietrich WD, et al. Photochemically induced spinal cord injury in the rat. *Brain Res*. 1986;367(1–2):296–300.

14. Johnson EM Jr, Deckwerth TL, Deshmukh M. Neuronal death in developmental models: possible implications in neuropathology. *Brain Pathol*. 1996;6(4):397–409.

15. Schwab ME, Bartholdi D. Degeneration and regeneration of axons in the lesioned spinal cord. *Physiol Rev*. 1996;76(2):319–370.

16. Tator C. Update on the pathophysiology and pathology of acute spinal cord injury. *Brain Pathol*. 1995;5:407–413.

17. Tator CH. Experimental and clinical studies of the pathophysiology and management of acute spinal cord injury. *J Spinal Cord Med*. 1996;19(4):206–214.

18. Tator C. Biology of neurological recovery and functional restoration after spinal cord injury. *Neurosurgery*. 1998;42(4):696–707.

19. Tator C, Fehlings M. Review of the secondary injury theory of acute spinal cord trauma with emphasis on vascular mechanisms. *J Neurosurg*. 1991;75:15–26.

20. Kwon BK, Tetzlaff W, Grauer JN, et al. Pathophysiology and pharmacologic treatment of acute spinal cord injury. *Spine J*. 2004;4(4):451–464.

21. Lemke M, Faden AI. Edema development and ion changes in rat spinal cord after impact trauma: injury dose-response studies. *J Neurotrauma*. 1990;7(1):41–54.

22. Merola A, O'Brien MF, Castro BA, et al. Histologic characterization of acute spinal cord injury treated with intravenous methylprednisolone. *J Orthop Trauma*. 2002;16(3):155–161.

23. Fujiki M, Kobayashi H, Inoue R, et al. Electrical preconditioning attenuates progressive necrosis and cavitation following spinal cord injury. *J Neurotrauma*. 2004;21(4):459–470.

24. Winkler T, Sharma HS, Gordh T, et al. Topical application of dynorphin A (1-17) antiserum attenuates trauma induced alterations in spinal cord evoked potentials, microvascular permeability disturbances, edema formation and cell injury: an experimental study in the rat using electrophysiological and morphological approaches. *Amino Acids*. 2002;23(1–3):273–281.

25. Hiersemenzel LP, Curt A, Dietz V. From spinal shock to spasticity: neuronal adaptations to a spinal cord injury. *Neurology*. 2000;54(8):1574–1582.

26. Ditunno JF, Little JW, Tessler A, et al. Spinal shock revisited: a four-phase model. *Spinal Cord*. 2004;42(7):383–395.

27. Diamantopoulos E, Zander Olsen P. Excitability of motor neurones in spinal shock in man. *J Neurol Neurosurg Psychiatry*. 1967;30(5):427–431.

28. Ashby P, Verrier M, Lightfoot E. Segmental reflex pathways in spinal shock and spinal spasticity in man. *J Neurol Neurosurg Psychiatry*. 1974;37(12):1352–1360.

29. Schadt JC, Barnes CD. Motoneuron membrane changes associated with spinal shock and the Schiff-Sherrington phenomenon. *Brain Res*. 1980;201(2):373-383.

30. Leis AA, Zhou HH, Mehta M, et al. Behavior of the H-reflex in humans following mechanical perturbation or injury to rostral spinal cord. *Muscle Nerve*. 1996;19(11):1373–1382.

31. Grillner S, Dubuc R. Control of locomotion in vertebrates: spinal and supraspinal mechanisms. *Adv Neurol*. 1988;47:425–453.

32. Grillner S. Neurobiological bases of rhythmic motor acts in vertebrates. *Science*. 1985;228:143–148.

33. Kiehn O, Hultborn H, Conway B. Spinal locomotor activity in acutely spinalized cats induced by intrathecal application of noradrenaline. *Neurosci Lett*. 1992;143:243–246.

34. Tator CH, Koyanagi I. Vascular mechanisms in the pathophysiology of human spinal cord injury. *J Neurosurg*. 1997;86(3):483–492.

35. Lu K, Liang CL, Chen HJ, et al. Injury severity and cell death mechanisms: effects of concomitant hypovolemic hypotension on spinal cord ischemia-reperfusion in rats. *Exp Neurol*. 2004;185(1):120–132.

36. Sapru HN. Spinal cord: anatomy, physiology, and pathophysiology. In: Kirshblum S, Campagnolo D, DeLisa J, eds. *Spinal Cord Medicine*. Philadelphia: Lippincott Williams & Wilkins; 2002:5–26.

37. Young W, Koreh I. Potassium and calcium changes in injured spinal cords. *Brain Res*. 1986;365(1):42–53.

38. Moriya T, Hassan AZ, Young W, et al. Dynamics of extracellular calcium activity following contusion of the rat spinal cord. *J Neurotrauma*. 1994;11(3):255–263.

39. Young W, Flamm ES. Effect of high-dose corticosteroid therapy on blood flow, evoked potentials, and extracellular calcium in experimental spinal injury. *J Neurosurg*. 1982;57(5):667–673.

40. Rasmussen H. The calcium messenger system (1). *N Engl J Med*. 1986;314(17):1094–1101.

41. Xu J, Hsu CY, Junker H, et al. Kininogen and kinin in experimental spinal cord injury. *J Neurochem*. 1991;57(3):975–980.

42. Demediuk P, Saunders RD, Clendenon NR, et al. Changes in lipid metabolism in traumatized spinal cord. *Prog Brain Res*. 1985;63:211–226.

43. Resnick DK, Nguyen P, Cechvala CF. Regional and temporal changes in prostaglandin E2 and thromboxane B2 concentrations after spinal cord injury. *Spine J*. 2001;1(6):432–436.

44. Tempel GE, Martin HF III. The beneficial effects of a thromboxane receptor antagonist on spinal cord perfusion following experimental cord injury. *J Neurol Sci*. 1992;109(2):162–167.

45. Braughler JM, Hall ED. Central nervous system trauma and stroke. I. biochemical considerations for oxygen radical formation and lipid peroxidation. *Free Radic Biol Med*. 1989;6(3):289–301.

46. Phillis JW. A "radical" view of cerebral ischemic injury. *Prog Neurobiol*. 1994;42(4):441–448.

47. Basu S, Hellberg A, Ulus AT, et al. Biomarkers of free radical injury during spinal cord ischemia. *FEBS Lett*. 2001;508(1):36–38.

48. Lukacova N, Halat G, Chavko M, et al. Ischemia-reperfusion injury in the spinal cord of rabbits strongly enhances lipid peroxidation and modifies phospholipid profiles. *Neurochem Res*. 1996;21(8):869–873.

49. Kakulas BA. The clinical neuropathology of spinal cord injury: a guide to the future. *Paraplegia*. 1987;25(3):212–216.

50. Kakulas BA. The applied neuropathology of human spinal cord injury. *Spinal Cord*. 1999;37(2):79–88.

51. Fehlings MG, Tator CH. The relationships among the severity of spinal cord injury, residual neurological function,

axon counts, and counts of retrogradely labeled neurons after experimental spinal cord injury. *Exp Neurol.* 1995;132: 220–228.

52. Eidelberg E, Straehley D, Erspamer R, et al. Relationship between residual hindlimb-assisted locomotion and surviving axons after incomplete spinal cord injuries. *Exp Neurol.* 1977;56(2):312–322.

53. Blight AR. Cellular morphology of chronic spinal cord injury in the cat: analysis of myelinated axons by line-sampling. *Neuroscience.* 1983;10(2):521–543.

54. Balentine JD. Pathology of experimental spinal cord trauma. II. ultrastructure of axons and myelin. *Lab Invest.* 1978;39(3):254–266.

55. Balentine JD. Pathology of experimental spinal cord trauma. I. the necrotic lesion as a function of vascular injury. *Lab Invest.* 1978;39(3):236–253.

56. Griffiths IR, McCulloch MC. Nerve fibres in spinal cord impact injuries. Part 1. changes in the myelin sheath during the initial 5 weeks. *J Neurol Sci.* 1983;58(3):335–349.

57. Lampert PW, Cressman MR. Fine-structural changes of myelin sheaths after axonal degeneration in the spinal cord of rats. *Am J Pathol.* 1966;49(6):1139–1155.

58. Klusman I, Schwab ME. Effects of pro-inflammatory cytokines in experimental spinal cord injury. *Brain Res.* 1997;762:173–184.

59. Bartholdi D, Schwab ME. Expression of pro-inflammatory cytokine and chemokine mRNA upon experimental spinal cord injury in mouse: an in situ hybridization study. *Eur J Neurosci.* 1997;9(7):1422–1438.

60. Yan P, Li Q, Kim GM, et al. Cellular localization of tumor necrosis factor-alpha following acute spinal cord injury in adult rats. *J Neurotrauma.* 2001;18(5):563–568.

61. Bethea JR, Nagashima H, Acosta MC, et al. Systemically administered interleukin-10 reduces tumor necrosis factor-alpha production and significantly improves functional recovery following traumatic spinal cord injury in rats. *J Neurotrauma.* 1999;16(10):851–863.

62. Lavine SD, Hofman FM, Zlokovic BV. Circulating antibody against tumor necrosis factor-alpha protects rat brain from reperfusion injury. *J Cereb Blood Flow Metab.* 1998;18(1): 52–58.

63. Kim GM, Xu J, Song SK, et al. Tumor necrosis factor receptor deletion reduces nuclear factor-kappaB activation, cellular inhibitor of apoptosis protein 2 expression, and functional recovery after traumatic spinal cord injury. *J Neurosci.* 2001;21(17):6617–6625.

64. Knoblach SM, Faden AI. Interleukin-10 improves outcome and alters proinflammatory cytokine expression after experimental traumatic brain injury. *Exp Neurol.* 1998; 153(1):143–151.

65. Brewer KL, Bethea JR, Yezierski RP. Neuroprotective effects of interleukin-10 following excitotoxic spinal cord injury. *Exp Neurol.* 1999;159(2):484–493.

66. Jones LL, Sajed D, Tuszynski MH. Axonal regeneration through regions of chondroitin sulfate proteoglycan deposition after spinal cord injury: a balance of permissiveness and inhibition. *J Neurosci.* 2003;23(28):9276–9288.

67. De Felipe C, Jenkins R, O'Shea R, et al. The role of immediate early genes in the regeneration of the central nervous system. *Adv Neurol.* 1993;59:263–271.

68. Hull M, Bahr M. Regulation of immediate-early gene expression in rat retinal ganglion cells after axotomy and during regeneration through a peripheral nerve graft. *J Neurobiol.* 1994;25(1):92–105.

69. Jenkins R, Tetzlaff W, Hunt SP. Differential expression of immediate early genes in rubrospinal neurons following axotomy in rat. *Eur J Neurosci.* 1993;5(3):203–209.

70. Herdegen T, Skene P, Bahr M. The c-Jun transcription factor-bipotential mediator of neuronal death, survival and regeneration. *Trends Neurosci.* 1997;20(5):227–231.

71. Schmitt AB, Breuer S, Polat L, et al. Retrograde reactions of Clarke's nucleus neurons after human spinal cord injury. *Ann Neurol.* 2003;54(4):534–539.

72. Kobayashi NR, Fan DP, Giehl KM, et al. BDNF and NT-4/5 prevent atrophy of rat rubrospinal neurons after cervical axotomy, stimulate GAP-43 and Tα1-tubulin mRNA expression, and promote axonal regeneration. *J Neurosci.* 1997;17(24):9583–9595.

73. Houle JD, Schramm P, Herdegen T. Trophic factor modulation of c-Jun expression in supraspinal neurons after chronic spinal cord injury. *Exp Neurol.* 1998;154(2):602–611.

74. Broude E, McAtee M, Kelley MS, et al. Fetal spinal cord transplants and exogenous neurotrophic support enhance c-Jun expression in mature axotomized neurons after spinal cord injury. *Exp Neurol.* 1999;155(1):65–78.

75. Houle JD, Ye JH. Changes occur in the ability to promote axonal regeneration as the post-injury period increases. *Neuroreport.* 1997;8(3):751–755.

76. Pallini R, Fernandez E, Sbriccoli A. Retrograde degeneration of corticospinal axons following transection of the spinal cord in rats. A quantitative study with anterogradely transported horseradish peroxidase. *J Neurosurg.* 1988; 68(1):124–128.

77. Mori F, Himes BT, Kowada M, et al. Fetal spinal cord transplants rescue some axotomized rubrospinal neurons from retrograde cell death in adult rats. *Exp Neurol.* 1997;143:45–60.

78. Houle JD, Jin Y. Chronically injured supraspinal neurons exhibit only modest axonal dieback in response to a cervical hemisection lesion. *Exp Neurol.* 2001;169(1):208–217.

79. Kapfhammer JP, Schwab ME. Increased expression of the growth-associated protein GAP-43 in the myelin-free rat spinal cord. *Eur J Neurosci.* 1994;6(3):403–411.

80. Schreyer DJ, Skene JH. Fate of GAP-43 in ascending spinal axons of DRG neurons after peripheral nerve injury: delayed accumulation and correlation with regenerative potential. *J Neurosci.* 1991;11(12):3738–3751.

81. Ramer LM, Ramer MS, Steeves JD. Setting the stage for functional repair of spinal cord injuries: a cast of thousands. *Spinal Cord.* 2005;43(3):134–161.

82. Wang KC, Kim JA, Sivasankaran R, et al. P75 interacts with the Nogo receptor as a co-receptor for Nogo, MAG and OMgp. *Nature.* 2002;420(6911):74–78.

83. Wong ST, Henley JR, Kanning KC, et al. A p75(NTR) and Nogo receptor complex mediates repulsive signaling by myelin-associated glycoprotein. *Nat Neurosci.* 2002;5(12): 1302–1308.

84. Kwon BK, Borisoff JF, Tetzlaff W. Molecular targets for therapeutic intervention after spinal cord injury. *Mol Interv.* 2002;2(4):244–258.

85. Buss A, Brook GA, Kakulas B, et al. Gradual loss of myelin and formation of an astrocytic scar during Wallerian degeneration in the human spinal cord. *Brain.* 2004;127(pt 1): 34–44.

86. Nashmi R, Fehlings MG. Changes in axonal physiology and morphology after chronic compressive injury of the rat thoracic spinal cord. *Neuroscience.* 2001;104(1):235–251.

87. Aloisi F, Ria F, Columba-Cabezas S, et al. Relative efficiency of microglia, astrocytes, dendritic cells and B cells in naive CD4+ T-cell priming and Th1/Th2 cell restimulation. *Eur J Immunol.* 1999;29(9):2705–2714.

88. Reier PJ, Houle JD, Tessler A, et al. Astrogliosis and regeneration: new perspectives on an old hypothesis. In: Norenberg MD, Hertz L, Schousboe A, eds. *The Biochemical Pathology of Astrocytes.* New York: Alan R Liss; 1988:107–122.

89. McGraw J, Hiebert GW, Steeves JD. Modulating astrogliosis after neurotrauma. *J Neurosci Res.* 2001;63(2):109–115.

90. McPhail LT, Plunet WT, Das P, et al. The astrocytic barrier to axonal regeneration at the dorsal root entry zone is induced by rhizotomy. *Eur J Neurosci.* 2005;21(1):267–270.

91. Davies SJA, Fitch MT, Memberg SP, et al. Regeneration of adult axons in white matter tracts of the central nervous system. *Nature.* 1997;390:680–683.

92. Niederost BP, Zimmermann DR, Schwab ME, et al. Bovine CNS myelin contains neurite growth-inhibitory activity associated with chondroitin sulfate proteoglycans. *J Neurosci.* 1999;19(20):8979–8989.

93. Pasterkamp RJ, Verhaagen J. Emerging roles for semaphorins in neural regeneration. *Brain Res Rev*. 2001;35:36–54.
94. Carbonell AL, Boya J. Ultrastructural study on meningeal regeneration and meningo-glial relationships after cerebral stab wound in the adult rat. *Brain Res*. 1988;439(1-2): 337–344.
95. Hayashi T, Sakurai M, Abe K, et al. Expression of angiogenic factors in rabbit spinal cord after transient ischaemia. *Neuropathol Appl Neurobiol*. 1999;25(1):63–71.
96. Folkman J, Klagsbrun M. Angiogenic factors. *Science*. 1987;235(4787):442–447.
97. Blight AR. Morphometric analysis of a model of spinal cord injury in guinea pigs, with behavioral evidence of delayed secondary pathology. *J Neurol Sci*. 1991;103(2):156–171.
98. Li Y, Raisman G. Schwann cells induce sprouting in motor and sensory axons in the adult rat spinal cord. *J Neuroscience*. 1994;14(7):4050–4063.
99. Beattie MS, Bresnahan JC, Komon J, et al. Endogenous repair after spinal cord contusion injuries in the rat. *Exp Neurol*. 1997;148(2):453–463.
100. Frisen J, Johansson CB, Torok C, et al. Rapid, widespread, and long lasting induction of nestin contributes to the generation of glial scar tissue after CNS injury. *J Cell Biol*. 1995;131(2):453–464.
101. Benn SC, Woolf CJ. Adult neuron survival strategies—slamming on the brakes. *Nat Rev Neurosci*. 2004;5(9):686–700.
102. Himes BT, Goldberger ME, Tessler A. Grafts of fetal central nervous system tissue rescue axotomized Clarke's nucleus neurons in adult and neonatal operates. *J Comp Neurol*. 1994;339(1):117–131.
103. Liu Y, Himes BT, Murray M, et al. Grafts of BDNF-producing fibroblasts rescue axotomized rubrospinal neurons and prevent their atrophy. *Exp Neurol*. 2002;178(2):150–164.
104. Merline M, Kalil K. Cell death of corticospinal neurons is induced by axotomy before but not after innervation of spinal targets. *J Comp Neurol*. 1990;296:506–516.
105. Pruitt JN II, Feringa ER, McBride RL. Corticospinal axons persist in cervical and high thoracic regions 10 weeks after a T-9 spinal cord transection. *Neurology*. 1988;38(6):946–950.
106. Giehl KM, Tetzlaff W. BDNF and NT-3, but not NGF, prevent axotomy-induced death of rat corticospinal neurons in vivo. *Eur J Neurosci*. 1996;8:1167–1175.
107. Liu PH, Tsai HY, Chung YW, et al. The proximity of the lesion to cell bodies determines the free radical risk induced in rat rubrospinal neurons subjected to axonal injury. *Anat Embryol (Berl)*. 2004;207(6):439–451.
108. Stout AK, Raphael HM, Kanterewicz BI, et al. Glutamate-induced neuron death requires mitochondrial calcium uptake. *Nat Neurosci*. 1998;1(5):366–373.
109. Sei Y, Fossom L, Goping G, et al. Quinolinic acid protects rat cerebellar granule cells from glutamate-induced apoptosis. *Neurosci Lett*. 1998;241(2-3):180–184.
110. Lindholm D. Role of neurotrophins in preventing glutamate induced neuronal cell death. *J Neurol*. 1994;242(suppl 1): S16–18.
111. Groves MJ, Christopherson T, Giometto B, et al. Axotomy-induced apoptosis in adult rat primary sensory neurons. *J Neurocytol*. 1997;26:615–624.
112. Garcia-Valenzuela E, Gorczyca W, Darzynkiewicz Z, et al. Apoptosis in adult retinal ganglion cells after axotomy. *J Neurobiol*. 1993;25(4):431–438.
113. Rossiter JP, Riopelle RJ, Bisby MA. Axotomy-induced apoptotic cell death of neonatal rat facial motoneurons: time course analysis and relation to NADPH-diaphorase activity. *Exp Neurol*. 1996;138(1):33–44.
114. Burek MJ, Oppenheim RW. Programmed cell death in the nervous system. *Brain Pathol*. 1996;6:427–446.
115. Himes BT, Tessler A. Neuroprotection from cell death following axotomy. In: Ingoglia N, Murray M, eds. *Axonal Regeneration in the Central Nervous System*. New York: Marcel Dekker; 2000:477–503.
116. Kakulas BA, Taylor JR. Pathology of injuries of the vertebral column and spinal cord. In: Vinken PJ, Bruyn PJ, Klauwens HL, et al., eds. *Handbook of Clinical Neurology. Spinal Cord Trauma*. Amsterdam: Elsevier; 1992:21–51.
117. Hughes JT. *Pathology of the Spinal Cord*. 2nd ed. Philadelphia: Saunders; 1978.
118. Waller A. Experiments on the section of glossopharyngeal and hypoglossal nerves of the frog and observations of the alternatives produced thereby in the structure of their primitive fibres. *Phil Trans R Soc Lond*. 1850;140:423–429.
119. Madsen PW III, Yezierski RP, Holets VR. Syringomyelia: clinical observations and experimental studies. *J Neurotrauma*. 1994;11(3):241–254.
120. Brodbelt AR, Stoodley MA. Post-traumatic syringomyelia: a review. *J Clin Neurosci*. 2003;10(4):401–408.
121. Smith KA, Rekate HL. Delayed postoperative tethering of the cervical spinal cord. *J Neurosurg*. 1994;81(2):196–201.
122. Ragnarsson TS, Durward QJ, Nordgren RE. Spinal cord tethering after traumatic paraplegia with late neurological deterioration. *J Neurosurg*. 1986;64(3):397–401.
123. Little JW, Burns SP. Neuromusculoskeletal complications of spinal cord injury. In: Kirshblum S, Campagnolo D, DeLisa J, eds. *Spinal Cord Medicine*. Philadelphia: Lippincott Williams & Wilkins; 2002:241–252.
124. Biyani A, el Masry WS. Post-traumatic syringomyelia: a review of the literature. *Paraplegia*. 1994;32(11):723–731.
125. Burchiel KJ, Hsu FP. Pain and spasticity after spinal cord injury: mechanisms and treatment. *Spine*. 2001;26(24 suppl):S146–160.
126. Vierck CJ Jr, Siddall P, Yezierski RP. Pain following spinal cord injury: animal models and mechanistic studies. *Pain*. 2000;89(1):1–5.
127. Finnerup NB, Gyldensted C, Nielsen E, et al. MRI in chronic spinal cord injury patients with and without central pain. *Neurology*. 2003;61(11):1569–1575.
128. Siddall P, Xu CL, Cousins M. Allodynia following traumatic spinal cord injury in the rat. *Neuroreport*. 1995;6(9): 1241–1244.
129. Siddall PJ, Taylor DA, McClelland JM, et al. Pain report and the relationship of pain to physical factors in the first 6 months following spinal cord injury. *Pain*. 1999;81(1–2): 187–197.
130. Bennett AD, Everhart AW, Hulsebosch CE. Intrathecal administration of an NMDA or a non-NMDA receptor antagonist reduces mechanical but not thermal allodynia in a rodent model of chronic central pain after spinal cord injury. *Brain Res*. 2000;859(1):72–82.
131. Woolf CJ, Thompson SW. The induction and maintenance of central sensitization is dependent on *N*-methyl-D-aspartic acid receptor activation; implications for the treatment of post-injury pain hypersensitivity states. *Pain*. 1991;44(3): 293–299.
132. Hains BC, Everhart AW, Fullwood SD, et al. Changes in serotonin, serotonin transporter expression and serotonin denervation supersensitivity: involvement in chronic central pain after spinal hemisection in the rat. *Exp Neurol*. 2002;175(2):347–362.
133. Mills CD, Johnson KM, Hulsebosch CE. Group I metabotropic glutamate receptors in spinal cord injury: roles in neuroprotection and the development of chronic central pain. *J Neurotrauma*. 2002;19(1):23–42.
134. Vierck CJ, Cannon RL, Stevens KA, et al. Mechanisms of increased pain sensitivity within dermatomes remote from an injured segment of the spinal cord. In: Yezierski RP, Burchiel KJ, eds. *Spinal Cord Injury Pain: Assessment, Mechanisms, Management*. Seattle: IASP Press; 2002: 155–173.
135. Fu SY, Gordon T. The cellular and molecular basis of peripheral nerve regeneration. *Mol Neurobiol*. 1997;14(1–2): 67–116.
136. Sunderland S. *Nerve Injuries and Their Repair*. Edinburgh: Churchill Livingstone; 1991.
137. Fernandes KJL, Tetzlaff WG. Gene expression in axotomized neurons: identifying the intrinsic determinants of axonal growth. In: Ingoglia N, Murray M, eds. *Axonal

Regeneration in the Central Nervous System. New York: Marcel Dekker; 2001:219–266.

138. Gordon T, Fu SY. Long-term response to nerve injury. *Adv Neurol.* 1997;72:185–199.

139. Sulaiman OA, Gordon T. Effects of short- and long-term Schwann cell denervation on peripheral nerve regeneration, myelination, and size. *Glia.* 2000;32(3):234–246.

140. Hoke A, Gordon T, Zochodne DW, et al. A decline in glial cell-line-derived neurotrophic factor expression is associated with impaired regeneration after long-term Schwann cell denervation. *Exp Neurol.* 2002;173(1):77–85.

141. Constantini S, Young W. The effects of methylprednisolone and the ganglioside GM1 on acute spinal cord injury in rats. *J Neurosurg.* 1994;80(1):97–111.

Chapter 2

The Neurological Evaluation and Medical Management of Acute Spinal Cord Injury

Anthony S. Burns and Ralph J. Marino

Spinal cord injury (SCI) is a devastating, life-altering event. Approximately 11,000 new injuries occur annually in the United States (1), and currently there are approximately 225,000 to 288,000 individuals living in the United States with the sequelae of SCI including permanent paralysis. Not surprisingly, the costs to society of SCI are staggering and in 1998 were estimated at $9.7 billion per year (2). The lifetime *direct* costs of a high tetraplegic injured at age 25 can exceed $2.8 million (1).

Males are disproportionately affected with a 4:1 male-to-female ratio, and the majority of injuries occur between the ages of 16 and 30. Mirroring the increasing age of the US general population, the average age at injury has increased from 28.7 years of age in the mid-1970s to 37.6 years since 2000. During this same period, the percentage of individuals age 60 or greater at the time of injury increased from 4.7% to 10.9%. The leading causes of SCI are motor vehicle accidents (47.5%) followed by falls (22.9%), violence (13.8%), and sports (8.9%) (1). The remaining injury etiologies account for

6.8% of injuries. The incidence of falls is increasing while sports-related injuries are decreasing. Injuries due to violence are primarily from firearms, with a smaller percentage due to stab wounds and miscellaneous mechanisms. Interestingly, acts of violence as a cause of SCI increased from 13.3% before 1980 to a peak of 24.8% between 1990 and 1999, before falling to their current levels.

HISTORY OF SPINAL CORD INJURY MEDICINE

The Edwin Smith Surgical Papyrus, dating from ancient Egypt (2500 BC), referred to SCI as "an ailment not to be treated" (3). For centuries, the prognosis continued to be dismal and the medical profession was paralyzed by pessimism and apathy. During World War I, mortality in patients with severe SCI was estimated at 80%, and even up to 1934, the death rate for American paraplegics exceeded 80% (4). The majority of patients succumbed within 6 to 8 weeks to sepsis associated with urinary tract infections and pressure ulcers. In addition, individuals who survived were largely relegated to institutional care with little hope of reintegration into the community. Unfortunately, there was little improvement until World War II.

In February 1944, the National Spinal Injuries Centre was established at Stoke Mandeville Hospital in Aylesbury, England. The SCI unit at Stoke Mandeville employed a comprehensive, multidisciplinary approach as a response to the large number of injured servicemen and ex-servicemen. Sir Ludwig Guttmann was the first director and is considered by many to be the father of SCI medicine. He had been one of Germany's leading neurosurgeons at the Jewish Hospital in Breslau before he fled to England in 1939. Guttmann espoused some fundamental principles for SCI units (4).

a. Management of a unit by an experienced physician who is prepared to give up part or all of his own specialty.
b. Sufficient allied health professionals, such as nurses and therapists, to cope with details of care.
c. Technical facilities to establish workshops and vocational outlets.
d. Attention to social, domestic, and industrial resettlement.
e. Regular aftercare, or extended care, over the lifetime of each individual.

Employing these principles, Stoke Mandeville enjoyed great success and served as an example for the rest of the world.

In 1945, The US Department of Veterans Affairs followed suit and established eight SCI units. In 1952, Dr. Donald Munro, with the sponsorship of the Liberty Mutual Insurance Company, established the first civilian SCI unit in the United States at Boston University Hospital. He was able to demonstrate a 200% to 300% reduction in medical and hospital costs (4). In 1972, the first model SCI system was awarded by the US Rehabilitation Services Administration to Good Samaritan Hospital in Phoenix, Arizona. The success of this demonstration project led to the establishment of six additional centers in 1972. The Model SCI Systems (MSCIS) program is now administered by the National Institute on Disability and Rehabilitation Research (NIDRR) within the Office of Special Education and Rehabilitation Services in the US Department of Education. The program has included 27 SCI centers over the years and for the 2000–2005 grant cycle there were 16 designated regional centers. MSCIS programs are capable of providing the entire continuum of care, from acute medical management to rehabilitation and lifelong follow-up. Grantees also contribute data to the National Spinal Cord Injury

Database. As a result of these efforts, life expectancy has increased substantially. For an individual injured at age 20, life expectancy ranges from 45.3 years for complete paraplegia to 16.4 years for ventilator-dependent tetraplegia.

In 1980, the US Department of Veterans Affairs established fellowship programs for SCI. In 1996, the Accreditation Council for Graduate Medical Education (ACGME) approved SCI medicine as a subspecialty, and the first examination was subsequently given in October 1998. As of November 2005, there were 21 ACGME accredited SCI fellowships. Subspecialty certification is conferred through the American Board of Physical Medicine and Rehabilitation; however, any current diplomate in good standing with a member Board of the American Board of Medical Specialties (ABMS) is eligible, if they otherwise meeting training requirements.

INITIAL CARE OF TRAUMATIC SPINAL CORD INJURY

Treatment of acute SCI begins with the resuscitation, medical stabilization, and neurological assessment of the patient. In the setting of a suspected SCI, the importance of an accurate neurological examination cannot be overemphasized. Diagnostic and treatment decisions are made in part based on the neurological examination. First, it is important to determine whether the patient has sustained a SCI, since certain interventions are only effective if started soon after injury. For example, high dose methylprednisolone must be started within 8 hours of SCI; otherwise, treatment initiated after 8 hours can result in less recovery compared to placebo (5). Careful examination can also reveal additional spinal or spinal cord injuries distant from the suspected site, as noncontiguous spine fractures occur in up to 10% to 15% of individuals with spine trauma (6,7). Surgical treatment is also influenced by neurological status. Surgical decompression and stabilization may be scheduled sooner for someone with an incomplete injury or with deteriorating neurological status, even though surgery has not been shown to improve neurological outcome.

Often the initial neurological assessment is limited by the need for urgent medical and surgical interventions as well as factors affecting patient cooperation such as pain, analgesic medications, drugs and alcohol, or intubation (8). It is therefore felt that an examination performed 3 to 7 days after injury is a better indicator of prognosis than the initial examination (9,10). Neurological examinations should be conducted periodically to monitor progress, establish goals for rehabilitation, and detect late deterioration or improvement (11).

NEUROLOGICAL EXAMINATION AND CLASSIFICATION OF SPINAL CORD INJURY

As the care we provide individuals with SCI has improved, so has our understanding of prognosis. In order to interpret the literature on recovery and prognosis after SCI, it is necessary to understand the terminology used to describe the level and severity of SCI. Classification of SCI is based upon a standardized examination, conducted according to the methods described in the *International Standards for Neurological Classification of Spinal Cord Injury* (12) and the accompanying *Reference Manual* (13), the gold standard for classification of SCI. The neurological assessment for traumatic SCI involves three parts: the sensory, motor, and rectal ("sacral sparing") examinations.

Sensory function is assessed by testing light touch and pinprick sensation for 28 dermatomes on the right and left sides of the body. Light touch is tested using a piece of cotton pulled away from the cotton applicator stick. Pinprick sensation is generally tested using the sharp and dull ends of a safety pin. Sensation for each individual dermatome is graded on a three-point scale, with 0 for absent, 1 for impaired, and 2 for normal (Fig. 2-1). Impaired means that the quality of sensation when the affected area is touched is different compared to the face, or if necessary, another uninvolved body part. For pinprick sensation, this includes areas of allodynia (a dull stimulus is interpreted as sharp) or hyperpathia (pinprick is sharper than the normal reference point). Also for pinprick, absent means absence of sharpness, or inability to distinguish the sharp and dull ends of the safety pin, not the absence of all sensation.

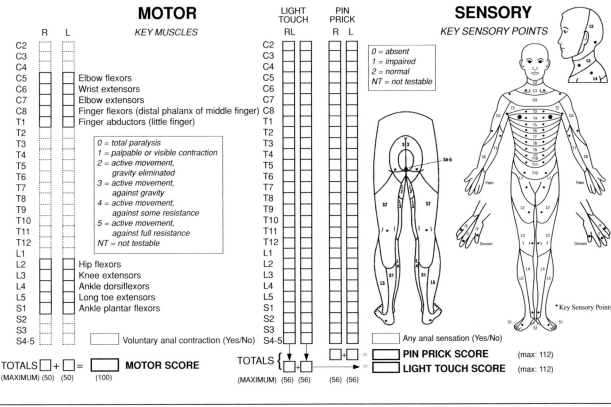

FIGURE 2-1. Standard neurological classification form for spinal cord injury. From: American Spinal Injury Association. *International Standards for Neurological Classification of Spinal Cord Injury, Revised 2002.* Chicago: American Spinal Injury Association, with permission.

The motor examination involves manual strength testing of five key muscles in each extremity, graded on a 6-point scale from 0 to 5 (Figs. 2-1 and 2-2). These muscles represent the C5-T1 and L2-S1 myotomes respectively. The rectal examination is performed to determine whether there is any sparing of sensory or motor function in sacral segments. Sacral sparing is confirmed by the presence of any of the following: pinprick or light-touch sensation at the anal mucocutaneous junction, deep anal sensation with the finger in the rectum, or the ability to voluntarily contract the anal sphincter. If there is uncer-

tainty regarding the presence or absence of sacral sparing, this portion of the exam should be repeated several times. The presence or absence of the bulbocavernosus and anal wink reflexes are also documented. There are a number of optional elements to the examination, such as testing for proprioception and evaluating additional muscles such as the deltoid or hip extensors, but they are not needed to classify patients (13).

With information obtained from the examination described above, one is able to classify the level and severity of injury. Sensory, motor, and neurological levels are

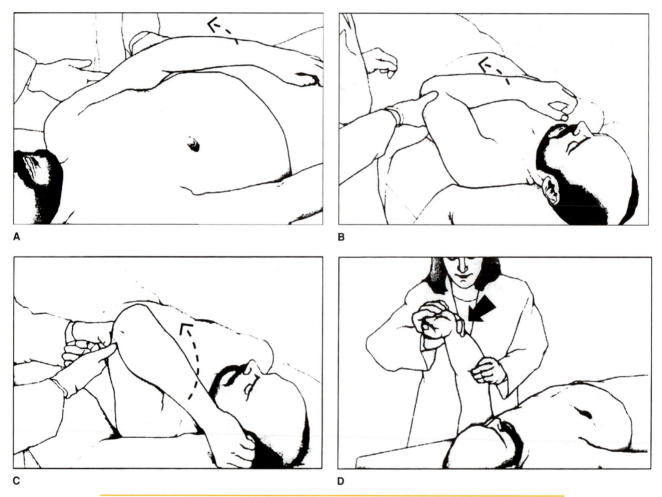

FIGURE 2-2. Test positions for various muscle grades of the elbow extensor (triceps) muscle. **A:** muscle grades 0 and 1, the triceps is being palpated for a volitional contraction in the gravity eliminated position, with grade 0 characterized by the absence of contraction and grade 1 characterized by trace contraction. **B:** Muscle grade 2, the triceps is being assessed in the gravity eliminated position for the ability to actively extend through a full range-of-motion. **C:** Muscle grade 3, the triceps is being assessed for the ability to actively extend through a full range of motion against gravity. **D:** Muscle grades 4 and 5, the triceps is being assessed for the amount of resistance (strength) present during extension against gravity, grade 4 defined as the ability to provide some resistance but less than normal, and grade 5 being normal. From: American Spinal Injury Association. *Reference Manual for the International Standards for Neurological Classification of Spinal Cord Injury.* Chicago: American Spinal Injury Association; 2003, pp. 28–30, with permission.

determined and represent the last levels with normal spinal cord function on both sides of the body. Sensory and motor levels can also be subdivided for the right and left sides respectively. The sensory level, specifically, is defined as the most caudal segment with normal sensory function, light–touch, and pinprick. For example, if sensation from rostral to caudal becomes abnormal at the C6 dermatome, then the sensory level is C5. Likewise, the motor level refers to the most caudal segment of the spinal cord with normal motor function. Normal motor function in this context means a motor grade of 3 or higher with all the above motor levels being grade 5. Again, it should be emphasized that to assign a sensory or motor level, all preceding rostral levels need to be normal for the modality being assessed. The neurological level of injury (NLI) is defined as the most caudal segment of the spinal cord with normal sensory and motor function on both sides of the body. It is therefore the same as the most rostral of the right and left motor and sensory levels. The zone of partial preservation (ZPP) refers to those dermatomes and myotomes caudal to the NLI that remain partially innervated and demonstrate partial preservation of function. The term is applicable only for complete injuries.

Severity of injury is graded by the ASIA Impairment Scale (AIS), a 5-point ordinal scale from A to E (Table 2-1). An AIS grade of A represents a complete injury, while grades B through E represent varying degrees of incomplete injuries. A complete injury is defined by the absence of sacral sparing as reviewed above, namely no sensation in the S4-5 segment or the inability to voluntarily contract the anal sphincter. This has been shown to be the

most reliable and clinically useful definition (14). An AIS grade of B represents an injury that is sensory incomplete (preserved sensation alone in the S4-5 segment), while grades C and D represent motor incomplete injuries. An AIS grade of E is given to a person who has recovered all sensory and motor function in the tested elements.

PROGNOSIS FOLLOWING TRAUMATIC SPINAL CORD INJURY

Much of the literature on prognosis after traumatic SCI in the United States comes from the MSCIS and its national database. Currently there are 16 centers throughout the United States, and data collected by individual centers is compiled in a common database maintained by the National Spinal Cord Injury Statistical Center, currently located at the University of Alabama at Birmingham (www.spinalcord.uab.edu/). The MSCIS database contains information on over 30,000 subjects with SCI (15).

Below we will review prognosis for neurological recovery according to the AIS grade. People with complete SCI are classified as AIS grade A. In this subset of patients, recovery of motor function distal to the zone of injury is relatively rare, and when it does occur tends to be minimal and nonfunctional. The MSCIS database indicates that about 15% of all AIS grade-A patients admitted within 1 week of injury convert to incomplete status by 1 year. However, only 2.3% of initially complete patients regain significant motor function below the injury level, that is, to AIS grade D (16). Other studies have reported complete to incomplete conversion rates ranging from 4% to 34% (9,14,17–19). Part of the reason for this wide range is the difficulty associated with performing an accurate neurological assessment during the early phase of injury. Factors that can impact reliability include those affecting cognition (traumatic brain injury, drug effects, and psychological disorders) as well as communication (ventilator dependency, language barrier) (8). Burns et al. (8) recently reported an overall conversion rate from complete (AIS A) to incomplete of 11.3% (6/53) by 1-year postinjury with three subjects regaining only sensation (AIS B) and three subjects having some volitional motor function. However, when analysis excluded subjects with factors affecting reliability, only 2 of 30 individuals (6.7%) converted from complete to incomplete, with both subjects improving to AIS grade B with no motor function below the zone of injury. In comparison, for subjects with factors affecting reliability, 4 of 23 (17.4%) individuals converted from complete to incomplete. Three of these subjects developed volitional motor function (AIS grade C or D) by 1 year.

▶ **TABLE 2-1** **The ASIA Impairment Scale**

Grade	Definition
A	Complete. No sensory or motor function is preserved in the sacral segments S4-S5.
B	Incomplete. Sensory but not motor function is preserved below the neurological level and includes the sacral segments S4-5.
C	Incomplete. Motor function is preserved below the neurological level, and more than half of the key muscles below the neurological level have a muscle grade <3 (grades 0 to 2).
D	Incomplete. Motor function is preserved below the neurological level, and at least half of the key muscles below the neurological level have a muscle grade ≥3.
E	Normal. Sensory and motor function are normal.

From: American Spinal Injury Association. *Reference Manual for the International Standards for Neurological Classification of Spinal Cord Injury.* Chicago: American Spinal Injury Association; 2003, with permission.

In contrast to recovery below the zone of injury, most people with complete tetraplegia have some local recovery within the ZPP. The majority of individuals with complete tetraplegia gain a motor level, although there are differences dependent on the initial level. If the initial motor level is C4, 70% will gain C5 motor function; the corresponding rates for C5 to C6 and C6 to C7 are 75% and 85%, respectively (20). Recovery more than two levels below the most caudal level with motor function is rare, being seen in only 1% of cases (18). In comparison to tetraplegia, neurological status following complete paraplegia changes little. Waters et al. (19) reported that in 73% (108/148) of patients, the neurologic level of injury did not change at 1 year. Only two patients recovered greater than two levels. None of the patients with an initial neurological level above T9 regained any lower extremity motor function.

Recovery in motor complete, sensory incomplete injuries (AIS grade B) is mixed, with about 50% attaining ambulatory status (11,21). Individuals with an AIS grade-B injury have some initial preservation of distal sensation, including the S4-5 dermatomes, but no accompanying motor function. Continuity of sensory preservation between the NLI and S4-5 is not required. It is known that type of sensory sparing influences prognosis—those with sacral or lower extremity pinprick sensation have a better chance of walking than those with only light touch sensation (21–25). Crozier et al. (24) found that eight of nine subjects with partial sparing of pinprick sensation at presentation walked compared to only two of 18 without pinprick preservation. Katoh and el Masry (25) also found that magnitude of pinprick preservation was a favorable prognostic indicator for motor recovery. In the largest series ($n = 131$) to date, Oleson et al. (21) recently performed a secondary analysis of the database from the Sygen (GM1-ganglioside) study (26). They also found a favorable association between sparing of pinprick sensation and recovery of ambulation, although the association was weaker than that of Crozier et al., 40% versus 67% for household ambulation and 16% versus 40% for community ambulation. Currently, the functional independence measure (FIM) defines community ambulation as the ability to ambulate a minimum of 150 feet.

Recovery in motor incomplete injuries (AIS grades C and D) is generally good, although this is influenced by the degree of motor deficit and the age of the patient. For AIS grade C patients younger than 50 years of age at the time of injury, the chance of walking exceeds 90%, while those over age 50 have only a 42% chance of walking (27). Up to 95% of individuals with AIS grade-D injuries will recover the ability to ambulate (11). Waters et al. (22,28,29) have looked at recovery of ambulation based on lower extremity strength at 1 month after injury. The investigators studied the predictive value of lower extremity motor scores obtained by adding the scores of the ten

key muscles in the legs (Fig. 2-1). All incomplete paraplegic injuries with a lower extremity motor score ≥ 10 (maximum possible score = 50) walked. For incomplete tetraplegic injuries, a score of at least 20 was required to ensure eventual ambulation.

The majority of neurological recovery in SCI patients occurs during the first 6 to 9 months (18,19,22,28–30). Afterward, the rate of improvement rapidly drops off with a plateau being reached 12 to 18 months postinjury with little additional improvement. Early improvement in neurological status is associated with greater recovery than slow improvement (31). Late recovery following complete SCI, defined as motor recovery >1 year after injury, is rare but can occur. Kirshblum et al. (32) evaluated changes in neurological status between 1 and 5 years postinjury and found approximately 2% of subjects converted from complete to motor incomplete status (AIS C or D) later than 1 year postinjury.

MAGNETIC RESONANCE IMAGING AND PROGNOSIS

Injury severity following traumatic SCI is reflected in the abnormalities visualized with magnetic resonance imaging (MRI). Characteristics shown to be related to prognosis have included the presence of intramedullary hemorrhage, presence of edema, length of edema, and cord compression. Early studies found that the presence of hemorrhage was associated with complete or motor complete injuries (33,34). A more recent study indicated that while the presence of hemorrhage is a negative prognostic factor, it may also be present in motor incomplete lesions. Flanders et al. (35) reported subjects with spinal cord hemorrhage regained only 9% of the resulting lower extremity motor deficit, while those without hemorrhage recovered 55% of lost motor function. In the absence of hemorrhage, edema extending greater than one spinal segment in length is associated with a poorer prognosis than more focal edema (33). Ishida et al. (31) demonstrated that lack of abnormal cord signal on MRI was a favorable prognostic indicator in cervical central cord injury.

In addition to the association with neurological recovery, findings on MRI are related to functional capabilities following SCI. In a study comparing early MRI findings (within 72 hours) with functional improvement after cervical SCI, patients without intramedullary hemorrhage had greater gains in self-care and mobility than patients with hemorrhage (36). Length of edema also had a negative correlation with self-care and mobility status at both rehabilitation admission and discharge. In addition, the rostral limit of edema was related to self-care and mobility scores, with lower levels of cervical edema corresponding to better function. Newer imaging techniques, including functional MRI (37), and more powerful magnets should increase the value of MRI in traumatic SCI.

ACUTE MEDICAL MANAGEMENT

Management of Cardiovascular Complications

The occurrence of deep vein thromboses (DVT) and pulmonary emboli (PE) are among the most feared complications during the acute period. In fact, individuals with acute SCI have a higher incidence of DVT than any other patient group (38). Without prophylaxis, 47% to 100% of individuals with acute SCI will develop a DVT (38,39), and PE is the third leading cause of death (40). Once adequate hemostasis is achieved, pharmacologic prophylaxis should be initiated as soon as possible, preferably within 72 hours of injury.

Clinical practice guidelines for the prevention of thromboembolism have recently been published by the Consortium for Spinal Cord Medicine (CSCM), sponsored by the Paralyzed Veterans of America (PVA) (39), as well as the American College of Chest Physicians (38). The second edition of the CSCM guidelines is currently available for purchase at the PVA website (www.pva.org/pvastore/). Individuals with partial motor paralysis should receive prophylactic subcutaneous or low-molecular-weight (LMW) heparin. In the setting of complete motor paralysis, LMW heparin is desirable due to its improved pharmacologic properties. Recently, daily (40 mg) and twice daily (30 mg) dosing of the LMW heparin enoxaparin have been reported to be equally efficacious for acute SCI (41). Prophylaxis should continue for either the duration of inpatient hospitalization, including rehabilitation, or alternatively 2 months in uncomplicated cases. Treatment should be extended to 3 months in the setting of additional risk factors, which include lower limb fractures, prior thrombosis, cancer, heart failure, obesity, and age >70.

Pharmacologic therapy should also be supplemented with mechanical prophylaxis. We suggest sequential compression devices for the first 2 weeks followed by a transition to antithrombotic compression stockings for the remainder of the hospitalization. If prophylaxis has been delayed more than 72 hours, the presence of leg thrombi should be excluded prior to the placement of compression devices. If contraindications preclude pharmacologic prophylaxis, weekly screening with lower extremity ultrasound is reasonable and consideration should be given to the placement of an inferior vena cava filter in cases felt to be at particularly high risk. Despite being a common practice in many trauma centers, the literature does not support the routine use of inferior vena cava filters as prophylaxis for PE in SCI (38). Following the diagnosis of a DVT, the patient should be on bedrest until 48 to 72 hours after the initiation of appropriate therapy to reduce the risk of pulmonary embolism.

Management of Autonomic Dysfunction

Patients with a neurological level at and above T6 are also at risk for a life-threatening complication called autonomic dysreflexia (AD). It is characterized by the abrupt onset of malignant hypertension. Any noxious stimulus can trigger episodes but the leading causes are bladder distention and bowel impaction (42,43). Other possible causes are listed in Table 2-2. Noxious afferent impulses are conducted to the spinal cord below the lesion resulting in the stimulation of sympathetic neurons in the intermediolateral gray matter and massive sympathetic efferent outflow through the splanchnic pathways (T6 through L2). Descending inhibition that normally originates above T6 is blocked, which leads to unopposed sympathetic outflow and malignant hypertension. Other signs and symptoms include severe headache, increased spasticity, sweating, blurred vision, nasal congestion, cutis anserina (goose bumps), piloerection, facial flushing, bradycardia, and general apprehension (43). Bradycardia and facial flushing are the result of parasympathetic activity to the heart and neurological levels above the injury, which remains intact via the vagal nerve. It should be noted that individuals with SCI can have a normal systolic blood pressure in the 90 to 110 mm Hg range; therefore, a blood pressure 20 to 40 mm Hg above baseline can be a sign of AD in the proper clinical context. Treatment is centered on performing a systematic survey of the patient to identify and treat the precipitating noxious stimuli, with special emphasis placed on bowel and bladder function. If the cause is not readily apparent, hypertension should be treated while the diagnostic evaluation to identify more uncommon causes (i.e., intra-abdominal and gynecological pathology) continues. Topical nitrates (i.e., ointment or paste) are often helpful because they can be easily removed following the resolution of the episode. Clinical practice guidelines have been published for AD (43). It is also reasonable to admit the patient and observe overnight for the recurrence of AD. In the setting of labor/delivery associated with post-SCI pregnancy, AD occurs predictably and can be prevented with epidural or spinal anesthesia (44).

Severe cervical injuries lead to an autonomic imbalance of the internal organs, such as the heart, which is characterized by parasympathetic predominance. This is due to the interruption of sympathetic pathways in the setting of an intact vagal nerve. The clinical manifestation is a susceptibility to vagal episodes with symptomatic bradycardia or even transient second- or third-degree heart block or asystole. Such episodes are often triggered by benign events such as endotracheal suctioning or repositioning the patient. Atropine readily reverses the vagal

▶ **TABLE 2-2** **Possible Causes of Autonomic Dysreflexia in Spinal Cord Injury**

Acute and Postacute:

- Bladder distention
- Urinary tract infection
- Epididymitis or scrotal compression
- Bowel distention
- Bowel impaction
- Gallstones
- Gastric ulcers or gastritis
- Invasive testing
- Hemorrhoids
- Gastrocolic irritation
- Appendicitis or other intra-abdominal pathology
- Menstruation
- Vaginitis
- Deep vein thrombosis
- Pulmonary emboli
- Pressure ulcers
- Blisters
- Contact with hard or sharp objects
- Fractures or other trauma
- Surgical procedures
- Pain
- Temperature fluctuations
- Any painful or irritating stimuli below the level of injury

Postacute:

- Cystoscopy, urodynamics, or detrusor sphincter dyssynergia
- Gastrocolic irritation
- Menstruation
- Pregnancy (labor and delivery)
- Sexual intercourse
- Ejaculation
- Ingrown toenail
- Burns or sunburn
- Blisters
- Insect bites
- Constrictive clothing, shoes, or appliances
- Heterotopic bone

Sources: Kuric J, Hixon AK. *Clinical Practice Guidelines: Autonomic Dysreflexia.* Jackson Heights, N.Y.: Eastern Paralyzed Veterans Association; 1996; Consortium for Spinal Cord Medicine. Acute management of autonomic dysreflexia: individuals with spinal cord injury presenting to health-care facilities. *J Spinal Cord Med.* 2002;25 (suppl 1):S67–S88.

symptomatology and should be kept at the bedside. In severe cases, temporary pacer pads can be maintained on the patient. The predilection to such episodes rarely persists beyond 2 to 6 weeks after injury, resolving by 2 weeks in the majority of cases (45). In the rare event that such episodes become life threatening or persist, a cardiology evaluation for pacemaker implantation can be helpful.

The predominance of parasympathetic tone can also lead to marked hypotension during the initial weeks. This is attributed to the elimination of sympathetic arteriolar tone, and like bradycardia, tends to gradually resolve. Acutely, it can be effectively addressed with intravenous vasoconstrictors (i.e., dopamine) (45). Weaning from intravenous medications can be facilitated by the addition of oral medications such as midodrine, an alpha$_1$-agonist, or fludrocortisone acetate, a potent mineralocorticoid.

Management of Respiratory Complications

Overall, respiratory complications are the leading cause of mortality during the first year postinjury as well as during long-term follow-up (40). Proper pulmonary care following a traumatic cervical SCI begins with the performance of an initial history and physical. Relevant issues that the health care provider should be aware of include a prior history of lung disease, smoking history, current medications, substance abuse, extent of neurological impairment, and coexisting injuries. Pneumonia, atelectasis, and other respiratory complications can occur in 40% to 70% of tetraplegics (46–51). The primary muscle of respiration, the diaphragm, is innervated by C3-C4-C5 via the phrenic nerve. In the absence of pre-existing disease or other medical complications, the majority of individuals with complete SCI and neurological levels at and below C4 can be expected to be ventilator independent. Long-term respiratory status is less clear with C3 injuries while the majority of individuals with a level of C2 and above can be expected to be ventilator dependent (52).

Despite the above, many individuals who will eventually wean require temporary ventilator support. Cervical injuries that are not initially intubated should be followed closely with serial vital capacities (VC) and negative inspiratory forces (NIF), which in the first few days could be as frequently as every 6 to 8 hours. Trends in addition to absolute values are important. The goal is to identify early deterioration in pulmonary function before it becomes clinically urgent. Other signs and symptoms which should prompt further investigation include fevers, an increased respiratory rate and shortness of breath, increased anxiety, and changes in secretion characteristics such as increased volume, increased tenacity, or more frequent suctioning. Consideration should be given to elective intubation for rapidly diminishing NIFs or VCs or values consistently below −30 to −40 for the NIF or 10 to 15 cc/kg of ideal body weight for the VC. In some patients, assistance can be provided and intubation avoided through the utilization of continuous positive airway pressure (CPAP) or bilevel positive airway pressure (BiPAP), with either a face mask or mouthpiece. During the early stages, an abdominal binder is often employed in the sitting position. This has been shown to increase vital capacity in tetraplegics patients (53–55), and is felt to work by increasing intra-abdominal pressure thereby displacing abdominal contents upward and maintaining the diaphragm in an ideal dome-shaped configuration.

For patients requiring mechanical ventilation, higher tidal volumes than typically used in hospitalized patients have been advocated (51,56). Peterson et al. (51) reported a lower incidence of atelectasis, shorter weaning times, and the absence of complications such as barotrauma or pneumothoraces when higher tidal volumes were used. Unlike other patient populations, individuals sustaining a SCI usually have healthy lungs and respiratory failure is purely a consequence of neuromuscular weakness. In this setting, primary goals include recruiting and maintaining aeration of alveoli, thereby preventing atelectasis and secondary complications such as secretion retention and superimposed pneumonia. Protocols for gradually increasing tidal volumes to 20 to 25 cc/kg ideal body weight are available in the recent PVA sponsored *Clinical Practice Guidelines for Respiratory Management following Spinal Cord Injury* (57) as well as earlier publications (58).

Maintaining secretion clearance requires constant vigilance. Pneumonia and atelectasis occur more often in the left than right lung (59). This has been attributed to the acute angle of takeoff of the left main stem bronchus, resulting in difficulty in accessing this airway for suctioning and secretion clearance. In cervical and high thoracic injuries, expiratory flow rates are inadequate for coughing due to the absence of volitional abdominal contractions. Expiratory capacity can be documented and followed with peak expiratory flow rates (60). Sympathetic innervation to the lungs is commonly compromised but parasympathetic innervation via the vagal nerve remains intact. This results in airway hyperreactivity and increased secretion production. Due to the above, scheduled bronchodilators and mucolytic agents (i.e., guaifenesin) are indicated. Chest physiotherapy and assisted coughing also help to mobilize secretions effectively. The latter involves either compressing the costophrenic margin bilaterally or exerting upward pressure inferior to the xyphoid process in a timed fashion with expiration. These maneuvers augment expiratory airflow and substitute for paralyzed abdominal muscles. The CoughAssist in-exsufflator (JH Emerson Co, Cambridge, Mass) is a device that rapidly generates positive pressures up to +40 mm Hg followed by a rapid reversal of airflow to 40 mm Hg accompanied by the removal of airway secretions. Most patients prefer it to endotracheal suctioning, as it avoids irritation associated with endotracheal suctioning, and it can be attached to a tracheotomy or alternatively utilized with a mouthpiece. At times, bronchoscopy can be performed for recalcitrant secretion retention ("mucous plugging"). Incentive spirometry should also be routinely employed in the ventilator independent patient.

Pressure Ulcer Prevention

Pressure ulcers are a devastating complication that occur in up to 40% of SCI patients during the initial hospitalization (61). They are also largely preventable with proper care. It is helpful to assess risk at admission utilizing a standardized scale such as the Braden scale (score range 6 to 23) (Fig. 2-3) (62–65). Patients with complete paralysis will score as high risk (≤12 points) and warrant prophylactic use of a specialized surface (i.e., low air loss mattress). Regardless of the mattress surface, patients need to be turned/repositioned every 2 hours to prevent the formation of pressure ulcers (61,66). Special attention needs to be paid to dependent areas such as the heels, sacrum, scapulae, occiput, and the greater trochanters when side lying. Adequate nutrition is crucial and weekly determination of parameters such as albumin/prealbumin can help direct therapy. Additional recommendations are outlined in recently published practice guidelines (61). Once a pressure ulcer is present, consultation should be promptly obtained from a wound care specialist. Untreated pressure ulcers can lead to sepsis, osteomyelitis, and even death.

Neurogenic Bowel and Bladder Dysfunction

SCI significantly impacts bowel function. Because of autonomic dysfunction and immobility, gut transit times are prolonged (67), which in turn can predispose to severe constipation or impaction. In addition, volitional control of defecation is often absent with severe injuries. The long-term goal will be to devise a program to stimulate bowel movements at the desired time with resulting continence the remainder of the day. The management of neurogenic bowel dysfunction in the chronic setting is beyond the scope of this chapter; however, clinical practice guidelines are available (68). In the acute setting, a neurogenic bowel program should be initiated when enteral nutrition is started. A reasonable program could include one capsule of docusate sodium (stool softener) two to three times a day, two capsules or 15 mL liquid senna (promotility agent) at noon, and a bisacodyl suppository nightly. The suppository stimulates the rectocolic reflex and coincides with the peak activity of senna, which is approximately 8 hours after ingestion. The stool softener can be excluded in subjects on liquid nutrition (i.e., gastrostomy tube) and an enema can be substituted for the suppository if more than 2 days have passed without a significant stool. In patients with cauda equina or conus medullaris injuries, an enema should be routinely substituted for the suppository. Stress ulcer prophylaxis also needs to be administered during the acute hospitalization.

Urinary retention is the primary voiding abnormality during the acute phase of SCI. Because of the need to closely monitor urine output and the unfamiliarity of acute care staff with implementing neurogenic bladder programs, it is prudent to maintain an indwelling catheter until the patient is transferred to a rehabilitation setting. When the neurological deficits are minimal and the

Braden Risk Assessment Scale

NOTE: Bed and chairbound individuals or those with impaired ability to reposition should be assessed upon admission for their risk of developing pressure ulcers. Patients with established pressure ulcers should be reassessed periodically.

Patient Name: _____   Room Number:_____   Date: _____

Sensory Perception	**1. Completely Limited**	**2. Very Limited**	**3. Slightly Limited**	**4. No Impairment**	*Indicate Appropriate Numbers Below*
Ability to respond meaningfully to pressure-related discomfort	Unresponsive (does not moan, flinch or grasp) to painful stimuli, due to diminished level of consciousness or sedation. OR limited ability to feel pain over most of body surface.	Responds only to painful stimuli. Cannot communicate discomfort except by moaning or restlessness. OR has a sensory impairment which limits the ability to feel pain or discomfort over 1/2 of body.	Responds to verbal commands, but cannot always communicate discomfort or need to be turned. OR has some sensory impairment which limits ability to feel pain or discomfort in 1 or 2 extremities.	Responds to verbal commands. Has no sensory deficit which would limit ability to feel or voice pain or discomfort.	
Moisture	**1. Constantly Moist**	**2. Very Moist**	**3. Occasionally Moist**	**4. Rarely Moist**	
Degree to which skin is exposed to moisture	Skin is kept moist almost constantly by perspiration, urine, etc. Dampness is detected every time patient is moved or turned.	Skin is often, but not always, moist. Linen must be changed at least once a shift.	Skin is occasionally moist, requiring an extra linen change approximately once a day.	Skin is usually dry. Linen only requires changing at routine intervals.	
Activity	**1. Bedfast**	**2. Chairfast**	**3. Walks Occasionally**	**4. Walks Frequently**	
Degree of physical activity	Confined to bed.	Ability to walk severely limited or non-existent. Cannot bear own weight and/or must be assisted into chair or wheelchair	Walks occasionally during day, but for very short distances, with or without assistance. Spends majority of each shift in bed or chair	Walks outside the room at least twice a day and inside room at least once every 2 hours during waking hours.	
Mobility	**1. Completely Immobile**	**2. Very Limited**	**3. Slightly Limited**	**4. No Limitations**	
Ability to change and control body position	Does not make even slight changes in body or extremity position without assistance.	Makes occasional slight changes in body or extremity position but unable to make frequent or significant changes independently	Makes frequent though slight changes in body or extremity position independently	Makes major and frequent changes in position without assistance	
Nutrition	**1. Very Poor**	**2. Probably Inadequate**	**3. Adequate**	**4. Excellent**	
Usual food intake pattern	Never eats a complete meal. Rarely eats more than 1/3 of any food offered. Eats 2 servings or less of protein (meat or dairy products) per day. Takes fluids poorly. Does not take a liquid dietary supplement. OR is NPO and/or maintained on clear liquids or I.V.'s for more than 5 days.	Rarely eats a complete meal and generally eats only about 1/2 of any food offered. Protein intake includes only 3 servings of meat or dairy products per day. Occasionally will take a dietary supplement. OR receives less than optimum amount of liquid diet or tube feeding.	Eats over half of most meals. Eats a total of 4 servings of protein (meat, dairy products) each day. Occasionally will refuse a meal, but will usually take a supplement if offered. OR is on a tube feeding or TPN regimen which probably meets most of nutritional needs.	Eats most of every meal. Never refuses a meal. Usually eats a total of 4 or more servings of meat and dairy products. Occasionally eats between meals. Does not require supplementation.	
Friction and Shear	**1. Problem**	**2. Potential Problem**	**3. No Apparent Problem**		
	Requires moderate to maximum assistance in moving. Complete lifting without sliding against sheets is impossible Frequently slides down in bed or chair, requiring frequent repositioning with maximum assistance. Spasticity, contractures or agitation lead to almost constant friction.	Moves feebly or requires minimum assistance. During a move, skin probably slides to some extent against sheets, chair restraints, or other devices. Maintains relatively good position in chair or bed most of the time, but occasionally slides down.	Moves in bed and in chair independently and has sufficient muscle strength to lift up completely during move. Maintains good position in bed or chair at all times.		

NOTE: Patients with a total score of 16 or less are considered to be at risk of developing pressure ulcers.
(15 or 16 = low risk; 13 or 14 = moderate risk; 12 or less = high risk)
© Copyright Barbara Braden and Nancy Bergstrom, 1988

Total Score:

FIGURE 2-3. Braden scale for assessing pressure ulcer risk. From: Copyright Barbara Braden and Nancy Bergstrom, 1988. Reprinted with permission.

patient will be discharged, it is important to document adequate bladder emptying by checking postvoid residuals 2 to 3 times. This can be accomplished noninvasively using a portable ultrasound device such as the Bladder Scan (Diagnostic Ultrasound, Bothell, Wash).

CURRENT EFFORTS TO TREAT AND IMPACT OUTCOMES FOLLOWING ACUTE SPINAL CORD INJURY

Before David and Aguayo (69) utilized peripheral nerve grafts to bridge a spinal cord lesion in an animal model, achieving axonal regeneration and restoring communication, following SCI, seemed largely unattainable. Since this report, our understanding of the underlying pathophysiology and associated barriers to recovery has increased exponentially. As a result, today's clinical and basic science investigators are actively challenging themselves to find new strategies for improving function following SCI. Potential therapeutic strategies include neuroprotection to limit secondary injury, cell replacement through transplantation, manipulation of the lesion environment to promote axon regeneration, and the utilization of rehabilitation strategies that promote neuroplasticity ("rewiring") by spared pathways in order to compensate for lost pathways.

Despite ongoing efforts, to date, there has been a paucity of trials performed for acute SCI in human subjects. Only methylprednisolone is routinely administered in the clinical setting, and recently, the efficacy of methylprednisolone has become the subject of intense, ongoing debate. Instead, efforts have focused on (a) rehabilitative strategies (occupational and physical therapy) that teach patients and caregivers compensatory strategies for neurological impairments and (b) optimizing medical management to prevent secondary complications and maximize overall health.

The Administration of Steroids

For the treatment of traumatic SCI, high-dose methylprednisolone (MP) therapy is the only pharmacological therapy reported to have efficacy in phase III randomized trials; the National Acute Spinal Cord Injury Study (NASCIS) II trial in 1990 and NASCIS III trial in 1997 respectively (70–73). Subsequently, MP administration for acute SCI has become widespread in the United States. The primary mechanism of action is likely the prevention of lipid peroxidation in neuronal membranes with anti-inflammatory and vasoactive effects also playing a role (74–76). Recently the efficacy of this treatment has been questioned and currently is the subject of ongoing debate (77–86). Much of the debate has centered on whether the magnitude of reported improvement with MP is clinically important.

Despite this, the majority of trauma centers in the United States continue to administer the drug. It is indicated if the patient presents with a neurological deficit within 8 hours of injury and is administered as an intravenous bolus (30 mg/kg) over 15 minutes followed by a 45-minute pause then a continuous drip (5.4 mg/kg/h) for 23 hours. This regimen was tolerated in the majority of NASCIS II subjects without significant side effects. The NASCIS III trial advocated extending the drip to 48 hours for individuals presenting within the 3- to 8-hour window following injury, but this practice is not as widespread and is clearly at the discretion of the individual trauma center. There was a significantly higher incidence of pneumonia and a trend toward an increased occurrence of severe sepsis in individuals receiving the extended drip (72). MP administration is not recommended outside the 8-hour postinjury window or in the setting of penetrating SCI.

Prior, Current, and Future Clinical Trials

The controversy regarding the utilization of MP highlights the critical need for new treatment strategies. To date, the treatment of acute SCI has been characterized, unfortunately, by the paucity of clinical trials. In 1991, a small, randomized clinical trial ($n = 37$ subjects) of GM-1 ganglioside reported an improvement in neurological recovery following SCI (87). GM-1 ganglioside was felt to have both neuroprotective and neuroregenerative effects (88,89). These encouraging results led to a multicenter, randomized clinical trial. Results were reported in 2001 and initially showed more rapid recovery in the interventional arm; however, by 26 weeks neurological outcomes were similar in both arms (26,90,91). One pilot study suggested a possible therapeutic effect of thyrotropin-releasing hormone (TRH) in patients with traumatic SCI; however, it was hampered by a small number of subjects and limited 12-month follow-up (92).

The issue of whether one should do early or delayed surgical decompression has also been actively debated, and there is an urgent need for clinical trials to definitively answer this question (93). Not surprisingly, in the absence of such studies, practice patterns vary widely (94). As reviewed by Fehlings et al. (93), animal studies suggest that early decompression following SCI can improve neurological outcomes.

Another exciting, new intervention that involves physical retraining is body weight support gait training. It is known that cats with completely transected spinal cords at the thoracic level can recover a functional, hind limb stepping pattern with weight supported treadmill training (95,96). The explanation for how this might work is based on the theoretical existence of a secondary central pattern generator (CPG) in the lumbar spinal cord. Based on animal and human work, it has been postulated that training this pattern generator with body weight support might

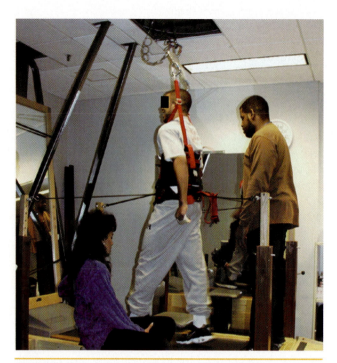

FIGURE 2-4. Subject with incomplete spinal cord injury undergoing bodyweight supported treadmill training.

facilitate the recovery of walking (Fig. 2-4) (97–101). Recently, a National Institutes of Health (NIH) funded multicenter study to evaluate its potential efficacy in humans concluded and the results are pending publication. Initial results, presented at the 2003 joint conference of the American Congress of Rehabilitation Medicine/American Society of Neurorehabilitation, found no difference in ambulation status in subjects with incomplete SCI randomized to body-weight support versus traditional physical therapy. In the future, methods that utilize the concept of activity-dependent neuroplasticity will likely play an increasing role in the rehabilitation of SCI patients.

Currently a phase II clinical trial is under way in North America based on immune-mediated mechanisms that have shown promise in animal models of SCI (102–105). The trial is sponsored by Proneuron Biotechnologies Inc., and employs autologous activated macrophages. The macrophages are isolated from the patient's own blood, activated through a proprietary process, and then injected directly into the injured spinal cord at the site of the lesion. The mechanism of action is not completely understood but is thought to involve the secretion of growth factors by the macrophages and the initiation of a controlled immune response that promotes healing. In an earlier phase I study conducted in Israel and Belgium, the company (www.spinalcordtrial.com/faq.html) reported that 4 of 16 subjects converted from complete to incomplete status. Results for the eight subjects from the

Israeli arm were recently published (106). Optimism for additional clinical trials of new therapies in the near future has been bolstered by rapid advancements in the laboratory.

Mobilization and Goals for Initial Rehabilitation

Neuropathic pain and spasticity are usually more of an issue during postacute rehabilitation; however, occasionally therapy needs be initiated during the acute phase of injury. Gabapentin has rapidly become the initial treatment of choice for neuropathic pain and is well tolerated in the majority of patients (107–112). In the inpatient setting, the drug can be started at 100 mg every 8 hours and titrated up every 2 to 3 days to 3,600 mg/day dosed three to four times a day. Widely used options for spasticity include oral baclofen, a γ–aminobutyric acid (GABA) agonist, and tizanidine, an α–adrenergic agonist, but their use can be complicated by central nervous system (CNS) side effects such as sedation and confusion. Dantrolene, which blocks the release of calcium from the sarcoplasmic reticulum muscle, is a peripheral acting agent that avoids the CNS side effects of other agents. Hepatoxicity is the primary side effect; therefore, liver function tests should be checked prior to initiation of therapy then periodically afterward. In those patients whose spasticity cannot be controlled with oral agents, intrathecal baclofen delivered via an implantable pump may be effective. Because much lower doses of baclofen are required when the drug is delivered intrathecally, many of the side effects of oral administration are avoided. As with oral baclofen, abrupt cessation of intrathecal baclofen should be avoided, as withdrawal may cause confusion, seizures, and even death (113–122).

Physical therapy (PT) and occupational therapy (OT) should be consulted as soon as range-of-motion (ROM) exercises for the extremities are medically feasible, even in the intensive care unit. Early involvement by PT/OT also provides ongoing education to the patient and family regarding the injury and the rehabilitation process. Upright positioning in bed and sitting should be initiated as soon as adequate spine stabilization is achieved. It is important that the spine surgeon provide specific instructions regarding precautions. This is particularly important when bracing is involved (e.g., "Is the brace required when supine or sitting in bed?"). Specific precautions, such as allowed ROM and weightbearing, also need to be clear for accompanying extremity injuries.

To avoid orthostatic hypotension, the head of the bed should be gradually elevated to 70 to 90 degrees while monitoring blood pressure before sitting or standing. Compression stockings (thigh- or knee-high) or elastic wrappings diminish blood pooling in the lower extremities. An elastic abdominal binder can be employed in early stages to counteract pooling in splanchnic vessels. If conservative measures fail, midodrine, an alpha agonist, or fludrocortisone, an aldosterone-like mineral corticoid can be used.

Early consultation should be obtained from a medical rehabilitation specialist, who can assist with assessing injury severity, managing medical issues specific to SCI, and rehabilitation decision making. Most patients will benefit from inpatient rehabilitation in a Commission on the Accreditation of Rehabilitation Facilities (CARF) accredited SCI program. Less intensive options are subacute and skilled nursing facilities. Following inpatient rehabilitation, outpatient follow-up is important. CARF accredited programs must have a mechanism for long-term follow-up. Individuals with cervical or high thoracic injuries are at increased risk for pulmonary complications and should be vaccinated for pneumococcus every 10 years and influenza annually.

Expected Outcomes following Rehabilitation

In 1955, Long (123) was the first to relate functional capacity to level of injury. His astute observations have stood the test of time and have served as a guide for estimating functional capacity based on the neurological level. Other investigators have also examined the impact of injury level on function (124–127). The Consortium for Spinal Cord Medicine (11) recently published an excellent set of clinical practice guidelines on expected outcomes following traumatic SCI. For this discussion, level of injury refers to motor level. It has been previously shown that motor level correlates better with self-care than the neurological level, which incorporates sensory function (128).

C1-4 patients are dependent for activities of daily living (ADLs), bed mobility, and transfers. They can often utilize a motorized wheelchair with specialized control mechanisms such as sip-and-puff. C1-3 patients are also usually permanently dependent on mechanical ventilation (52). C5 patients have active elbow flexion and can perform some simple ADLs with set-up and special hand devices. This group of patients is otherwise dependent on an attendant for ADLs and transfers. They are unable to rollover or come to a sitting position in bed without additional adaptive devices. They can utilize a motorized wheelchair with hand controls, but they are unable to propel themselves in a manual wheelchair.

C6 patients have full innervation of the rotator cuff musculature and added shoulder stability. More importantly, active wrist extension is possible utilizing the extensor carpi radialis. Active wrist extension is accompanied by passive finger flexion and opposition of the second digit with the thumb. This passive grip is referred to as a tenodesis grip and can be developed with appropriate occupational therapy to grasp and manipulate objects. Tenodesis grip can be strengthened using a wrist-driven flexor-hinge orthosis. Nevertheless, most of these patients still require assistance for ADLs, bed mobility, and transfers. Wheelchair propulsion is also possible for short distances on smooth, level surfaces. Hand rim projections (knobs) can facilitate this.

C7 patients gain functional strength in the triceps. The ability to forcefully extend the elbow allows the patient to lift his or her bodyweight. These patients can roll over, sit up in bed, and move about in the sitting position. Motivated patients can also transfer independently. Some assistance may still be required for toileting and dressing activities, particularly for the lower extremities. Eating can be done independently except for cutting. Independent wheelchair propulsion is possible for long distances on smooth surfaces.

C8 and T1 patients gain increasingly greater intrinsic hand function, which results in improved grasp strength and dexterity. This patient should be independent with bed mobility and transfers. Individuals with levels of C8 and below should also be independent with ADLs. Patients with injuries below T1 are at a minimum independent using a wheelchair. Prospects for meaningful ambulation depend on the variables discussed above. Sitting balance progressively improves with lower thoracic levels.

CONCLUSION

The care of individuals following traumatic SCI has improved dramatically since pre–World War II when mortality was 60% to 80% within months of injury. This has been facilitated largely by the development of specialized SCI centers predicated on providing interdisciplinary, comprehensive care. With proper medical management, secondary complications are largely preventable and many individuals now lead healthy, productive lives following injury. Unfortunately, our ability to impact the extent of neurorecovery following the most severe injuries remains limited, and rehabilitation to a large extent focuses on teaching compensatory strategies to deal with resulting impairments. Although the number of clinical trials has been limited to date, the future holds great promise and it is with great anticipation that we await the challenge of translating exciting laboratory advancements to the clinical care of our patients.

REFERENCES

1. National Spinal Cord Injury Statistical Center. Spinal Cord Injury: Facts and Figures at a Glance. Available at: www. spinalcord.uab.edu. Accessed June 2, 2005.

2. Berkowitz M, O'Leary P, Kruse D, et al. *Spinal Cord Injury: An Analysis of Medical and Social Costs*. New York: Demos Medical Publishing; 1998.

3. Lifshutz J, Colohan A. A brief history of therapy for traumatic spinal cord injury. *Neurosurg Focus*. 2004;16(1):1–8.

4. Bedbrook GM. The development and care of spinal cord paralysis (1918 to 1986). *Paraplegia*. 1987;25(3):172–184.

5. Bracken MB, Holford TR. Effects of timing of methylprednisolone or naloxone administration on recovery of segmental and long-tract neurologic function in NASCIS 2. *J Neurosurg*. 1993;79(4):500–507.

6. Henderson RL, Reid DC, Saboe LA. Multiple noncontiguous spine fractures. *Spine*. 1991;16(2):128–131.

7. Vaccaro AR, An HS, Lin S, et al. Noncontiguous injuries of the spine. *J Spinal Disord*. 1992;5(3):320–329.

8. Burns AS, Lee BS, Ditunno JF Jr, et al. Patient selection for clinical trials: the reliability of the early spinal cord injury examination. *J Neurotrauma*. 2003;20(5):477–482.

9. Maynard FM, Reynolds GG, Fountain S, et al. Neurological prognosis after traumatic quadriplegia. Three-year experience of California Regional Spinal Cord Injury Care System. *J Neurosurg*. 1979;50(5):611–616.

10. Brown PJ, Marino RJ, Herbison GJ, et al. The 72-hour examination as a predictor of recovery in motor complete quadriplegia. *Arch Phys Med Rehabil*. 1991;72(8):546–548.

11. Consortium for Spinal Cord Medicine. *Outcomes Following Traumatic Spinal Cord Injury: Clinical Practice Guidelines for Health-care Professionals*. Washington, D.C.: Paralyzed Veterans of America; 1999.

12. American Spinal Injury Association. *International Standards for the Neurological Classification of Spinal Cord Injury*. Chicago: American Spinal Injury Association; 2002.

13. American Spinal Injury Association. *Reference Manual for the International Standards for Neurological Classification of Spinal Cord Injury*. Chicago: American Spinal Injury Association; 2003.

14. Waters RL, Adkins RH, Yakura JS. Definition of complete spinal cord injury. *Paraplegia*. 1991;29(9):573–581.

15. Lammertse DP, Jackson AB, Sipski ML. Research from the Model Spinal Cord Injury Systems: findings from the current 5-year grant cycle. *Arch Phys Med Rehabil*. 2004;85(11):1737–1739.

16. Marino RJ, Ditunno JF Jr, Donovan WH, et al. Neurologic recovery after traumatic spinal cord injury: data from the Model Spinal Cord Injury Systems. *Arch Phys Med Rehabil*. 1999;80(11):1391–1396.

17. Frankel HL, Hancock DO, Hyslop G, et al. The value of postural reduction in the initial management of closed injuries of the spine with paraplegia and tetraplegia. I. *Paraplegia*. 1969;7(3):179–192.

18. Waters RL, Adkins RH, Yakura JS, et al. Motor and sensory recovery following complete tetraplegia. *Arch Phys Med Rehabil*. 1993;74(3):242–247.

19. Waters RL, Yakura JS, Adkins RH, et al. Recovery following complete paraplegia. *Arch Phys Med Rehabil*. 1992;73(9):784–789.

20. Ditunno JFJ, Cohen ME, Hauck WW, et al. Recovery of upper-extremity strength in complete and incomplete tetraplegia: a multicenter study. *Arch Phys Med Rehabil*. 2000;81(4):389–393.

21. Oleson CV, Burns AS, Ditunno JF, et al. Prognostic value of pinprick preservation in motor complete, sensory incomplete spinal cord injury. *Arch Phys Med Rehabil*. 2005;86(5):988–992.

22. Waters RL, Adkins RH, Yakura JS, et al. Motor and sensory recovery following incomplete paraplegia. *Arch Phys Med Rehabil*. 1994;75(1):67–72.

23. Foo D, Subrahmanyan TS, Rossier AB. Post-traumatic acute anterior spinal cord syndrome. *Paraplegia*. 1981;19(4):201–205.

24. Crozier KS, Graziani V, Ditunno JFJ, et al. Spinal cord injury: prognosis for ambulation based on sensory examination in patients who are initially motor complete. *Arch Phys Med Rehabil*. 1991;72(2):119-121.

25. Katoh S, el Masry WS. Motor recovery of patients presenting with motor paralysis and sensory sparing following cervical spinal cord injuries. *Paraplegia*. 1995;33(9):506–509.

26. Geisler FH, Coleman WP, Grieco G, et al. The Sygen multicenter acute spinal cord injury study. *Spine*. 2001;26(suppl 24):S87–S98.

27. Burns SP, Golding DG, Rolle WAJ, et al. Recovery of ambulation in motor-incomplete tetraplegia. *Arch Phys Med Rehabil*. 1992;78(11):1169–1172.

28. Waters RL, Adkins RH, Yakura JS, et al. Motor and sensory recovery following incomplete tetraplegia. *Arch Phys Med Rehabil*. 1994;75(3):306–311.

29. Waters RL, Adkins R, Yakura J, et al. Donal Munro Lecture: Functional and neurologic recovery following acute SCI. *J Spinal Cord Med*. 1998;21(3):195–199.

30. Ditunno JFJ, Stover SL, Freed MM, et al. Motor recovery of the upper extremities in traumatic quadriplegia: a multicenter study. *Arch Phys Med Rehabil*. 1992;73(5):431–436.

31. Ishida Y, Tominaga T. Predictors of neurologic recovery in acute central cervical cord injury with only upper extremity impairment. *Spine*. 2002;27(15):1652–1658; discussion 1658.

32. Kirshblum S, Millis S, McKinley W, et al. Late neurologic recovery after traumatic spinal cord injury. *Arch Phys Med Rehabil*. 2004;85(11):1811–1817.

33. Schaefer DM, Flanders A, Northrup BE, et al. Magnetic resonance imaging of acute cervical spine trauma: correlation with severity of neurologic injury. *Spine*. 1989;14(10):1090–1095.

34. Flanders AE, Schaefer DM, Doan HT, et al. Acute cervical spine trauma: correlation of MR imaging findings with degree of neurologic deficit. *Radiology*. 1990;177(1):25–33.

35. Flanders AE, Spettell CM, Tartaglino LM, et al. Forecasting motor recovery after cervical spinal cord injury: value of MR imaging. *Radiology*. 1996;201(3):649–655.

36. Flanders AE, Spettell CM, Friedman DP, et al. The relationship between the functional abilities of patients with cervical spinal cord injury and the severity of damage revealed by MR imaging. *AJNR Am J Neuroradiol*. 1999;20(5):926–934.

37. Stroman PW, Kornelsen J, Bergman A, et al. Noninvasive assessment of the injured human spinal cord by means of functional magnetic resonance imaging. *Spinal Cord*. 2004;42(2):59–66.

38. Geerts WH, Pineo GF, Heit JA, et al. Prevention of venous thromboembolism: the seventh ACCP conference on antithrombotic and thrombolytic therapy. *Chest*. 2004;126 (suppl 3):338S–400S.

39. Consortium for Spinal Cord Medicine Clinical Practice Guidelines. Prevention of thromboembolism in spinal cord injury. *J Spinal Cord Med*. 1997;20(3):259–283.

40. DeVivo MJ, Krause JS, Lammertse DP. Recent trends in mortality and causes of death among persons with spinal cord injury. *Arch Phys Med Rehabil*. 1999;80(11):1411–1419.

41. Hebbeler SL, Marciniak CM, Crandall S, et al. Daily vs twice daily enoxaparin in the prevention of venous thromboembolic disorders during rehabilitation following acute spinal cord injury. *J Spinal Cord Med*. 2004;27(3):236–240.

42. Kuric J, Hixon AK. *Clinical Practice Guidelines: Autonomic Dysreflexia*. Jackson Heights, N.Y.: Eastern Paralyzed Veterans Association; 1996.

43. Consortium for Spinal Cord Medicine. Acute management of autonomic dysreflexia: individuals with spinal cord injury presenting to health-care facilities. *J Spinal Cord Med*. 2002;25(suppl 1):S67–S88.

44. Burns AS, Jackson AB. Gynecologic and reproductive issues in women with spinal cord injury. *Phys Med Rehabil Clin N Am*. 2001;12(1):183–199.

45. Lehmann KG, Lane JG, Piepmeier JM, et al. Cardiovascular abnormalities accompanying acute spinal cord injury in

humans: incidence, time course and severity. *J Am Coll Cardiol*. 1987;10(1):46–52.

46. Jackson AB, Groomes TE. Incidence of respiratory complications following spinal cord injury. *Arch Phys Med Rehabil*. 1994;75(3):270–275.

47. Bellamy R, Pitts FW, Stauffer ES, et al. Respiratory complications in traumatic quadriplegia: analysis of 20 years' experience. *J Neurosurg*. 1973;39(5):596–600.

48. Carter RE. Respiratory aspects of spinal cord injury management. *Paraplegia*. 1987;25(3):262–266.

49. Kiwerski J. Respiratory problems in patients with high lesion quadriplegia. *Int J Rehabil Res*. 1992;15(1):49–52.

50. Reines HD, Harris RC. Pulmonary complications of acute spinal cord injuries. *Neurosurgery*. 1987;21(2):193–196.

51. Peterson WP, Barbalata L, Brooks CA, et al. The effect of tidal volumes on the time to wean persons with high tetraplegia from ventilators. *Spinal Cord*. 1999;37(4):284–288.

52. Wicks AB, Menter RR. Long-term outlook in quadriplegic patients with initial ventilator dependency. *Chest*. 1986; 90(3):406–410.

53. Fugl-Meyer AR, Grimby G. Ventilatory function in tetraplegic patients. *Scand J Rehabil Med*. 1971;3(4):151–160.

54. Fugl-Meyer AR. Effects of respiratory muscle paralysis in tetraplegic and paraplegic patients. *Scand J Rehabil Med*. 1971;3(4):141–150.

55. Estenne M, De Troyer A. Mechanism of the postural dependence of vital capacity in tetraplegic subjects. *Am Rev Respir Dis*. 1987;135(2):367–371.

56. Peterson W, Charlifue W, Gerhart A, et al. Two methods of weaning persons with quadriplegia from mechanical ventilators. *Paraplegia*. 1994;32(2):98–103.

57. Consortium for Spinal Cord Medicine. *Respiratory Management Following Spinal Cord Injury: A Clinical Practice Guideline for Health-care Professionals*. Washington, D.C.: Paralyzed Veterans of America; 2005.

58. Peterson WP, Brooks CA, Mellick D. Protocol for ventilator management in high tetraplegia. *Top Spinal Cord Inj Rehabil*. 1997; 2(3):101-106.

59. Fishburn MJ, Marino RJ, Ditunno JF. Atelectasis and pneumonia in acute spinal cord injury. *Arch Phys Med Rehabil*. 1990;71(3):197–200.

60. Wang AY, Jaeger RJ, Yarkony GM, et al. Cough in spinal cord injured patients: the relationship between motor level and peak expiratory flow. *Spinal Cord*. 1997;35(5):299–302.

61. Consortium for Spinal Cord Medicine Clinical Practice Guidelines. Pressure ulcer prevention and treatment following spinal cord injury: a clinical practice guideline for health-care professionals. *J Spinal Cord Med*. 2001;24(suppl1): S40–101.

62. Bergstrom N, Braden BJ, Laguzza A, et al. The Braden scale for predicting pressure sore risk. *Nurs Res*. 1987;36(4): 205–210.

63. Bergstrom N, Braden B. A prospective study of pressure sore risk among institutionalized elderly. *J Am Geriatr Soc*. 1992;40(8):747–758.

64. Bergstrom N, Braden B, Boynton P, et al. Using a research-based assessment scale in clinical practice. *Nurs Clin N Am*. 1995;30(3):539–551.

65. Braden BJ, Bergstrom N. Risk assessment and risk-based programs of prevention in various settings. *Ostomy Wound Manage*. 1996;42(suppl 10A):6S–12S.

66. Salcido R. Patient turning schedules: why and how often? *Adv Skin Wound Care*. 2004;17(4 Pt 1):156.

67. Nino-Murcia M, Stone JM, Chang PJ, et al. Colonic transit in spinal cord-injured patients. *Invest Radiol*. 1990;25(2): 109–112.

68. Consortium for Spinal Cord Medicine. *Neurogenic Bowel Management in Adults with Spinal Cord Injury: Clinical Practice Guidelines*. Washington, D.C.: Paralyzed Veterans of America; 1998.

69. David S, Aguayo AJ. Axonal elongation into peripheral nervous system "bridges" after central nervous system injury in adult rats. *Science*. 1981;214(4523):931–933.

70. Bracken MB, Shepard MJ, Collins WF, et al. A randomized, controlled trial of methylprednisolone or naloxone in the treatment of acute spinal-cord injury: results of the Second National Acute Spinal Cord Injury Study. *N Engl J Med*. 1990;322(20):1405–1411.

71. Bracken MB, Shepard MJ, Collins WF Jr, et al. Methylprednisolone or naloxone treatment after acute spinal cord injury: 1-year follow-up data: results of the second National Acute Spinal Cord Injury Study. *J Neurosurg*. 1992;76(1): 23–31.

72. Bracken MB, Shepard MJ, Holford TR, et al. Administration of methylprednisolone for 24 or 48 hours or tirilazad mesylate for 48 hours in the treatment of acute spinal cord injury: results of the Third National Acute Spinal Cord Injury Randomized Controlled Trial. National Acute Spinal Cord Injury Study. *JAMA*. 1997;277(20):1597–1604.

73. Bracken MB, Shepard MJ, Holford TR, et al. Methylprednisolone or tirilazad mesylate administration after acute spinal cord injury: 1-year follow-up. Results of the third National Acute Spinal Cord Injury randomized controlled trial. *J Neurosurg*. 1998;89(5):699–706.

74. Hall ED. The effects of glucocorticoid and nonglucocorticoid steroids on acute neuronal degeneration. *Adv Neurol*. 1993;59:241–248.

75. Hall ED. The neuroprotective pharmacology of methylprednisolone. *J Neurosurg*. 1992;76(1):13–22.

76. Amar AP, Levy ML. Pathogenesis and pharmacological strategies for mitigating secondary damage in acute spinal cord injury. *Neurosurgery*. 1999;44(5):1027–1039; discussion 1039–1040.

77. Nesathurai S. Steroids and spinal cord injury: revisiting the NASCIS 2 and NASCIS 3 trials. *J Trauma*. 1998;45(6): 1088–1093.

78. Bracken MB. Methylprednisolone and acute spinal cord injury: an update of the randomized evidence. *Spine*. 2001;26(suppl 24):S47–S54.

79. Hurlbert RJ. Methylprednisolone for acute spinal cord injury: an inappropriate standard of care. *J Neurosurg*. 2000;93(suppl 1):1–7.

80. Hurlbert RJ, Moulton R, Hurlbert RJ, et al. Why do you prescribe methylprednisolone for acute spinal cord injury? a Canadian perspective and a position statement. *Can J Neurol Sci*. 2002;29(3):236–239.

81. Hurlbert RJ. The role of steroids in acute spinal cord injury: an evidence-based analysis. *Spine*. 2001;26(24S):S39–S46.

82. Bracken MB. Methylprednisolone and spinal cord injury. *J Neurosurg*. 2000;93(suppl 1):175–179.

83. Bracken MB, Holford TR. Neurological and functional status 1 year after acute spinal cord injury: estimates of functional recovery in National Acute Spinal Cord Injury Study II from results modeled in National Acute Spinal Cord Injury Study III. *J Neurosurg*. 2002;96(suppl 3):259–266.

84. Bracken MB. Steroids for acute spinal cord injury. [update of *Cochrane Database Syst Rev*. 2000;(2):CD001046; PMID: 10796741]. *Cochrane Database Syst Rev*. 2002;(3):CD001046.

85. Short DJ, El Masry WS, Jones PW. High dose methylprednisolone in the management of acute spinal cord injury—a systematic review from a clinical perspective. *Spinal Cord*. 2000;38(5):273–286.

86. Coleman WP, Benzel D, Cahill DW, et al. A critical appraisal of the reporting of the National Acute Spinal Cord Injury Studies (II and III) of methylprednisolone in acute spinal cord injury. *J Spinal Disord*. 2000;13(3):185–199.

87. Geisler FH, Dorsey FC, Coleman WP. Recovery of motor function after spinal-cord injury—a randomized, placebo-controlled trial with GM-1 ganglioside. *N Engl J Med*. 1991;324(26):1829–1838.

88. Bose B, Osterholm JL, Kalia M. Ganglioside-induced regeneration and reestablishment of axonal continuity in spinal cord-transected rats. *Neurosci Lett*. 1986;63(2):165–169.

89. Oliveira AL, Langone F. GM-1 ganglioside treatment reduces motoneuron death after ventral root avulsion in adult rats. *Neurosci Lett*. 2000;293(2):131–134.

90. Geisler FH, Coleman WP, Grieco G, et al. Measurements and recovery patterns in a multicenter study of acute spinal cord injury. *Spine*. 2001;26(suppl 24):S68–S86.

91. Geisler FH, Coleman WP, Grieco G, et al. Recruitment and early treatment in a multicenter study of acute spinal cord injury. [comment]. *Spine*. 2001;26(suppl 24):S58–S67.

92. Pitts LH, Ross A, Chase GA, et al. Treatment with thyrotropin-releasing hormone (TRH) in patients with traumatic spinal cord injuries. *J Neurotrauma*. 1995;12(3): 235–243.

93. Fehlings MG, Sekhon LH, Tator C. The role and timing of decompression in acute spinal cord injury: what do we know? what should we do? *Spine*. 2001;26(suppl 24):S101–S110.

94. Tator CH, Fehlings MG, Thorpe K, et al. Current use and timing of spinal surgery for management of acute spinal surgery for management of acute spinal cord injury in North America: results of a retrospective multicenter study. *J Neurosurg*. 1999;91(suppl 1):12–18.

95. Barbeau H, Rossignol S. Recovery of locomotion after chronic spinalization in the adult cat. *Brain Res*. 1987; 412(1):84–95.

96. Barbeau H, McCrea DA, O'Donovan MJ, et al. Tapping into spinal circuits to restore motor function. *Brain Res Rev*. 1999;30(1):27–51.

97. De Leon RD, Hodgson JA, Roy RR, et al. Locomotor capacity attributable to step training versus spontaneous recovery after spinalization in adult cats. *J Neurophysiol*. 1998; 79(3):1329–1340.

98. Dietz V, Harkema SJ. Locomotor activity in spinal cord-injured persons. *J Appl Physiol*. 2004;96(5):1954–1960.

99. Edgerton VR, de Leon RD, Tillakaratne N, et al. Use-dependent plasticity in spinal stepping and standing. *Adv Neurol*. 1997; 72:233–247.

100. Wernig A, Muller S, Nanassy A, et al. Laufband therapy based on "rules of spinal locomotion" is effective in spinal cord injured persons. *Eur J Neurosci*. 1995;7(4):823–829.

101. Wickelgren I. Teaching the spinal cord to walk. *Science*. 1998;279(5349):319–321.

102. Rapalino O, Lazarov-Spiegler O, Agranov E, et al. Implantation of stimulated homologous macrophages results in partial recovery of paraplegic rats. *Nat Med*. 1998;4(7):814–821.

103. Schwartz M, Lazarov-Spiegler O, Rapalino O, et al. Potential repair of rat spinal cord injuries using stimulated homologous macrophages. *Neurosurg*. 1999;44(5):1041–1045.

104. Schwartz M. Macrophages and microglia in central nervous system injury: are they helpful or harmful? *J Cereb Blood Flow Metab*. 2003;23(4):385–394.

105. Bomstein Y, Marder JB, Vitner K, et al. Features of skin-coincubated macrophages that promote recovery from spinal cord injury. *J Neuroimmunol*. 2003;142(1–2):10–16.

106. Knoller N, Auerbach G, Fulga V, et al. Clinical experience using incubated autologous macrophages as a treatment for complete spinal cord injury: phase I study results. *J Neurosurg Spine*. 2005;3(3):173–181.

107. Ahn SH, Park HW, Lee BS, et al. Gabapentin effect on neuropathic pain compared among patients with spinal cord injury and different durations of symptoms. *Spine*. 2003;28 (4):341–346; discussion 346–347.

108. Haller H, Leblhuber F, Trenkler J, et al. Treatment of chronic neuropathic pain after traumatic central cervical cord lesion with gabapentin. *J Neural Transm*. 2003;110(9): 977–981.

109. Levendoglu F, Ogun CO, Ozerbil O, et al. Gabapentin is a first line drug for the treatment of neuropathic pain in spinal cord injury. *Spine*. 2004;29(7):743–751.

110. Putzke JD, Richards JS, Kezar L, et al. Long-term use of gabapentin for treatment of pain after traumatic spinal cord injury. *Clin J Pain*. 2002;18(2):116–121.

111. Tai Q, Kirshblum S, Chen B, et al. Gabapentin in the treatment of neuropathic pain after spinal cord injury: a prospective, randomized, double-blind, crossover trial. *J Spinal Cord Med*. 2002;25(2):100–105.

112. To TP, Lim TC, Hill ST, et al. Gabapentin for neuropathic pain following spinal cord injury. *Spinal Cord*. 2002; 40(6):282–285.

113. Alden TD, Lytle RA, Park TS, et al. Intrathecal baclofen withdrawal: a case report and review of the literature. *Childs Nerv Syst*. 2002;18(9–10):522–525.

114. Gooch JL, Oberg WA, Grams B, et al. Complications of intrathecal baclofen pumps in children. *Pediatr Neurosurg*. 2003;39(1):1–6.

115. Hyser CL, Drake ME Jr. Status epilepticus after baclofen withdrawal. *J Natl Med Assoc*. 1984;76(5):533, 537–538.

116. Kao LW, Amin Y, Kirk MA, et al. Intrathecal baclofen withdrawal mimicking sepsis. *J Emerg Med*. 2003;24(4):423–427.

117. Kofler M, Arturo LA. Prolonged seizure activity after baclofen withdrawal. *Neurology*. 1992;42(3):697–698.

118. Mohammed I, Hussain A. Intrathecal baclofen withdrawal syndrome: a life-threatening complication of baclofen pump: a case report. *BMC Clin Pharml*. 2004;4(1):6.

119. Rivas DA, Chancellor MB, Hill K, et al. Neurological manifestations of baclofen withdrawal. *J Urol*. 1993;150(6): 1903–1905.

120. Sampathkumar P, Scanlon PD, Plevak DJ. Baclofen withdrawal presenting as multiorgan system failure. *Anesth Analg*. 1998;87(3):562–563.

121. Santiago-Palma J, Hord ED, Vallejo R, et al. Respiratory distress after intrathecal baclofen withdrawal. *Anesth Analg*. 2004;99(1):227–229.

122. Terrence CF, Fromm GH. Complications of baclofen withdrawal. *Arch Neurol*. 1981;38(9):588–589.

123. Long C. Functional significance of spinal cord lesion level. *Arch Phys Med Rehabil*. 1955;36:249–255.

124. Welch RD, Lobley SJ, O'Sullivan SB, et al. Functional independence in quadriplegia: critical levels. *Arch Phys Med Rehabil*. 1986;67(4):235–240.

125. Yarkony GM, Roth EJ, Heinemann AW, et al. Rehabilitation outcomes in C6 tetraplegia. *Paraplegia*. 1988;26(3):177–185.

126. Yarkony GM, Roth E, Lovell L, et al. Rehabilitation outcomes in complete C5 quadriplegia. *Am J Phys Med Rehabil*. 1988;67(2):73–76.

127. Zafonte RD, Demangone DA, Herbison GJ. Daily self-care in quadriplegic subjects. *Neurol Rehabil*. 1991;1:17–24.

128. Marino RJ, Rider-Foster D, Maissel G, et al. Superiority of motor level over single neurological level in categorizing tetraplegia. *Paraplegia*. 1995;33(9):510–513.

Chapter 3

Surgical Treatment of Spinal Injury

Daniel R. Fassett and James S. Harrop

Traumatic injuries to the spinal column are common events, with more than 50,000 fractures to the spinal column occurring annually in the United States (1). Spinal injury remains a heterogeneous group of injuries and therefore various strategies are employed in their treatment. Multiple clinical variables must be addressed, including the degree of ligamentous and bony injury, the presence of neurologic deficits, perceived patient compliance, and overall health status; these factors are used to determine how the injuries are treated. Treatment can range from simple limitation in activity to external orthosis to open reduction and internal fixation with spinal instrumentation. The goal of treating these injuries is to utilize the least invasive surgical technique to stabilize the injured segment while limiting the potential for subsequent catastrophic neurologic injury, progression of a deformity, and chronic pain conditions. These surgical goals are also tempered by other medical management issues that focus on minimizing hospitalization and immobilization and maximizing the benefits of early and aggressive rehabilitation.

HISTORICAL PERSPECTIVE OF SPINAL INJURY TREATMENT

Treatment of traumatic spinal injuries was first recorded by Hippocrates (460–370 BCE) who used traction devices to obtain spinal reduction and advocated external stabilization and immobilization. Surgery was not considered a viable option at this time because of the high mortality of surgical techniques, and the presence of neurologic deficits in the setting of spinal trauma was deemed universally fatal. Surgical decompression for the treatment of traumatic spinal cord injury was initially popularized by Paulus of Aegina (625–690 CE) but was not universally accepted because of very poor surgical outcomes at the time. In 1646, Fabricius Hildanus performed the first documented open reduction of a spinal fracture (2–7).

It was not until the advent of spinal instrumentation in the 1950s that a more aggressive surgical approach was favored in the treatment of spinal column injuries. Before the development of spinal instrumentation, there was a bias toward conservative treatment, which often involved long periods of immobilization (4 to 8 weeks commonly) typically with traction to restore the spinal alignment and allow the fractures time to heal (8). These long periods of immobilization were associated with significant medical complications including pneumonia, deep vein thrombosis, and decubitus ulcers. The use of spinal instrumentation provided surgeons the ability to restore immediate stability to the spinal column, thus allowing for earlier mobilization and fewer complications from prolonged immobilization. In addition, spinal instrumentation theoretically improved fusion rates by providing a stable environment of bone healing, thus reducing the risks of late neurologic deterioration due to spinal instability, progressive spinal deformity, and associated axial back pain syndromes. Even with improvements in instrumentation, it was realized that all instrumentation will fail eventually unless a bony fusion is achieved and, therefore, arthrodesis remains a critical part of all spinal stabilization surgeries (4,6).

CLINICAL AND RADIOGRAPHIC EVALUATION OF THE TRAUMA PATIENT

The treatment of spinal trauma consists of an assessment of the traumatic injury through a detailed neurologic examination, physical examination, and then a radiographic evaluation. Radiographic evaluation often begins with plain radiographs followed by supplemental imaging of questionable areas of injury. Although modern imaging techniques have greatly aided in the diagnosis of fractures, determination of ligamentous instability with imaging alone is still unproven even with techniques designed to evaluate the soft tissues such as magnetic resonance imaging (MRI) (9).

Cervical Spine Evaluation

Any trauma patient should immediately be placed in cervical spine immobilization when assessed by emergency medical services (EMS) in the field. Any nonintoxicated patient without neck pain, neurologic deficits, and distracting injuries (injuries to other portions of the body that could potentially mask the pain associated with spinal injury) can be cleared of cervical spine injury with a normal clinical examination alone (i.e., showing no neck pain over a full range of motion of the cervical spine) (10). Neurologically intact patients with neck pain or tenderness are usually assessed with three view (anteroposterior [AP], lateral, and open-mouth odontoid views) plain radiographs as initial assessment (11). If these plain radiographs are normal, these patients are often kept in cervical collar immobilization for 1 to 2 weeks and then should have delayed passive cervical flexion and extension

imaging to assess for potential occult ligamentous injury. Although the prevalence of occult ligamentous injury in the setting of normal radiographs is small, the delay in the follow-up flexion/extension imaging can minimize false negative results by allowing muscle spasm to subside. In the neurologically intact patient with *severe* neck pain and normal plain radiographs, computed tomography (CT), and possibly MRI should be considered to rule out an occult fracture or herniated disc not seen on the plain radiographs (11).

In comatose, obtunded, or intoxicated/sedated patients, where an adequate neurologic examination cannot be obtained, plain radiographs or CT scan are standard in most trauma protocols. With the increase in speed and resolution of multidetector helical CT scanning, this modality is becoming more popular for evaluating multitrauma patients in a time-efficient manner. If these patients remain comatose, dynamic flexion/extension studies with fluoroscopic guidance or a normal cervical spine MRI within 48 hours of injury is sometimes performed for cervical spine clearance, although the inherent value of either method for the exclusion of occult soft tissue injury is questionable (9,11).

Patients with neurologic deficits that are clinically attributable to a spinal cord injury deserve rapid radiographic assessment possibly including plain films, CT scanning, and MRI. In the setting of an obvious cervical spine deformity with neurologic deficits, some surgeons may immediately institute reduction measures such as cervical traction. Other surgeons may insist upon further evaluation with CT and MRI before initiating any reduction measures. The extent of radiographic workup in the setting of spinal cord injury will depend on the preferences of the individual surgeon, the unique characteristics of the fracture being evaluated, and the character of neurologic examination. Patients with incomplete spinal cord injuries, where there is some neurologic function below the level of the spinal cord injury, may warrant an emergent MRI examination to assess integrity of the spinal canal and rule out herniated discs as an explanation for the neurologic deficits. The patient with a progressive, incomplete neurologic deficit requires immediate assessment and treatment as these patients have the greatest potential to permanently lose function with treatment delay.

Thoracic and Lumbar Spine Evaluation

Awake, neurologically intact patients can have thoracic and lumbar spine precautions discontinued if they do not have any pain suggestive of spinal injury and do not have distracting injuries. Neurologically intact patients that complain of pain localizing to the spine or who harbor a distracting injury should be evaluated radiographically with a minimum of AP and lateral plain radiographs.

Depending upon the severity of their symptoms, CT or MRI imaging may be warranted. Comatose, obtunded, or sedated/intoxicated patients should always be evaluated with plain films or CT scanning. Multisystem trauma patients often require routine CT imaging of the chest, abdomen, and pelvis. It has been suggested that limited resolution imaging of the thoracic and lumbar spine can be extracted from these data sets and used as a substitute for radiographs of these areas (12).

In patients with neurologic deficits where there is a high suspicion for spinal injury, CT scans with coronal and sagittal reconstructions are often the initial imaging modality to improve the sensitivity for diagnosis of spinal injury and also provide better anatomic details about the specific fracture. A patient with a persistent neurologic deficit and a "normal" CT scan warrants performance of an emergent MRI both to visualize the spinal cord and cauda equina and to rule out soft tissue etiologies of spinal column compromise such as herniated discs or epidural hematoma that may be not visualized with CT scanning. Some surgeons may wish to obtain emergent MRI in patients with obvious fractures diagnosed with CT, since the MRI can help locate the level of the conus medullaris, assess the integrity of the intervertebral discs, and better appreciate the extent of ligamentous injury. All of these factors may impact the treatment of the patient by providing the surgeon with a better appreciation of the anatomy of the spinal injury.

CURRENT TREATMENT OPTIONS

External Orthosis

Numerous external orthosis (spinal braces) options are available for the treatment of spinal injuries. The principle of bracing is to reduce motion at the injured spinal area in order to improve the likelihood of healing and reduce the potential for neurologic injury as a result of spinal instability. In general it is felt that maximal reduction in motion will result in better healing of the injured spinal segment, but literature is lacking in regard to how much motion is "too much" when considering bracing. Indications for external orthosis following spinal injury can vary significantly among individual surgeons since there are limited guidelines in the surgical literature for this type of treatment. Some fractures may not require any bracing as they are deemed to be very low risk for spinal instability and other fractures may be stabilized surgically, thus eliminating the need for external orthosis.

For the cervical spine, options ranging from least to most restrictive are soft and hard cervical collars (Philadelphia, Aspen, Miami J), cervical bracing with the addition of a thoracic vest (SOMI and Minerva braces),

and halo-vest immobilization (Fig. 3-1). A cervical collar is the least cumbersome of the cervical spine orthosis options; however, this comes at the cost of it offering the least support in terms of limiting range of motion. Studies have shown that cervical hard collars allow for over 30 degrees of flexion-extension motion in the cervical spine and provide minimal support at the lower cervical spine (13). Braces that add a thoracic vest immobilize the cervical spine and cervicothoracic junction better but still allow for significant motion at the craniocervical junction (Fig. 3-1B) (14,15). Halo-vest immobilization (Fig. 3-1C) accomplishes the most rigid immobilization by fixating a halo-ring around the head (pins into the skull) and securing the halo-ring to a thoracic vest by rods. Although halo immobilization provides the most support and may improve fusion rates, it may be associated with complications ranging from pin loosening, pin site infections, to swallowing dysfunction, reduced immobilization, and cerebral abscesses attributable to intracranial penetration of fixation pins. Halo immobilization also tends to limit motion of the upper cervical spine with greater efficiency than the middle and lower cervical spine. Even with halo immobilization, studies have shown that 2 to 10 degrees of motion can take place at the craniocervical junction, and the lower cervical spine and cervicothoracic junction may not be adequately mobilized (14). In addition, immobilization in a halo can cause limited motion at the ends of the spine (craniocervical and cervicothoracic) with exaggerated motion in the subaxial spine, referred to as snaking (14).

In the thoracic spine, the rib cage provides some natural support for thoracic spine fractures. The upper thoracic region (T5 and above) is a very difficult region to immobilize with external orthosis, unless the patient is immobilized with a halo orthosis with a long thoracic vest. Spinal fractures from T6 to L2 are typically braced with a custom molded, hard-shell orthosis (thoracolumbar-sacral orthosis [TLSO]) or with more versatile, adjustable-fit braces (e.g., Jewitt, Aspen) (Fig. 3-2A) or clamshell brace (Fig. 3-2B). Below L3, a lumbosacral orthosis is used for support. In addition, to increase the immobilization at the lumbosacral junction, a leg extension can be fitted to the orthosis to assist in limiting motion across the pelvis. Casting (Fig. 3-2C) is another option for lumbar and thoracolumbar fractures and can provide better support and eliminate concerns of noncompliance.

Surgical Options for Traumatic Spinal Injuries

Controversy persists in the surgical community regarding the optimal treatment of many traumatic spinal injuries, especially regarding timing of surgical intervention and type of surgical approach. Surgical intervention is often

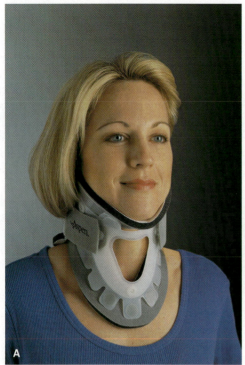
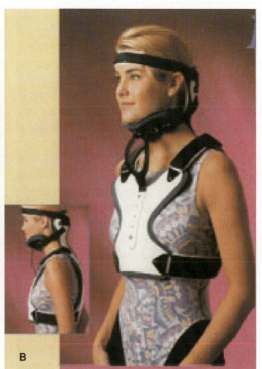
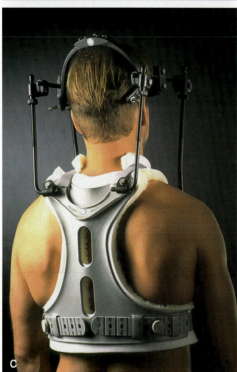

FIGURE 3-1. A wide variety of spinal orthoses are available to treat cervical spine injuries including: **(A)** cervical collars (Aspen cervical collar shown), **(B)** cervical brace with thoracic vest (Minerva brace shown), and **(C)** halo-vest immobilization (Bremer Halo Crown and AirFlo vest by DePuy Spine, A Johnson & Johnson Company).

advocated to (a) decompress the neural elements in cases of neurologic deficit; (b) prevent possible late neurologic injury in unstable fractures; (c) correct and prevent deformity that could result in chronic axial (back) pain or neurologic loss; and (d) provide for early mobilization, thus avoiding the complications of prolonged bed rest.

Anterior (ventral), posterior (dorsal), and combined anterior and posterior approaches can be used to treat traumatic spinal instability. The surgical approach selected may depend on the fracture pattern, the neurologic status of the patient, and the individual preference of the surgeon. Anterior approaches may be favored in situations

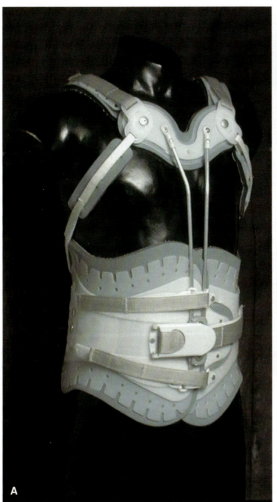

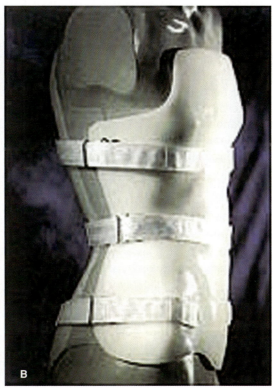

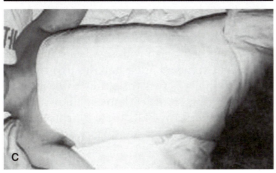

FIGURE 3-2. Thoracolumbar fractures can be braced with **(A)** adjustable-fit thoracolumbar sacral orthosis (Aspen TLSO shown), **(B)** custom-fit hard-shell braces (clam shell), and **(C)** casting.

where a herniated disc or bone fragment is causing ventral compression on the spinal cord. In addition, fracture patterns where the integrity of the anterior column of the spine is significantly compromised (unstable spine) may be best addressed by an anterior approach to restore the structural stability of the anterior spinal column. In either case, the surgical approach also includes some form of *instrumentation. Spinal instrumentation* is a method of straightening and stabilizing the spine after spinal fusion, by surgically attaching hooks, rods, and

wire to the spine in a way that redistributes the stresses on the bones and keeps them in proper alignment.

Posterior surgical approaches and instrumentation typically allow for better reduction when deformities are present and may benefit in restoring the *posterior tension band* in distraction-type injuries where there is disruption of the posterior ligamentous structures. The posterior ligamentous structures (ligamentum flavum, interspinous ligaments, supraspinous ligaments, and so forth) serve to hold the spine in normal alignment and since they are under tension in most parts of the spine they are referred to collectively as the *posterior tension band*. Injury to these ligamentous structures can allow the spine to deform into a more kyphotic posture. With posterior instrumentation, there is restoration of the biomechanical forces needed to hold the spine in normal alignment. In terms of restoration of alignment, posterior instrumentation (lateral mass screws) typically provides better fixation and mechanical advantage that can be used in spinal reduction maneuvers to better restore spinal alignment.

In translation injuries (fracture-dislocations), when there is severe, circumferential disruption of the spinal column, combined anterior-posterior instrumentation procedures may be used to maximize stability of the spinal column and increase the fusion rates. Circumferential spinal instrumentation (anterior and posterior combined operations) is more commonly utilized in areas of high biomechanical stress, such as the cervicothoracic junction and thoracolumbar junction, where the biomechanical forces on the spine are greater and make these areas more prone to failure of stabilization procedures.

There is no single preferred approach to many types of spinal fractures; frequently the preferences of the individual surgeon take precedence. Despite the maturation of surgical techniques and development of sophisticated spinal instrumentation devices, there is a lack of good guidelines for the treatment of many fractures. In general, posterior approaches to the thoracic and lumbar spine are often favored because of the ease and familiarity of approach. Anterior approaches to the thoracic and lumbar spine tend to be more technically challenging (mobilizing the lung, viscera, and great vessels) and may require the assistance of a general or thoracic surgeon to aid with the approach to the spine.

TREATMENT OF CERVICAL SPINE INJURIES

Occipital Condyle Fractures

Occiptial condyle fracture is an uncommon injury occurring in less than 3% of patients with blunt craniovertebral trauma (16,17). CT is required to diagnose this injury as there is less than 3% diagnostic sensitivity with plain radiographs (18). These fractures were first classified by Anderson and Montesano (19) into (a) Type I—comminuted due to axial compression, (b) Type II—extension of a basilar skull fracture through the occipital condyle, and (c) Type III—an avulsion of the occipital condyle likely due to a rotational force that avulses a portion of the occipital condyle with the alar ligament (Fig. 3-3). There is a lack of adequate studies to determine the optimum

treatment strategy for these fractures. Most surgeons consider type I and II fractures stable injuries and will recommend cervical collar immobilization alone as an option to reduce pain associated with this injury.

Type III occipital condyle fractures are considered to be mechanically unstable and have been associated with development of lower cranial nerve deficits if untreated. Translation >1 mm between the occipital condyles and lateral masses of C1 at the occipital-C1 joint is considered abnormal. Most unilateral type III fractures are treated with cervical collar immobilization, but some surgeons advocate halo immobilization for fractures that have features of instability such as marked fracture displacement or abnormal craniocervical alignment. There are no specific guidelines or measurements that predict which unilateral type III fractures are at risk for long-term instability. After a period of immobilization, unilateral fractures can be evaluated in follow-up with CT scanning to assess for the extent of bone union across the fractured segment, and flexion/extension radiographs can be useful to assess for stability at the occipitocervical junction. Gross instability at the occipitocervical junction is presumed for the rare bilateral type III occipital condyle fractures, and atlanto-occipital dislocation (AOD) can be a component of this injury. When the features of AOD are present, an occipital cervical fusion is the preferred method of treatment or in any patient that continues to have instability despite conservative therapy with external immobilization. (20,21).

Atlanto-Occipital Dislocation

AOD has a significantly high fatality rate as a result of the significant forces required to create this injury. AOD is commonly associated with significant intracranial injury as well as vertebral artery injuries as a result of this distraction injury across the craniocervical junction. With improvements in the early recognition and stabilization of spinal injuries by EMS, more patients are surviving this injury. As a result of the tremendous distractive forces associated with the AOD, the tectorial membrane, posterior ligamentous structures, and facet capsules between the atlas and occipital condyles are injured, yet surprisingly these injuries can be difficult to detect on radiography and a high degree of vigilance is required. Several diagnostic criteria exist to help diagnose this injury on lateral radiographs including (a) the Powers ratio (22), (b) basion-dens distances, (such as Harris's rule of 12) (23–25), (c) distances from posterior mandible to anterior arch of C1 or dens (Dublin method) (26), and (d) Lee's X-line method (27) (Table 3-1). Of these diagnostic options, Harris's rule of 12 appears to be the most sensitive means of diagnosing this injury on plain films or sagittal reformatted CT images (Fig. 3-4A). MRI potentially can also be

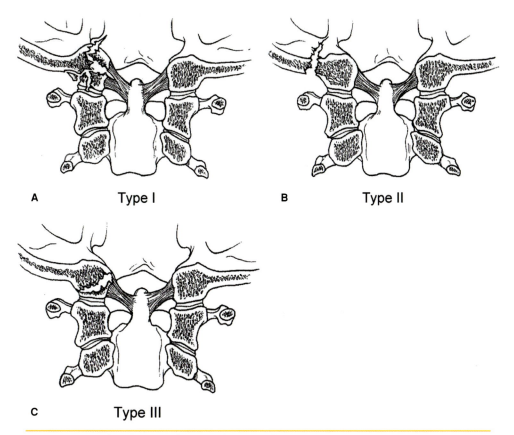

A   Type I   B   Type II

C   Type III

FIGURE 3-3. Classification of occipital condyle fractures according to Anderson and Montesano (1). **A:** Type I fractures may occur with axial loading. (Anderson PA, Montesano PX. Morphology and treatment of occipital condyle fractures. *Spine.* 1988;13(7):731–736.) **B:** Type II fractures are extensions of a basilar cranial fracture. **C:** Type III fractures may result from an avulsion of the condyle during rotation, lateral bending, or a combination of mechanisms. (From Jackson RS, Banit DM, Rhyne AL III, et al. Upper cervical spine injuries. *J Am Acad Orthop Surg.* 2002;10(4):271–280, with permission.)

very beneficial by showing the ligamentous disruption at the craniocervical junction.

AOD is considered highly unstable because of the extent of ligamentous injury and requires surgical stabilization with occipitocervical fusion procedures that instrument bridge across the occiput and upper cervical spine via a posterior approach (Fig. 3-4B).

Jefferson Fracture

Bilateral fractures through the ring of C1 (classic Jefferson fracture) (Fig. 3-5A) and other fractures of C1 can typically be treated with conservative measures (collar or halo immobilization) because of the high rate of spontaneous fusion and limited ligamentous instability. Integrity of the transverse ligament is used as a determinant of stability and the need for possible surgical stabilization. The most common means of evaluating the integrity of the transverse ligament is with an open-mouth odontoid view radiograph to assess the alignment of the lateral masses

of C1 and C2 using the rule of Spence (28). Greater than 7 mm of combined lateral overhang of the lateral masses of C1 on C2 constitutes violation of the rule of Spence and suggests likely transverse ligament rupture (Fig. 3-5B). The transverse ligament may also be evaluated on MRI, but the application of MRI in detecting transverse ligament rupture is unproven (29). Flexion-extension plain films can also be used to assess for possible C1-2 instability. In the presence of C1-2 instability from transverse ligament rupture, C1-2 arthrodesis is recommended via wiring techniques, transarticular screws, or other C1 and C2 screw techniques (Fig. 3-6). Various rods, plates, and wire loop (Fig. 3-6A) constructs are available to stabilize the craniocervical junction. These systems generally provide screw fixation into the posterior occiput at the cephalad end. For fixation at the caudal end, a variety of devices can be used, including atlantoaxial transarticular screws (screws placed through the C2 pars interarticularis, across the C1-2 lateral mass articulation, and into the lateral mass of C1) (Fig. 3-6B), C2 pars interarticularis or

▶ **TABLE 3-1** **Criteria Used to Diagnose Atlanto-Occipital Dislocation on Plain Lateral Radiographs**

1. Powers Ratio
- Ratio of the distances from basion to the anterior wall of the posterior arch of C1 divided by the distance from the opisthion (posterior lip of the foramen magnum) to the posterior wall of the anterior arch of C1.
- Normal ≤0.9, Indeterminate 0.9–1.0, Abnormal >1.0
- Only sensitive for diagnosing anteriorly directed dislocations.

2. Harris Rule of 12s
- Two distances are measured: (a) distance from the base of the dens to the clivus and (b) distance from a line draw from the posterior wall of the dens to the clivus.
- It is considered abnormal if the clivus is >12 mm above the tip of the dens or 12 mm anterior to the posterior dens line; therefore, the basis for rule of 12s. If the clivus is >4 mm posteriorly displaced behind the posterior dens line, this is also consider abnormal and likely represents a posteriorly directed dislocation.
- Considered the most sensitive rule to diagnose all directions of dislocation.

3. Dublin method
- Measures the distance from the posterior ramus of the mandible to the ventral aspect of the anterior ring of C1 and the ventral aspect of the base of the dens.
- A distance from the posterior ramus of the mandible to the anterior arch of C1 >9 mm and >17 mm from the mandible to the base of the dens are both abnormal and concerning for AOD.
- Care must be taken to take radiographs with the mouth in closed position because opening the mandible shortens these distances and can provide false-negative results.

4. X-line method
- Utilizes two lines drawn from the foramen magnum to C2 vertebral landmarks.
- The first line is drawn from the basion to the inferior aspect of the axis spinolaminar junction. If any portion of this line intersects with portions of C2 body or dens, then this is considered abnormal.
- The second line is drawn from the opisthion to the posterior inferior corner of the body of C2. If any portion of this line intersects C1, then this is abnormal and a concern for AOD.

pedicle screws, and C2 laminar screws (Fig. 3-6C). Extension of the construct to the subaxial spine with lateral mass screws can provide improved fixation in some cases where bone quality or poor screw purchase is a concern.

Odontoid Fractures

Odontoid fractures have been classified into three types by Anderson and D'Alonzo (30) based on the anatomic level of the fracture. Type I fractures, avulsion fractures of the tip of the odontoid at the attachment of the apical ligament, are exceedingly rare. The most common odontoid fracture, type II fractures, occur through the base of the dens at the intersection with the body of C2 but do not extend into the facets. Type III fractures involve the body of C2. Most odontoid fractures, particularly type III, can be treated nonoperatively through immobilization. Type III fractures have a high spontaneous fusion rate with halo immobilization attributable to the large surface area of type III fractures and good blood supply to the bone in the area of the fracture. In contrast, type II fractures have the lowest fusion rate because of the small fusion area and poor vascularity of this region. Certain groups of patients with type II fractures have been shown to have an even higher risk for nonunion, including those in patients older than 40 to 60 years old, posteriorly displaced fractures, and fractures displaced greater than 4 to 6 mm (31–34).

There are two surgical approaches for the treatment of type II odontoid fractures (Fig. 3-7): odontoid screw fixation (osteosynthesis), or a posterior C1-2 fusion technique. Odontoid screw fixation involves placement of a lag screw across the fracture in the plane of the dens. A lag screw is a smooth shaft screw that is threaded only at a short portion at the tip of the screw. This technique with a lag screw *pulls* the fractured dens fragment back into position with the body of C2 to promote bone healing through compression and stabilization. Initially when this technique was developed, some surgeons recommended placing two screws into the odontoid; however, this two-screw technique has not proven to be superior to one-screw techniques in biomechanical and clinical studies (35,36). The direct odontoid screw is typically limited to recent fractures <6 months old because fractures older than 6 months show a lower rate of fusion. The theoretical benefit of odontoid screw fixation is preservation of motion at the C1-2 articulation; however, this benefit is debated because there can be a significant loss in range of motion attributable to the traumatic injury of the C1-2 articulations at the time of the initial event. Another benefit of odontoid screw fixation is that the anterior approach is usually very well tolerated with minimal pain in comparison with posterior approaches to the cervical spine; however, severe dysphagia has been known to occur commonly in older patients and can last for months after surgery (37,38).

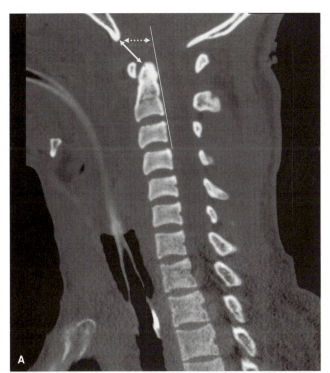

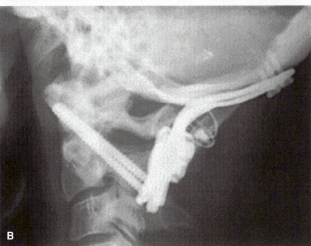

FIGURE 3-4. Atlanto-occipital dislocation (AOD). **A:** Sagittal reformatted CT image showing loss of normal orientation of the skull base to the upper cervical spine from an acute AOD with increased distance between the basion and tip of the odontoid process. The distance between the basion and the tip of the dens is the basion-dental interval (BDI; *double arrow*). The distance between the basion and the posterior spinal line extension from C2 is the basion-axial interval (BAI; *dotted line*). Distances >12 mm are considered abnormal. **B:** Occipital-cervical instrumentation used to treat a 32-year-old male with atlanto-occipital dislocation (AOD). Occipital-cervical loop construct attached to the occiput with three screws centered on the midline occipital keel and attached to C2 with C1-2 transarticular screws.

Posterior approaches to immobilize the C1-2 joints can be performed using C1-2 transarticular screws (Fig. 3-6), a C1-2 screw and rod instrumentation technique, or posterior wiring stand-alone techniques (Gallie, Brooks, and Sonntag techniques). These posterior fusion techniques address the C1-2 instability caused by an odontoid fracture but at the expense of motion at C1-2. The C1-2 articulation accounts for approximately 50% of rotation in the cervical spine, which will be lost with a successful posterior fusion procedure, but patients with an intact subaxial spine typically are able to compensate for this loss of rotation at C1-2 and function without significant lifestyle changes.

The earliest method for posterior C1-2 fusion, which used a loop of wire to transfix the posterior arches of C1 and C2, was first introduced by Cone and Turner (39) in 1937, and improved by Gallie (40) in 1939. Subsequent modifications were made to Gallie's technique by Brooks and then Sonntag (Fig. 6A) (41,42). All of these techniques had adequate fusion rates (~80%) but required external orthosis, usually in the form of halo immobilization, for 6 months. In 1976, Grob and Magerl (43) introduced C1-2 transarticular screws, which provide immediate stability to the C1-2 articulation and in most cases eliminate the need for rigid external orthosis. The use of C1-2 transarticular screws involves placing a screw (or bilateral screws) through the pars interarticularis of C2, across the C1-2 lateral mass articulation, and into the lateral mass of C1 (Fig. 3-6B). This is a technically challenging procedure because of the small size of the C2 pars interarticularis and due to the close proximity of the vertebral artery to the trajectory of the screws. In up to 10% of cases, an aberrant vertebral artery encroaches into the pars interarticularis of C2 and does not provide sufficient space to pass a transarticular screw safely. With the limitations of transarticular screws, a newer technique was developed where screws are inserted directly into the C1 lateral masses and additional screws into C2 pars interarticularis or C2 pedicle with stabilization accomplished by attaching a rod between these two screws (Fig. 3-6C) (44). This procedure significantly reduces the risk of vertebral artery injury and can be safely used in a larger percentage of cases than transarticular screws. In addition, this technique allows the fracture to be directly manipulated and reduced intraoperatively. Both of these screw techniques have increased fusion rates to almost 95% and have reduced the need for external orthosis.

Hangman Fracture

Bilateral fractures through the pars interarticularis of C2, the so-called hangman fracture, can be successfully treated with immobilization in over 90% of cases. Two classification schemes, the Francis and Effendi classifications, use fracture displacement (>3.5 mm) and angulation (>11

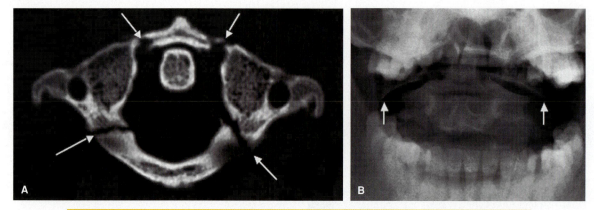

FIGURE 3-5. **A:** Axial CT and **(B)** open-mouth odontoid view of a 30-year-old male with a Jefferson fracture of C1. The axial CT shows bilateral fractures through the anterior and posterior rings of C1 (arrows). The open-mouth odontoid view shows the lateral masses of C1 overhanging laterally on the lateral masses of C2 by >7 mm (11 mm total overhang in this patient) indicating likely transverse ligament rupture (arrows).

degrees ventral angulation) to help predict which fractures may require surgical stabilization (45,46). Fractures without significant angulation (<11 degrees) or subluxation (<3.5 mm) can be treated with just cervical collar and close observation. Fractures with significant subluxation or angulation that can be reduced are typically treated with halo immobilization. Surgical stabilization is usually reserved for nonreducible fractures or fractures with recurrent subluxation despite immobilization. Surgical stabilization can be accomplished by either C2-3 anterior cervical discectomy and fusion (ACDF), C1-2 transarticular screws, C1 lateral mass and C2 screws, or C2 pars screws to reapproximate the fracture (47).

Subaxial Cervical Spine Injuries

Anterior column (spinal elements that are ventral to posterior longitudinal ligament) fractures, isolated posterior element injuries, and fracture-dislocations are all relatively common traumatic subaxial cervical spine injuries. Isolated injury to the anterior spinal column may be treated with conservative measures (collar, cervicothoracic orthosis, or halo) but occasionally these injuries will require surgical stabilization. Although there are no established guidelines for surgical intervention of isolated anterior column injury, in general, neurologic deficits with ventral spinal cord compression, >50% loss of vertebral body height, kyphosis >11 degrees, sagittal plane translation >3.5 mm, and persistent neck pain in the presence of deformity are all indications for surgical stabilization (Table 3-2) (48,49). Once a kyphotic deformity is present, it typically will progress because the weight-bearing axis of the spine is shifted to a position ventral to the vertebral body, promoting further kyphotic progression (50). For this reason, kyphotic deformities in the cervical spine that

▶ **TABLE 3-2** **General Indications for Surgical Intervention for Isolated Anterior Column Injuries to the Subaxial Cervical Spine**

- Neurologic deficits with ventral spinal cord compression
- Vertebral body height loss >50%
- Kyphosis >11 degrees
- Sagittal plane translation of 3.5 mm or greater between adjacent vertebral bodies
- Persistent neck pain in the presence of deformity

are treated with conservative measures deserve close observation to prevent loss of stability.

Isolated anterior-column injuries to the cervical spine that need surgical stabilization are most commonly approached anteriorly to perform corpectomy (removal of vertebral body) and place strut bone graft (usually iliac crest *autograft* or *allograft*). *Autograft* is obtaining by harvesting a small piece of the patient's iliac crest and *allograft* has been harvested from a cadaveric donor. Titanium mesh cages are an alternative to structural grafts to restore structural stability to the anterior column (Fig. 3-8A). These cages can be filled with mixtures of autograft, allograft, and other osteoconductive and -inductive agents (e.g., bone morphogenic protein). Anterior plating (Fig. 3-8B,C) is often used to provide additional structural support, which improves fusion rates, decreases postoperative pain, and allows for an earlier return to more normal activities (51). Newer anterior cervical plating systems, termed "dynamic plates" (Fig. 3-8C), provide for settling to take place between the adjacent vertebrae, keeping the interbody bone grafts under compression and, in theory, improving bone formation (52). Static plates (Fig. 3-8B), which do not allow for settling, are criticized for carrying all of the

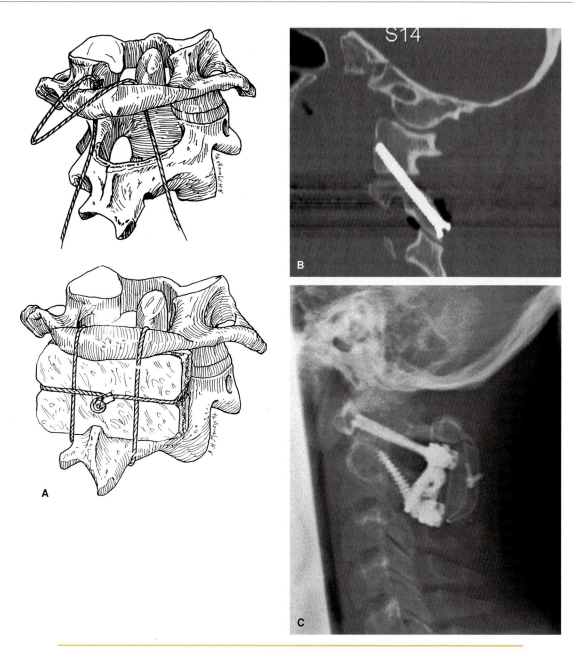

FIGURE 3-6. Posterior instrumentation used to treat C1-2 instability. **A:** Posterior wiring and bone graft technique (Sonntag fusion) where cables are placed around the C1 posterior ring and spinous process of C2 with custom fit bone grafts placed between C1 and C2 to improve stability and promote arthrodesis. (From Weinstein SL. *Pediatric Spine Surgery.* 2nd ed. Philadelphia: Lippincott Williams & Wilkins; 2001:143, with permission.) **B:** CT scan sagittal reconstruction showing C1-2 transarticular screws placed through the pars interarticularis of C2, across the C1-2 lateral mass articulation, and into the lateral mass of C1. **C:** Lateral radiograph showing C1-2 screw and rod construct, which involves placing bilateral screws into the lateral mass of C1 and pedicle or pars of C2. Bilateral rods are placed within C1 and C2 screws to stabilize the motion segment. Both transarticular screws and C1-2 screw with rod constructs are usually supplemented with posterior bone grafting and wiring to promote arthrodesis.

axial load through the plate and screws, thus "stress shielding" the interbody graft and possibly leading to pseudoarthrosis formation. In the setting of trauma, static plates are favored by many surgeons as they may provide more structural stability than dynamic plates, but this remains controversial. The inherent mechanisms of dynamic plates may permit more motion and less stability than static cervical plates, and this is hypothesized to be more pronounced in the setting of traumatic instability.

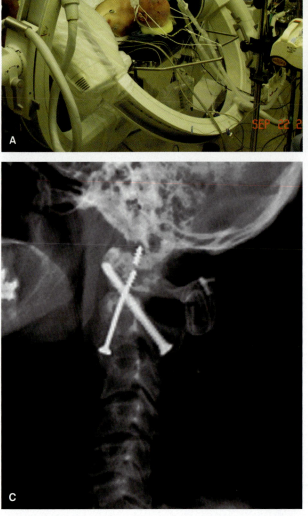

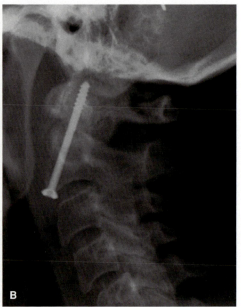

FIGURE 3-7. Odontoid fractures can be surgically stabilized by anterior (odontoid screw fixation) or posterior (C1-2 arthrodesis procedures). Odontoid screw fixation is performed by placing a lag (smooth shaft screw threaded only at end) screw through the inferior portion of the C2 body in a trajectory parallel to the odontoid to pull the fractured dens into normal alignment to promote bone healing. **A:** This procedure if performed with the aid of biplane fluoroscopy to determine screw trajectory. In theory, direct odontoid screw fixation preserves motion at the C1-2 articulation. **B:** The posterior lateral radiograph shows an odontoid screw placed to treat a type 2 odontoid fracture. **C:** Posterior procedures, such as the transarticular screws shown, that were placed after odontoid nonunion and odontoid screw fracture, stabilize the C1-2 articulation and are usually supplemented with posterior bone graft and wiring to promote fusion.

In more severe injuries, such as fracture-dislocations, the amount of ligamentous and intravertebral disc injury is often greater than the bony involvement. When posttraumatic deformity is present, such as cases of unilateral or bilateral jumped facets, these injuries are often initially treated with traction in an attempt to achieve reduction to normal anatomic alignment (Fig. 3-9). The value of obtaining of a prereduction MRI in an awake and cooperative patient is frequently debated by the spine surgeons. Some surgeons argue that there is potential for cord injury from a herniated disc impinging on the spinal cord during reduction; and a priori knowledge of this fact is relevant before attempting a closed reduction. However, most surgeons agree that prereduction MRI is not needed in an awake patient, in which serial neurologic exams can be performed during the closed reduction. Moreover, in patients with complete or near-complete spinal cord injuries, the misaligned spine should be reduced as soon as possible without the inherent delay in performing MRI because the potential benefits of early reduction far outweigh the risks of neurologic decline. Comatose, anesthetized, or noncooperative

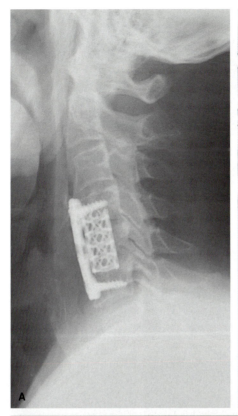
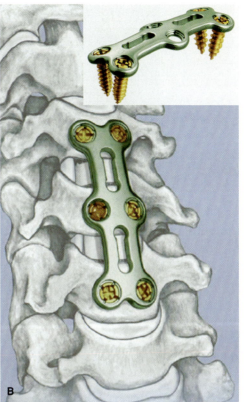
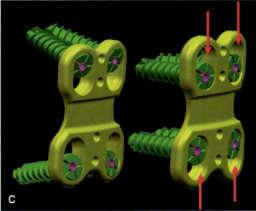

FIGURE 3-8. Subaxial spine injuries can be addressed by anterior, posterior, or combined anterior-posterior approaches. **A:** Lateral radiograph of a C5 burst fracture that was treated with C5 corpectomy, interpositional titanium cage, and anterior cervical fusion. **B:** Static anterior cervical plate (CSLP plate, Synthes Corp). **C:** Dynamic anterior cervical plate (ABC plate, Aesculap) allows for load sharing and settling of the interbody graft by allowing for the fixation screws to slide within the slots on the plate.

patients with minimal to no neurologic deficits should have an MRI before reduction (53).

Once a dislocation has been reduced, the injury must be stabilized with either an anterior or posterior fusion procedure, but often repair will necessitate a combination (i.e., both an anterior and posterior) of procedures (Fig. 3-10) to restore the integrity of the anterior spinal column and the posterior tension band. Posterior instrumentation in the subaxial spine is most commonly accomplished using lateral mass screws (Fig. 3-11A) in C3, C4, and C5. Depending on the anatomy and experience of the surgeon, C6 screw fixation can be accomplished with lateral mass screws or pedicle screws (Fig. 3-11B,C). To counteract the increase biomechanical stress at the cervical-thoracic junction, instrumentation failure is reduced by the use of pedicle screws at the lower limb of the metallic construct instead of lateral mass screws, which provides more secure anchoring.

THORACIC AND LUMBAR SPINE INJURIES

Classification Schemes for Thoracic and Lumbar Trauma

Multiple classification schemes (Table 3-3) have been proposed to help define thoracolumbar spinal injuries and improve consistency of communication between

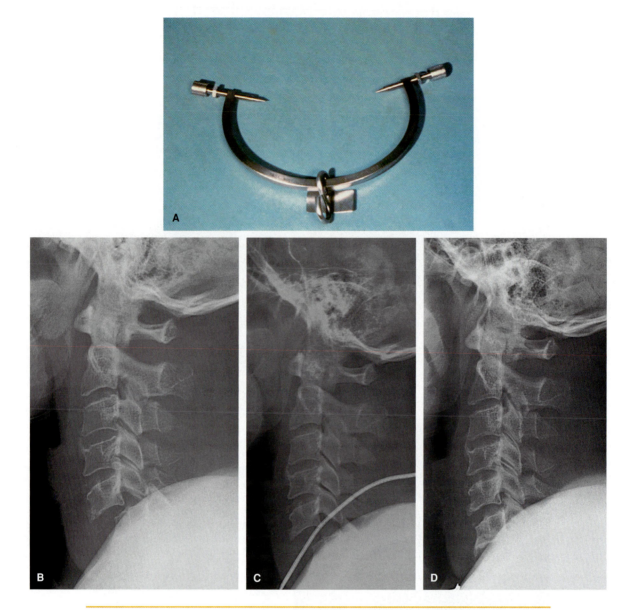

FIGURE 3-9. Cervical traction is often used to reduce spinal fractures prior to surgical stabilization. **A:** Garder-Wells tongs are fixated into the skull and weights are applied to these tongs to provide traction. **B,C,D:** A 35-year-old male who was involved in a motor vehicle accident and suffered a spinal cord injury as a result of subluxation with C5-6 bilateral jumped facets. B: The initial lateral radiograph shows greater than 50% subluxation of C6 on C7 and bilateral jumped facets at this level. C: The patient was placed in 35 pounds of cervical traction and the C5-6 interspace is widening. D: At 50 pounds of cervical traction, the facets and the subluxation were reduced.

physicians. There is still no general consensus on which schema to use. In 1968, Holdsworth (54) was one of the first to classify traumatic thoracolumbar fractures. He proposed a two-column model (Fig. 3-12), dividing the spine into anterior and posterior columns, and placed emphasis on the integrity of the posterior longitudinal ligament (PLL) and posterior elements for predicting stability. In Holdsworth's two-column model all the elements ventral to the PLL are considered the anterior column and the elements posterior to the PLL are the posterior column.

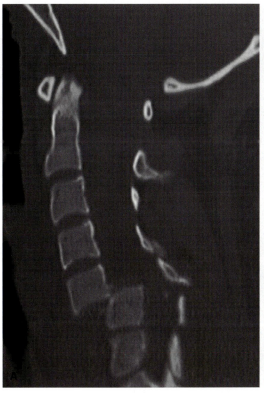
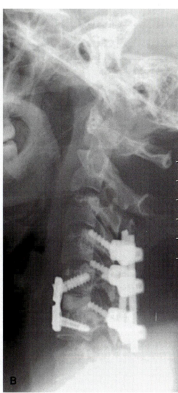

FIGURE 3-10. Severe C5-6 traumatic dislocation in a 21-year-old female. **A:** Initial CT sagittal reconstruction shows >100 % anterior subluxation of C5 on C6. **B:** Following closed reduction to re-establish alignment, this injury was treated with anterior (plating at C5 to C6) and posterior instrumentation from C4 to C6 (lateral mass screws) due to the extensive instability of this injury.

Mechanistically, Holdsworth's classification divided fractures into flexion, flexion and rotation, extension, and compression injuries. Whitesides (55) further expanded on the two-column model of Holdsworth by classifying these fractures based upon their inherent stability (i.e., stable or unstable), and also emphasized the importance of the posterior ligamentous complex in determining stability. According to Whitesides, stable fractures included simple compression fractures and burst fractures with intact posterior elements. Unstable fractures included slice fractures,

▶ **TABLE 3-3** Classification Schemes Used to Characterize Thoracolumbar Fractures

Name	*Fracture Classifications*
Holdsworth	Flexion, Flexion and Rotation, Extension, and Compression injuries
Whitesides	Stable
	■ Compression and burst fractures with intact posterior elements
	Unstable
	■ Burst with posterior element injury, slice fractures, flexion-distraction injuries, extension injuries
Denis	Compression, Burst, Seat belt-type, and Fracture Dislocation
McAfee	Wedge-Compression, Stable Burst, Unstable Burst, Chance fractures, Flexion–Distraction Injuries, and Translational Injuries
Gaines	Subclassified burst fractures based on the amount of comminution, apposition of fragments, and the amount of preoperative kyphosis to predict which fractures would fail short-segment posterior fixation.
AO (Magerl)	Fractures are classified into 3 basic categories: Type A: compression, Type B: distraction, Type C: multidirectional with translation. There is increased risk of instability and neurologic insult as injuries progress from Type A to Type C fractures, and each type of fracture is further subdivided based on the severity.

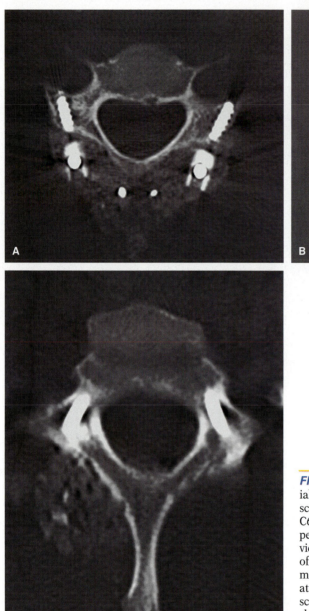

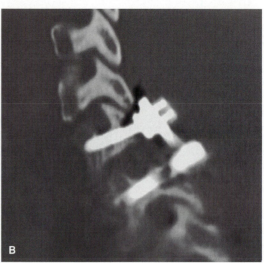

FIGURE 3-11. Posterior screw fixation in the subaxial spine is usually accomplished with lateral mass screws at C3, C4, and C5. The posterior elements of C6 can accommodate either lateral mass screws or pedicles screws. A pedicle screw will typically provide stronger pullout strength but at C6 there is risk of vertebral artery injury with pedicle screw placement. At C7, pedicle screws are used for posterior fixation. **A:** Axial CT showing bilateral lateral mass screws into C5. **B:** Sagittal CT reconstructed images showing C7 and T1 pedicle screws and an **(C)** axial CT image showing C7 pedicle screws.

burst fractures with posterior element disruption, flexion-distraction injuries, and extension injuries.

In 1983, Denis (56) proposed the three-column model (Fig. 3-12) for thoracolumbar fractures based on axial CT scan images and classified these fractures into four categories: *compression*, *burst*, *seat-belt type*, and *fracture dislocation*. In contrast to previous authors who emphasized the importance of the posterior column in predicting stability, Denis's three-column model underscores the importance of the middle column. The middle column consists of the posterior portion of the vertebral body, the posterior annulus fibrosus, and the posterior longitudinal ligament. Denis believed that involvement of two of the three

columns resulted in unstable fractures (56). McAfee et al. (57) agreed with the three-column model of Denis, but suggested that Denis's classification scheme was too complex. They proposed a new classification scheme with more emphasis on the mechanism of injury and categorized fractures into the following groups: *wedge-compression*, *stable burst*, *unstable burst*, *Chance fractures*, *flexion–distraction injuries*, and *translational injuries*. Stable and unstable burst fractures were differentiated by the competence of the posterior elements.

In 1994 McCormack et al. (58) proposed a classification for burst fractures to help predict which patients would fail with short-segment (i.e., fewer adjacent levels)

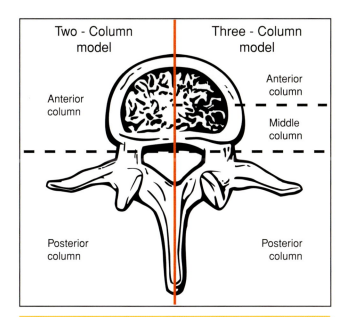

FIGURE 3-12. Two- and three-column models have been used to characterize spinal injuries and help gauge instability with the respective columns shown in this illustration. In the two-column model (left of red vertical line), all structures located ventral to the posterior longitudinal ligament (*dashed line*) are part of the anterior column. In the three-column model of Denis (right of red vertical line), the anterior column structures are divided into an anterior and middle column roughly divided by the middle of the vertebral body.

posterior pedicle screw instrumentation alone. This classification characterizes burst fractures with a point scale (3 to 9) based on the amount of comminution, apposition of fragments, and the amount of preoperative kyphosis. Burst fractures with seven or more points on this scale appear to be more prone to instrumentation failure with short-segment posterior fixation alone. This is generally attributed to failure of the anterior column to provide structural support and, thus, this scale may be useful in determining in which instances an additional anterior procedure may be warranted.

The Modified Comprehensive Classification (Arbeitsgemeinschaft für Osteosynthesefragen/Association for the Study of Internal Fixation [AO/ASIF]), originally described by Magerl et al. (59) and then modified by Gertzbein (60), is currently the most commonly used classification system for thoraco-lumbar fractures. This classification system divides fractures into three main types: *A, compression; B, distraction;* and *C, multidirectional with translation* (Fig. 3-13). The utility of this system is the orderly manner in which it ranks fractures based on severity. There is increased risk of instability and neurologic insult as injuries progress from type A to type C fractures, and each type of fracture is further subdivided based on the severity. Despite the orderly classification of fractures within this system, difficulties can arise with the AO/ASIF classification system because of the complexity of its 27 subtypes. Many surgeons use

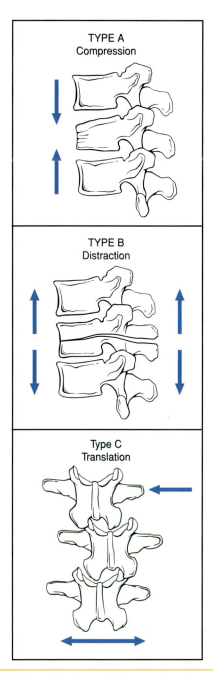

FIGURE 3-13. Modified Comprehensive Classification System (AO/ASIF). Type A: Compression injury to the anterior and middle columns, Type B: Distraction injuries involving posterior column, Type C: Translation (fracture-dislocation) injuries.

this classification system, but few use all 27 subtypes within this classification system.

Influence of Spinal Level on Surgical Approach in the Thoracic Spine

The fracture location within the thoracic and lumbar spine can have a significant influence on the surgical approach taken. Traumatic injuries to the upper thoracic spine

(T1-5) can be very difficult to treat. In addition to the difficulty with bracing this area of the spine, surgical stabilization of the upper thoracic spine is challenging because of the limited intraoperative visualization of this area. Anterior surgical approaches in the upper thoracic spine can be especially difficult, often requiring measures like sternotomy to gain adequate exposure of the ventral spine. There is also a lack of instrumentation designed specifically to address this area of the spine. In addition, posterior instrumentation constructs that cross the cervicothoracic junction are limited. Posterior approaches with pedicle screw fixation are most commonly used to treat traumatic instability in this area; however, the pedicles in the upper thoracic spine can be very small, especially the T4, T5, and T6 pedicles, making pedicle screw fixation technically more challenging to perform. Laminar hooks and transverse process hooks can be used for additional stability when the anatomy does not favor use of pedicle screw fixation.

Middle thoracic spine injuries (T6 to T10) can accommodate immobilization better than upper thoracic injuries and, with the added support of the rib cage, they can be managed more conservatively than other thoracolumbar fractures. Both anterior and posterior instrumentation approaches are available to treat fractures in this area. Anterior approaches have the benefit of allowing for reconstruction of the anterior spinal column, but a thoracotomy is required and therefore this approach incurs the additional potential complications of operating within the thoracic cavity. Anterior instrumentation for use in this area has evolved to lower profile systems that minimize the risk of injury to the thoracic viscera. Newer endoscopic approaches are now being performed that not only have a lower morbidity of an open procedure but have the added benefit for quicker recovery from surgery. Early anterior thoracic and lumbar instrumentation, like the Kaneda device (Fig. 3-14A), used anterior screws placed into the vertebral bodies from a lateral trajectory and rods connecting the screws for stabilization. Newer plating systems (Fig. 3-14B), which have a lower profile (i.e., no protrusion of screw heads above the level of the plates), also use screw fixation into the vertebral bodies. Expandable cages (Fig. 3-14C) can be used in the thoracic and lumbar spine to provide immediate structural stability to the anterior column after a corpectomy or vertebrectomy. These devices produce sufficient anterior distraction and deformity correction.

Posterior instrumentation in the thoracic and lumbar spine has evolved from early rod and wiring, such as Harrington rods and hook-and-rod constructs, to pedicle screws (Fig. 3-15) that produce stronger three-column spinal fixation. Posterior pedicle screw placement creates immediate stabilization through the posterior, middle, and anterior columns, which allows greater forces to be used for fracture or deformity reduction and correction.

Traumatic injuries at the thoracolumbar junction (T11-L2) are among the more common spinal injuries because of the unique biomechanics of this area. The transition between the rigid thoracic spinal column and the relatively mobile lumbar spine creates a fulcrum at the thoracolumbar junction. There is a transfer of energy up the lordotic lumbar spine and down the kyphotic thoracic spine, creating maximum stress at the thoracolumbar junction. As a result, up to 75% of fractures in the thoracic and lumbar spine occur at the thoracolumbar junction, and it is the second most common site for spinal fractures after the cervical spine. Management of these fractures can be complex and many of the strategies remain controversial, with some physicians favoring more aggressive surgical treatment because of the high biomechanical forces exerted on this area of the spine and the sensitivity of the conus medullaris to compression. Like other areas of the thoracic and lumbar spine, there may be a bias toward posterior instrumentation because of the ease and familiarity of the approach. Transthoracic and thoracoscopic approaches, with possible splitting of the diaphragm, may be used to access the ventral vertebral column down to L2.

There is a general tendency to treat the remainder of the lumbar spine (L3 and below) more conservatively than thoracolumbar junction fractures because the biomechanical stresses are not as substantial as in other areas and the cauda equina is more tolerant to compression than the spinal cord. When surgery is contemplated, the posterior approaches are often favored, as general surgery assistance may be needed by some spinal surgeons for anterior approaches to this area of the spine via retroperitoneal or transperitoneal approaches.

Surgical Treatment of Specific Thoracolumbar Fracture Patterns

Most thoracolumbar (compression/wedge/burst fractures) can be treated conservatively with bracing; in general, only severe burst fractures in this class of injuries require surgical stabilization. Neurologic deficits in the setting of canal compromise are one surgical indication for decompression and stabilization. Another general indication for surgical stabilization of burst fractures includes loss or disruption of the posterior ligamentous complex, which can be inferred from >25 degrees of kyphosis on radiographs or direct visualization of disruption of the posterior ligamentous complex on fat-suppressed sagittal T2-weighted MRI. There has been a trend over the past decade toward short-segment fixation at the thoracolumbar junction in an effort to preserve motion at adjacent levels. The McCormack et al. (58) classification may be used to determine which burst fractures will fail short-segment instrumentation and require further anterior column reconstruction.

Distraction injuries, seat belt-type injuries, and Chance fractures, where there is loss of integrity of the posterior

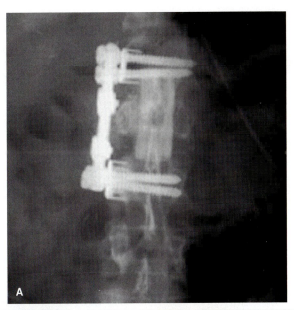

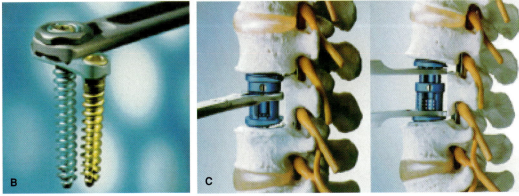

FIGURE 3-14. Anterior instrumentation has become more popular in the thoracic and lumbar spine. **A:** AP radiograph showing Kaneda device (Depuy Spine) stabilizing a corpectomy. **B:** MACS-TL (Aesculap) is a new, lower profile system in which the screw heads are flush with the fixation plate can be placed thoracoscopically. **C:** Expandable cages (Synex cage, Synthes Corp) have been designed for the thoracic and lumbar spine to restore integrity of the anterior column and provide distraction to help correct deformities.

column, may be managed conservatively but often require posterior instrumentation to restore the posterior tension band. Translation injuries or rotational fractures are the most unstable fractures and have the highest risk for neurologic injury; they therefore almost always require surgical stabilization. Severe translation injuries often require a combined anterior-posterior approach to restore stability to the spinal column.

USE OF INTRAOPERATIVE IMAGING

Intraoperative imaging is often used by surgeons to confirm the appropriate level for surgery and improve the accuracy of spinal instrumentation placement. Fluoroscopy and plain films can each be used to confirm the

level of surgery, but fluoroscopy has the added flexibility of real-time images for guidance. Lateral fluoroscopy is used most commonly, but AP, oblique, and biplanar (one AP and one lateral) (Fig. 3-7A) fluoroscopy each have roles depending on the surgical need. Careful attention should be made to obtain "true" lateral or AP images by adjusting the fluoroscope to eliminate obliquity, which can lead to errors in perception. In the cervical spine, aligning the facet joints so they are superimposed on each other serves as a good guide for obtaining the true lateral view. In the thoracic and lumbar spine, the vertebral body endplates can serve this same function for obtaining perfect lateral alignment on the fluoroscope. In the AP plane, the pedicles and spinous processes serve as good landmarks for adjusting the fluoroscope to eliminate obliquity.

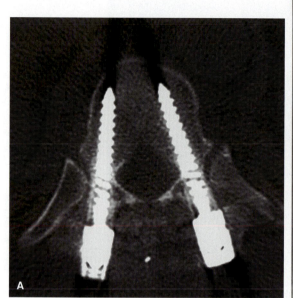
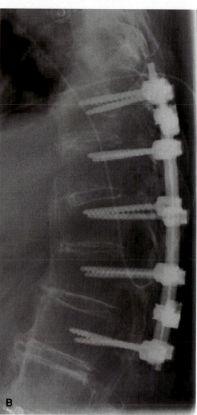

FIGURE 3-15. Posterior thoracic and lumbar instrumentation. Pedicle screws are the most commonly used instrumentation in the thoracic and lumbar spine and can usually be placed throughout the thoracic and lumbar spine depending on the individuals anatomy and size of pedicles (T4-6 typically have smallest pedicles). **A:** The axial CT scan shows a pedicle screw placed through the pedicle into the vertebral body. **B:** Lateral plain radiograph showing rods connected to pedicle screws.

The cervicothoracic junction is typically the most difficult area to visualize with intraoperative fluoroscopy. Maneuvers to pull the shoulders toward the feet (taping or traction) can help maximize visualization at the lower cervical spine. Collimating the fluoroscopic beam to the site of interest can also improve visualization and reduce radiation exposure. In obese patients, fluoroscopic visualization may be marginal throughout the spine but can be improved with these same maneuvers.

Counting vertebral levels to localize the appropriate surgical level can be very difficult in the thoracic region. It is often best to count up from a known level in the lumbar region rather than counting down from the cervicothoracic junction, which is often poorly visualized. If localization is a concern, a skin marker or subcutaneously implanted marker can help significantly with localization when correlated with preoperative studies. More complex stereotactic navigation systems using preoperative CT scans or sophisticated intraoperative fluoroscopy are also available to help with intraoperative localization and hardware placement, but image quality and accuracy are often suboptimal with current technology.

SUMMARY

Although the surgical techniques and instrumentation for repair of spinal fractures have progressed substantially, there is a relative lack of uniformity in the surgical management of spinal trauma because of a lack of good class I evidence and guidelines for a majority of spinal injuries. The surgical indications and approaches taken to manage spinal trauma vary greatly among spine surgeons. Instrumentation continues to have a significant role in the stabilization of some unstable fractures. Continued evolution of instrumentation that more faithfully reproduces the biomechanics of the normal tissues is expected, and new minimally invasive surgical techniques that will minimize perioperative morbidity and length of hospitalization overall are being developed.

REFERENCES

1. Vaccaro AR, Silber JS. Post-traumatic spinal deformity. *Spine*. 2001;26(24 suppl):S111–118.
2. Lifshutz J, Colohan A. A brief history of therapy for traumatic spinal cord injury. *Neurosurg Focus*. 2004;16(1):1–8.
3. Markham J. Surgery of the spinal cord and vertebral column. In: Walker, A, ed. *A History of Neurological Surgery*. New York: Hafner; 1967:364–392.
4. Omeis I, DeMattia JA, Hillard VH, et al. History of instrumentation for stabilization of the subaxial cervical spine. *Neurosurg Focus*. 2004;16(1):1–6.
5. Deshaies E, DiRisio D, Popp J. Medieval management of spinal injuries: parallels between Theodoric of Bologna and contemporary spine surgeons. *Neurosurg Focus*. 2004;16(1):1–3.
6. Singh H, Rahimi SY, Yeh DJ, et al. History of posterior thoracic instrumentation. *Neurosurg Focus*. 2004;16(1):1–4.
7. Goodrich J. History of spine surgery in ancient and medieval worlds. *Neurosurg Focus*. 2004;16(1):1–13.
8. Frankel HL, Hancock DO, Hyslop G, et al. The value of postural reduction in the initial management of closed injuries of the spine with paraplegia and tetraplegia. I. *Paraplegia*. 1969;7(3):179–192.
9. Silker CW, Mirvis SE, Shanmuganathan K. Assessing cervical spine stability in obtunded blunt trauma patients: review of medical literature. *Radiology*. 2005;234:733–739.
10. Radiographic assessment of the cervical spine in asymptomatic trauma patients. *Neurosurgery*. 2002;50(3 suppl):S30–35.
11. Radiographic assessment of the cervical spine in symptomatic trauma patients. *Neurosurgery*. 2002;50(3 suppl): S36–43.
12. Roos JE, Hilfiker P, Platz A, et al. MDCT in emergency radiology: is a standardized chest or abdominal protocol sufficient for evaluation of thoracic and lumbar spine trauma? *AJR*. 2004;183:959–968.
13. Hughes SJ. How effective is the Newport/Aspen collar? A prospective radiographic evaluation in healthy adult volunteers. *J Trauma*. 1998;45(2):374–378.
14. Benzel EC, Hadden TA, Saulsberg CM. A comparison of the Minerva and halo jackets for stabilization of the cervical spine. *J Neurosurg*. 1989;70(3):411–414.
15. Sharpe KP, Rao S, Ziogas A. Evaluation of the effectiveness of the Minerva cervicothoracic orthosis. *Spine*. 1995;20(13): 1475–1459.
16. Noble ER, Smoker WR. The forgotten condyle: the appearance, morphology, and classification of occipital condyle fractures. *AJNR Am J Neuroradiol*. 1996;17(3):507–513.
17. Leone A, Cerase A, Colosimo C, et al. Occipital condylar fractures: a review. *Radiology*. 2000;216(3):635–644.
18. Occipital condyle fractures. *Neurosurgery*. 2002;50(3 suppl): S114–119.
19. Anderson PA, Montesano PX. Morphology and treatment of occipital condyle fractures. *Spine*. 1988;13(7):731–736.
20. Vaccaro AR, Lim MR, Lee JY. Indications for surgery and stabilization techniques of the occipito-cervical junction. *Injury*. 2005;36(suppl 2):B44–53.
21. Hanson JA, Deliganis AV, Baxter AB, et al. Radiologic and clinical spectrum of occipital condyle fractures: retrospective review of 107 consecutive fractures in 95 patients. *AJR Am J Roentgenol*. 2002;178(5): 1261–1268.
22. Powers B, Miller MD, Kramer RS, et al. Traumatic anterior atlanto-occipital dislocation. *Neurosurgery*. 1979;4(1):12–17.
23. Wholey MH, Bruwer AJ, Baker, HL Jr. The lateral roentgenogram of the neck; with comments on the atlanto-odontoid-basion relationship. *Radiology*. 1958;71(3):350–356.
24. Harris JH Jr, Carson GC, Wagner LK, et al. Radiologic diagnosis of traumatic occipitovertebral dissociation: 2. Comparison of three methods of detecting occipitovertebral relationships on lateral radiographs of supine subjects. *AJR Am J Roentgenol*. 1994; 162(4):887–892.
25. Harris JH, Carson GC, Wagner LK. Radiologic diagnosis of traumatic occipitovertebral dissociation: 1. Normal occipitovertebral relationships on lateral radiographs of supine subjects. *AJR Am J Roentgenol*. 1994;162(4):881–886.
26. Dublin AB, Marks WM, Weinstock D, et al. Traumatic dislocation of the atlanto-occipital articulation (AOA) with short-term survival. With a radiographic method of measuring the AOA. *J Neurosurg*. 1980;52(4):541–546.
27. Lee C, Woodring JH, Goldstein SJ, et al. Evaluation of traumatic atlantooccipital dislocations. *AJNR Am J Neuroradiol*. 1987;8(1):19–26.
28. Spence KF Jr, Decker S, Sell KW. Bursting atlantal fracture associated with rupture of the transverse ligament. *J Bone Joint Surg Am*. 1970;52(3):543–549.
29. Dickman CA, Mamourian A, Sonntag VK, et al. Magnetic resonance imaging of the transverse atlantal ligament for the evaluation of atlantoaxial instability. *J Neurosurg*. 1991;75(2):221–227.
30. Anderson LD, D'Alonzo, RT. Fractures of the odontoid process of the axis. *J Bone Joint Surg Am*. 1974;56(8):1663–1674.
31. Sonntag VK, Hadley MN. Nonoperative management of cervical spine injuries. *Clin Neurosurg*. 1988;34:630–649.
32. Apuzzo ML, Heiden JS, Weiss MH, et al. Acute fractures of the odontoid process. An analysis of 45 cases. *J Neurosurg*. 1978; 48(1):85–91.
33. Ekong CE, Schwartz ML, Tator CH, et al. Odontoid fracture: management with early mobilization using the halo device. *Neurosurgery*. 1981; 9(6):631–637.
34. Hadley MN, Dickman CA, Browner CM, et al. Acute axis fractures: a review of 229 cases. *J Neurosurg*. 1989;71(5 pt 1):642–647.
35. Jenkins JD, Coric D, Branch CL Jr. A clinical comparison of one- and two-screw odontoid fixation. *J Neurosurg*. 1998; 89(3):366–370.
36. McBride AD, Mukherjee DP, Kruse RN, et al. Anterior screw fixation of type II odontoid fractures. A biomechanical study. *Spine*. 1995;20(17):1855–1860; discussion 1859–1860.
37. Bohler J. [Screw-osteosynthesis of fractures of the dens axis]. *Unfallheilkunde*. 1981;84(6):221–223.
38. Apfelbaum RI, Lonser RR, Veres R, et al. Direct anterior screw fixation for recent and remote odontoid fractures. *J Neurosurg Spine*. 2000; 93(2):227–236.
39. Cone W, Turner WG. The treatment of fracture-dislocations of the cervical vertebrae by skeletal traction and fusion. *J Bone Joint Surg*. 1937;19:584–602.
40. Gallie W. Fractures and dislocations of the cervical spine. *Am J Surg*. 1939;46:495–499.
41. Dickman CA, Sonntag VK, Papadopoulos SM, et al. The interspinous method of posterior atlantoaxial arthrodesis. *J Neurosurg*. 1991;74(2):190–198.
42. Brooks AL, Jenkins EB. Atlanto-axial arthrodesis by the wedge compression method. *J Bone Joint Surg Am*. 1978; 60(3):279–284.
43. Grob D, Magerl F. [Surgical stabilization of C1 and C2 fractures]. *Orthopade*. 1987;16(1):46–54.
44. Harms J, Melcher RP. Posterior C1-C2 fusion with polyaxial screw and rod fixation. *Spine*. 2001;26(22):2467–2471.
45. Francis WR, Fielding JW, Hawkins RJ, et al. Traumatic spondylolisthesis of the axis. *J Bone Joint Surg Br*. 1981;63B (3):313–318.
46. Effendi B, Roy D, Cornish B, et al. Fractures of the ring of the axis. A classification based on the analysis of 131 cases. *J Bone Joint Surg Br*. 1981;63B(3):319–327.
47. Greene KA, Dickman CA, Marciano FF, et al. Acute axis fractures. Analysis of management and outcome in 340 consecutive cases. *Spine*. 1997;22(16):1843–1852.
48. White AA III, Southwick WO, Panjabi MM. Clinical instability in the lower cervical spine: a review of past and current concepts. *Spine*. 1976;1(1):15–27.
49. White AA III, Johnson RM, Panjabi MM, et al. Biomechanical analysis of clinical stability in the cervical spine. *Clin Orthop Relat Res*. 1975(109): 85–96.
50. Panjabi MM, White AA III, Johnson RM. Cervical spine mechanics as a function of transection of components. *J Biomech*. 1975;8(5):327–336.
51. Caspar W, Barbier DD, Klara PM. Anterior cervical fusion and Caspar plate stabilization for cervical trauma. *Neurosurgery*. 1989;25(4):491–502.

52. Epstein NE. Anterior cervical dynamic ABC plating with single level corpectomy and fusion in forty-two patients. *Spinal Cord*. 2003;41(3):153–158.

53. Initial closed reduction of cervical spine fracture-dislocation injuries. *Neurosurgery*. 2002;50(3 suppl):S44–50.

54. Holdsworth FW. Diagnosis and treatment of fractures of the spine. *Manit Med Rev*. 1968;48(1):13–15.

55. Whitesides TE Jr. Traumatic kyphosis of the thoracolumbar spine. *Clin Orthop*. 1977(128):78–92.

56. Denis F. The three column spine and its significance in the classification of acute thoracolumbar spinal injuries. *Spine*. 1983;8(8):817–831.

57. McAfee PC, Yuan HA, Fredrickson BE, et al. The value of computed tomography in thoracolumbar fractures. An analysis of one hundred consecutive cases and a new classification. *J Bone Joint Surg Am*. 1983;65(4):461–473.

58. McCormack T, Karaikovic E, Gaines RW. The load sharing classification of spine fractures. *Spine*. 1994;19(15): 1741–1744.

59. Magerl F, Aebi M, Gertzbein SD, et al. A comprehensive classification of thoracic and lumbar injuries. *Eur Spine J*. 1994;3(4):184–201.

60. Gertzbein SD. Spine update. Classification of thoracic and lumbar fractures. *Spine*. 1994;19(5):626–628.

Imaging

Chapter 4

Controversies in Clearing the Spine

C. Craig Blackmore and Ken F. Linnau

There are approximately 11,000 cases of spinal cord injury per year in the United States with an incidence of 40 cases per million persons per year (1). According to the National Spinal Cord Injury Database, overall, approximately 250,000 persons in the United States currently are living with spinal cord injury. Reflecting the general trauma population, the majority (81%) are males and the average age is relatively young at 32.8 years. Approximately half the spinal cord injuries occur from motor vehicle crashes. Falls from >10 feet, gunshot wounds, motorcycle crashes, crush injuries, and medical/surgical complications account for most of the remaining cases (1).

Spinal cord injury involves a great burden to society as well as to the individual. First-year medical costs for subjects with spinal cord injury range from $200,000 to $680,000, depending on the level of injury (2,3). The lifetime costs of care for a person with spinal cord injury averages $2 million, with variation based on whether an injury is complete and the level of injury (1–3). Expenditures in the United States per year are approximately $6 billion on the detection, treatment, and rehabilitation for spinal cord injury patients. This does not include an additional $57,000 per year per person on indirect costs such as lost wages and productivity (1). In addition to the obvious quality-of-life implications of such injuries, life expectancy is also affected,

being approximately half of that of otherwise matched individuals (1,4,5).

CERVICAL SPINE INJURY

Who Should Undergo Cervical Spine Imaging in the Acute Setting?

The majority of cervical spinal cord injury occurs from unstable cervical spine fracture. Unfortunately, unstable cervical spine fractures may be clinically unapparent upon presentation to the emergency department. Only one third of spinal trauma patients present initially with a neurological deficit (6,7). Moreover, important clinical features such as pain from injury may be masked by other injuries, medication, and drug and alcohol intoxication. Patients who have spine fractures but are neurologically intact at the time of presentation to the emergency department may progress and develop neurologic compromise (8–10). In an early study by Rogers (11) in the 1950s, progression to neurologic deficit occurred in 50% of subjects with cervical spine fracture who were initially neurologically intact. With modern field and emergency department spine immobilization techniques, this rate is much lower. However, based on a longitudinal study of 253 spine fracture patients in Alberta, Reid reported that progression to neurologic deficit in patients with initially missed cervical spine fractures is as high as 10% (8). Accordingly, the current consensus recommendations of the American College of Surgeons *Advanced Trauma Life Support* (12) and the Appropriateness Criteria of the American College of Radiology (13) advise imaging of the spine in patients who are at risk for fracture.

Defining the group of subjects who are at risk for cervical spine fracture and therefore in whom imaging is appropriate remains challenging. Cervical spine imaging is one of the most common imaging exams performed on trauma patients in many trauma centers throughout the United States and other developed nations. The yield from such imaging however is very low with only 0.9% to 2.8% of imaging studies demonstrating fractures (14–16). Although cervical spine imaging itself is not an expensive procedure, the frequency of performance makes it a high-cost item for trauma care (17,18).

Efforts to define optimal imaging selection criteria have centered on the development and validation of clinical prediction rules. Clinical prediction rules are decision-making tools consisting of several factors that suggest a course of action or provide a probability of a disease or injury (19). Clinical prediction rules composed of clinical factors can be used to determine the probability of injury or can be applicable in selecting subjects appropriately for imaging. In order to be useful, clinical prediction rules must be easy to use, strongly predictive, and yield consistent results with multiple users and diverse populations. The process of determining a clinical prediction rule involves developing a possible set of clinical criteria, testing interobserver reliability, and validating the clinical prediction rule in a second set of subjects (19,20).

In the past decade, two large prospective multicenter investigations have been performed to define clinical prediction rules for selection of appropriate subjects for cervical spine imaging after trauma. The first of these was the National Emergency X-Ray Utilization Study (NEXUS) in the United States, published in 2000 (15). The NEXUS study was a prospective validation of clinical criteria that were already in place at emergency departments throughout the United States. The NEXUS investigators developed a collaboration of 21 emergency departments and enrolled a total of 34,069 trauma subjects in whom imaging was requested. Eight hundred eighteen (2.4%) of the subjects had cervical spine fractures. The NEXUS study group applied an a priori prediction rule of clinical criteria that specified when imaging was indicated, and it used the radiologist's interpretation of the imaging results as the gold standard for evaluating the effectiveness of the criteria. The NEXUS criteria for *not* imaging (Table 4-1) included normal neurologic examination, absence of posterior midline tenderness, and a normal level of alertness without intoxication or painful distracting injuries. The NEXUS study did not affect the ongoing clinical care of the study subjects, so imaging

▶ **TABLE 4-1** NEXUS Criteria for Appropriate Cervical Spine Imaging

The NEXUS study indicates that cervical spine imaging is *not* necessary in trauma patients who meet *all* of the following five criteria:

1. No midline cervical spine tenderness
2. No focal neurological deficit
3. Normal level of alertness
4. No intoxication
5. No painful distracting injury

Source: Hoffman J, Mower W, Wolfson A, et al. Validity of a set of clinical criteria to rule out injury to the cervical spine in patients with blunt trauma. *N Eng J Med.* 2000;343:94–99.

consisted primarily of radiography, supplemented by computed tomography (CT) and magnetic resonance imaging (MRI) as dictated by the clinical status of each patient and by local practice patterns. The NEXUS group found that their clinical prediction rule could adequately identify subjects at risk of fracture, with a sensitivity of 99.6%. In addition, interobserver agreement was excellent (kappa = 0.73) (15).

Unfortunately, while the sensitivity of the NEXUS criteria was high, the specificity was rather low (12.6%), indicating that the number of unnecessary normal radiographic studies that use of the NEXUS rule would eliminate was small (15). Because the NEXUS study relied principally on imaging criteria that pre-existed at participating centers, there was no measurable impact on imaging utilization.

Important strengths of the NEXUS study were its large sample size and inclusion of multiple emergency departments from a range of sizes and types of facilities, including academic centers, community hospitals, level-one trauma centers, as well as low-volume trauma centers. The broad representation in the study sample suggests that, at least in the United States, the guidelines set forth by the NEXUS study can be applied to a wide range of hospital settings.

Subsequent to the NEXUS study, the Canadian cervical spine study group performed their own separate validation of clinical prediction rules in determining when imaging is appropriate in cervical spine trauma (21). The first phase of the Canadian study was the prospective development of a clinical prediction rule from 8,924 subjects who were evaluated at ten hospitals in Ontario. Investigators used 20 unique clinical predictors of cervical spine injury that were not commonly relied on in standard clinical practice. The Canadian study differs from the NEXUS study primarily due to its usage of different clinical parameters to qualify appropriate usage of imaging in cervical spine trauma. From this initial development study, the Canadian investigators identified criteria that had 100% sensitivity and 42.5% specificity for detection of acute cervical spine injury (Table 4-2). The second

▶ **TABLE 4-2** **Canadian Cervical Spine Clinical Prediction Rule**

Imaging of the cervical spine is *not* necessary if patients are alert (GCS 15) and *all* of the conditions detailed below are met.

1. No high-risk factor present, including:
　Age 65 or more years
　Dangerous mechanism, including:
　　Fall from >3 meters/5 stairs
　　Axial load to head (diving)
　　High-speed vehicular crash (60 mph, rollover, ejection)
　　Bicycle crash
　　Motorized recreational vehicle crash
　Paresthesias in extremities
2. Any low-risk factor is present, including:
　Simple rear-end vehicular crash mechanism, excluding:
　　Pushed into oncoming traffic
　　Hit by bus/large truck
　　Rollover
　　Hit by high-speed vehicle
　Sitting position in emergency department
　Ambulatory at any time
　Delayed onset of neck pain
　Absence of midline cervical tenderness
3. Able to actively rotate neck (45 degrees left and right)

Source: Stiell I, Wells G, Vandemheen K, et al. The Canadian C-spine rule for radiography in alert and stable trauma patients. *JAMA.* 2001;286: 1841–1848.

portion of the Canadian study was a validation of the criteria developed in the first portion of the study. This was performed in the same ten hospitals on another 8,283 trauma patients. The results of this validation study found that the clinical prediction rule had a 99.4% sensitivity and a 45.1% specificity for predicting when a cervical spine injury was present with the additional benefit of a high interobserver agreement (14,21).

It is difficult to draw direct comparisons between the NEXUS and the Canadian Cervical Spine results because of differences in the study populations on which they were validated. The Canadian study only included subjects who had a Glasgow coma scale (GCS) score of 15 (i.e., normal) and who were hemodynamically stable (21). The NEXUS included trauma patients regardless of GCS scores and hemodynamic instability, although the decreased mental status was one of the criteria for performance of radiography (15,22). In addition, the Canadian study included all subjects in whom cervical spine injury was suspected due to mechanism and other defined clinical criteria with the treating physician's decision to order radiography having no bearing on enrollment (21), while NEXUS was limited to subjects who underwent imaging with the decision to perform radiography left to the physician's discretion (15,22).

Perhaps the most important difference between the two studies is the specificity of the prediction rules. The

higher specificity of the Canadian C-Spine Rule (42.5%), as compared to the NEXUS rule (12.9%), implies that the Canadian C-Spine Rule may have a greater impact on utilization by decreasing unnecessary ordering of cervical radiographs by a greater proportion. However, this higher specificity may also be explained by differences in study group selection between the Canadian and NEXUS cohort (23). To date, no data have been published on the actual effect of either rule on imaging ordering behavior in practice or on any changes in the performance of unnecessary imaging. A concern with the Canadian cervical spine rule is that the criteria are perceived to be much more complex than the NEXUS rule, and it includes provocative testing for symptoms (e.g., head turning and flexion), a practice with which some US physicians may not be comfortable. A lively debate has emerged between the two research groups, but no clear advantage of one clinical prediction rule over the other has been demonstrated (14,23–26). In an attempt to provide standards for practice, the American Association of Neurological Surgeons/Congress of Neurological Surgeons (AANS/CNS) reviewed the literature and recommended that radiographic assessment is not necessary for those asymptomatic patients who are "awake, alert, and not intoxicated, who are without neck pain or tenderness, and who do not have significant associated injuries that detract from their general evaluation" (27).

What Imaging Approach Is Appropriate for Subjects at Different Levels of Risk for Cervical Spine Fracture?

Subjects identified as at risk for cervical spine imaging by either the NEXUS or Canadian cervical spine rule represent a large and heterogeneous group. Further, different imaging technologies may be appropriate in different patients. The traditional initial approach for evaluation of the acutely injured cervical spine has been with radiography. As of early 2005, the three-view radiography series (anteroposterior, lateral, and open mouth) is still the imaging modality of choice recommended by the American College of Radiology Appropriateness Criteria (13) and the *Advanced Trauma Life Support* (ATLS) course of the American College of Surgeons (12). The AANS/CNS recommends this three-view radiograph series as the initial study for symptomatic patients (27). Based on a critical literature review in 1997, the pooled estimate of the sensitivity of traditional cervical radiography for fracture is 94% (28). However, this sensitivity may be much lower in major multisystem trauma victims (29,30). In addition, the specificity is affected by the characteristics of the patient being imaged (31). In patients with major trauma and multiple injuries, the probability of obtaining adequate cervical spine radiographs of diagnostic quality is diminished. For example, one study found that in subjects with head injury, adequate cervical spine radiographs will only be obtained in 89% of patients, and in subjects with head injury from high-energy mechanisms such as motor vehicle and motorcycle crashes, adequate radiographs can only be obtained 78% to 84% of the time (31). In addition, in a study of multitrauma, intensive care unit patients in Alberta, Canada, radiographs were inadequate in 82% (32). Factors that degrade the quality of radiographs include the use of devices that obscure portions of the spine and soft tissues such as backboards or endotracheal tubes, the presence of other immobilizing injuries (such as upper extremity fractures precluding use of the swimmer's view), and impairment of the patient's cognitive status from drugs, cerebral injury, or hypoxia. The continued value of cervical radiography in the primary evaluation of trauma patients is due its wide availability at virtually all trauma centers, as well as the widespread experience in interpretation of radiography.

Use of helical CT scanning, first proposed by Núñez et al. (33,34) in the mid-1990s, has gained acceptance as a more accurate alternative to radiography for initial evaluation of the cervical spine (29,32,35,36). Single detector CT scan has a sensitivity of 98% to 99% for fracture with a specificity of 93% (29,34,37). In addition to being more accurate, CT of the cervical spine may also be acquired more rapidly than radiography when performed on subjects who are to undergo CT of other body regions. In patients with minor injury, radiography may require only 10 minutes on average, but this time increases up to an hour in subjects with multiple injuries from major trauma (17). Núñez et al. (33) reported that time in the emergency department for major trauma patients was decreased when CT was used as the initial cervical spine imaging approach. Subsequent investigations have supported the time advantage of CT (35,38).

Blackmore et al. (19,28,37,39) provide a definition of appropriate subjects for use of CT through a combination of a clinical prediction rule and cost effectiveness analysis. Cost-effectiveness analysis is a health policy tool that balances the outcomes and dollar costs of differing approaches to patient care. Cost-effectiveness analysis is usually based on a theoretical computer model that includes all of the possible outcomes from a medical care decision, with the associated short- and long-term costs (40,41). For the cervical spine, the cost-effectiveness model incorporates the choice between CT and radiography, with the probability that an injury is present, the probability that the injury will be missed by each imaging approach, and the effect on the patient of missed injury. In addition, the model considers the costs of the initial imaging, the costs of any further imaging tests induced by false positive studies, and the costs of any adverse outcomes resulting from missed injury (28).

From the cost-effectiveness analysis, when all short- and long-term costs and outcomes are considered, CT is a more cost effective method for initial cervical spine imaging than radiography in high risk patients. CT was only cost effective if the probability of cervical spine fracture was greater than 4%. The cost effectiveness of CT is related in part to the high frequency of inadequate radiographs, which lead to additional imaging. Also, the higher inherent sensitivity of CT for fractures leads to fewer missed injuries and better patient outcomes. Although the probability of development of neurologic deficit from missed fracture is relatively low, the consequences of such a missed injury may be catastrophic both in terms of costs and of outcome. Cost-effectiveness analysis suggests that use of CT in a hypothetical cohort of 100,000 trauma patients with a 10% fracture risk could prevent 23 cases of paralysis and save $3.4 million when compared to use of radiography. Therefore, CT as the initial imaging evaluation is most appropriate in high-risk patients (28).

The definition of "high risk" has been retrospectively developed by a clinical prediction rule and subsequently prospectively validated at the Harborview Medical Center (a large level-one trauma center in Seattle, Washington) (39,42). Subjects at high probability of cervical spine fracture met any of the following criteria: focal neurologic deficit, a severe head injury (intracranial hemorrhage, skull fracture, or persistent unconsciousness), or a high-energy mechanism (Table 4-3). In a prospective CT validation study applying these criteria to a cohort of almost 5,000 patients, these Harborview High Risk Cervical Spine Criteria found a incidence of fracture of 12.8% (42). These findings indicated that the applied CT criteria should be cost effective, as the incidence exceeds the 4% threshold for cost effectiveness. Based on the single center development study, agreement on the clinical predictors was excellent (average kappa = 0.80) (39). The prediction rule, however, has not been validated at other centers.

▶ **TABLE 4-3 Harborview High Risk Cervical Spine Criteria**

Subjects are at high risk of cervical spine injury (>10%) and CT would be the optimal initial imaging approach in subjects who meet *any* of the following criteria:

1. High-energy injury mechanism
   High-speed (>35 mph) motor vehicle or motorcycle crash
   Motor vehicle crash with death at scene
   Fall from height >10 feet
2. High-risk clinical parameter
   Significant head injury, including intracranial hemorrhage or persistent unconsciousness in emergency department
   Neurological signs or symptoms referable to the cervical spine
   Pelvic or multiple extremity fractures

Source: Hanson JA, Blackmore CC, Mann FA, et al. Cervical spine screening: a decision rule can identify high risk patients to undergo screening helical CT of the cervical spine. *AJR Am J Roentgenol.* 2000;174:713–718.

New technologies for multidetector CT are rapidly advancing and most of the accuracy and cost effectiveness data relate to either single detector helical or at most four detector CT scanners. With the new generation of 16 and up to 64 detector scanners, it is likely that CT today is more accurate and more cost effective than the published literature supports. This remains to be evaluated in future investigations.

In summary, despite the aforementioned consensus recommendations, the weight of the evidence of recent year has shifted to primary use of CT to screening cervical spine in high-risk patients, such as those defined by the Harborview High Risk Cervical Spine Criteria (42), particularly if CT is also to be used to evaluate the subject's head. Radiography remains appropriate in low-risk subjects, as well as in those situations where CT is not available.

SPECIAL POPULATIONS

Flexion-Extension Radiography in Patients with Focal Pain

Many physicians believe that a normal static radiographic imaging evaluation of the cervical spine on trauma patients does not preclude potentially unstable ligamentous injuries; however, this position is controversial. The incidence of cervical spine injury due to blunt trauma among imaged patients is approximately 2.4% (15). Pure ligamentous cervical spine injury (without fracture) is rare, with a prevalence of only 0.6%. This prevalence does not vary substantially between patients with reliable and unreliable clinical evaluations (i.e., obtunded, head injured, intoxicated subjects), despite a higher mortality rate in the "unreliable" group (43). However, because of the possibility of unstable ligamentous injury, many guidelines, including the American College of Surgeons Advanced Trauma Life Support Course, recommend active flexion-extension radiographs for awake, alert, and unintoxicated patients (GCS of 15) with persistent posterior, midline point tenderness (12). Similarly, the American College of Radiology Appropriateness Criteria (13) considers flexion-extension radiography studies most appropriate for symptomatic patients (severe pain without neurologic symptoms) with normal static radiographs, if ligamentous injury is suspected. The AANS/CNS note as an option that cervical spine immobilization may be discontinued if "normal and adequate" flexion-extension radiographs are obtained in an awake patient with normal radiographs or CT in the presence of neck pain or tenderness; however, this guideline also notes that, in the same population, a normal MRI within 48 hours would be adequate for cervical spine clearance (27).

Flexion-extension radiographs of the cervical spine have been used since the 1930s (44) and have been advocated in the acute setting after blunt trauma since the 1960s (45). Flexion-extension cervical radiography can theoretically aid in the identification of unstable ligamentous cervical spine injury or very subtle but unstable fractures. The presumption is that there are radiographic signs on flexion-extension studies that allow identification of instability, including listhesis and focal kyphosis. Unfortunately, data supporting the use of flexion-extension radiography is limited. No large scientific clinical studies have identified and conclusively validated specific measurable criteria to determine what imaging criteria constitute an abnormal flexion-extension radiographic study (46). The usual practice is to assess intervertebral body motion (subluxation and relative kyphosis) to determine presence or absence of an unstable cervical spine injury. The criteria used are mostly derived from cadaver models and validation data from clinical studies is still very limited (46).

Individual differences in the degree of physiologic range of motion between cervical vertebrae have been recognized and substantial variation in normal cervical spine motion with respect to gender and age was described (47,48). In addition, a wide individual variation can be found in the appearance of the cervical curvature on flexion-extension radiographs of normal subjects (46). The normal behavior of cervical spine motion between flexion and extension position is found to differ at various levels of the cervical spine. C4-5 normally is the level with the highest degree of mobility and the C2-3 segment is least mobile in the normal cervical spine (47). Based on limited evidence from whiplash patients with chronic injury, translation of one vertebral body relative to the one below of >2 mm may be a useful radiographic parameter. However, clinical validation for this criterion is also lacking (20,44,46).

In addition, there are currently no established clinical decision rules that specifically address the appropriate use of flexion-extension radiographs for the cervical spine trauma. The yield from flexion-extension radiography has been low in reported series (45,49–52), most of which were retrospective in nature. As summarized in a recent structured review of the literature, flexion-extension radiography is unlikely to be abnormal in children (53) and adds little to the evaluation of adults with neck pain after blunt trauma (54). Moreover, the small number of subjects with injury in these clinical series limits the calculation of sensitivity within an acceptably narrow confidence interval (55).

In summary, no reliable evidence exists regarding the appropriate role for flexion-extension radiography in the acute evaluation of cervical spine trauma.

Imaging in Obtunded Patients

Concern for occult ligamentous injuries that remains undetected on initial imaging may lead to performance of additional imaging on unreliable or obtunded patients. For example, the Eastern Association for the Surgery of Trauma (EAST) recommends that patients with altered mental status who are not anticipated to regain normal mental status within 48 hours undergo physician assisted flexion-extension fluoroscopy to clear the cervical spine (56). This procedure can be both technically challenging and potentially dangerous in the obtunded patient who harbors an occult unstable injury. Some centers advocate the use of MRI to exclude occult soft tissue injury to the intervertebral discs, ligamentous complexes, and spinal cord (13).

There is absence of scientific support for use of either flexion extension fluoroscopy or MRI to clear the injured cervical spine for instability. The practice of flexion-extension fluoroscopy is based on limited case series data (57–61). No rigorous studies with unbiased inclusion criteria and outcome measures exist, and no studies have been performed to determine if dynamic fluoroscopy identifies any injuries missed with initial CT. In addition, cases of iatrogenic complications due to physician-assisted flexion-extension fluoroscopy have been reported, with one patient becoming paralyzed following a false-negative exam and removal of cervical collar (61). The authors of two recent series (including one of the original proponents of dynamic fluoroscopy) conclude that dynamic fluoroscopy is not routinely necessary to clear the cervical spine of unconscious patients (61,62), because isolated ligamentous injury without radiographic evidence of fracture is extremely rare (0.04%–0.08%) (61,63) and inadequate flexion-extension studies are common (27%) (62).

At our institution flexion-extension fluoroscopy is rarely used for evaluating unreliable subjects. If a question of cervical instability remains after performance of a satisfactory clinical examination and CT of the cervical spine, the cervical spine of clinically unreliable patients is cleared with upright lateral radiography with the patient in a soft cervical collar. If no displacement is shown on the upright lateral radiograph, the soft collar is removed while the patient is recumbent (to reduce the incidence of cervical collar–related pressure ulcers (64) and replaced when patients are moved into a more upright position (e.g., for pulmonary toilet and physical therapy). This protocol is maintained until patients regain consciousness. This approach is based only on our own experience, without published supporting evidence.

MRI is believed to be highly sensitive for soft tissue abnormality of the acutely injured cervical spine (65–68) and MRI abnormalities may be identified in approximately 25% of obtunded patients (69,70). However, the importance of injuries identified on MRI and the specificity of MRI is unclear (71,72). A recent review of the literature found that only 5.6% of subjects with ligamentous abnormality seen on MRI required surgery or treatment with halo immobilization (73). In biomechanical studies on cadavers, only 60% to 79% of MRI abnormalities had anatomic correlates; in the cervical spine disruption of the anterior and posterior longitudinal ligaments were most conspicuous (100% sensitivity) with injury to the ligamentum flavum, capsular ligaments, and interspinous ligaments identified less reliably (50%–75% sensitivity) (74,75). Hogan et al. (76) evaluated the capability of multidetector CT in predicting soft tissue injury in 366 obtunded cervical trauma patients. MR imaging was negative for 354 patients of this group; however, 12 patients had abnormalities on MRI including: four with ligamentous injury, three with intervertebral disc injury, seven with spinal cord contusion, and one with a combined injury. Multidetector CT had a negative predictive value of 98.9% for ligamentous injury and 100% predictive value for unstable cervical spine injury. The authors concluded that a normal multidetector CT study in the obtunded or unreliable blunt cervical trauma patient is sufficient to exclude unstable injury in this setting and that routine use of MRI is not warranted.

Most subjects with isolated paraspinal MR signal abnormalities (i.e., signal changes in the posterior ligamentous complex) will be managed nonoperatively, and it is not clear if any clinically important injuries will be missed by CT and detected by MRI. Further, MRI criteria associated with or predictive of clinical instability have not been conclusively established. At present, there is not sufficient evidence to recommend routine use of MRI to exclude cervical spine injury over standard modalities. MRI is a superior method to evaluate the soft tissue component of injury (77). MRI is warranted when changes of posttraumatic myelopathy are present.

Finally, most current recommendations for supplemental imaging to exclude ligamentous injury are predicated upon radiography as the initial screen procedure (56). The higher sensitivity and anatomic detail of CT may make other imaging, flexion-extension radiographs and MRI, for occult ligamentous injury even less necessary.

Imaging in Elderly Subjects

The biomechanics of injury in the elderly differ from younger adults due to three factors. First, osteopenia, which is ubiquitous in this population, leads to a lower energy threshold for fracture and affects fracture location (78,79). In addition, biomechanically, the spine in elderly patients is altered by degenerative fusion usually in the lower cervical segments, which leads to marked decrease in motion in the lower cervical spine (78,80–82). Finally, the mechanism of cervical spine injury in the elderly is substantially different than in younger adults with low-velocity falls being more common in the elderly, and high-energy motor vehicle crashes more common in younger subjects (78,82). As a consequence, patterns of injury in the elderly differ from those in younger subjects (82–85). Lomoschitz et al. (86) identified that fractures of the upper cervical spine, particularly C2, are more common in subjects over 65 years of age than in younger subjects. The predilection of C2 injuries become even more striking if one considers the very elderly, those of age 75 or greater. In these very elderly subjects, C2 account for nearly 50% of all fractures that are identified. Injuries to the lower cervical segments become increasingly uncommon as patients age.

Osteopenia and degenerative changes in the elderly spine combined with difficulties in positioning such patients may make radiography more challenging to perform and interpret. There are no good data on the accuracy of radiography for detection of fracture in the elderly subjects, however, it has been reported that cervical spine fractures in the elderly may be overlooked in the initial radiographic evaluation in 15% to 40% of subjects (78,85,87).

Bub et al. (88) investigated clinical predictors of cervical spine fracture in the elderly with a view toward identifying subjects in whom it would be appropriate to use CT scan. Using a case control study design, the investigators concluded that the risk factors for cervical injury were the same for elderly subjects as for those of younger age. Presence of other injuries, including head injury and neurologic deficit, as well as high-energy mechanisms, were criteria that identified high-risk subjects in elderly patients. However, in contrast to the younger population, fall from standing height, a low energy mechanism, was sufficiently common to account for 11% of all fractures in the elderly population, despite the fact that this was not a high-risk criterion. Fall from standing height resulted most frequently in fractures at C2 and were missed by the clinical prediction rule in the elderly. Bub et al. concluded that the same clinical prediction rule should be applied in the elderly as in younger subjects, but that particular vigilance was necessary at the C2 level on both clinical examination and interpretation of radiographs. There is no published cost-effectiveness analysis available on appropriate imaging in the elderly.

Imaging in Children

Cervical spine fractures are uncommon in children. The overall incidence of spinal fractures in pediatric trauma patients is <1% (89,90). In addition, the injury patterns are different, with cranio-cervical junction injuries being more prevalent in this group (90). Clinical prediction rules applied to adults have not been adequately tested on children and are likely not to be relevant due to different biomechanics and injury patterns. The NEXUS study did include pediatric subjects, but only four subjects with fractures were identified who were <9 years old, obviating the possibility of drawing conclusion for this age group (89). No validated method exists to identify pediatric subjects who are of high risk for fracture.

The pediatric population also poses special consideration regarding radiation dose due to the inherent radiosensitivity of developing tissues in children compared to adults (91). Moreover, if exposed to radiation

early in life, longer induction times in children may predispose them to cancer later in life. Accordingly, the higher radiation dose of multiple detector CT is a relative contraindication to use of this technology in children. A study by Adelgais et al. (92) demonstrated that imaging costs and radiation doses were increased if children were imaged with CT without a reduction in sedation usage or time in the emergency department. No methodologically rigorous data are available on either CT or radiography in younger age groups. Given the absence of evidence demonstrating benefit or cost effectiveness in the pediatric population, we believe that the higher radiation dose mitigates against initial use of CT in this population. At our institution, we rely on anteroposterior (AP) and lateral radiographs under the age of 4, AP lateral and open mouth radiographs from 4 to 8 years old, and children at 9 years of age and older are imaged with the adult protocol. This is the approximate age at which the fracture patterns revert to the adult patterns (90). CT is reserved for those subjects in whom an abnormality is identified on radiography.

THORACOLUMBAR SPINE

Who Should Undergo Imaging of the Thoracolumbar Spine in Acute Trauma?

Fractures of the thoracic and lumbar spine are more common than fractures of the cervical spine, with an incidence of 640 to 1,170 per million person years (93,94). The majority of these fractures, however, are pathologic fractures that occur in the elderly as a consequence of minor trauma and due to underlying osteoporosis. These osteoporotic fractures tend to be biomechanically stable, and though accompanied by pain and a tendency to be debilitating, they do not generally lead to neurologic deficit. Osteoporotic and pathologic fractures will not be covered in this chapter. Nonpathological traumatic fractures of the thoracolumbar spine do occur in approximately 2% to 6% of admitted trauma patients (95,96). The most common sites of injury are the T12 to L4 (97). Data on outcome and costs of such injuries are limited.

There are few studies that suggest guidelines for appropriate thoracolumbar spine imaging in the trauma setting. There is a single prospective validation study of a clinical prediction rule (Table 4-4) performed at a single center on 2,404 consecutive subjects with 142 (6.3%) fractures. All subjects had AP and lateral radiography, with additional radiography, CT, and MRI performed at the discretion of the radiologist. The criteria had a sensitivity of 100% for fracture; however, the specificity was only 3.9%, suggesting that use of the suggested clinical prediction rule had little value in excluding fractures. Other studies have suggested guidelines, but without prospective validation (98).

▶ **TABLE 4-4** **Thoracolumbar Spine Imaging Criteria**

Thoracolumbar spine imaging *is* indicated in subjects who meet *any* of the following criteria:

1. Complaint of thoracolumbar spine pain
2. Thoracolumbar spine midline tenderness
3. Decreased level of consciousness
4. Abnormal peripheral nerve examination
5. Painful distracting injury
6. Intoxication with ethanol or drugs.

Source: Holmes JF, Panacek EA, Miller PQ, et al. Prospective evaluation of criteria for obtaining thoracolumbar radiographs in trauma patients. *J Emerg Med.* 2003;24:1–7.

What Thoracolumbar Spine Imaging Approach Is Appropriate?

Radiographs have been the standard approach to imaging the thoracolumbar spine for decades. More recently, however, with the use of multidetector CT to evaluate the chest, abdominal, and pelvic viscera, the thoracolumbar spine has also been imaged with CT (99–102). Multidetector scanners enable multiplanar reconstruction often with isotropic image voxels. The use of CT images reconstructed from visceral CT has been shown in several small studies to obviate the need for dedicated thoracolumbar spine imaging with radiography (99–102). Such CT reconstructions are demonstrated to be more sensitive than radiography, although the few studies that exist are limited by verification and selection biases. The current studies all include <100 subjects with fracture, and report sensitivity for fracture of 95% to 98%. CT spine reconstructions from visceral CT can be performed at minimal additional cost and avoid additional radiation exposure, although no formal cost-effectiveness analyses have yet been reported (102). Agreement in interpretation of reconstructed thoracolumbar CT is also high (102). The current rapid evolution of multidetector CT scanners with increased numbers of detectors and higher spatial resolution is expected to increase accuracy of such reconstructions. In addition, continued development of rapid image processing algorithms and increased availability of multidetector scanners should lead to increased use of this technology. However, while retrospective spine reconstructions from an abdominal data set may have the equivalent sensitivity to spine radiography, it should be recognized that retrospective spine reconstructions obtained from a large field-of-view thick slice partition CT data set are of substantially lower quality than dedicated spine CT acquired at high resolution. Therefore, the quality of the acquired data will always need to be considered when excluding spinal fractures.

One current challenge is understanding the clinical significance of some subtle or incomplete injuries visible on CT but not radiography. Fractures isolated to the transverse process, lamina, articular pillar, or spinous process, as well as minimal anterior compression fractures may have little clinical significance, but may be detected with increased frequency when CT screening is utilized.

In summary, even with incomplete evidence, at this time CT reconstructions from an abdominal CT data set can be considered an adequate substitute for thoracolumbar spine radiographs for trauma patients. At our institution, we routinely reconstruct the thoracic and lumbar spine from visceral CT scans when these are available. Otherwise, we employ AP and lateral radiography as the initial imaging evaluation of the thoracic and lumbar spine. Any suspicious findings on this "screening" CT evaluation must be subsequently assessed with a dedicated CT study of the spine.

REFERENCES

1. *Annual Report for the Model Spinal Cord Injury Care Systems.* National Spinal Cord Injury Center. Birmingham: University of Alabama; 2005.
2. Berkowitz M. Assessing the socioeconomic impact of improved treatment of head and spinal cord injuries. *J Emerg Med.* 1993;1:63–67.
3. Kalsbeek WD, McLaurin RL, Harris BSd, et al. The National Head and Spinal Cord Injury Survey: major findings. *J Neurosurg.* 1980;31:S19–31.
4. Waters RL, Sie IH, Adkins RH. Rehabilitation of the patient with a spinal cord injury. *Orthop Clin North Am.* 1995;26: 117–122.
5. Webb SB Jr, Berzins E, Wingardner TS, et al. Spinal cord injury: epidemiologic implications, costs and patterns of care in 85 patients. *Arch Phys Med Rehabil.* 1979;60:335–340.
6. Bracken MB, Freeman DH, Hellenbrand K. Incidence of acute traumatic hospitalized spinal cord injury in the United States, 1970–1977. *Am J Epidemiol.* 1981;113:615–622.
7. Fine PR, Kuhlemeier KV, DeVivo MJ, et al. Spinal cord injury: an epidemiologic perspective. *Paraplegia.* 1979;17: 237–250.
8. Reid DC, Henderson R, Saboe L, et al. Etiology and clinical course of missed spine fractures. *J Trauma.* 1987;27:980–986.
9. Davis JW, Phreaner DL, Hoyt DB, et al. The etiology of missed cervical spine injuries. *J Trauma.* 1993;34:342–346.
10. Gerrelts BD, Petersen EU, Mabry J, et al. Delayed diagnosis of cervical spine injuries. *J Trauma.* 1991;31:1622–1626.
11. Rogers WA. Fractures and dislocations of the cervical spine: an end-result study. *J Bone Joint Surg.* 1957;39-A:341–376.
12. *Advanced Trauma Life Support.* Chicago: American College of Surgeons; 1997.
13. American College of Radiology ACR Appropriateness Criteria. Available at: http://www.acr.org/ac pda. Accessed Aug. 4, 2006.
14. Stiell IG, Clement CM, McKnight RD, et al. The Canadian C-spine rule versus the NEXUS low-risk criteria in patients with trauma. *N Eng J Med.* 2003;349:2510–2518.
15. Hoffman J, Mower W, Wolfson A, et al. Validity of a set of clinical criteria to rule out injury to the cervical spine in patients with blunt trauma. *N Eng J Med.* 2000;343:94–99.
16. Kreipke DL, Gillespie KR, McCarthy MC, et al. Reliability of indications for cervical spine films in trauma patients. *J Trauma.* 1989;29:1438–1439.
17. Blackmore CC, Zelman WN, Glick ND. Resource cost analysis of cervical spine trauma radiography. *Radiology.* 2001; 220:581–587.
18. Maloney TW, Rogers DE. Medical technology: a different view of the contentious debate over costs. *N Engl J Med.* 1979;301(26):1413–1419.

19. Blackmore C. Clinical prediction rules in trauma imaging: who, how and why? *Radiology*. 2005;235:371–374.

20. Laupacis A, Seklar N, Stiell IG. Clinical prediction rules: a review and suggested modifications of methodological standards. *JAMA*. 1997;277:488–494.

21. Stiell I, Wells G, Vandemheen K, et al. The Canadian C-spine rule for radiography in alert and stable trauma patients. *JAMA*. 2001;286:1841–1848.

22. Hoffman J, Wolfson A, Todd K, et al. Selective cervical spine radiography in blunt trauma: methodology of the National Emergency X-Radiography Utilization Study (NEXUS). *Ann Emerg Med*. 1998;32:461-469.

23. Yealy DM, Auble TE. Choosing between clinical prediction rules. *N Engl J Med*. 2003;349:2553–2555.

24. Dickinson G, Stiell IG, Schull M, et al. Retrospective application of the NEXUS low-risk criteria for cervical spine radiography in Canadian emergency departments. *Ann Emerg Med*. 2004;43:507–514.

25. Mower WR, Wolfson AB, Hoffman JR, et al. The Canadian C-spine rule [letter]. *N Eng J Med*. 2004;350:1467–1468.

26. Mower WR, Hoffman J. Comparison of the Canadian C-Spine Rule and the NEXUS decision instrument in evaluating blunt trauma patients for cervical spine injury. *Ann Emerg Med*. 2004;43:515–517.

27. Radiographic assessment of the cervical spine in asymptomatic trauma patients. *Neurosurgery*. 2002;50:S30–35.

28. Blackmore CC, Ramsey SD, Mann FA, et al. Cervical spine screening with CT in trauma patients: a cost-effectiveness analysis. *Radiology*. 1999;212:117–125.

29. Holmes JF, Akkinepalli R. Computed tomography versus plain radiography to screen for cervical spine injury: a meta-analysis. *J Trauma*. 2005;58:902–905.

30. Diaz JJ, Gillman C, Morris JA, et al. Are five view plain films of the cervical spine unreliable? A prospective evaluation in blunt trauma patients with altered mental status. *J Trauma*. 2003;55:658–664.

31. Blackmore CC, Deyo RA. Specificity of cervical spine radiography: importance of clinical scenario. *Emerg Radiol*. 1997;4:283–286.

32. Widder S, Doig C, Burrowes P, et al. Prospective evaluation of computed tomographic scanning for the spinal clearance of obtunded patients: preliminary results. *J Trauma*. 2004;56:1179–1184.

33. Núñez DB, Ahmad AA, Coin CG, et al. Clearing the cervical spine in multiple trauma victims: a time-effective protocol using helical computed tomography. *Emerg Radiol*. 1994;1:273–278.

34. Núñez DB, Zuluaga A, Fuentes-Bernardo DA, et al. Cervical spine trauma: how much do we learn by routinely using helical CT? *Radiographics*. 1996;16:1307–1318.

35. Barba CA, Taggert J, Morgan AS, et al. A new cervical spine clearance protocol using computed tomography. *J Trauma*. 2001;51:652–656; discussion 656–657.

36. Griffen MM, Frykberg ER, Kerwin AJ, et al. Radiographic clearance of blunt cervical spine injury: plain radiograph or computed tomography scan? *J Trauma*. 2003;55:222–227; discussion 226–227.

37. Hanson JA, Blackmore CC, Mann FA, et al. Cervical spine injury: accuracy of helical CT as a screening technique. *Emerg Radiol*. 2000;7:31–35.

38. Daffner RH. Helical CT of the cervical spine for trauma patients: a time study. *AJR Am J Roentgenol*. 2001;177:677–679.

39. Blackmore CC, Emerson SS, Mann FA, et al. Cervical spine imaging in patients with trauma: determination of fracture risk to optimize use. *Radiology*. 1999;211:759–765.

40. Detsky AS, Naglie IG. A clinician's guide to cost-effectiveness analysis. *Ann Intern Med*. 1990;113:147–154.

41. Gold MR, Siegel JE, Russell LB, et al. *Cost-effectiveness in Health and Medicine*. New York: Oxford University Press; 1996.

42. Hanson JA, Blackmore CC, Mann FA, et al. Cervical spine screening: a decision rule can identify high risk patients to undergo screening helical CT of the cervical spine. *AJR Am J Roentgenol*. 2000;174:713–718.

43. Chiu W, Haan J, Cushing B, et al. Ligamentous injuries of the cervical spine in unreliable blunt trauma patients: incidence, evaluation, and outcome. *J Trauma*. 2001;50:457–464.

44. Dvorak J, Punjabi MM, Grob D, et al. Clinical validation of functional flexion/extension radiographs of the cervical spine. *Spine*. 1993;18:120–127.

45. Brady WJ, Moghtader J, Cutcher D, et al. ED use of flexion-extension cervical spine radiography in the evaluation of blunt trauma. *Am J Emerg Med*. 1999;17:504–508.

46. Knopp R, Parker J, Tashjian J, et al. Defining radiographic criteria for flexion-extension studies of the cervical spine. *Ann Emerg Med*. 2001;38:31–35.

47. Lin RM, Tsai KH, Chu LP, et al. Characteristics of sagittal vertebral alignment in flexion determined by dynamic radiographs of the cervical spine. *Spine*. 2001;26:256–261.

48. Kuhns LR. *Imaging of Spinal Trauma in Children*. Hamilton, Ontario: BC Decker; 1998.

49. Insko EK, Gracias VH, Gupta R, et al. Utility of flexion and extension radiographs of the cervical spine in the acute evaluation of blunt trauma. *J Trauma*. 2002;53:426–429.

50. Lewis LM, Docherty M, Ruoff BE, et al. Flexion-extension views in the evaluation of cervical spine injuries. *Ann Emerg Med*. 1991;20:117–121.

51. Pollack CV, Hendey GW, Martin DR, et al. Use of flexion-extension radiographs of the cervical spine in blunt trauma. *Ann Emerg Med*. 2001;38:8–11.

52. Wang JC, Hatch JD, Sandhu HS, et al. Cervical flexion and extension radiographs in acutely injured patients. *Clin Orthop Relat Res*. 1999;365:111–116.

53. Pitt E, Thakore S. Best evidence topic report: role of flexion extension radiography in paediatric neck injuries. *Emerg Med J*. 2005;22:192–193.

54. Pitt E, Thakore S. Best evidence topic report: role of flexion/extension radiography in neck injuries in adults. *Emerg Med J*. 2004;21:587–588.

55. Stiell IG. Clinical decision rules in the emergency department. *CMAJ*. 2000;163:1465–1466.

56. Marion D, Domeier R, Dunham CM, et al. Determination of cervical spine stability in trauma patients. *Eastern Assoc Surg Trauma*. 2000;1–6.

57. Sees D, Rodriguez C, Flaherty S, et al. The use of bedside fluoroscopy to evaluate the cervical spine in obtunded trauma patients. *J Trauma*. 1998;45:768–771.

58. Davis JW, Parks SN, Detlefs CL, et al. Clearing the cervical spine in obtunded patients: the use of dynamic fluoroscopy. *J Trauma*. 1995;39:435–438.

59. Griffiths HJ, Wagner J, Anglen J, et al. The use of forced flexion/extension views in the obtunded trauma patient. *Skeletal Radiol*. 2002;31:587–591.

60. Brooks RA, Willett KM. Evaluation of the Oxford protocol for total spine clearance in the unconscious trauma patient. *J Trauma*. 2001;50:862–867.

61. Davis JW, Kaups KL, Cunningham MA, et al. Routine evaluation of the cervical spine in head-injured patients with dynamic fluoroscopy: a reappraisal. *J Trauma*. 2001;50:1044–1047.

62. Anglen J, Metzler M, Bunn P, et al. Flexion and extension views are not cost-effective in a cervical spine clearance protocol for obtunded trauma patients. *J Trauma*. 2002;52:54–59.

63. Hendey GW, Wolfson AB, Mower WR, et al. Spinal cord injury without radiographic abnormality: results of the National Emergency X-Radiography Utilization Study in blunt cervical trauma. *J Trauma*. 2002;53:1–4.

64. Webber-Jones JE, Thomas CA, Bordeaux RE Jr. The management and prevention of rigid cervical collar complications. *Orthop Nurs*. July–August 2002;21(4):19–25.

65. Hall AJ, Wagle VG, Raycroft J, et al. Magnetic resonance imaging in cervical spine trauma. *J Trauma*. 1993;34:21–26.

66. Davis SJ, Teresi LM, Bradley WG, et al. Cervical spine hyperextension injuries: MR findings. *Radiology*. 1991;180:245–251.

67. El Khoury GY, Kathol MH, Daniel WW. Imaging of acute injuries of the cervical spine: value of plain radiography, CT, and MR imaging. *AJR Am J Roentgenol*. 1995;164:43–50.

68. Saifuddin A. MRI of acute spinal trauma. *Skeletal Radiol.* 2001;30:237–246.
69. Albrecht RM, Kingsley D, Schermer CR, et al. Evaluation of cervical spine in intensive care patients following blunt trauma. *World J Surg.* 2001;25:1089–1096.
70. D'Alise MD, Benzel EC, Hart BL. Magnetic resonance imaging evaluation of the cervical spine in the comatose or obtunded trauma patient. *J Neurosurg.* 1999;91:54–59.
71. Williams RL, Hardman JA, Lyons K. MR imaging of suspected acute spinal instability. *Injury.* 1998;29:109–113.
72. Keiper MD, Zimmerman RA, Bilaniuk LT. MRI in the assessment of the supporting soft tissues of the cervical spine in acute trauma in children. *Neuroradiology.* 1998;40: 359–363.
73. Sliker CW, Mirvis SE, Shanmuganathan K. Assessing cervical spine stability in obtunded blunt trauma patients. *Radiology.* 2005;234:733–739.
74. Kliewer MA, Gray L, Paver J, et al. Acute spinal ligament disruption: MR imaging with anatomic correlation. *J Magn Reson Imaging.* 1993;3:855–861.
75. Obenauer S, Herold T, Fischer U, et al. The evaluation of experimentally induced injuries to the upper cervical spine with a digital x-ray technic, computed tomography and magnetic resonance tomography. *Rofo.* 1999;171:473–479.
76. Hogan GJ, Mirvis SE, Shanmuganathan K, et al. Exclusion of unstable cervical spine injury in obtunded patients with blunt trauma: is MR imaging needed when multidetector row CT findings are normal? *Radiology.* 2005;237:106–113.
77. Katzberg, RW, Benedetti PF, Drake CM, et al. Acute cervical spine injuries: prospective MR imaging assessment at a level 1 trauma center. *Radiology.* 1999;213:203–212.
78. Mann FA, Kubal WS, Blackmore CC. Improving the diagnosis of cervical spine injury in the elderly: implications of the epidemiology of injury. *Emerg Radiol.* 2000;7:36–41.
79. Amling M, Wening VJ, Posl M, et al. Structure of the axis-Key to the etiology of the dens fracture. *Chirurg.* 1994;65: 964–969.
80. Lee C, Woodring JH, Rogers LF, et al. The radiographic distinction of degenerative slippage (spondylolisthesis and retrolisthesis) from traumatic slippage of the cervical spine. *Skeletal Radiol.* 1986;15:439–443.
81. White A, Panjabi M. *Clinical Biomechanics of the Spine.* Philadelphia: Lippincott; 1978.
82. Regenbogen VS, Rogers LF, Atlas SW, et al. Cervical spinal cord injuries in patients with cervical spondylosis. *AJR Am J Roentgenol.* 1986;146:277–284.
83. Liebermann IH, Webb JK. Cervical spine injuries in the elderly. *J Bone Joint Surg Br.* 1994;76:877–881.
84. Olerud C, Anderson S, Svensson B, et al. Cervical spine fractures in the elderly. *Acta Orthop Scand.* 1999;70:509–513.
85. Spivak JM, Weiss MA, Cotler JM, et al. Cervical spine injuries in patients 65 and older. *Spine.* 1994;19:2302–2306.
86. Lomoschitz F, Blackmore C, Mirza S, et al. Cervical spine injuries in patients 65 years old and older: epidemiological analysis regarding the effects of age and injury mechanism on distribution, type, and stability of injury. *AJR Am J Roentgenol.* 2002;178:573–577.
87. Daffner RH, Goldberg AL, Evans TC, et al. Cervical vertebral injuries in the elderly: a ten year study. *Emerg Radiol.* 1998;5:38–42.
88. Bub L, Blackmore C, Mann F, et al. Cervical spine fractures in patients 65 years old: a clinical prediction rule for blunt trauma. *Radiology.* 2005;234:143–149.
89. Viccellio P, Simon H, Pressman B, et al. A prospective multicenter study of cervical spine injury in children. *Pediatrics.* 2001;108:E20.
90. Kokoska E, Keller M, Rallo M, et al. Characteristics of pediatric cervical spine injuries. *J Pediatric Surg.* 2001;36:100–105.
91. National Research Council. *Health Effects of Exposure to Low Levels of Ionizing Radiation: BEIR V.* Washington, D.C.: National Academy Press, 1990.
92. Adelgais KM, Grossman DC, Langer SG, et al. Use of helical computed tomography for imaging the pediatric cervical spine. *Acad Emerg Med.* 2004;11:228–236.
93. Hu R, Mustard CA, Burns C. Epidemiology of incident spinal injury in a complete population. *Spine.* 1996;4:492–499.
94. Cooper C, Atkinson EJ, O'Fallon WM, et al. Incidence of clinically diagnosed vertebral injuries: a population based study in Rochester, Minnesota, 1985–1989. *J Bone Miner Res.* 1992;7: 221–227.
95. Frankel HL, Rozycki GS, Ochsner GM, et al. Indications for obtaining surveillance thoracic and lumbar spine radiographs. *J Trauma.* 1994;37:673–676.
96. Holmes JF, Panacek EA, Miller PQ, et al. Prospective evaluation of criteria for obtaining thoracolumbar radiographs in trauma patients. *J Emerg Med.* 2003;24:1–7.
97. Holmes JF, Miller PQ, Panacek EA, et al. Epidemiology of thoracolumbar spine injury in blunt trauma. *Acad Emerg Med.* 2001;8:866–872.
98. Hsu JM, Joseph T, Ellis AM. Thoracolumbar fracture in blunt trauma patients: guidelines for diagnosis and imaging. *Injury.* 2003;34:426–433.
99. Sheridan P, Peralta R, Rhea J, et al. Reformatted visceral protocol helical computed tomographic scanning allows conventional radiographs of the thoracic and lumbar spine to be eliminated in the evaluation of blunt trauma patients. *J Trauma.* 2003;55:665–669.
100. Roos JE, Hilfiker P, Platz A, et al. MDCT in emergency radiology: is a standardized chest or abdominal protocol sufficient for evaluation of thoracic and lumbar spine trauma? *AJR Am J Roentgenol.* 2004;183:959–968.
101. Hauser CJ, Visvikis G, Hinrichs C, et al. Prospective validation of computed tomographic screening of the thoracolumbar spine in trauma. *J Trauma.* 2003;55:228–234.
102. Wintermark M, Mouhsine E, Theumann N, et al. Thoracolumbar spine fractures in patients who have sustained severe trauma: Depiction with multi-detector row CT. *Radiology.* 2003;227:681–689.

Plain Film Radiography and Computed Tomography of the Cervical Spine: Part I. Normal Anatomy and Spinal Injury Identification

Alejandro Zuluaga and Diego B. Núñez, Jr.

Evaluation of suspected spine injuries has become one of the most controversial and challenging issues in radiology. In the past decade, there have been a large number of reports in medical literature addressing this problem. Diagnostic imaging of the cervical spine is the definitive method for determining the presence, location, extent, and nature of injury to the cord and vertebral column. Efficient and economic application of diagnostic imaging for spinal trauma, however, requires thorough knowledge of the indications for, and limitations of, various imaging techniques.

As quoted by the American College of Radiology (1) expert panel on musculoskeletal imaging regarding patients with suspected cervical spine injury: "In recent years, there has been a profound change in the way in which patients suspected of having cervical spine injuries are evaluated. Foremost among this change has been a significant body of evidence within the radiologic literature supporting a more prominent role of helical computed tomography (CT) as a screening tool for these

patients. Initial reports in the early 1990s, particularly by Núñez et al (2,3), demonstrated how much more efficient helical CT was in identifying fractures. Their conclusions were supported by those of other investigators, who validated the initial observations in larger scale studies."

Single and multidetector helical CT has begun replacing plain radiography as the method of choice for cervical trauma screening in most large US trauma centers (2–9). There are many reasons why CT has superseded plain radiography, including ease of performance, speed of study, and, most importantly, its greater ability than plain radiography to detect fractures. Thus several questions arise regarding cervical spine plain radiography: Should it still be done? And if so, how many views are needed? (10) Traditionally, a three-view series has been performed including anteroposterior (AP), lateral, and open-mouth odontoid views. In the past, supine oblique views were also used to look at the articular pillars and pedicles and to evaluate the cervico-thoracic junction. In many centers, a lateral swimmer's view was also obtained.

Unfortunately, obtaining such series is time consuming. In a time study, Daffner (11) found that the average time for obtaining six views was 22 minutes with 79% of patients requiring one or more views to be repeated. In contrast, examination times with CT were much shorter and a cervical spine study may be obtained when the patient undergoes cranial CT; at Daffner's institution, screening the patient and viewing the images require the patient to remain on the CT table for an average of only 12 additional minutes (11). Blackmore et al. (5) at the University of Washington, developed a new set of guidelines (decision rule) for the use of helical CT (4). In addition, they showed that using helical CT for routine screening of cervical injuries in high-risk multitrauma victims is cost effective (5).

In this chapter we will review the relative merits of radiography and multidetector CT (MDCT) for the assessment of suspected cervical spine trauma. Additionally, we will discuss the normal radiographic and CT anatomy of the cervical spine, as well as radiographic and CT evidence of spinal injury. In the next chapter, we will present common patterns of traumatic lesions that result from the various mechanisms that exceed the normal range of motion of the cervical spine.

STRENGTHS AND WEAKNESS OF PLAIN FILM RADIOGRAPHY AND COMPUTED TOMOGRAPHY

Plain Radiography

Plain film radiography is readily available in all emergency centers; it is a reliable and quick method that can be performed with portable and fixed equipment. Plain radiography provides a very good overview of the extent and magnitude of injury and can make a definitive and specific diagnosis in certain spinal injuries. Plain radiography has been considered the standard initial "screening" examination used to evaluate patients with suspected spine trauma. In fact, plain film radiography remains the mainstay for evaluation of trauma patients worldwide who do not have ready access to CT.

Cross-table lateral radiographs have been used for years for the initial evaluation of the cervical spine trauma. However, the generally accepted opinion is that lateral radiographs are inadequate to exclude cervical spine injury because of the high number of false positives and false negatives, and because the reported predictive value of a study with negative findings is not sufficient for the study to be used as the only screening examination (12). An additional limitation is the frequent incomplete visualization of the cervicothoracic and cranio-cervical junctions in unconscious and uncooperative multiple-trauma victims, which can result in significant delay.

Repeated exposures are frequently necessary before adequate radiographs are obtained in this subset of obtunded and uncooperative patients.

Overall, plain radiography remains accepted as the technique of choice for initial evaluation of an injured cervical spine. This practice is supported by the fact that if the results of an adequately exposed and properly positioned radiographic series of the spine are normal, then it is unlikely that CT will reveal a fracture. However, there is sufficient evidence that a significant number of fractures can be missed if the evaluation of the cervical spine relies exclusively on plain radiography. These claims are particularly valid for the subset of patients who meet multiple trauma criteria, for whom plain radiography has a limited value. Woodring and Lee (13) reported the limitations of plain radiography in detecting fractures, using a retrospective review of radiographs and CT scans in 216 patients with cervical spine fractures. They determined prospectively that plain radiography did not detect fractures in 23% of their patients and that the cervical spine injuries were unstable in 50% of the cases. Our own experience indicates that plain radiography can miss up to 57% of fractures (2,3). In a series by Acheson et al. (14), only 47% of fractures were seen or suspected on initial screening radiographs when compared with those ultimately detected by CT.

Supine oblique views are no longer necessary in patients who are undergoing cervical CT examination. Oblique views, although useful in patients with unilateral locked facet, are most valuable in adding two more views of the cervicothoracic junction in patients with equivocal lateral or swimmer's views that are not undergoing CT examination (low risk, obese short-necked patients). Both of these functions, however, can now be accomplished with the use of CT (1).

Flexion-extension radiographs are not very helpful in the acute setting because muscle spasm in acutely injured patients precludes an adequate examination. Insko et al. (15), in a review of 106 consecutive cases of blunt trauma evaluated with flexion and extension radiographs of the cervical spine obtained in the acute setting at a level-one trauma center, reported that when adequate motion was present on flexion and extension radiographs, the false-negative rate was zero. However, in the acute setting, 30% of the examinations were limited by inadequate motion. A higher percentage of injury (12.5%) was detected by subsequent cross-sectional imaging in these patients. Limited flexion and extension motion on physical examination should preclude the use of flexion and extension radiographs, as they are of limited diagnostic utility. Cross-sectional imaging may be warranted in this high-risk group of patients (15). Flexion-extension radiographs are best reserved for follow-up of symptomatic patients with suspected ligamentous instability, usually 7 to 10 days after muscle spasm has subsided; in these patients, however, magnetic resonance imagery (MRI) is the procedure of choice. Flexion-extension radiographs are also helpful for ensuring that minor degrees of anterolisthesis or retrolisthesis in patients with cervical spondylosis are fixed deformities (1,16,17).

Some authors have suggested the use of passive flexion and extension imaging under fluoroscopic guidance for patients in whom one cannot obtain a reliable physical examination (5,18–20). Almost all patients studied in this manner have been normal, as would be expected from the extremely low pretest probability of unstable injury. The limited data available do not provide sufficient evidence to support routine use of this technique. A number of cervical injuries will not be detected by this method, including herniated intervertebral discs and extradural hemorrhage. These lesions may cause spinal cord compression that creates or worsens a neurologic deficit without evidence of overt subluxation on fluoroscopy. Davis et al. (21) performed fluoroscopic examinations on 301 patients. There were 297 true-negative examinations, two true-positive examinations (stable injuries), one false-negative examination, and one false-positive examination. The incidence of ligamentous injury identified by fluoroscopy in this study was two of 301 (0.7%). Unstable cervical spine ligamentous injuries were identified in only 0.02% of all trauma patients. Complications of this procedure have also been reported with one patient developing quadriplegia when fluoroscopic evaluation was performed (21).

Helical and Multidetector Computed Tomography

The introduction of helical scanning has expanded the clinical applications of CT. The advantage of helical CT and MDCT over single-section CT is faster acquisition of a volumetric data set, which results in shorter examination time. Motion and misregistration artifacts are minimized, and high-quality reconstructed images can be obtained. In many instances, additional scanning after the initial acquisition is avoided by the ability to retrospectively generate overlapping interscan images using original data. These advantages are particularly relevant in acutely ill and multiple-trauma victims who require rapid and accurate imaging assessment. CT may reveal more fractures than plain films and may allow evaluation of the cervicothoracic and cranio-cervical junctions, areas traditionally poorly visualized on plain films.

With the development of MDCT, an increased tube output, and a reduction of the rotation time, it became possible to cover larger scan ranges in z-direction with a collimation of 0.5 to –4 mm and a reasonable acquisition time (22). As compared to single detector helical CT, MDCT results in improved image quality, such as decreased stairstep artifacts, when generating images in planes different

from the one of data acquisition (multiplanar reformations [MPRs]) (23). The major improvement for generating MPRs, however, is the ability to achieve near isotropic voxels, as predicted by Kalender (24) in 1995. Isotropic imaging permits calculation of MPRs with an image quality close to that of the transverse images calculated from the raw data set (25–27). On the other hand, these advances have lead to what Rubin (28) terms a data explosion. Processing this vast amount of data is now the challenge of multidetector-row CT technology (28,29). To reduce the large number of images, Begemann et al. (29) retrospectively assessed the value of coronal and sagittal reformations alone in the diagnosis of acute vertebral fractures and evaluated whether it still remains necessary to examine the axial images. In 244 vertebral bodies, 70/70 fractured vertebrae were diagnosed on reviewing MPRs alone. There were no false positive cases. In 2/70 fractures, the anatomically exact diagnosis was complemented by examination of the axial images. Forty-two of 43 unstable fractures were correctly diagnosed on MPRs alone. With preferential MPR reading, the total number of images to be analyzed was significantly reduced (P <0.01). Their preliminary results indicate that examination of the MPRs alone is a feasible approach for assessment of vertebral fractures that can also accurately classify them as either stable and unstable (provided the MPRs are done properly). The transverse images must be read complementarily in cases of complex fractures, in osteopenic patients, in cases of CT scans with artifacts, or if any questions arise about the exact type of the fracture.

Horizontal fractures that are oriented in the plane of the scan, such as transverse odontoid fractures, may not always be demonstrated by CT. However, helical and MDCT have been useful in overcoming this diagnostic problem secondary to overlapping imaging of contiguous segments. Furthermore, these injuries are more likely to be demonstrated in sagittal and coronal reformations.

What is the cost of CT versus plain radiography? Cost should not be based on charges but should be based on the actual cost to operate the equipment per hour (10). This includes the technologist's time, film cost, time required for the study, and, most importantly, the accuracy of diagnosis (5,30–32). When these parameters are used, CT has been shown to be more cost effective than plain radiography (5). There is one additional "cost" to be considered with using CT: radiation exposure. It is generally acknowledged that helical CT, and especially multidetector CT examinations, carries a higher radiation dose than plain radiography (33). However, work is currently under way to determine methods of decreasing this radiation exposure, primary via lowering the milliamperage setting needed for diagnostic quality examinations.

INDICATIONS FOR COMPUTED TOMOGRAPHY TECHNIQUES

The indications for cervical spine plain film and CT examination are listed in Tables 5-1, 5-2, and 5-3. The protocols for single and MD helical CT are given in Tables 5-4 and 5-5.

Three-dimensional Computed Tomography Techniques

In essence, three-dimensional (3D) CT software programs transform existing axial CT data into a 3D rendering of the portion of the spinal skeleton being examined. The 3D display increases neither examination time nor patient radiation dosage. The 3D volume images can then be manipulated in real time to find the preferred angle of viewing or perspective to enhance appreciation of pathology. As described in prior studies (34–36), 3D CT reformations do not reveal a significant number of unsuspected traumatic lesions but they do provide improved definition

▶ **TABLE 5-1** Indications for Plain Films

As quoted by the ACR expert panel on musculoskeletal imaging, there is agreement among most investigators that patients who are alert, have never lost consciousness, are not under the influence of alcohol and/or drugs, have no distracting injuries, have no cervical tenderness, and have no neurologic findings need no imaging (1). Patients who do not fall into this category should have as a minimum a three-view cervical radiographic series followed in some cases by helical CT (1,2,3,4). In many instances the cervical CT examination will be performed immediately after a cranial CT, while the patient is still in the CT suite. This is both time effective as well as cost effective (5). Adapted from the ACR expert panel on musculoskeletal imaging (1).

Suspected Cervical Spine Trauma

1. Asymptomatic and alert, no cervical tenderness, no neurologic findings, no distracting injury, with or without cervical collar.
   Radiologic exam: No imaging.

2. Alert, cervical tenderness, no neurologic findings, no distracting injury.
   Radiologic exam: AP, lateral, and open mouth radiographs.

3. Limited CT scan with motion artifact.
   Radiologic exam: AP, lateral, and open mouth radiographs.

1. American College of Radiology. *Expert Panel on Musculoskeletal Imaging ACR Appropriateness Criteria for Suspected Cervical Spine Trauma.* Reston, Va.: ACR; 2003.
2. Berne JD, Velmahos GC, el-Tawil Q, et al. Value of complete cervical helical computed tomographic scanning in identifying cervical spine injury in the unevaluable blunt trauma patient with multiple injuries: a prospective study. *J Trauma.* 1999;47:896–903.
3. Daffner RH. Cervical radiography for trauma patients: a time effective technique? *AJR Am J Roentgenol.* 2000;175:1308–1311.
4. Davis JW, Phreaner DL, Hoyt DB, et al. The etiology of missed cervical spine injuries. *J Trauma.* 1993;34(3):342–346.
5. Daffner RH. Cervical helical CT for trauma patients: a time analysis. *AJR Am J Roentgenol.* 2001;177:677–679.

▶ **TABLE 5-2** Indications for CT

Suspected Cervical Spine Trauma

1. Alert, cervical tenderness, paresthesias in hands or feet.
   Radiologic exam: Screening CT of the complete cervical spine with sagittal and coronal reformations supplemented by the lateral radiograph. MRI following CT, if indicated.

2. Unconscious.
   Radiologic exam: Screening CT of the complete cervical spine with sagittal and coronal reformations supplemented by the lateral radiograph.

3. Impaired sensorium (including alcohol and/or drugs).
   Radiologic exam: Screening CT of the complete cervical spine with sagittal and coronal reformations supplemented by the lateral radiograph.

4. Impaired sensorium (alcohol and/or drugs), neurologic findings.
   Radiologic exam: Screening CT of the complete cervical spine with sagittal and coronal reformations supplemented by the lateral radiograph. MRI following CT, if indicated.

Adapted from American College of Radiology. *Expert Panel on Musculoskeletal Imaging ACR Appropriateness Criteria for Suspected Cervical Spine Trauma.* Reston, Va.: ACR; 2003, with permission.

▶ **TABLE 5-3** Other Indications for CT

1. Uncertain plain radiographic findings:
   Radiologic exam: CT of the involved segment with sagittal and coronal reformations.

2. In the presence of osseous injury by plain films: to provide details and aid in surgical planning.
   Radiologic exam: CT of the complete cervical spine with sagittal and coronal reformations

3. Inadequate visualization of the cervical spine by plain films:
   Radiologic exam: CT of the involved segment with sagittal and coronal reformations.

4. Localize foreign bodies and bone fragments in relation to neural elements:
   Radiologic exam: CT of the complete cervical spine with sagittal and coronal reformations.

5. Patients with high risk of having cervical spine injury (1) [High speed accident (>35 mph, 55 km/h), death at crash scene, fall >10 feet (3 m), closed head injury and pelvic or multiple extremity fractures].
   Radiologic exam: Screening CT of the complete cervical spine with sagittal and coronal reformations supplemented by the lateral radiograph.

6. Patients with neurologic findings (suspected nerve root injury), negative plain films, and negative noncontrast CT in which MRI is not feasible.
   Radiologic exam: CT Myelogram.

1. Hanson JA, Blackmore CC, Mann FA, et al. Cervical spine injury: clinical decision rule to identify high risk patients for helical CT screening. *AJR Am J Roentgenol.* 2000;174:713–717.

▶ **TABLE 5-4** Cervical Spine Screening

Single Detector Helical CT:

- Collimation: 3 mm
- Pitch: 1.5
- A KVp of 140/120 with mAs of 280/170 for the upper thoracic/cervical spine segments, respectively.
- From the occiput to T4

Multidetector CT (4 slice):

- 4 × 1.5 mm collimation
- 3-mm thick sections
- 1.5-mm overlap
- Pitch: 0.875
- From the occiput to T4
- Transverse image reconstruction 1 mm
- Multiplanar reformations (sagittal and coronal reformations) were reformatted to 2-mm thickness every 2 mm through the entire spine.

Multidetector CT (16 slice):

- 16 × 0.75 mm collimation
- 2 mm thick sections
- 1-mm overlap
- Pitch: 0.663
- From the occiput to T4
- Transverse image reconstruction 1 mm
- Three contiguous sections were fused for review and storage on a picture archiving and communication system (PACS)
- Multiplanar reformations (sagittal and coronal reformations) were reformatted to 2-mm thickness every 2 mm through the entire spine.

▶ **TABLE 5-5** Patients with Known or Suspected Cervical Spine Injury

Noncontiguous fractures are commonly underdiagnosed at conventional radiography. They are reported to occur in 5% to 20% of patients with spinal fractures. Because multilevel fractures are considered biomechanically unstable, a cautious search for multiple fractures throughout the spine is critical (Fig. 5-1).

Single Detector Helical CT:

- Collimation: 1 mm
- Pitch: 1.5
- A KVp of 140/120 with mAs of 280/170 for the upper thoracic/cervical spine segments, respectively.
- From the occiput to T4

Multidetector CT (4 slice):

- 4 × 1.5 mm collimation
- 3-mm thick sections
- 1.5-mm overlap
- Pitch: 0.875
- From the occiput to T4
- Transverse image reconstruction 1 mm
- Multiplanar reformations (sagittal and coronal reformations) were reformatted to 2-mm thickness every 2 mm through the entire spine.

Multidetector CT (16 slice):

- 16 × 0.75 mm collimation
- 2-mm thick sections
- 1-mm overlap
- Pitch: 0.663
- From the occiput to T4
- Transverse image reconstruction 1 mm
- Three contiguous sections were fused for review and storage on a picture archiving and communication system (PACS)
- Multiplanar reformations (sagittal and coronal reformations) were reformatted to 2-mm thickness every 2 mm through the entire spine.

and comprehension of the extent and nature of detected injuries. Advantages of 3D CT imaging includes: (a) ability to synthesize multiple 2D image information, especially in areas with complex anatomy, (b) visualization of complex injuries presenting vertebral rotation or dislocation and loss of alignment, (c) a more comprehensive assessment of cases requiring surgical planning, and (d) better demonstration of displaced fractures (37). The most commonly used 3D techniques include surface rendering, maximum intensity projection (MIP), and volume rendering (38).

Surface Rendering

Surface-rendering, or shaded surface display (SSD), 3D algorithms require the user to set a threshold Hounsfield unit value, and the first voxel encountered along a projection ray that exceeds the threshold value is displayed as the bone surface (Fig. 5-2). No other CT information along that projection contributes to the viewed image. The surface is typically modeled as overlapping polygons with 3D cues created by using a virtual light source (38).

Depending on the choice of threshold level, however, small fractures may be undetected, or spurious holes may appear in other bones (37).

Maximum Intensity Projection

MIP is a 3D rendering technique that selects the maximum voxel value along a line projecting from the viewer's eye (Fig. 5-3). As opposed to the surface-rendering technique, no predetermined Hounsfield unit value needs to be specified as a threshold. As the displayed pixel will represent only the highest intensity material along the projected view, calcifications in the soft tissue may obscure bone surface, although this limitation can be overcome by editing, or trimming, the volume of data to be analyzed.

(text continues on page 79)

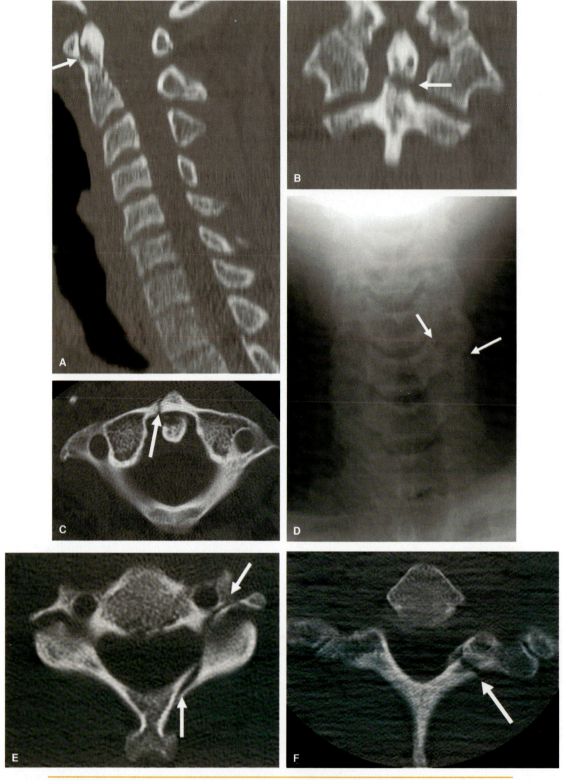

FIGURE 5-1. Combined cervical spine injuries. **A–C:** CT MPRs in midsagittal (A) and coronal (B) planes, as well as axial CT image (C), demonstrate a minimally displaced type II odontoid fracture (*white arrow in A and B*). Note associated nondisplaced fracture of the right anterior atlas arch (*white arrow in C*). **D–F:** AP radiograph (D) and axial CT image (E) show a left C5 pedicolaminar fracture (*white arrows in D and E*). Another axial CT image (F) at T1 demonstrates a left laminar fracture (*white arrow in F*).

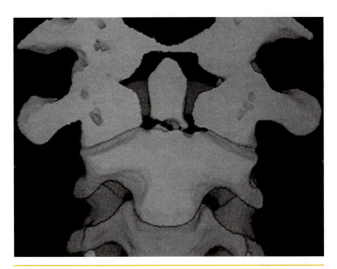

FIGURE 5-2. Surface rendering of a type II odontoid fracture. Surface rendering, or shaded surface display (SSD), uses a preselected threshold Hounsfield unit value and the first voxel encountered is displayed as bone surface. As this technique converts data from a volume to a surface, it discards data resulting in faster editing.

Volume Rendering

Although surface rendering and MIP use approximately 10% of the data to create 3D images, volume rendering incorporates information from all voxels encountered along a projection ray, thus conveying more information than the other techniques (Fig. 5-4) (38). In addition, experience with cadaveric models suggests that volume-rendered images accurately detect fractures even when

they are not displaced, whereas surface-rendered images do not accurately detect small fractures (39). Volume-rendered images can also eliminate streak artifact from surgical hardware and bullet fragments. This technique, however, requires more powerful computers to render images at a reasonable speed. The normal anatomy of the cervical spine as depicted by plain film radiography and CT is shown in Figures 5-5 through 5-18.

COMPUTED TOMOGRAPHY AND RADIOGRAPHIC EVIDENCE OF INJURY

In the evaluation of radiographs and CT images, specific signs have been shown to be suggestive of spinal injury. Some of the more commonly utilized findings are: the "Ring of C2" and "Fat C2" signs (Figs. 5-19, 5-20, 5-21), abnormal spinolaminar line (Table 5-6 and Figs. 5-22, 5-23, 5-24), and the apophyseal joint and "hamburger bun" (Figs. 5-25 and 5-26).

PREVERTEBRAL SOFT TISSUE EDEMA

An increase in the size of the prevertebral soft tissues caused by hemorrhage or edema is a sign of underlying cervical spine injury. Unfortunately, this is only partially true. Because of the broad range of measurements and considerable overlap between normal and abnormal, it is

(text continues on page 89)

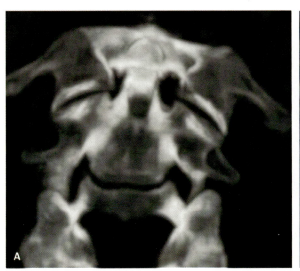
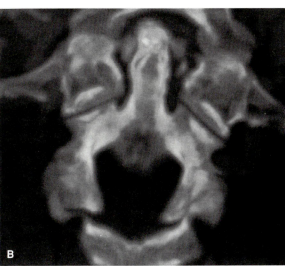

FIGURE 5-3. Maximum intensity projection (MIP) of the C1-2 articulation. MIP technique determines the maximum voxel value along line through volume. Volume editing helps reduce artifacts from conflicting high densities. The volume that is analyzed (also called the slab) can be manipulated to evaluate the different components of the C1-2 articulation **(A,B)**. Generally, 3D cues, such as surface shading, are not used with MIP images, making 3D assessment more difficult.

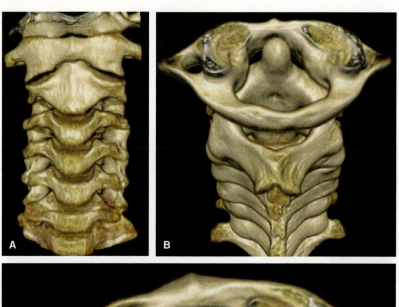

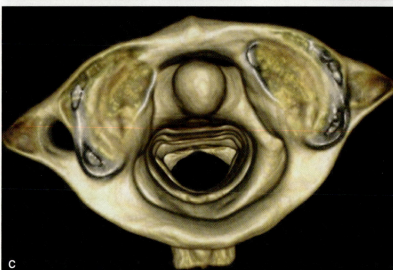

FIGURE 5-4. Volume rendering of the cervical spine. A–C: Volume rendering uses information from all the voxels along the projection ray and displays the resulting composite for each pixel. By adjusting opacity levels, foreground and background can be discriminated. This technique, however, requires more powerful computers to display images at a reasonable speed as compared to surface rendering or MIP.

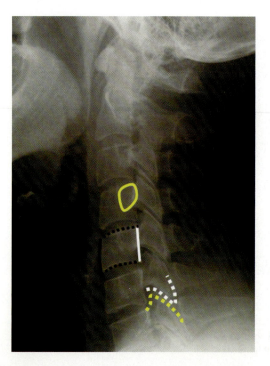

FIGURE 5-5. Lateral radiograph of a normal cervical spine in neutral position. The anterior cortex of the vertebral body of C5 is indicated by a black line, the posterior cortex by a white line, and the superior and inferior end plates of C5 by black discontinuous lines. The pedicle of C4 is indicated by the yellow line, the inferior facet of C6 by a white discontinuous line, and the superior facet of C7 by a yellow discontinuous line.

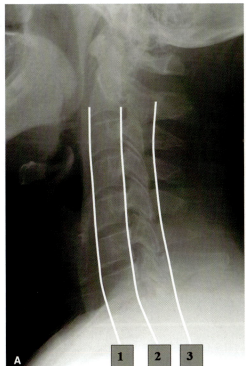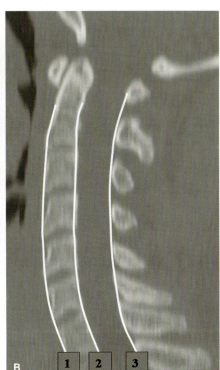

FIGURE 5-6. Lateral radiograph **(A)** and sagittal CT multiplanar reformation **(B)** of a normal cervical spine. The vertebrae are aligned in a gentle lordotic configuration. The lines connecting the anterior margin of the vertebral bodies (1), the posterior cortical margins of the vertebral bodies (2), and the anterior margins of the junctions of the spinous processes and laminae (spinolaminar line) (3) should form three parallel gentle convex curves with no steps or discontinuities. The spacing between these lines is uniform.

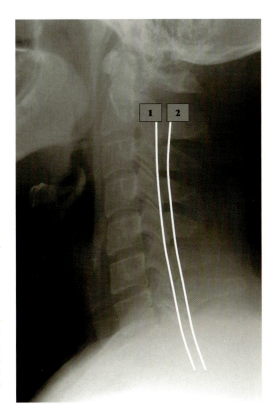

FIGURE 5-7. Normal laminar space. The laminar space is the distance from the posterior aspect of the articular pillars (1) to the spinolaminar line (2). When a true lateral view is obtained, the laminar space is uniform between adjacent levels. Young et al. (44) have described use of the "laminar space" to indicate rotational injuries of the cervical spine; injury is suggested when there is abrupt alteration of the laminar space between two adjacent levels.

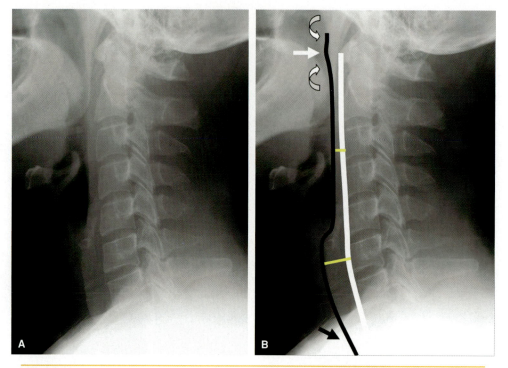

FIGURE 5-8. Normal prevertebral soft tissues. Normal lateral radiographs **(A,B)**. The prevertebral soft tissue is normal in thickness (*yellow lines, C3 <7 mm and C6 <20 mm*) and contour (*black line*). Note slight convex bulge anterior to C1 anterior tubercle (*white arrow*) and concavity caudal and rostral to the tubercle (*curved arrows*). At the cervicothoracic level the soft tissue shadow contour (*black arrow*) is normally near parallel to the arc formed by the anterior cortices of the lower cervical and upper thoracic vertebral bodies.

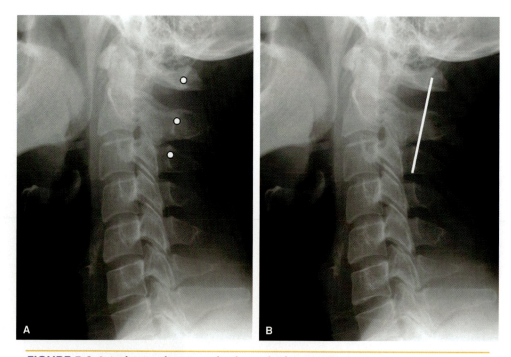

FIGURE 5-9. Spinolaminar line. Lateral radiograph of a normal cervical spine in neutral position **(A,B)**. The spinolaminar line (*white line in B*) is an important anatomical landmark easily visualized on the lateral radiograph of the cervical spine. Any displacement in this line may be an indication of subtle traumatic vertebral injury/dislocation. This is particularly relevant to the upper cervical spine, where the complex anatomy and frequent absence of associated neurological deficit make diagnosis difficult. A line (*white line in B*) drawn through C1-3 spinolaminar lines (*white dots in A*) should intercept the C2 spinolaminar line. A displacement of the C2 spinolaminar line of more than 2 mm, compared with a line drawn between the spinolaminar lines of C1 and C3, is abnormal.

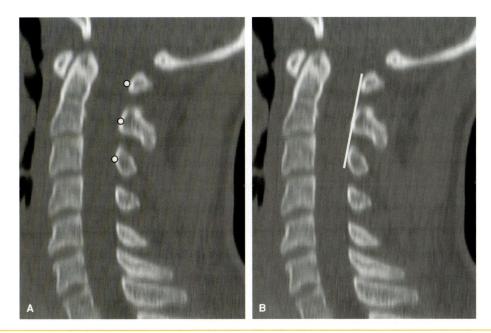

FIGURE 5-10. Spinolaminar line. **A,B:** Sagittal multiplanar CT reformations of a normal cervical spine in neutral position. The spinolaminar line (*white line in B*) is an important anatomical landmark easily visualized on the lateral radiograph of the cervical spine. Any displacement in this line may be an indication of subtle traumatic vertebral injury/dislocation. This is particularly relevant at the upper cervical spine, where the complex anatomy and frequent absence of associated neurological deficit make diagnosis difficult. A line (*white line in B*) drawn through the C1-3 spinolaminar lines (*white dots in A*) should intercept the C2 spinolaminar line. A displacement of the C2 spinolaminar line of more than 2 mm, compared with a line drawn between the spinolaminar line of C1 and C3, is abnormal.

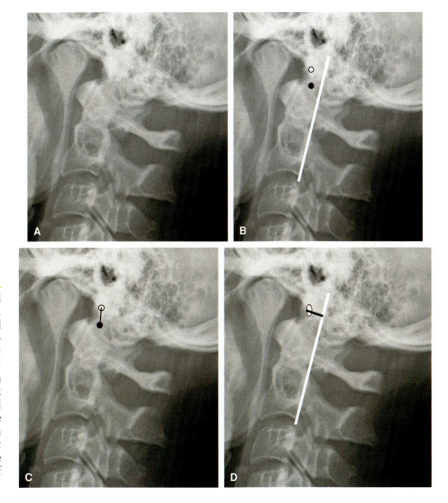

FIGURE 5-11. Normal atlantooccipital alignment as described by Harris et al. (45,46). **A,B:** Lateral radiograph of a normal cervical spine in neutral position B. Landmarks: Inferior tip of the clivus (*white dot in B*), top of the odontoid process (*black dot in B*), and the posterior axial line (PAL), which is a line extended along the posterior cortex of the axis (*white line in B*). **C:** Basion dental interval (BDI), the distance between the basion (*white dot*) should lie within 12 mm of the top of the odontoid process (*black dot*). **D:** The basion-axial interval (BAI), the PAL (*white line*) should lie within 12 mm of the basion (*white dot*). (*continued*)

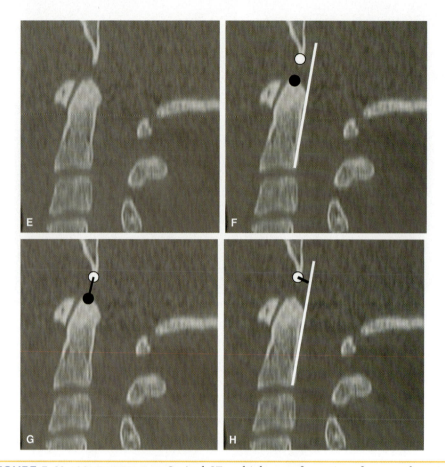

FIGURE 5-11. (*CONTINUED*) **E–H:** Sagittal CT multiplanar reformation of a normal cervical spine in neutral position. **F:** Landmarks: Inferior tip of the clivus (*white dot in F*), top of the odontoid process (*black dot in F*), and the posterior axial line PAL (a line extended along the posterior cortex of the axis) (*white line in F*). **G:** Basion dental interval (BDI): the distance between the basion (*white dot*) should lie within 12 mm of the top of the odontoid process (*black dot*). **H:** The basion-axial interval (BAI): the PAL (*white line*) should lie within 12 mm of the basion (*white dot*).

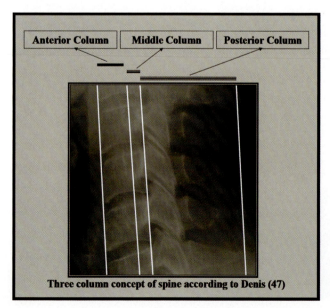

Three column concept of spine according to Denis (47)

FIGURE 5-12. Three-column concept of the spine according to Denis (47). Although the three-column concept initially evolved from a retrospective review of 412 thoracolumbar spine injuries and observation of spinal instability, it has also been applied to the cervical spine. The posterior column consists of what Holdsworth described as the posterior ligamentous complex. The middle column includes the posterior longitudinal ligament, posterior annulus fibrosus, and posterior wall of the vertebral body. The anterior column consists of the anterior vertebral body, anterior annulus fibrosus, and anterior longitudinal ligament.

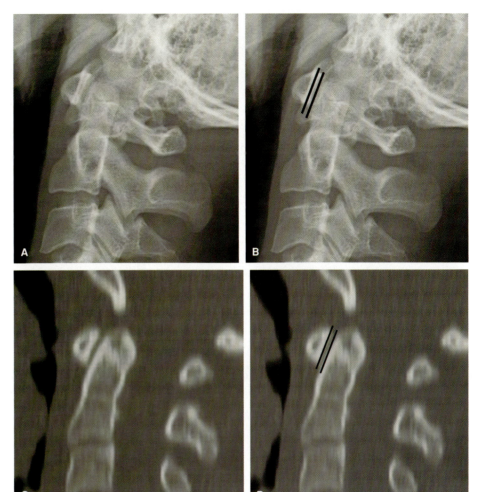

FIGURE 5-13. Normal anterior atlanto-dental interval (AADI). Lateral radiographs **(A,B)** and sagittal multiplanar reformation **(C,D)** of a normal cervical spine in neutral position. The width of the space between the anterior arch of C1 and the dens (*space between black lines in B and D*) does not normally exceed 3 mm in adults and 5 mm in children. In adults, because of maturity of the transverse atlantal ligament, the AADI remains constant in flexion and extension. In infants and children until the age of approximately 8 years, the AADI varies in width in flexion and extension.

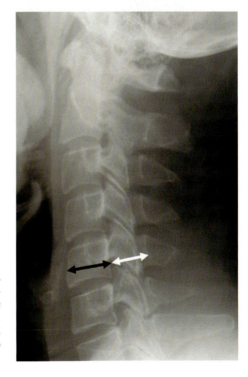

FIGURE 5-14. Diameter of the spinal canal. The normal AP diameter of the cervical canal is stated to be 12 to 21 mm. There are some difficulties in making accurate measurements secondary to differences in magnification or focal spot-film distance. This problem can be overcome by comparing the anteroposterior width of the canal with that of the vertebral body. The normal ratio of the spinal canal (*white arrow*) to the vertebral body (*black arrow*) is 0.8 or more.

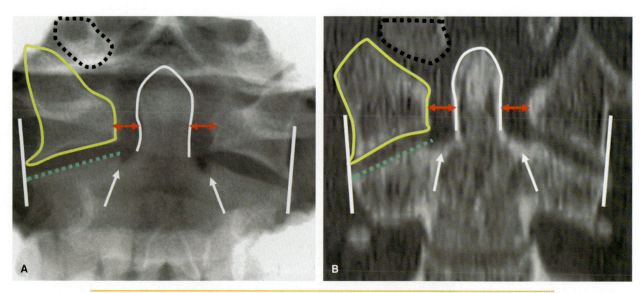

FIGURE 5-15. The normal atlantoaxial articulation seen in the neutral open-mouth odontoid view **(A)** and coronal CT multiplanar reformation **(B)**. Landmarks: right lateral mass of C1 (*yellow line*); dens (*white line*); right superior facet of C2 (*interrupted green line*); lateral atlanto-dental intervals (*red arrows in A and B*). Right occipital condyle (*interrupted black line*). The dens is centrally located between the lateral masses of the axis with symmetric lateral atlanto-dental intervals in neutral position (*red arrows in A and B*). The lateral margins of the lateral atlantoaxial joints are symmetric and are on essentially the same vertical plane, plus or minus 1 mm (*vertical white lines*). Note the normal notches at the base of the dens (*white arrows*). The C1 lateral masses articulate with the superior facet of C2 and with the occipital condyles.

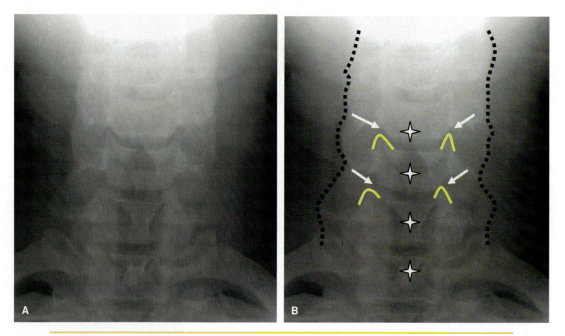

FIGURE 5-16. **A,B:** Anteroposterior (AP) radiographs of a normal cervical spine in neutral position. The spinous processes are normally midline structures (*white stars*) that should be aligned or gradually offset due to head turning. The joints of Luschka (*white arrows in B*), including the uncinate processes (*yellow lines in B*) should be symmetrically and vertically aligned at all levels. The lateral cortical margins (*interrupted black lines in B*) of the lateral columns, which represent the lateral cortex of the anatomically superimposed articular masses, appear as smooth and gently undulating, intact linear densities without disruptions. Note that the vertebral bodies are equal in height and that the apposing cortical margins of the intervertebral disc space are parallel. (*continued*)

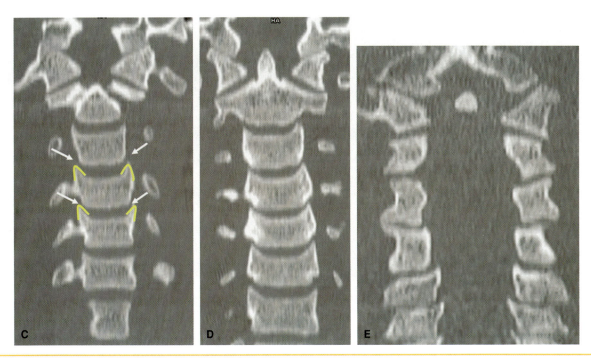

FIGURE 5-16. *(CONTINUED)* **C,D:** Normal coronal CT multiplanar reformations. The joints of Luschka (*white arrows in C*), including the uncinate processes (*yellow lines in C*) should be symmetrically and vertically aligned at all levels. **E:** As with the AP radiograph, the vertebral bodies are equal in height and the apposing cortical margins of the intervertebral disc space are parallel.

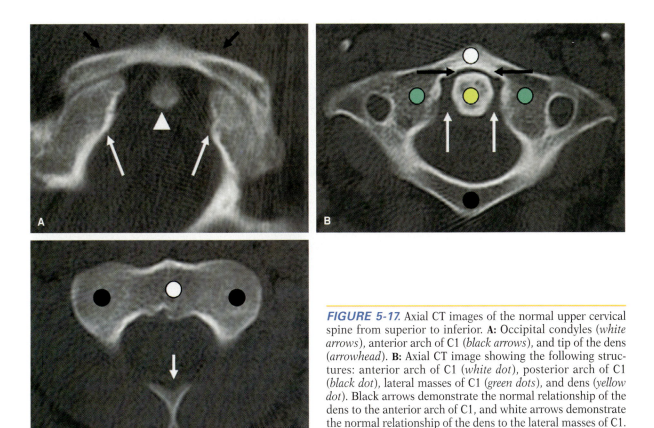

FIGURE 5-17. Axial CT images of the normal upper cervical spine from superior to inferior. **A:** Occipital condyles (*white arrows*), anterior arch of C1 (*black arrows*), and tip of the dens (*arrowhead*). **B:** Axial CT image showing the following structures: anterior arch of C1 (*white dot*), posterior arch of C1 (*black dot*), lateral masses of C1 (*green dots*), and dens (*yellow dot*). Black arrows demonstrate the normal relationship of the dens to the anterior arch of C1, and white arrows demonstrate the normal relationship of the dens to the lateral masses of C1. **C:** Body of C2 (*white dot*), lateral masses of C2 (*black dots*), and posterior arch of C1 (*white arrow*).

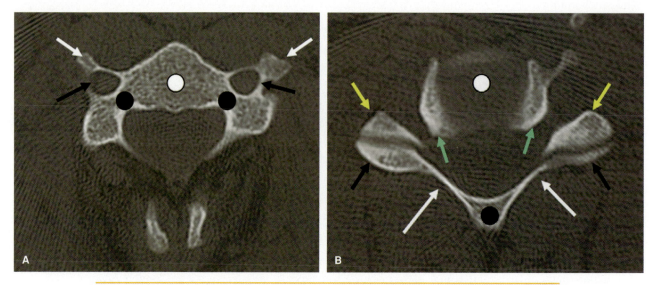

FIGURE 5-18. Axial CT images of the normal lower cervical spine vertebrae. **A:** Vertebral body (*white dot*), transverse process (*white arrows*), foramen transversarium (*black arrows*), pedicles (*black dots*). **B:** Disc space (*white dot*), laminae (*white arrows*), spinous process (*black dot*), superior articular process of the subjacent vertebra (*yellow arrows*), inferior articular process of the vertebra above (*black arrow*), and uncinate processes of the subjacent vertebra (*green arrows*).

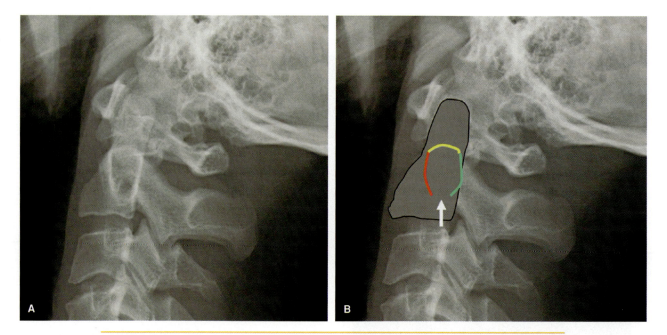

FIGURE 5-19. "Ring of C2." **A,B:** Lateral radiograph of a normal cervical spine in neutral position. The anterior arch (*red line in B*) represents the anterior cortices of the axis pedicles. The superior arc (*yellow line in B*) is a composite shadow produced by the cortex of the notch at the base of the dens and that portion of the superior articulating facets tangent to the central x-ray beam. The posterior arc (*green line in B*) is formed by the posterior cortex of the axis body (*posterior axial line*). The "ring of C2" has a normal interruption at the inferior aspect (*white arrow*) due to the foramen transversarium.

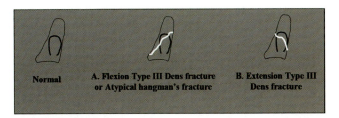

FIGURE 5-20. "Ring of C2" sign of fracture. Diagram of C2. Note disruption of the "ring of C2" and typical course of fracture lines in flexion type III dens fracture/atypical hangman fracture (**A**) and in extension type III dens fracture (**B**).

▶ **TABLE 5-6 Abnormal Spinolaminar Line**

1. Anterior or posterior C1 spinolaminar line displacement (Figs. 5-22 and 5-23):
   - Type II dens fracture with atlanto-axial dislocation (anterior or posterior).
   - Transverse atlantal ligament (TAL) injury (anterior).
2. Anterior or posterior C2 spinolaminar line displacement (Fig. 5-24):
   - Hangman fracture (posterior).
   - C2-3 dislocation (anterior or posterior).

impossible to establish absolute values that consistently discriminate between normal and abnormal.

Although the exact temporal relationship between injury and the appearance of prevertebral soft tissue edema is unknown, hematomas may not be evident on immediate postinjury examinations (performed within 2 hours of injury), but they may appear subsequently. Most hematomas resolve and measurements return to normal within 5 to 14 days of injury. Injuries involving anterior structures are more likely to cause an increase in the size of the prevertebral soft tissues than those limited to the posterior elements. Penning (40) has suggested the following measurements for prevertebral soft tissues as the upper limits of normal in adults: 10 mm anterior to the arch of C1, 7 mm anterior to C3, and 20 mm anterior

to C6 (Fig. 5-8). However, absolute measurements of the prevertebral soft tissues are not particularly accurate indicators of injury and can vary with head position, body habitus, and phase of inspiration, among other factors (41,42). Herr et al. (41) evaluated prevertebral soft tissue measurements at the C3 level in 212 blunt trauma patients using 4 mm as the upper limit of normal. They found that a measurement of greater than 4 mm was only 64% sensitive for detecting cervical spine fractures involving the anterior, posterior, upper, or lower cervical spine. Harris (43) has shown that the contour of the craniocervical prevertebral soft tissues can be particularly useful in detecting subtle upper cervical spine injuries. The normal contour of the prevertebral soft tissues from C2 to the base of the skull may be described as being posteriorly concave in front of the dens and inferior to the atlas tubercle, anteriorly convex anterior to the C1 tubercle, and again posteriorly concave above the tubercle (Fig. 5-8).

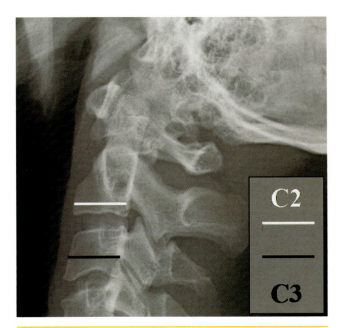

FIGURE 5-21. "Fat C2" sign. Normal relationship between C2 and C3. Lateral radiograph of a normal cervical spine in neutral position. The anteroposterior width of C2 (*white line*) equals that of C3 (*black line*). In C2 body fractures the width of C2 exceeds that of C3 (positive "Fat C2 sign").

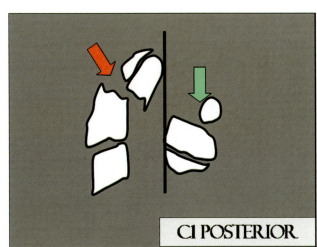

CI POSTERIOR

FIGURE 5-22. Posterior C1 spinolaminar line displacement (*green arrow*): displaced type II dens fracture (*red arrow*) with posterior atlanto-axial dislocation. Compare to the normal position of the spinolaminar line in Figures 5-9 and 5-10.

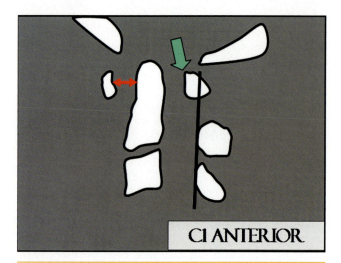

FIGURE 5-23. Anterior C1 spinolaminar line displacement (*green arrow*): transverse atlantal ligament (TAL) injury with abnormal anterior atlanto-dental interval (*red arrow*) and anterior displacement of C1.

ABNORMALITIES OF VERTEBRAL BODY HEIGHT

Variations in height of the vertebral body consist of varying degrees of anterior wedging. The height of the cervical fourth and fifth vertebral bodies may be less than that of the adjacent third and sixth vertebral bodies. If the anterior height of the vertebral body is less than the posterior height by 3 mm or more, then a fracture of the vertebral body can be assumed.

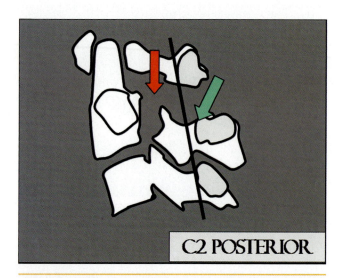

FIGURE 5-24. Posterior C2 spinolaminar line displacement (*green arrow*): hangman fracture (*red arrow*).

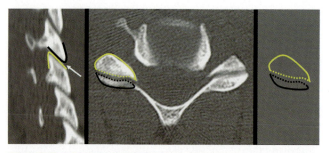

FIGURE 5-25. The normal apophysial (facet, facetal, interfacetal) joint. **A:** Right parasagittal CT multiplanar reformation. The facetal joint (*white arrow*) is the space between the superior articular process (anterior) of the subjacent vertebra (*yellow line*) and the inferior articular process of the vertebra above (*black line*). The apophysial joints are normally angled approximately 35 degrees caudally. **B:** Axial CT image. **C:** Right facet joint diagram. The superior facet (anterior) of the subjacent vertebra is rounded anteriorly (*yellow line*) and straight posteriorly (*interrupted yellow line*) at the joint surface, whereas the opposite is true of the inferior facet of the vertebra above (posterior), which is flat anteriorly (*interrupted black line*) at the joint surface and rounded posteriorly (*black line*). When the joints are normal, the flattened joint surfaces face each other. Normal facet joints are oriented on axial CT examination so that they resemble the sides of a "hamburger bun" (C).

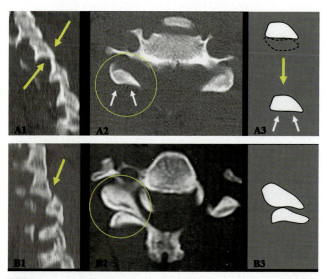

FIGURE 5-26. Abnormal apophysial (interfacetal) joint. **A:** Right perched facet. (1) Right parasagittal CT multiplanar reformation shows the right perched facet (*yellow arrows*). (2) In perched facets there is complete uncovering of the articulating facet surfaces. The naked facet sign refers to the axial computed tomographic (CT) appearance of uncovered articulating processes. On axial CT images, the involved level will reveal nonarticulating facet with loss of the joint space (*white arrow*) (48). (3) Naked facet sign illustration (*white arrows*). **B:** Right facet joint dislocation. (1) Right parasagittal CT multiplanar reformation shows the right facet dislocation (*yellow arrow*). (2) Axial CT image. (3) Illustration. With facet dislocation the superior vertebra undergoes forward translation, there is anterior displacement of the corresponding inferior articulating facet on the superior articulating facet of the vertebra below, and the rounded surfaces face each other. Facet dislocation reverses the orientation of the "hamburger bun" (rounded) halves to each other (49) (compare to a normal facet joint in Fig. 5-25).

ALIGNMENT OF CERVICAL SPINE

Alignment of the cervical spine is evaluated on the lateral radiograph by means of three separate anteriorly convex lines (Fig. 5-6). The degree of convexity of these lines is reduced by muscle spasm and the position of the chin. The curves are increased when the head is extended and reduced when the head is flexed.

CONCLUSION

In this chapter we have summarized the indications and various techniques available for the radiographic and CT evaluation of the cervical spine following trauma. Radiography is still preferred in low risk "reliable" (awake, alert, normal mental status, and no significant distracting pain) subjects. CT is the preferred imaging modality in subjects at high risk of injury, however, because of higher sensitivity and specificity. We have also reviewed the normal anatomy of the cervical spine and introduced signs of injury. In the following chapter, we will look at the classification of spinal injury as well as particular injury subtypes based on location.

REFERENCES

1. American College of Radiology. *Expert Panel on Musculoskeletal Imaging ACR Appropriateness Criteria for Suspected Cervical Spine Trauma.* Reston, Va.: ACR; 2003.
2. Núñez DB Jr, Ahmad AA, Coin GC, et al. Clearing the cervical spine in multiple trauma victims: a time-effective protocol using helical CT. *Emerg Radiol.* 1994;1:273–278.
3. Núñez DB Jr, Zuluaga A, Fuentes-Bernardo DA, et al. Cervical spine trauma: how much more do we learn by routinely using helical CT? *Radiographics.* 1996;16(6):1307–1318.
4. Hanson JA, Blackmore CC, Mann FA, et al. Cervical spine injury: clinical decision rule to identify highrisk patients for helical CT screening. *AJR Am J Roentgenol.* 2000;174: 713–717.
5. Blackmore CC, Ramsey ST, Mann FA, et al. Cervical spine screening with CT in trauma patients: a cost-effectiveness analysis. *Radiology.* 1999;212:117–125.
6. Berne JD, Velmahos GC, el-Tawil Q, et al. Value of complete cervical helical computed tomographic scanning in identifying cervical spine injury in the unevaluable blunt trauma patient with multiple injuries: a prospective study. *J Trauma.* 1999;47:896–903.
7. Lawrason JN, Novelline RA, Rhea JT, et al. Can CT eliminate the initial portable lateral cervical spine radiograph in the multiple trauma patient? a review of 200 cases. *Emerg Radiol.* 2001;8:272–275.
8. Li AE, Fishman EK. Cervical spine trauma: evaluation by multidetector CT and three-dimensional volume rendering. *Emerg Radiol.* 2003;10:34–39.
9. Ptak T, Kihiczak D, Lawrason JN. Screening for cervical spine trauma with helical CT: experience with 676 cases. *Emerg Radiol.* 2001;8:315–319.
10. Daffner RH. Controversies in cervical spine imaging in trauma patients. *Emerg Radiol.* 2004;11:2-8.
11. Daffner RH. Cervical radiography for trauma patients: a time effective technique? *AJR Am J Roentgenol.* 2000;175: 1308–1311.
12. Turetsky DB, Vines FS, Clayman DA, et al. Technique and use of supine oblique views in acute cervical spine trauma. *Ann Emerg Med.* 1993;22:685–689.
13. Woodring JH, Lee C. Limitations of cervical radiography in the evaluation of acute cervical trauma. *J Trauma.* 1993;34: 32–39.
14. Acheson MB, Livingston RR, Richardson ML, et al. High-resolution CT scanning in the evaluation of cervical spine fractures: Comparison with plain film examinations. *AJR Am J Roentgenol.* 1987;148:1179–1185.
15. Insko EK, Gracias VH, Gupta R, et al. Utility of flexion and extension radiographs of the cervical spine in the acute evaluation of blunt trauma. *J Trauma.* 2002;53(3):426–429.
16. Brady WJ, Moghtader J, Cutcher D, et al. ED use of flexion-extension cervical spine radiography in the evaluation of blunt trauma. *Am J Emerg Med.* 1999;17(6):504–508.
17. Dwek JR, Chung CB. Radiography of cervical spine injury in children: are flexion-extension radiographs useful for acute trauma? *AJR Am J Roentgenol.* 2000;174(6):1617–1619.
18. Davis JW, Kaups KL, Cunningham MA, et al. Cervical spine evaluation in obtunded patients: the use of dynamic fluoroscopy. *J Trauma.* 1995;39:435–438.
19. Scarrow AM, Levy EI, Resnick DV, et al. Cervical spine evaluation in obtunded or comatose pediatric trauma patients: a pilot study. *Pediatr Neurosurg.* 1999;30:169-175.
20. Sees DW, Rodriguez Cruz LR, Flaherty SF, et al. The use of bed side fluoroscopy to evaluate the cervical spine in obtunded trauma patients. *J Trauma.* 1998;45:768–771.
21. Davis JW, Kaups KL, Cunningham MA, et al. Routine evaluation of the cervical spine in head-injured patients with dynamic fluoroscopy: reappraisal. *J Trauma.* 2001;50:1044–1047.
22. Ohnesorge B, Flohr T, Schaller S, et al. The technical bases and uses of multi-slice CT. *Radiology.* 1999;39:923–931.
23. Fleischmann D, Rubin GD, Paik DS, et al. Stair-step artifacts with single versus multiple detector-row helical CT. *Radiology.* 2000;216:185–196.
24. Kalender WA. Thin-section three-dimensional spiral CT: is isotropic imaging possible? *Radiology.* 1995;197:578–580.
25. Flohr TH, Klingenbeck-Regn K, Ohnesorge B, et al. Multislice CT scanning with the SOMATOM Volume Zoom. In: Baker ME, ed. *Multislice CT—A Practical Guide.* Berlin, Heidelberg, New York: Springer; 2000:79–89
26. Mahesh M. Search for isotropic resolution in CT from conventional through multiple-row detector. *Radiographics.* 2002;22:949–962.
27. Honda O, Johkoh T, Yamamoto S, et al. Comparison of quality of multiplanar reconstructions and direct coronal multidetector CT scans of the lung. *AJR Am J Roentgenol.* 2002; 179:875–879.
28. Rubin GD. Data explosion: the challenge of multidetector-row CT. *Eur J Radiol.* 2000;36:74–80.
29. Begemann PG, Kemper JA, Gatzka C, et al. Value of multiplanar reformations (MPR) in multidetector CT (MDCT) of acute vertebral fractures: do we still have to read the transverse images? *J Compt Assist Tomogr.* 2004;28(4):572–580.
30. Saini S, Seltzer SE, Bramson RT. Technical cost of radiologic examinations: analysis across imaging modalities. *Radiology.* 2000;216:269–272.
31. Forman HP. Cost, value, and price: what is the difference and why care? *Radiology.* 2001;218:25–26.
32. Saini S, Sharma R, Levine LA, et al. Technical cost of CT examinations. *Radiology.* 2001;218:172–175.
33. Rybicki F, Nawfel RD, Judy PF, et al. Skin and thyroid dosimetry in cervical spine screening: two methods for evaluation and a comparison between a helical CT and radiographic trauma series. *AJR Am J Roentgenol.* 2002;179:933–937.
34. Domenicucci M, Preite R, Ramieri A, et al. Three-dimensional computed tomographic imaging in the diagnosis of vertebral column trauma: experience based on 21 patients and review of the literature. *J Trauma.* 1997;42(2):254–259.
35. Saeed M, Buitrago-Fellez CH, Ferst PF, et al: Three dimensional CT in the diagnosis of spinal trauma: comparison with plain film and two dimensional examinations. *Eur J Radiol.* 1994;4:161.

36. Lang P, Genant HK, Chafetz N, et al. Three dimensional computed tomography and multiplanar reformations in the assessment of pseudoarthrosis in posterior lumbar fusion patients. *Spine*. 1988;13:69–75.

37. Li AE, Fishman EK. Cervical spine trauma: evaluation by multidetector CT and three-dimensional volume rendering. *Emerg Radiol*. 2003;10:34–39.

38. Calhoun PS, Kuszyk BS, Heath DG, et al. Three-dimensional volume rendering of spiral CT data: theory and method. *Radiographics*. May–June 1999;19(3):745–764.

39. Drebin RA, Magid D, Robertson DD, et al. Fidelity of three-dimensional CT imaging for detecting fracture gaps. *J Comput Assist Tomogr*. 1989;13:487–489.

40. Penning L. Prevertebral hematoma in cervical spine injury: incidence and etiologic significance. *AJR Am J Roentgenol*. March 1981;136(3):553–561.

41. Herr CH, Ball PA, Sargent SK, et al. Sensitivity of prevertebral soft tissue measurement of C3 for detection of cervical spine fractures and dislocations. *Am J Emerg Med*. 1998;16: 346–349.

42. Templeton PA, Young JW, Mirvis SE, et al. The value of retropharyngeal soft tissue measurements in trauma of the adult cervical spine: cervical soft tissue measurements. *Skeletal Radiol*. 1987;16:98–104.

43. Harris JH Jr. Abnormal cervicocraneal retropharyngeal soft tissue contour in the detection of subtle acute cervicocranial injuries. *Emerg Radiol*. 2000;7:11.

44. Young JW, Resnik CS, DeCandido P, et al. The laminar space in the diagnosis of rotational flexion injuries of the cervical spine. *AJR Am J Roentgenol*. January 1989;152(1):103–107.

45. Harris JH, Carson GC, Wagner LK. Radiologic diagnosis of traumatic occipitovertebral dissociation: 1. Normal occipitovertebral relationships on lateral radiographs of supine subjects. *AJR Am J Roentgenol*. 1994;162:881–886.

46. Harris JH, Carson GC, Wagner LK, et al. Radiologic diagnosis of traumatic occipitovertebral dissociation: 2. Comparison of three methods of detecting occipitovertebral relationships on lateral radiographs of supine subjects. *AJR Am J Roentgenol*. 1994;162:887–892.

47. Denis F: Spinal instability as defined by the three-column spine concept in a acute spinal trauma. *Clin Orthop*. 1984; 189:65–76.

48. White AA III, Panjabi MM. *Clinical Biomechanics of the Spine*. 2nd ed. Philadelphia: JB Lippincott; 1991.

49. Daffner SD, Daffner RH. Computed tomography diagnosis of facet dislocations: the "hamburger bun" and "reverse hamburger bun" signs. *J Emerg Med*. November 2002;23(4): 387–394.

Plain Film Radiography and Computed Tomography of the Cervical Spine: Part II. Classification and Subtypes of Spinal Injury

Alejandro Zuluaga Santamaria and Diego B. Núñez, Jr.

It is helpful to consider injuries to the cervical spine in terms of their mechanism (1). These mechanisms include flexion, flexion rotation, extension, extension rotation, vertical compression, lateral flexion, and imprecisely understood mechanisms that may result in odontoid fractures and atlanto-occipital dislocation. As emphasized by Harris (1), however, it is also important

to note that different injuries may be caused by a single predominant force vector (2), and that there are groups of injuries that occur with each predominant force vector, with the magnitude of the force determining the extent of the injury. Cervical spine injuries can also be classified into upper and lower cervical injuries. Upper cervical injuries include injuries to the base of the skull (including the occipital condyles or C0), C1, and C2. Lower cervical injuries (subaxial) include injuries from C3 through C7. A classification of cervical spine injuries are presented based upon the predominant force vector (Table 6-1), however they will be discussed and illustrated from the perspective of their location (upper and lower cervical spine) in the remainder of the chapter.

STABILITY VERSUS INSTABILITY

Stable injuries resist movement in response to physiologic loading and do not create or worsen neurologic deficits. White and Punjabi (3) have defined "clinical instability" as "the loss of the ability of the spine under physiologic loads to maintain its pattern of displacement so that there is no initial or additional neurologic deficit, no major deformity, and no incapacitating pain." The three-column concept of Denis (4) is very important in understanding the concept of stability and the reciprocal movements of the spine that occur during both normal and pathologic flexion and extension (i.e., in flexion, the anterior column of the spine is compressed while the posterior column is reciprocally distracted). The anterior longitudinal ligament (ALL), the annulus, and the anterior two thirds of the vertebral body and disc constitute the anterior column; the posterior third of the vertebral body and disc, the posterior annulus, and the posterior longitudinal ligament (PLL) constitute the middle column; and everything posterior to that constitutes the posterior column (Fig. 5-12). When assessing stability in the spinal column, the three-column theory of Denis (4) suggests that if two columns have failed, the spinal column is unstable. In general, this requires failure of the middle column in conjunction with either the anterior or posterior column, as disruption of two contiguous columns decreases the load carrying capacity of the spine. Plain film and computed tomography (CT) signs of cervical spine instability are presented in Table 6-2, and potentially unstable fractures are listed in Table 6-3.

UPPER CERVICAL SPINE INJURIES (C0–C3)

Occipital Condyle Fractures

Occipital condyle fractures (OCF) were first reported in 1817 by Sir Charles Bell based on autopsy findings, and they were first described radiographically in 1962 and by CT in 1983 (5). OCF are rare, being found at postmortem examination in 1% to 5% of patients who had sustained trauma to the cervical spine and head (6). Clinical manifestations of OCF are highly variable, and such fractures are not typically shown with conventional radiography.

▶ **TABLE 6-1 Cervical Spine Injuries: Classification by Predominant Force Vector**

Flexion injury
Common injuries associated with a flexion mechanism include the following:

- Simple wedge compression fracture without posterior disruption
- Anterior subluxation
- Bilateral facet dislocation
- Flexion teardrop fracture
- Clay shoveler fracture
- Anterior atlantoaxial dislocation

Flexion-rotation injury
Common injuries associated with a flexion-rotation mechanism include:

- Unilateral facet dislocation
- Rotary atlantoaxial dislocation

Lateral flexion injury
Common injuries associated with a lateral flexion mechanism include:

- Unilateral fracture of the occipital condyle
- Lateral mass of C1
- Eccentric fracture of the superior articular process of C2
- Combination of the above mentioned injuries

Extension injury
Common injuries associated with an extension mechanism include:

- Hyperextension sprain dislocation
- Hyperextension fracture dislocation
- Laminar fracture
- Hangman fracture
- Extension teardrop fracture
- Avulsion horizontal fracture, anterior arch of C1
- Fracture of the posterior arch of C1 (posterior neural arch fracture of C1)
- Posterior atlantoaxial dislocation

Extension-rotation injury
Common injuries associated with an extension-rotation mechanism include:

- Pillar fracture
- Pedicolaminar fracture-separation

Vertical compression (axial loading) injury
Common injuries associated with a vertical compression mechanism include:

- Jefferson fracture (burst fracture of the ring of C1)
- Burst fracture (dispersion, axial loading)
- Atlas fracture
- Isolated fracture of the lateral mass of C1 (pillar fracture)

Multiple or complex injuries
Common injuries associated with multiple or complex mechanisms include:

- Odontoid fracture
- Fracture of the transverse process of C2 (lateral flexion)
- Atlanto-occipital dislocation (flexion or extension with a shearing component)
- Occipital condyle fracture (vertical compression with lateral bending)

▶ **TABLE 6-2 Plain Film and CT Signs of Instability**

Plain film lateral view and sagittal CT multiplanar reformation:

- Anterior translation of the vertebral body a distance >3.5 mm relative to the subjacent vertebra
- Vertebral body shows greater than 20 degrees of angulation relative to the adjacent vertebra
- Vertebral body shows >11 degrees of angulation relative to the adjacent vertebral body pairs
- Increase in atlantoaxial distance (>3 mm)
- Hangman fracture with >3 mm of fragment displacement or >a 15-degree angle at the fracture site
- Hangman fracture with abnormal C2-3 disc space or with C2-3 dislocation
- Anterior or posterior displacement of the C2 spinolaminar line of >2 mm relative to a line drawn between the spinolaminar lines of C1 and C3
- Basion-dental interval (BDI) >12 mm
- Basion-axial line interval (BAI) >12 mm
- Unilateral facet dislocation
- Bilateral facet dislocation

Open-mouth odontoid view and coronal CT multiplanar reformation:

- Sum of C1 lateral mass offset in excess of 7 mm (adding the amount of lateral displacement of each C1 lateral mass)
- Odontoid fracture type I or II
- Occipital condyle fracture type III

Plain film AP view and coronal CT multiplanar reformation:

- Widening of the uncovertebral joints

▶ **TABLE 6-3 Unstable or Potentially Unstable Cervical Spine Injuries**

Upper cervical spine
- Atlantooccipital dislocation
- Occipital condyle fracture, type III
- Atypical Jefferson fracture
- Atlanto-axial dissociation
- Hangman fracture types II, IIA, and III
- Atypical hangman fracture
- Odontoid fractures types I and II

Lower cervical spine
- Anterior subluxation: if displacement of the vertebral body anteriorly exceeds 3.5 mm, or if the body shows >20 degrees of angulation (or >11 degrees of angulation compared with the adjacent vertebral body pairs), the injury is considered unstable
- Hyperflexion fracture dislocation
- Bilateral facet dislocation
- Unilateral facet dislocation
- Hyperflexion teardrop fracture
- Hyperextension dislocation and hyperextension fracture dislocation
- Burst fracture
- Isolated articular pillar fracture

Potential clinical findings include persistent upper cervical pain despite an absence of a radiologic abnormality, spasmatic torticollis, limitation of skull mobility, dysphagia, and lower cervical nerve deficits. In severe cases, brainstem injury may occur, or there may be injury to the vertebral arteries (6–8). Since the introduction of CT imaging, numerous small series and case reports have appeared describing the mechanisms, clinical manifestations, and imaging features of OCF (6–10). CT has revealed that OCF are more common than was suspected before the CT era.

The classification mechanism most commonly used for OCF is the Anderson-Montesano system (Table 6-4) (11). Using this system, the type I OCF injury (Fig. 6-1) is a loading fracture of the occipital condyle, in which the condyle typically is fractured in a vertical sagittal plane, but where there is no fracture displacement or associated

▶ **TABLE 6-4 Occipital Condyle Fractures**

Plain film findings: Difficult diagnosis due to overlapping of the bony structures of the face, upper cervical spine, and skull base.

Lateral view:
- Prevertebral soft tissue swelling
- Usually not visible on lateral cervical spine radiograph, unless associated with occipito-atlantal dislocation

AP view:
- Usually not visible on AP cervical spine radiograph

Open-mouth odontoid view:
- May be visible in open-mouth views that include the condyles

CT findings:
- OCF are readily identified on axial or coronal reformatted CT

Axial images:
Anderson-Montesano classification system (11):

- Type I: Loading fracture of the occipital condyle, typically comminuted and in a vertical sagittal plane, but where there is no fracture displacement or associated craniocervical instability. (Fig. 6-1).
- Type II: Skull-base fracture that propagates into one or both occipital condyles (Figs. 6-2 and 6-3).
- Type III: Inferomedial avulsion fracture of the condyle by the intact alar ligament, with medial displacement of the fragment into the foramen magnum. Type III OCF are considered potentially unstable because of an avulsed alar ligament (Figs. 6-4, 6-5)

Coronal reconstruction:
- Assess condylar fracture and fragment displacement into the foramen magnum (Figs. 6-4, 6-5).

Sagittal reconstruction:
- Assess occipito-atlantal dislocation and condylar fracture (Fig. 6-2).

UNSTABLE:
- Occipital condyle fragment displacement >5 mm
- Occipito-atlantal dislocation
- Bilateral occipital condyle fractures

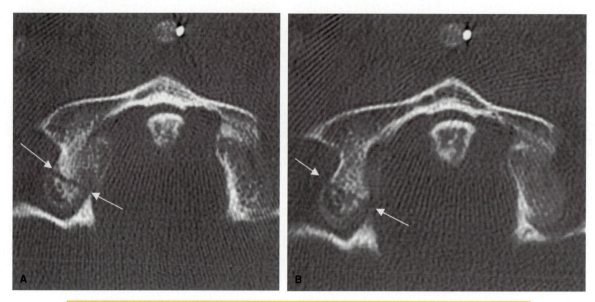

FIGURE 6-1. Type I occipital condyle fracture. **A,B:** Axial CT images show a right occipital condyle fracture (*arrows*) with minimal displacement.

cranio-cervical instability. Cranio-cervical instability is based primarily on the integrity of the alar ligaments and the tectorial membrane. The type II injury (Figs. 6-2, 6-3) is a skull-base fracture that propagates into one or both occipital condyles. The injury results from direct skull-base trauma and is usually stable at the cranio-cervical junction. Type III injuries (Figs. 6-4, 6-5) result in an inferomedial avulsion fracture of the condyle by the intact alar ligament, with medial displacement of the fragment into the foramen magnum. There is usually associated strain or tearing of the contralateral alar ligament and possible avulsion of the inferior tip of the clivus (Fig. 6-5). Type III OCF are considered potentially unstable because of an avulsed alar ligament.

CT is the diagnostic standard for occipital condyle fractures, and the base of the skull should be included in all CT examinations of the upper cervical spine. The presence of occipital condylar fractures must be excluded in all symptomatic elderly patients who have experienced trauma to the head and neck.

Atlanto-occipital Dislocation

Atlanto-occipital dislocation (AOD) is an uncommon injury that involves complete disruption of all ligamentous relationships between the occiput and the atlas (C1) (Fig. 6-6). Stability and function of the atlanto-occipital articulation are provided by the cruciate ligament, tectorial membrane, apical dental ligament, and paired alar ligaments, as well as the articular capsule ligaments. Death usually occurs immediately from stretching of the brainstem, which can result in respiratory arrest. Traumatic atlanto-occipital dislocation has been reported to occur in up to 31% of motor vehicle fatalities (12,13). Increasing numbers of survivors with satisfactory neurologic outcomes are attributed to improved on-scene resuscitation, spinal immobilization, transportation, new diagnostic techniques, and a higher index of suspicion. Patients who survive often have neurological impairment including lower cranial neuropathies, unilateral or bilateral weakness, or quadriplegia. Up to 50% of cases are overlooked on the initial conventional radiographic evaluation (12,13). Children are at relatively increased risk for this injury due to their relatively large head size, shallow C1-2 articulations, and ligament laxity (14). There are three principal forms of traumatic atlanto-occipital dislocation (15,16). The first and the most common pattern is an anterior and superior displacement of the cranium relative to C1. The second is a pure superior displacement (distraction) of the cranium. The third, and least frequent, is a posterior dislocation of the cranium in relation to the spine. The lateral cervical spine radiograph is most likely to reveal the injury; in this projection, the relationship of the dens and clivus and related structures can be established in several ways. The Powers and Lee-X-line require identification of the basion and opisthion that are often obscure on the lateral cervical radiograph (17–21). Harris et al. (17,18) have proposed two measurements that appear to have high sensitivity and specificity for the diagnosis of AOD and that are based on readily identified landmarks. By this method the basion-dental measurement (BDI) should not exceed 12 mm in the adult, and a

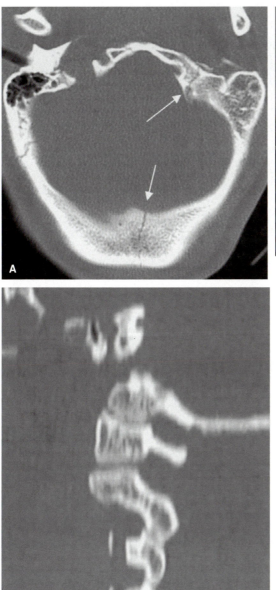

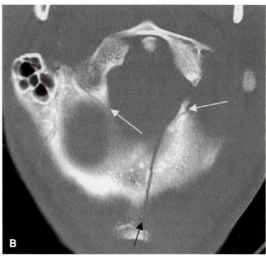

FIGURE 6-2. Type II occipital condyle fracture. **A:** Axial CT shows a left occipital fracture extending through the left occipital condyle (*arrows*). **B:** Axial CT of the same patient shows the left occipital fracture (*black arrow*) extending through the skull base bilaterally (*white arrows*). **C:** Left parasagittal CT multiplanar reformation shows no evidence of atlanto-occipital dislocation.

line drawn along the margin of the posterior axis (posterior axial line) extended cephalad to the basion should not be further than 12 mm distant (basion-axial line interval; BAI) (Fig. 5-11). A comparative study by Harris et al. (18) found a 60% sensitivity of the Power ratio, a 20% sensitivity of the Lee method, and 100% sensitivity of the BAI-BDI method among those in whom the required landmarks could be identified. Przybylski et al. (12) reported failure to diagnose AOD in two of five patients with the Power ratio, one of five patients with the X-line method, and in two of five with the BAI-BDI

method. No radiographic method reviewed has complete sensitivity. The BAI-BDI method proposed by Harris et al. is at present the most reliable means to diagnose AOD on a lateral cervical spine radiograph. The diagnosis of atlanto-occipital dislocation may not be easy. It must first be suspected on the basis of soft tissue swelling, craniocervical junction (12) posterior fossa (22) subarachnoid hemorrhage, or via questionable relationships at the atlanto-occipital junction. Sagittal CT reconstructions or sagittal magnetic resonance imaging (MRI) can allow for the diagnosis when plain radiography is inconclusive.

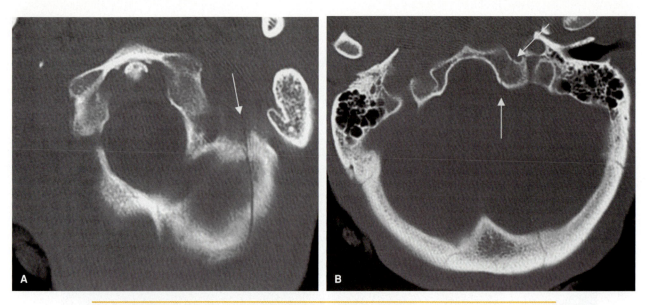

FIGURE 6-3. Type II occipital condyle fracture. **A:** Axial CT shows a left skull base fracture (*arrow*). **B:** Axial CT of the same patient shows the left skull base fracture extending through the left occipital condyle (*white arrows*).

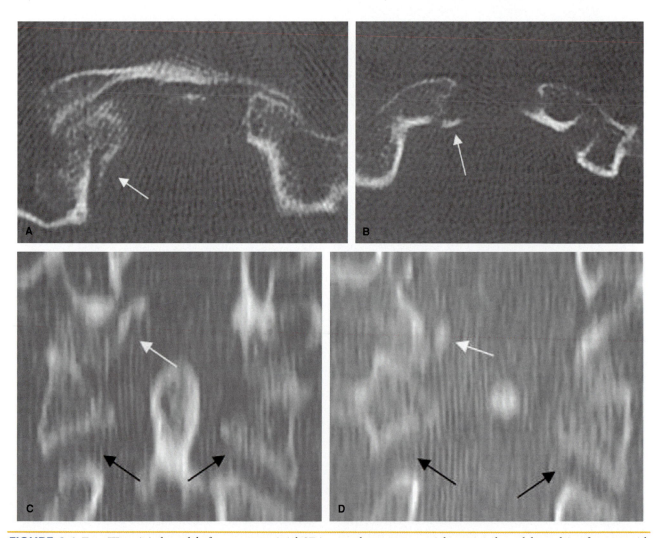

FIGURE 6-4. Type III occipital condyle fracture. **A,B:** Axial CT images demonstrate a right occipital condyle avulsion fracture with medial displacement of the fragment (*arrows*). **C,D:** Coronal CT multiplanar reformations show avulsion of the medial aspect of the right occipital condyle (*white arrows*). Note distraction between C1-2 (*black arrows*), indicating that the injury involves at least two levels.

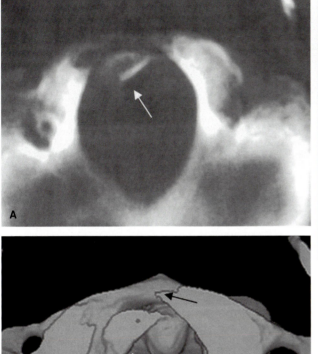

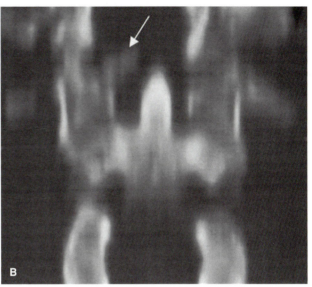

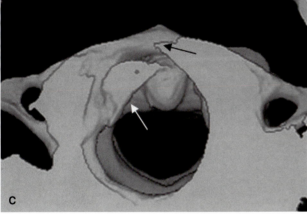

FIGURE 6-5. Type III occipital condyle fracture. **A:** Axial CT image demonstrates a right occipital condyle avulsion fracture with medial displacement of the fragment into the foramen magnum (*arrow*). **B:** Coronal CT multiplanar reformation shows avulsion of the medial aspect of the right occipital condyle (*arrow*) with >5 mm medial displacement of the avulsed fragment into the foramen magnum. **C:** Reformatted 3D-shaded surface superior axial view demonstrates the right condylar fracture with medial displacement of the avulsed fragment into the foramen magnum (*white arrow*). Note the extension of the fracture to the clivus (*black arrow*).

Atlas (C1) Fractures

Fractures of the first cervical vertebra ring are generally related to axial loading and commonly occur in association with other injuries, including those of the occipital condyle and the axis. Neurologic compromise is relatively infrequent with fractures of the cervical vertebra C1 ring, presumably because the axial compression mechanism results in a burst configuration with expansion of the spinal canal.

Jefferson Fracture

The classic Jefferson fracture (JF), described in 1920 (23), is a four-point injury with fractures occurring at the junctions of the anterior and posterior arches with the lateral masses, the weakest structural portions of the atlas (C1) (Figs. 6-7, 6-8). However, CT has shown that a JF requires

only one anterior and one posterior arch fracture, although any combination of anterior and posterior arch fractures may occur (24) (Fig. 6-7). Most commonly there are two fractures in the posterior arch (one on each side) and a single fracture in the anterior arch, off the midline (25). At times, there is a single fracture in each arch. A JF is created by sudden and direct axial loading on the vertex. The lateral articular masses of the atlas become compressed between the occipital condyles and the superior articular facets of the axis. By its nature, this is a decompressive injury because the bony fragments are displaced radially away from the neural structures (Figs. 6-9, 6-10). Although the typical JF behaves in a stable fashion, variant injuries patterns can be or are mechanically unstable (Fig. 6-12, Table 6-5). Lee and Woodring (26) described a group of patients with axial loading injuries with less than four-part fractures and with fractures through the ring in atypical locations.

▶ **TABLE 6-5** Jefferson Fracture

Plain film findings: The most significant findings are on the frontal projection of the atlas and axis.

Open-mouth odontoid view:
- Bilateral offset or spreading of the lateral articular masses of C1 in relation to the apposing articular surfaces of C2 (Figs. 6-9, 6-10).
- It is often difficult to visualize the lines of fracture per se, but the presence of the fracture may be implied from lateral displacement of the lateral masses of C1 relative to the peripheral margins of the superior facet of C2.

Lateral view: (difficult diagnosis on the lateral view)
- Occasionally, the fractures are demonstrated on the lateral projection (usually the posterior arch fracture) (Fig. 6-11)
- Increase in the atlantoaxial distance (>3 mm)
- Anterior or posterior displacement of the C1 spinolaminar line
- The retropharyngeal soft tissue may be abnormal in both contour and thickness (Fig. 6-11)

AP view:
- Usually not visible on AP cervical spine radiograph

UNSTABLE:
It has been suggested that the degree of offset distinguishes between stable and unstable Jefferson's fractures (103,104). An unstable JF is one in which the transverse ligament is disrupted.

- Total C1 lateral masses offset of both sides in excess of 7 mm (adding the amount of lateral displacement of each C1 lateral mass)
- Increase in the atlantoaxial distance (>3 mm)
- CT findings: CT very accurately identifies the injury and establishes the exact sites of fracture, fracture displacement, and associated injuries.

Axial images:
- Identify and establish the sites and number of C1 ring fractures (Figs. 6-8 and 6-12)
- Establish separation between fracture fragments of the atlas, if >7 mm the lesion is considered unstable

Coronal reconstruction:
- Assess offset or spreading of the lateral articular masses of C1 in relation to the apposing articular surfaces of C2

Sagittal reconstruction:
- Assess increase in the atlantoaxial distance (>3 mm) and anterior or posterior displacement of the C1 spinolaminar line

3D reconstructions (superior and frontal views):
- Establish separation between fracture fragments of the atlas (superior view) and spreading of the lateral articular masses of C1 (frontal view) in relation to the apposing articular surfaces of C2 (Fig. 6-8)

UNSTABLE:
It has been suggested that the degree of offset distinguishes between stable and unstable Jefferson fractures (103,104). An unstable JF is one in which the transverse ligament is disrupted.

Coronal reconstructions:
- Total C1 lateral masses offset of the two sides in excess of 7 mm (adding the amount of lateral displacement of each C1 lateral mass)

Sagittal reconstructions: Increase in the atlantoaxial distance (>3 mm)
Axial views: >7 mm separation between fracture fragments of the atlas
- Because multilevel fractures (C1 and C2) are considered unstable, a cautious search for contiguous fractures is critical (Fig. 6-35)

If there is a separation between the fracture fragments of the atlas by more than 6 to 7 mm, the injury is considered unstable because the separation implies disruption of the transverse atlantal ligament (TAL), which is a strong band that extend between the medial aspect of the C1 lateral masses and holds the dens against the anterior arch of C1. This fragment separation can be ascertained from the superior three-dimensional (3D) axial views, coronal CT reconstruction, or open-mouth anteroposterior (AP) odontoid view (Table 6-5). In all JF is important to carefully assess the atlanto-dental space to be sure that it does not exceed 3 mm in adult patients (Fig. 6-11). A greater distance would imply TAL tearing (27). JF are commonly associated with concurrent injuries of the

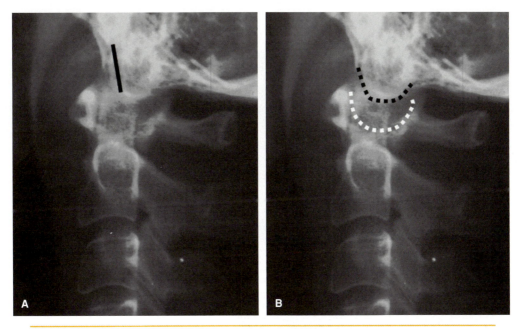

FIGURE 6-6. Atlanto-occipital distraction injury. **A,B:** lateral radiographs of the cervical spine show increased separation between the basion and superior tip of the odontoid (*black line in A*) exceeding 12 mm. The occipital condyles (*interrupted black line in B*) are superiorly dislocated with respect to the superior surfaces of C1 (*interrupted white line in B*).

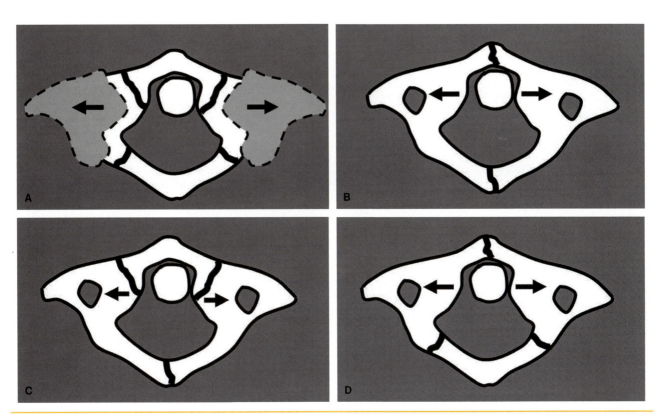

FIGURE 6-7. Jefferson fracture. The classic JF is a four-point injury with fractures occurring at the junctions of the anterior and posterior arches with the lateral masses, the weakest structural portions of the atlas (C1), with resultant bilateral offset or spreading of the lateral articular masses of C1 **(A)** (*arrows indicate offset of lateral masses*). However, CT has shown that JF require only one anterior and one posterior arch fractures **(B)**, although any combination of anterior and posterior arch fractures may occur **(C,D)**. Most commonly there are two fractures in the posterior arch (one on each side) and a single fracture in the anterior arch off the midline (D). (Harris JH. Jr, Mirvis SE. Vertical compression injuries. *The Radiology of Acute Cervical Spine Trauma*, 3rd ed. Baltimore: Williams & Wilkins; 1996:340–345; Landells CD, Van Pethegem PK. Fractures of the atlas: classification, treatment and morbidity. *Spine*. 1988;13:450–452.)

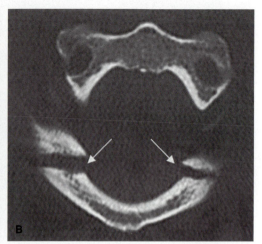

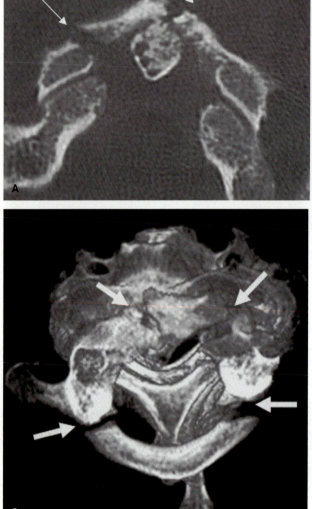

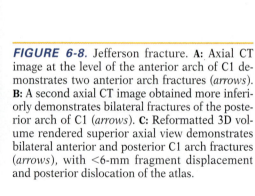

FIGURE 6-8. Jefferson fracture. **A:** Axial CT image at the level of the anterior arch of C1 demonstrates two anterior arch fractures (*arrows*). **B:** A second axial CT image obtained more inferiorly demonstrates bilateral fractures of the posterior arch of C1 (*arrows*). **C:** Reformatted 3D volume rendered superior axial view demonstrates bilateral anterior and posterior C1 arch fractures (*arrows*), with <6-mm fragment displacement and posterior dislocation of the atlas.

upper cervical spine, particularly the high and low dens fractures and hangman fracture.

Pitfalls in the diagnosis of the JF include clefts and aplasias in the atlas ring that simulate fractures; these are typically differentiated by smooth, well-defined corticated bone margins. In children younger than age 5, the ossification of the lateral mass of C1 often exceeds that of the ossification of C2, giving rise to what has been termed "pseudo spread" of C1 upon C2 (28,29).

Lateral Mass (C1) Fracture

Fractures of the lateral mass of C1 usually occur as a result of a lateral tilt or an eccentric axial loading (Fig. 6-13). The fracture may be limited to the lateral mass of C1, or more commonly, occurs in association with occipital condyle fractures and/or fracture of the articular process of C2. The C1 lateral mass fracture is usually visible on

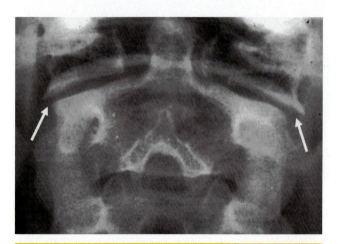

FIGURE 6-9. Jefferson fracture. AP open-mouth view demonstrates lateral displacement of the lateral masses of C1 bilaterally (*arrows*) in relation to the superior facets of C2 (compare to normal cervical spine in Fig. 5-15).

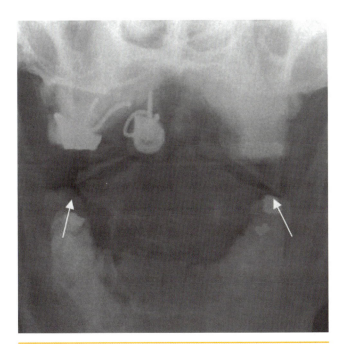

FIGURE 6-10. Jefferson fracture. AP open-mouth view demonstrates minimal asymmetric offset of C1 upon C2 bilaterally (*arrows*), left greater than right.

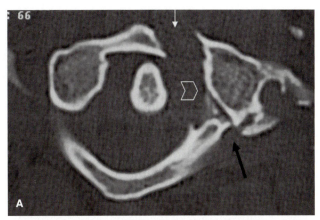

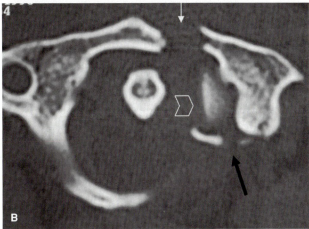

FIGURE 6-12. Atypical Jefferson fracture. **A,B:** Axial CT images show a displaced (>7 mm suggesting instability) single fracture of the left anterior arch of C1 (*white arrows*) and left lateral comminuted fracture of the posterior atlas ring (*black arrows*). Avulsed fragments from the medial surface of the left lateral mass of C1 by the transverse atlantal ligament (TAL) are noted (*open arrowhead*).

the open-mouth view; however, sometimes the abnormal cervico-cranial prevertebral soft tissue contour is the only sign of injury in plain films. A fracture of the lateral mass of C1 is considered unstable because the TAL is detached from the lateral mass.

Isolated Fractures of C1

Isolated fractures of the anterior or posterior arch of C1 are usually stable (Figs. 6-14, 6-15); these injuries should be distinguished from the Jefferson bursting fracture and its variants. The most common isolated fracture of C1 is a bilateral vertical fracture through the posterior neural arch (30–33). This type of fracture is caused by hyperextension of the head on the neck, which compresses the neural arch of C1 between the occiput and the neural arch of C2. It is best demonstrated on the lateral view. It carries no risk of neurologic deficit. This fracture must be distinguished from developmental defects (Fig. 6-16).

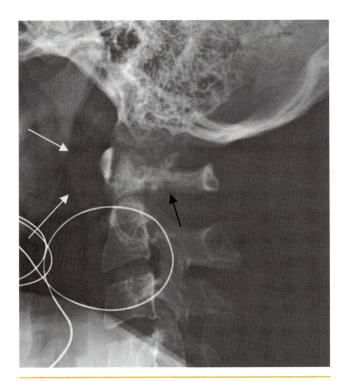

FIGURE 6-11. Jefferson fracture. Lateral radiograph shows soft tissue swelling anterior to C1 and the upper margin of C2 (*white arrows*). A fracture of the posterior C1 arch (*black arrow*), representing a part of a Jefferson fracture, is identified. Normal anterior atlantoaxial distance is noted.

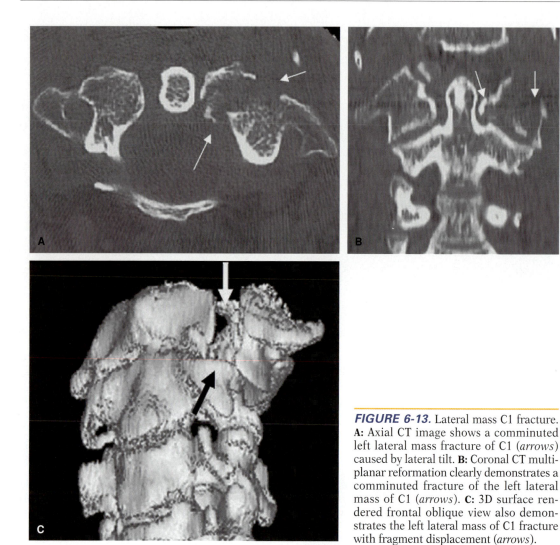

FIGURE 6-13. Lateral mass C1 fracture. **A:** Axial CT image shows a comminuted left lateral mass fracture of C1 (*arrows*) caused by lateral tilt. **B:** Coronal CT multiplanar reformation clearly demonstrates a comminuted fracture of the left lateral mass of C1 (*arrows*). **C:** 3D surface rendered frontal oblique view also demonstrates the left lateral mass of C1 fracture with fragment displacement (*arrows*).

FIGURE 6-14. Isolated fracture of the anterior arch of C1. **A:** Inferior-frontal and **(B)** frontal reformatted 3D CT. Shaded surface views demonstrate an isolated fracture of the anterior atlas arch (*arrows*).

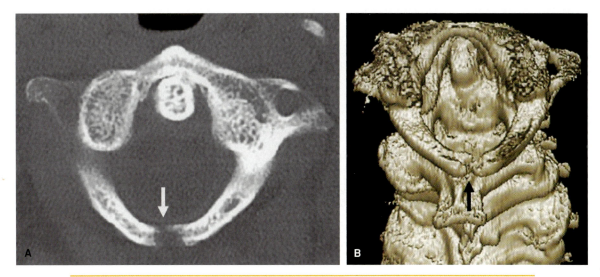

FIGURE 6-15. Isolated fracture of the posterior arch of C1. **A:** axial CT and **(B)** posterior-superior reformatted 3D CT. Shaded surface view demonstrate an isolated fracture of the posterior atlas ring (*arrows*).

Horizontal fractures of the anterior arch of the atlas have been described (Fig. 6-17) (34,35). These fractures are characteristically minimally displaced, best visualized on the lateral view, and often associated with dens fractures. Horizontal fractures result from avulsion mediated through the tendinous ligamentous insertion on the anterior tubercle by the anterior longitudinal ligament and the longus colli muscle. These lesions may be missed on axial CT images, but they are readily visualized on the lateral radiographs and sagittal CT reconstructions.

Axis (C2) Fractures

About 15% to 20% of cervical fractures involve the axis, 40% of which are associated with head injuries and

18% with other cervical spine injuries (36–39). Approximately 25% are hangman fractures, over half (58%) are odontoid fractures, and the remainder are miscellaneous fractures involving the body, lateral mass, or spinous process (32,40,41).

Hangman Fracture (Traumatic Spondylolisthesis of C2)

Hangman fractures are variously known as traumatic spondylolisthesis of the axis (C2), fractures of the neural arch of the axis, or fractures of the ring of the axis. Schneider et al. (42) noted that this injury is identical to that created by judicial hanging (43,44), and thus the designation of the hangman fracture (42,45,46). In actuality,

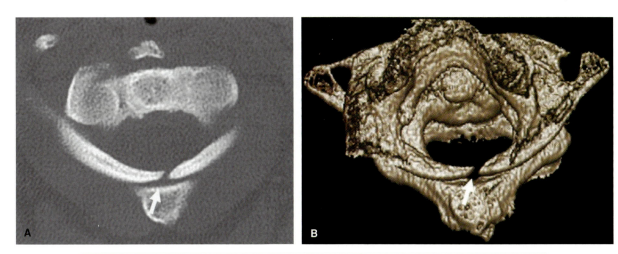

FIGURE 6-16. Partial nonossification of posterior atlas ring. **A:** Axial CT image and **(B)** volume rendered 3D reconstruction superior view show smooth margins of a partially nonossified posterior atlas ring (*arrows*).

▶ **TABLE 6-6 Hangman Fracture (Traumatic Spondylolisthesis of C2)**

Plain film findings: It is difficult to visualize the fracture on the anteroposterior view; it is best demonstrated on the lateral view.

Lateral view: The fracture usually is diagnosed readily on the lateral radiograph in >90% of cases unless nondisplaced.

- Prevertebral soft tissue swelling or hematoma related to the hyperextension mechanism may be apparent at C1 to C3 (Figs. 6-22, 6-23), but is often absent.
- Fractures are often anterior to the inferior facets. They are oblique, extending from superior/posterior to inferior/anterior (Figs. 6-18, 6-20, 6-22, 6-23).
- Positive axis ring sign (105,106), which will show posterior ring disruption from atypical fractures extending into the posterior C2 vertebral body cortex (Fig. 6-24 and Figs. 5-19 and 5-20).
- The axis body may appear widened in the AP dimension compared with that of C3 from an atypical fracture producing the "fat C2 sign" (Fig. 6-24) (105,106). In normal individuals the anteroposterior width of C2 equals that of C3 (Fig. 5-21).
- Posterior displacement of the C2 spinolaminar line of >2 mm, compared with a line drawn between the spinolaminar line of C1 and C3 (Figs. 6-18, 6-20, 6-22, 6-23 and Table 5-6 and Fig. 5-24).
- An avulsion fracture of the anterior margin of the axis or anterior superior margin at C3 is often present and identifies the site of rupture of the anterior longitudinal ligament (Fig. 6-23).

AP view: Usually not visible on AP cervical spine radiograph.

CT findings: CT is valuable to exclude or verify fracture line extension into the vertebral foramina or vertebral body, or to detect subtle concurrent adjacent injuries.

Axial images:
- Identify the sites of C2 ring fractures and extension into the vertebral foramina or vertebral body (Figs. 6-19 and 6-24).
- Establish separation between fracture fragments of the pars interarticularis of C2 (Figs. 6-19 and 6-24).

Coronal reconstruction:
- Usually provides no additional information as to the nature of the hangman fracture, but can be valuable to detect concurrent adjacent injuries.

Sagittal reconstruction:
- Assess the fractures lines and posterior displacement of the C2 spinolaminar line (Fig. 6-25)
- Assess C2-3 disc space
- Establish separation and angulation between fracture fragments of the pars interarticularis of C2 (Fig. 6-25).

UNSTABLE:
- More than 3 mm of fragment displacement or >15-degree angle at the fracture site
- Abnormal C2-3 disc space
- C2-3 dislocation
- Because multilevel fractures (C1 and C2) are considered unstable, a cautious search for contiguous fractures is critical.

the hangman fracture is a group of injuries with variable mechanisms that have different radiographic appearances (Table 6-6). The most common form of this injury results from extension combined with axial loading. The full force of acute hyperextension of the head on the neck is transmitted through the pedicles of C2 onto the apophyseal joints (45). The weakest points in this chain are the interarticular segments of the pedicle. Thus, the arch of C2 is fractured anterior to the inferior facet (45). These injuries are commonly sustained in automobile accidents as the chin or forehead encounters the steering wheel or dashboard, forcing the head into hyperextension. Hangman fracture is a bilateral fracture through the pars interarticularis of C2. The pars interarticularis is found between the superior and inferior articular processes of C2. Spinal cord damage is uncommon, despite frequent significant fracture displacement, due to the wide spinal canal at this level.

Effendi et al. (47) described a classification of the hangman fracture that includes three types. Type I fracture is defined as an isolated "hairline" fracture, with <3 mm fragment displacement, <15-degree angle at the fracture site, and normal C2-3 disc space (Figs. 6-18, 6-19, 6-20). The mechanism of this injury is hyperextension with concomitant axial loading and a force sufficient enough to cause the fracture but not enough to disrupt the ALL, PLL, or the C2-3 disc. These lesions are often subtle and easily missed radiographically. Commonly associated concomitant injuries are C1 posterior arch fractures, C1 lateral mass fractures, and odontoid fractures. Type II injuries are characterized by more than 3 mm of fragment displacement (Fig. 6-21) or more than a 15-degree angle at the fracture site and an abnormal C2-3 disc space. The mechanism of this injury is hyperextension with concomitant axial loading, followed by flexion with concomitant axial compression. The resultant injury pattern is bilateral pedicle fractures with slight disruption of the ALL and significant disruption of the PLL and C2-3 disc.

Levin and Edwards (48), modifying the work of Effendi et al. (47), introduced a new subtype of this fracture, type IIA (Fig. 6-22). Type IIA fractures demonstrate no anterior displacement but do show severe angulation. The mechanism for this injury is flexion with concomitant distraction. The resultant injury pattern is bilateral pedicle fractures with C2-3 disc disruption and some degree of insult to the PLL. This is an unstable fracture. Radiographs taken while the patient is in cervical traction demonstrate an increase in the C2-3 posterior disc space.

Type III consists of the changes that characterize type II injury plus a C2-3 articular facet dislocation (Fig. 6-23). In type III there is displacement of the body of the axis forward in the flexion position associated with disruption of the facet joints of C2-3, which are either dislocated or locked. In the series of Effendi et al. (47), 65% of hangman

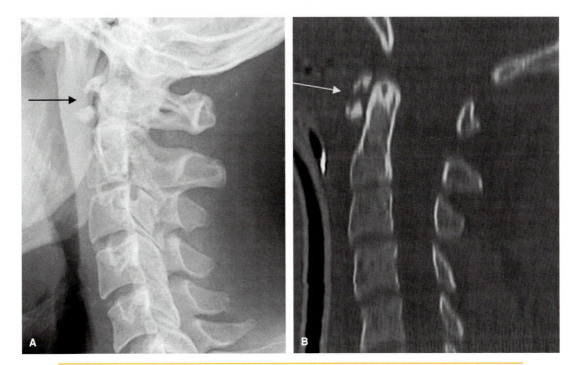

FIGURE 6-17. Hyperextension avulsion (horizontal) fracture of the anterior arch of C1. **A:** Lateral radiograph and **(B)** sagittal CT multiplanar reformation show an avulsion fracture of the anterior atlas arch (*arrows*) and prevertebral soft tissue swelling.

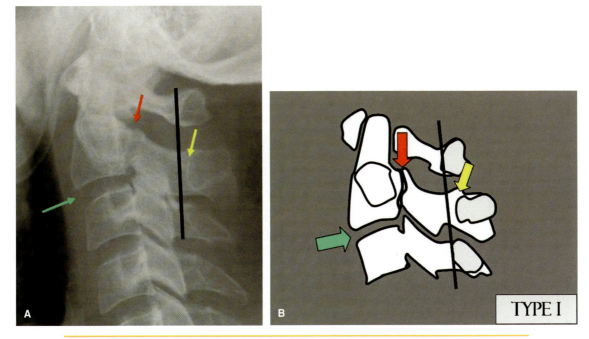

FIGURE 6-18. Type I hangman fracture. **A:** Lateral radiograph and **(B)** type I hangman fracture illustration demonstrate a nondisplaced subtle fracture line through the pars interarticularis of the axis (*red arrow*) and posterior offset of the C2 spinolaminar line (*black line/yellow arrow*). The second intervertebral disc is intact (*green arrow*).

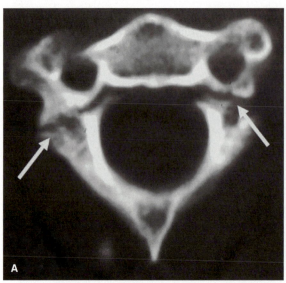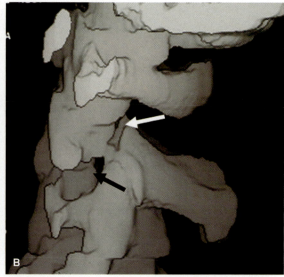

FIGURE 6-19. Type I hangman fracture. **A:** Axial CT demonstrates the bilateral pars fracture of C2 (*white arrows*) without significant fragment displacement. **B:** CT reformatted 3D surface rendered lateral view shows the nondisplaced subtle fracture line through the pars interarticularis of the axis (*white arrows*) and normal C2-3 disc space (*black arrow*).

fractures were type I, 28% were type II, and 7 % were type III. Type I injuries are considered stable, type II and III injuries are considered unstable (Table 6-6).

"Atypical" traumatic spondylolisthesis of C2, even though quite common, refers to a lesion in which one (uni-lateral) or both (bilateral) fractures occur in the coronal plane of the middle column of the axis body (5) (Figs. 6-24, 6-25). In this variant hangman fracture, the involved component of the posterior vertebral body may undergo retropulsion and may contribute to cord injury. The clinical significance of identifying the atypical hangman fracture relates to the approximately 30% higher incidence of paralysis than occurs with typical Effendi type I and II injuries.

Odontoid Fractures

Fractures of the odontoid process arise as a result of diverse mechanisms. The traditional classification of dens

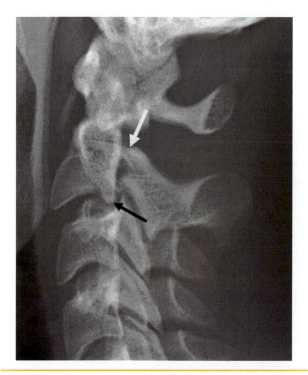

FIGURE 6-20. Type I hangman fracture. Lateral cervical radiograph demonstrates fracture through the pars interarticularis (*white arrow*) without extension to the "C2 ring." There is slight anterior displacement of the axis body without angulation (*black arrow*).

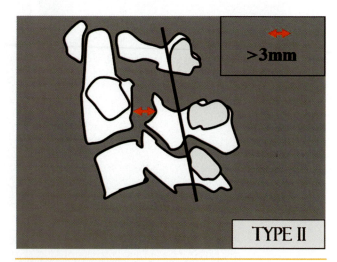

FIGURE 6-21. Type II hangman fracture. Illustration demonstrates >3 mm of fragment displacement and posterior offset of the C2 spinolaminar line.

▶ **TABLE 6-7** Odontoid Fractures

Plain film findings: The radiologic diagnosis of odontoid fractures usually is established using the lateral cervical and open-mouth odontoid view radiographs.

Open-mouth odontoid view: In types I and II dens fractures the diagnosis depends primarily on radiographic findings in the anteroposterior open-mouth projection.

- Radiographically, type I odontoid fractures are characterized by an oblique fracture of the superolateral odontoid process.
- Radiographically, type II odontoid fractures are characterized by a transverse or oblique transverse fracture through the lower portion of the dens. The fracture is confined to the dens only.
- The transverse fracture at the base of the dens must be differentiated from a developmental abnormality termed as os odontoideum (107). Os odontoideum is rounded, has a cortical margin around its entire surface, and is usually more widely separated from the base of the odontoid than a fracture. Nonunion odontoid fractures may be impossible to distinguish from an os odontoideum.
- A Mach effect is frequently seen at the base of the dens on the open-mouth odontoid view and is caused by either the inferior cortex of the posterior neural arch of the atlas or the superior cortex of the neural arch of the axis. Extension of the Mach lines beyond the dens or the axis body allows distinction from acute fractures.

Lateral view: (Difficult diagnosis on the lateral view) (Figs. 6-28, 6-34, 5-35, 6-36).

- The retropharyngeal soft tissue may be abnormal in both contour and thickness.
- Minimal displacement often precludes demonstration of the fracture line.
- The anterior and posterior cortical margins of the dens and body of C2 should be examined closely on the lateral projection for evidence of cortical disruption. Positive axis ring sign (105,106) will show posterior or anterior ring disruption in type III fractures.
- Type III fractures are almost always better visualized on the lateral projection and may not be evident on the anteroposterior view (Fig. 6-34).
- Anterior or posterior displacement of the C2 spinolaminar line of >2 mm, relative to a line drawn between the spinolaminar line of C1 and C3.
- The axis body may appear widened in AP dimension compared with that of C3 in type III fractures, producing the "fat C2 sign."

AP view: Usually not visible on AP cervical spine radiograph.

CT findings:

Axial images:
- A type II odontoid fracture oriented in the axial plane may not be demonstrated on axial CT images but should be demonstrated on sagittal and coronal reformations.
- Assess comminution in type II odontoid fracture.

Coronal reconstruction:
- Assess the odontoid fractures lines (Figs. 6-29, 6-30, 6-31, 6-33).
- Establish the lateral odontoid process/C1 displacement.

Sagittal reconstruction:
- Assess the odontoid fractures lines (Figs. 6-29, 6-31, 6-32, 6-33, 6-34, and 6-36).
- Establish the anterior or posterior odontoid process/C1 displacement (Fig. 6-32 and 6-36).
- The retropharyngeal soft tissue may be abnormal in both contour and thickness (Fig. 6-29).
- 3D reconstructions: (superior and frontal views) (Fig. 6-30, 6-35, and 6-36).
- 3D reconstructions synthesize 2D image information.
- 3D images are useful in complex odontoid fractures presenting with vertebral rotation or dislocation and loss of alignment.
- Easy to visualize the spatial relation between C1 and C2.

UNSTABLE:
- If the odontoid fragment is displaced by >5 mm, a 75% nonunion rate results (106). This increases to 86% with more than 6 mm of displacement (55).
- Odontoid fracture with anterior or posterior displacement of the C2 spinolaminar line of >2 mm relative to a line drawn between the spinolaminar line of C1 and C3.
- Because multilevel fractures (C1 and C2) are considered unstable, a cautious search for contiguous fractures is critical (Fig. 6-35 and Fig. 5-1).
- Odontoid fractures with atlanto-axial dissociation.

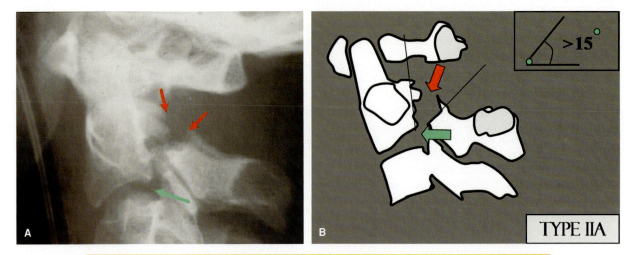

FIGURE 6-22. Type IIA hangman fracture. **A:** Lateral radiograph and **(B)** illustration demonstrate a hangman fracture with significant angulation (>15 degree) and displacement (>3 mm) at the fracture site (*red arrows*). Note the abnormal posterior widening of the C2-3 disc space (*green arrow*).

fractures proposed by Anderson and D'Alonso (49) consists of three types based upon the location of the fracture site with respect to the dens (Fig. 6-26, Table 6-7). Type I is described as an oblique fracture of the superior lateral aspect of the dens, avulsed by the alar ("check") ligament; this is an extremely uncommon injury, occurring in <4% of odontoid fractures (Fig. 6-27). Type I injuries may indicate atlanto-occipital dislocation and should be regarded as a sign of instability (50). The type II fracture, also referred to as a high odontoid fracture by Gehweiler et al. (51) and Alexander et al. (52), is a fracture at the base of the dens (Figs. 6-28, 6-29, 6-30, 6-31, 6-32, 6-33, 6-34, 6-35,

6-36) (Figs. 5-1 and 5-22). In 1988 Hadley et al. (53) introduced a comminuted subtype of this fracture, type IIA. Since then, several authors have recommended a more aggressive surgical approach in the treatment of this subtype. However, only a few cases of comminuted type II fractures have been reported. Koivikko et al. (54) in 2003 reviewed 26 type II fractures imaged by multislice CT. Subtle comminution of the fracture was observed in 12 of the cases. They concluded that subtle comminution in type II odontoid fractures is seen more commonly than previously reported in the literature when imaged by multislice CT. The type III fracture, also referred to as a low

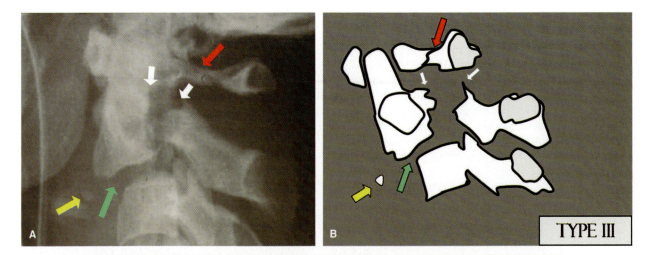

FIGURE 6-23. Type III hangman fracture. **A:** Lateral radiograph and **(B)** illustration demonstrate a hangman fracture with significant angulation (>15 degree) and displacement (>3 mm) at the fracture site (*white arrows*), bilateral interfacetal dislocation, disrupted C2-3 disc, posterior atlas ring fracture (*arrowhead*), massive prevertebral soft tissue swelling, and extension teardrop fracture of the axis (*black arrow*).

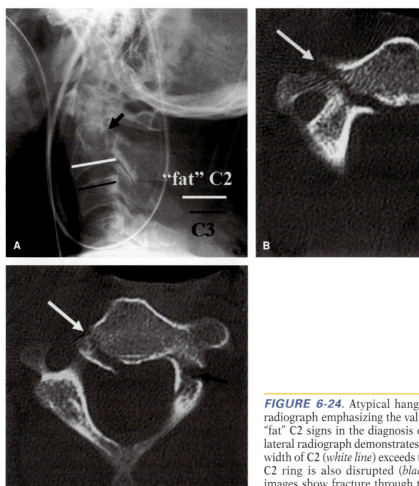

FIGURE 6-24. Atypical hangman fracture. **A:** Lateral radiograph emphasizing the value of the "ring of C2" and "fat" C2 signs in the diagnosis of C2 body fractures. The lateral radiograph demonstrates the "fat" C2; note that the width of C2 (*white line*) exceeds that of C3 (*black line*). The C2 ring is also disrupted (*black arrow*). **B,C:** Axial CT images show fracture through the right axis body (*white arrow*) and comminuted fracture involving the left pars interarticularis (*black arrow*).

odontoid fracture by Gehweiler et al. (51) and Alexander et al. (52), is an oblique fracture of the superior portion of the axis body caudal to its junction with the base of the dens (Figs. 6-33, 6-34). Type II injuries are the most common injury, comprising 60% of dens fractures (55). Both acute and un-united type II odontoid fractures result in atlantoaxial instability because the proximal (cephalad) fragment and the atlas constitute a single unit (Figs. 6-32, 6-36). Dens fractures are frequently associated with fractures of the face and mandible, Jefferson fractures (Fig. 6-35), and extension teardrop fractures. Weisskopf et al. (56) compared four different radiological diagnostic methods in the analysis of odontoid fractures. Thirty-one patients with odontoid fractures were investigated using standard anteroposterior and lateral radiographs, conventional tomography, axial computerized tomography, and two-dimensional reconstruction in the sagittal and the coronal planes. They found that CT examination with sagittal and coronal reconstructions was equivalent to conventional tomography in diagnostic accuracy and was also less time consuming. They concluded, therefore, that CT could replace conventional tomography.

C2 Lateral Body Fractures

An isolated C2 lateral body fracture is rare and is usually found incidentally when evaluating for other C2 traumatic pathology (Fig. 6-37). If a C2 lateral body fracture is found, other C-spine pathology must be sought (ipsilateral occipital condyle, C1 lateral mass, and lower cervical spine fractures). The mechanism of this fracture is axial compression with concomitant lateral bending. The isolated fracture may present with high neck pain and a normal neurological examination. Radiographic findings include impaction of the C2 component of the atlantoaxial articulation surface, asymmetry of C2 lateral body height, and lateral tilting of the arch of C1. Atlanto-occipital and atlantoaxial dissociation can be seen.

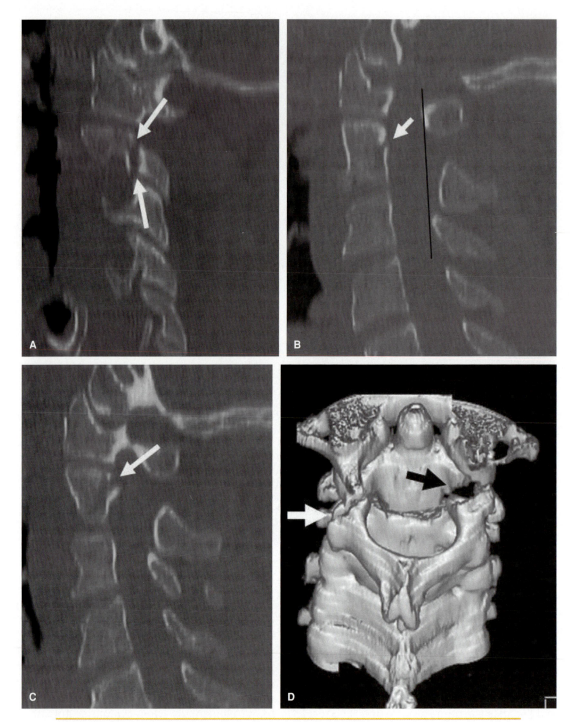

FIGURE 6-25. Atypical hangman fracture. **A:** Left parasagittal CT multiplanar reformation show the pars interarticularis fracture (*arrows*). **B,C:** Right parasagittal CT multiplanar reformations demonstrate a fracture line extending into the posterior axis body (*arrows*). Note the posterior offset of C2 spinolaminar line **(B)**. **D:** Reformatted 3D volume rendered cutaway posterior view establishes a pars fracture on the left (*white arrow*) and the atypical fracture through the right side of the axis body (*black arrow*). This is an Effendi type II lesion because of anterior translation of the anterior body fragment on the right side.

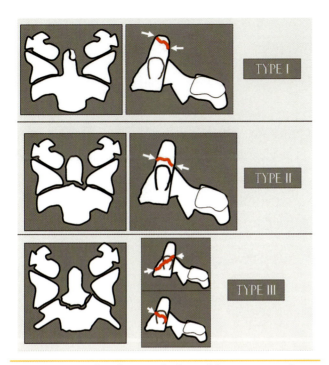

FIGURE 6-26. Classification of odontoid fractures according to Anderson and D'Alonso. (Anderson LD, D'Alonzo RT. Fractures of the odontoid process of the axis. *J Bone Joint Surg.* 1974;56A:1663–1674.)

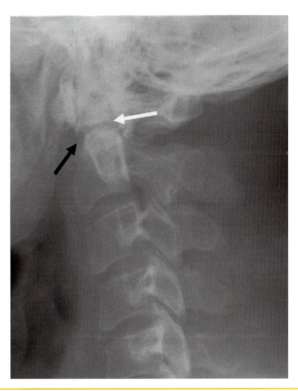

FIGURE 6-28. Type II odontoid fracture. Lateral cervical radiograph demonstrates a transverse fracture through the base of the odontoid (*white arrow*) with minimal anterior displacement of the cephalad fragment (cortical "step-off," *black arrow*).

Atlantoaxial Dissociation

Acute traumatic atlantoaxial dissociation (AAD) is a rare injury in which there is partial (subluxation) or complete (dislocation) derangement of the lateral atlantoaxial articulations. This is directly related to an acute traumatic event, and radiographic diagnosis may be difficult, particularly in the rotational forms. AAD is characterized by excessive movement at the junction between the atlas (C1) and axis (C2) due to either a bony or ligamentous abnormality. Neurologic symptoms occur when the spinal

(text continues on page 116)

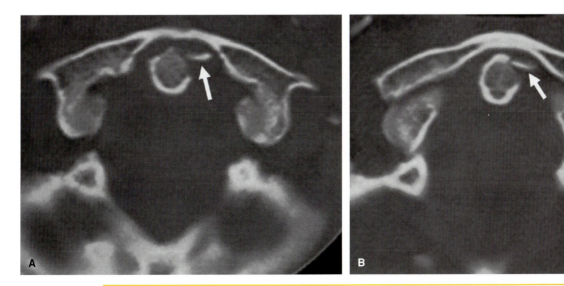

FIGURE 6-27. Type I odontoid fracture. **A,B:** Axial CT images. In both axial images a small fracture fragment (*white arrows*) is avulsed from the left superolateral aspect of the dens.

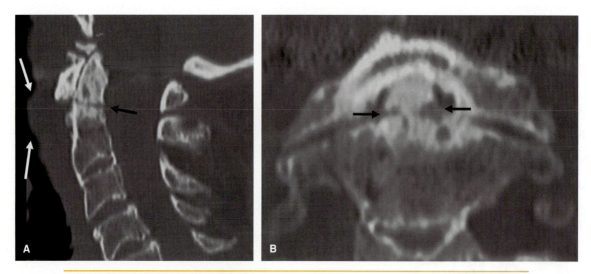

FIGURE 6-29. Type II odontoid fracture. **A:** sagittal and **(B)** coronal CT multiplanar reformations demonstrate a nondisplaced type II odontoid fracture (*black arrow*). Note the abnormal cervico-cranial prevertebral soft tissue contour in **(A)** (*white arrows*).

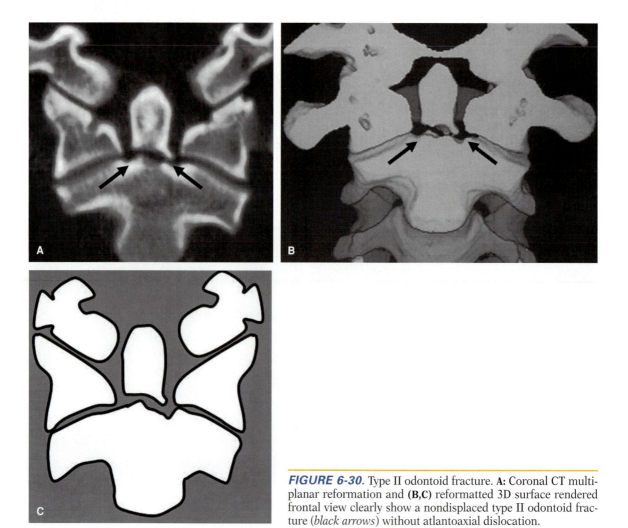

FIGURE 6-30. Type II odontoid fracture. **A:** Coronal CT multiplanar reformation and **(B,C)** reformatted 3D surface rendered frontal view clearly show a nondisplaced type II odontoid fracture (*black arrows*) without atlantoaxial dislocation.

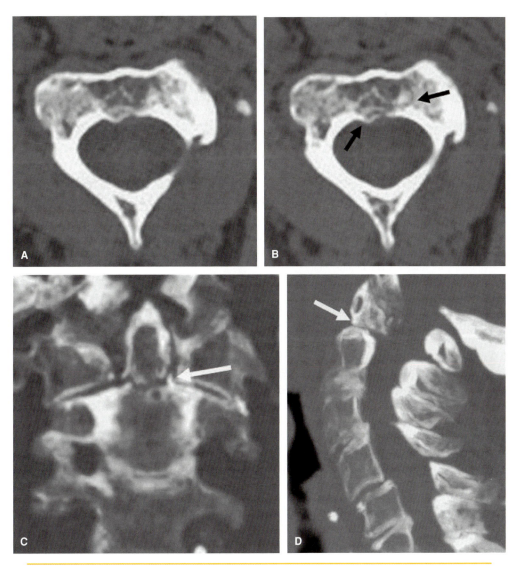

FIGURE 6-31. Subtle Type II odontoid fracture. **A,B:** Axial CT images through the odontoid were nondiagnostic, demonstrating a questionable fracture line (*black arrows*). **C:** Coronal and **(D)** lateral 3D MIP reformations reveal the minimally displaced type II odontoid fracture (*white arrows*).

cord is involved. Certain congenital conditions can be associated with AAD, including Down syndrome, osteogenesis imperfecta, neurofibromatosis, Morquio syndrome, spondyloepiphyseal dysplasia congenita, and chondrodysplasia punctata. In individuals with Down syndrome, the primary cause of AAD is the laxity of the transverse ligament (which holds the dens against the posterior border of the anterior arch).

The three mechanisms of AAD are flexion extension, distraction, and rotation. The most common abnormalities involve the transverse ligament or odontoid process. Fielding and Hawkins (57), in 1977, subdivided atlantoaxial rotatory fixation into four categories (Table 6-8).

Type I AAD: AAD with rotatory fixation without anterior displacement of the atlas. The odontoid acts as the pivot and the transverse and alar ligaments are intact. This is the most common type of rotatory fixation and occurs within the normal range of rotation of the atlantoaxial joint (Figs. 6-38, 6-39).

Type II AAD: Rotatory fixation with <5 mm of anterior displacement of the atlas. This is the second most common type and is associated with deficiency of the transverse ligament.

Type III AAD: Rotatory fixation with >5 mm of anterior displacement of the atlas. This degree of displacement implies deficiency of the TAL (Fig. 6-40).

▶ **TABLE 6-8** Rotatory Atlantoaxial Dissociation

Plain film findings: The "cock-robin" posture makes radiographic positioning difficult. The complex anatomy of the atlantoaxial region coupled with problems of positioning make radiographs difficult to interpret.

Open-mouth odontoid view:

- Shows asymmetry of the lateral masses of C1 with respect to the odontoid. The lateral mass that has rotated forward appears wider and closer to the midline. As the head is turned to the left, the right C1 lateral mass appears to increase in width, the lateral atlanto-dental space (LADS) narrows, and the joint space appears to widen, while the left lateral mass appears truncated, the left LADS increases, and joint space appears to narrow.
- The facet joints may be obscured because of apparent overlapping.
- The combined spread of the lateral masses of C1 on C2 should not exceed 7 mm. A number >7 mm would indicate rupture of the transverse ligament.
- Displacement of the spinous process of the axis from the midline in the direction opposite that of head rotation.
- In practice, the odontoid view is often extremely difficult to obtain in these patients.

Lateral view: (The lateral cervical spine radiograph is difficult to interpret because of head tilt.)

- The atlas may be obscured by the skull and appearances may simulate occipito-atlantal assimilation (61).
- Indistinctness of the anterior atlanto-dental space.
- Depending on the degree of rotation, one lateral mass of the atlas may be seen anterior to the odontoid on the lateral cervical radiograph.
- Because of head tilt, the right and left sides of the posterior arch of the atlas fail to superimpose.
- Asses anterior atlanto-dental interval (AADI): Normal <3 mm (adult patients), 3–5 mm with anterior displacement of C1 (TAL injury), >5 mm with anterior displacement of C1 (TAL and alar ligament injury).
- The retropharyngeal soft tissue may be abnormal in both contour and thickness.

UNSTABLE:

- Abnormal AADI: >3 mm (adult patients), implies transverse atlantal ligament (TAL) or alar ligament injury.
- On the open-mouth odontoid view, the combined spread of the lateral masses of C1 on C2 should not exceed 7 mm. A number greater than 7 mm would indicate rupture of the transverse ligament.
- Anterior or posterior displacement of the C2 spinolaminar line of >2 mm relative to a line drawn between the spinolaminar line of C1 and C3.

CT findings: Because of difficulties in obtaining and interpreting plain radiographs, CT is essential for imaging this condition.

Axial images:

- Demonstrate the rotated position of the atlas on the axis (Fig. 6-38). In subluxation or dislocation, the amount of maximal rotation of C1 relative to C2 typically exceeds the normal maximal 45 degrees (108) and may approach 90 degrees with dislocation.
- Associated forward (Fielding type II and III) or backward (Fielding type IV) displacement of the atlas may be appreciated.
- Fractures undetectable at plain radiography may be revealed (Fig. 6-38).

Coronal reconstruction:

- The combined spread of the lateral masses of C1 on C2 should not exceed 7 mm. A number >7 mm indicates rupture of the transverse ligament.
- Establish the lateral odontoid process/C1 displacement.
- 3D reconstructions (superior and frontal views):

Superior view:

- Demonstrates the rotated position of the atlas on the axis (Fig. 6-39).
- Associated forward (Fielding type II and III) or backward (Fielding type IV) displacement of the atlas may be appreciated (Fig. 6-36).

Frontal view:

- The combined spread of the lateral masses of C1 on C2 should not exceed 7 mm. A number >7 mm indicates rupture of the transverse ligament.
- Establish the lateral odontoid process/C1 displacement (Fig. 6-40).

Because static CT appearances in patients with type I rotatory AAD and torticollis are identical to normal subjects who have voluntarily turned their heads, a dynamic study is recommended (58–60). Patients are initially examined at rest and CT is subsequently repeated with maximal voluntary contralateral rotation of the head. In patients with rotatory fixation, CT demonstrates little or no motion of the atlas on the axis with this maneuver, whereas CT in normal volunteers shows a reduction or a reversal of the rotation (58,59).

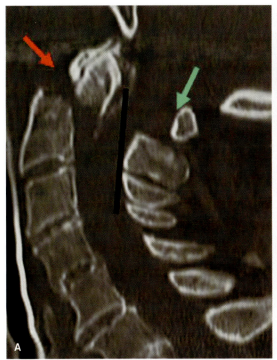

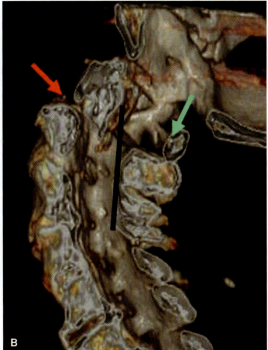

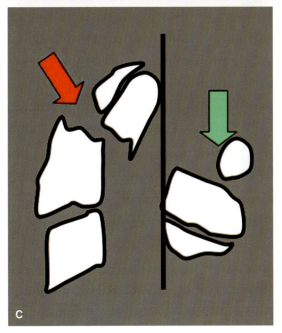

FIGURE 6-32. Displaced Type II odontoid fracture with posterior atlantoaxial dislocation. **A:** Sagittal CT multiplanar reformation and **(B)** reformatted 3D CT volume rendered cutaway lateral view show a displaced type II odontoid fracture (*red arrows*) with posterior atlantoaxial dislocation. **C:** Note the posterior offset of the C1 spinolaminar line (*green arrows*).

Type IV AAD: Rotatory fixation with posterior displacement of the atlas. This is the most uncommon type and occurs with deficiency of the dens, such as in type II odontoid process fractures (Fig. 6-36) or unstable os odontoideum (congenital or posttraumatic).

All of these injuries can be associated with concurrent fractures, neurological deficits, or vertebral artery injury that will, in part, determine the method of stabilization and need for internal fixation. AAD types II, III, and IV may compromise the spinal canal, resulting in cord compression and neurological signs; the prognosis is therefore graver than in type I (57).

Because static CT appearances in patients with type I rotatory AAD and torticollis are identical to normal subjects who have voluntarily turned their heads, a dynamic study is recommended (58–60). Patients are initially examined at rest and CT is subsequently repeated with

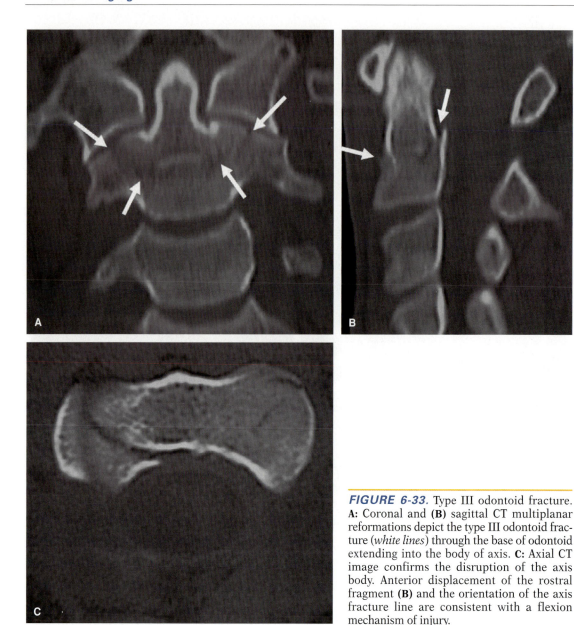

FIGURE 6-33. Type III odontoid fracture. **A:** Coronal and **(B)** sagittal CT multiplanar reformations depict the type III odontoid fracture (*white lines*) through the base of odontoid extending into the body of axis. **C:** Axial CT image confirms the disruption of the axis body. Anterior displacement of the rostral fragment **(B)** and the orientation of the axis fracture line are consistent with a flexion mechanism of injury.

maximal voluntary contralateral rotation of the head. In patients with rotatory fixation, CT demonstrates little or no motion of the atlas on the axis with this maneuver, whereas CT in normal volunteers shows a reduction or a reversal of the rotation (58,59).

DISRUPTION OF THE TRANSVERSE PORTION OF THE CRUCIATE LIGAMENT (TRANSVERSE ATLANTAL LIGAMENT)

Acute injuries involving the TAL include rupture of the ligament itself (Fig. 6-40) or detachment of the ligament from the lateral mass of C1 by virtue of an avulsion

fracture (Fig. 6-41). Acute traumatic rupture of the TAL may be associated with a Jefferson fracture or a fracture of the lateral mass of C1 caused by lateral tilt. On the open-mouth odontoid view, rupture of the TAL is indicated if the combined spread of the lateral masses of C1 on C2 exceeds 7 mm. On the lateral view, an anterior atlanto-dental interval (AADI) >3 mm indicates injury to the TAL. In most cases, the injury is purely ligamentous and unlikely to heal. Therefore, these injuries usually are treated with posterior C1-2 fusion. If CT scan reveals a bony avulsion injury as the source of failure, a trial of halo bracing may be indicated.

It must be remembered, however, that rheumatoid arthritis may widen the AADI due to erosion of the dens or attenuation of the TAL (Fig. 6-40).

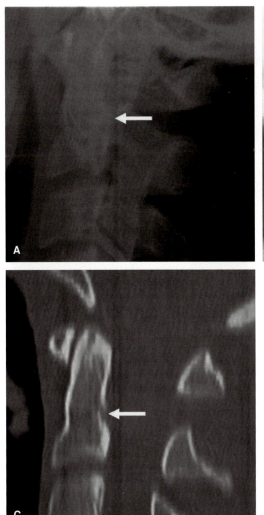

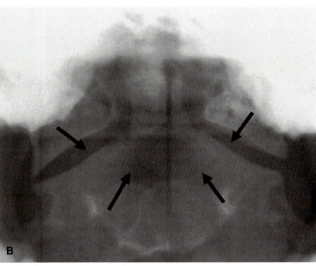

FIGURE 6-34. Subtle type III odontoid fracture. On the lateral radiograph **(A)**, the fracture is extremely subtle, being indicated by disruption of the posterior arc of the axis ring (*white arrow*) and "fat axis body" appearance. On the open-mouth projection **(B)**, the fracture line is barely visible (*black arrows*). Sagittal multiplanar CT reformation **(C)** confirms the type III dens fracture line (*white arrow*).

Torticollis

Atlantoaxial rotational injury must be distinguished from torticollis (Fig. 6-42). Torticollis, or "wry neck," is more precisely defined as "acute rotational displacement" and may be due to a variety of conditions. It is clinically manifested by simultaneous lateral tilt and rotation of the head. The causes of torticollis can be subdivided in two groups (61):

- Disorders of rotation of the atlantoaxial joint resulting in fixed or limited rotation of the neck. This may occur spontaneously, secondary to trauma, or in association with congenital anomalies or arthritides.
- Other disorders causing limited rotation of the neck without primarily involving the atlantoaxial joint, where the primary abnormality is in the sternocleidomastoid muscle (congenital fibrosis, lymphadenitis, tumors of the cervical spine, painful neck).

Rotatory subluxation is sometimes observed after upper respiratory infection or after head and neck surgery. Grisel syndrome is the occurrence of atlantoaxial subluxation (AAS) in association with inflammation of adjacent soft tissues. The etiology is not totally understood, but Parke et al. (62) demonstrated a direct connection between the periodontal venous plexus and the pharyngovertebral veins. This may provide a route for exudates to be transported to the cervical spine, creating a local inflammatory reaction. In addition, children appear to be more susceptible secondary to their steeper dens-facet angle and rich vascular folds in the atlantoaxial and lateral atlantoaxial joint.

Torticollis is usually self-limited and occurs mainly in children to young adolescents (58). The symptoms usually disappear in 4 to 5 days. Most cases resolve spontaneously, although in a few instances the rotatory deformity becomes fixed and irreducible. The fixation usually

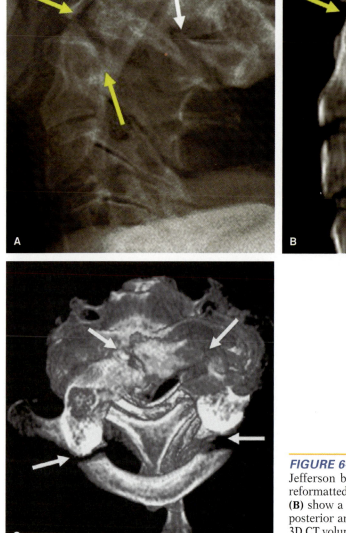

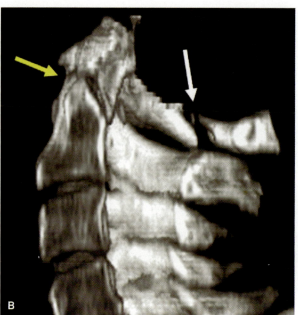

FIGURE 6-35. Type II odontoid fracture associated with a Jefferson bursting fracture. Lateral radiograph **(A)** and reformatted 3D CT volume rendered cutaway lateral view **(B)** show a type II odontoid fracture (*yellow arrows*) with posterior arch of C1 fracture (*white arrows*). Reformatted 3D CT volume rendered superior view **(C)** demonstrates the C1 anterior and posterior arch fractures (*white arrows*).

occurs within the normal range of rotation of the atlantoaxial joint. In some cases, however, true subluxation or dislocation occurs (59,61,63).

LOWER CERVICAL SPINE INJURIES (C3-7)

Flexion Injuries

When the predominant force vector is applied in flexion, compression of the anterior column and distraction of the posterior column occur. Injuries in this group include the following: clay-shoveler fracture, anterior subluxation, simple wedge compression fracture without posterior disruption, bilateral facet dislocation, and flexion teardrop fracture. Some of these injuries are purely ligamentous, some are purely bony, and some represent a combination of bony and ligamentous injuries.

Clay-shoveler Fracture

The clay-shoveler fracture is an avulsion injury of the spinous process of C6, C7, or T1 (in order of frequency). The fracture results from abrupt flexion of the head and

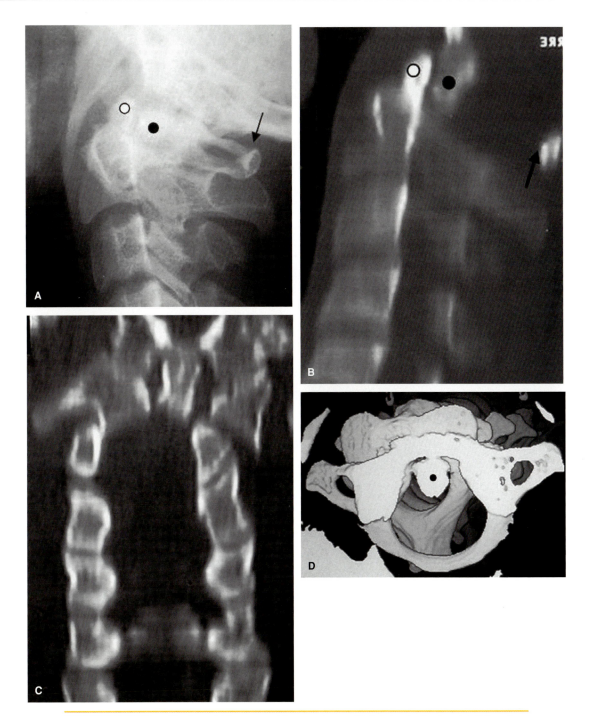

FIGURE 6-36. Type II odontoid fracture with posterior and left lateral atlantoaxial dislocation. **A:** Lateral cervical radiograph shows posterior displacement of the odontoid process (*black dot*) and the atlas vertebra. Note that the anterior arch of C1 (*white dot*) lies superior to the C2 vertebral body and there is posterior offset of the C1 spinolaminar line (*black arrow*). Sagittal **(B)** and coronal **(C)** multiplanar CT reformations demonstrate the type II odontoid fracture and the posterior **(B)** and left lateral **(C)** displacement of C1. **D:** Reformatted 3D CT surface rendered superior axial view shows posterior and left lateral displacement of C1 and the odontoid process (*black dot*), with minimal rotation of C1 to the left. Additionally, there is significant involvement of the spinal canal with narrowing of its AP and lateral diameters. The proximal (cephalad) dens fragment (*black dot*) and the atlas constitute a single unit. The anterior atlanto-dental interval (AADI) is normal.

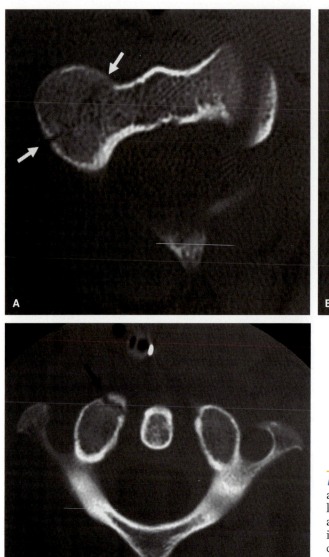

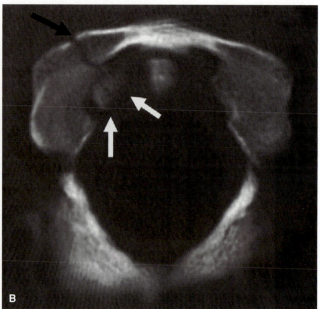

FIGURE 6-37. Right occipital condyle fracture associated with asymmetric atlas ring fracture and right lateral body of C2 from lateral flexion. **A:** Axial CT image shows a nondisplaced fracture across the right lateral body of C2 (*white arrows*). **B,C:** Axial CT images show a minimally displaced fracture of right occipital condyle (*white arrows*). Note associated fracture of the right anterior atlas arch (*black arrow in B*) extending into the medial right C1 lateral mass (*black arrow in C*).

neck against the tensed ligaments of the posterior aspect of the neck (64). The name is derived from the cervical spine injury sustained by Australian clay miners who, when attempting to throw a shovel full of clay from the mine floor, abruptly pulled their heads and necks into hyperflexion when the shovel stuck in the clay. It is the opposite of anterior subluxation in that the posterior longitudinal ligament remains intact, producing an avulsion fracture of the spinous process. The clay-shoveler fracture line has a characteristic oblique orientation and a typical location within the spinous process (Figs. 6-43, 6-44). The typical clay-shoveler fracture is both mechanically and neurologically stable. Atypically, the fracture may extend into the lamina, in which case the spinal canal is involved and there is potential for spinal cord injury (Fig. 6-45).

Anterior Subluxation (Hyperflexion Subluxation or Sprain)

Anterior subluxation (AS) in the cervical spine occurs when posterior ligamentous complexes (nuchal ligament, capsular ligaments, supraspinous and infraspinous ligaments, ligamenta flava, posterior longitudinal ligament) rupture and a minor tear of the annulus posteriorly, with varying degrees of extension into the posterior aspect of the disc (Table 6-9, Figs. 6-46, 6-47, 6-48, 6-49). The anterior longitudinal

(text continues on page 128)

▶ **TABLE 6-9** Anterior Subluxation (Hyperflexion Subluxation or Sprain)

Plain film findings:

Lateral view: The radiological diagnosis may be made from lateral views of the cervical spine in neutral position or from dynamic views. Dynamic views or MRI should be obtained when the diagnosis of anterior subluxation (AS) is equivocal on the neutral film. Optimally, dynamic projections should be made with the patient erect, with an experienced physician in attendance, and with an alert and cooperative patient. Removal of the cervical immobilization device requires prior clinical "clearance" and the absence of instability signs on the initial AP and lateral neutral position examinations (Table 6-2). Flexion and extension must be unassisted, with the patient limiting motion to the level of pain tolerance. The findings of AS seen in neutral position become exaggerated upon flexion and are reduced in extension.

- Abrupt hyperkyphotic angulation at the level of ligamentous injury. The abrupt angulation distinguishes AS from the smooth, continuous, uninterrupted physiologic reversal of cervical lordosis produced by the military position, recumbency, or muscle spasm (Figs. 6-46, 6-47, 6-48).
- Widening of the interspinous distance at one level ("fanning"), relative to adjacent levels (Fig. 6-46, 6-47, 6-48).
- Exposure of the superior facet joint surface of the vertebra below the lesion (Fig. 6-47).
- Incongruity of the contiguous facets of the affected apophyseal joints.
- Lack of parallelism of facets (Figs. 6-46 and 6-47).
- Disc space is widened posteriorly and narrowed anteriorly.
- Involved vertebra may be displaced (translated) slightly anteriorly (1–3 mm) (Fig. 6-49). Green et al. (109) state that anterior displacement of 1 mm to 3 mm indicates subluxation, while displacement in excess of 3.5 mm indicates frank dislocation or fracture. Abel (110) has referred to this displacement as sagging and has found it to be highly suggestive of instability of the posterior elements. It is important to be aware that AS can occur without anterior translation.
- Involved vertebra may be anteriorly rotated on its anteroinferior corner.
- Small anterior superior compression fractures of the subjacent vertebral body (Fig. 6-47).
- Increased thickness of the prevertebral soft tissues as a result of hematoma formation (evidence of disc and/or ligament damage).

AP view:
- Widening of the interspinous distance (Fig. 6-47). This sign represents the "fanning" seen on the lateral radiograph.
- Lateral dislocation (also called lateral translation) may occur without significant anterior or posterior displacement.

UNSTABLE:
- Anterior translation of the vertebral body >3.5 mm relative to the subjacent vertebra.
- Vertebral body angulation >20 degrees relative to the adjacent vertebra.
- Vertebral body angulation >11 degrees relative to the adjacent vertebral body pairs.

CT findings: CT is valuable for detection of radiographically occult fractures. CT is unlikely to be of significant value in the diagnosis of AS.

Axial images:
- Fractures undetectable at plain radiography may be revealed.
- Naked facet sign: In AS the superior vertebra subluxes forward and there is anterior displacement of its inferior articulating facet on the superior articulating facet of the vertebra below. This results in an uncovering of the articulating facet surfaces. The degree of facet uncovering varies. The naked facet sign refers to the CT appearance of uncovered articulating processes (Fig. 5-26). On axial CT images, the involved level will reveal bilateral solitary nonarticulating facets with loss of the joint space (111).

Sagittal reformation: The facet relationships may be better revealed in sagittal multiplanar reconstructions.
- Abrupt hyperkyphotic angulation at the level of ligamentous injury (Fig. 6-48).
- Widening of the interspinous distance at one level ("fanning") relative to adjacent levels (Fig. 6-48).
- Exposure of the superior facet joint surface of the vertebra below the lesion.
- Incongruity of contiguous facets of the affected apophyseal joints.
- Lack of parallelism of facets.
- Disc space is widened posteriorly and narrowed anteriorly.
- Involved vertebra may be displaced (translated) slightly anteriorly (1–3 mm). Abel (110) has referred to this displacement as "sagging" and has found it to be highly suggestive of instability of the posterior elements. It is important to be aware that AS can occur without anterior translation.
- Involved vertebra may be anteriorly rotated on its anteroinferior corner.
- Small anterior superior compression fractures of the subjacent vertebral body.
- Increased thickness of the prevertebral soft tissues as a result of hematoma formation (evidence of disc and/or ligament damage).

Coronal reformation:
- Lateral dislocation (also called lateral translation) may occur without significant anterior or posterior displacement.

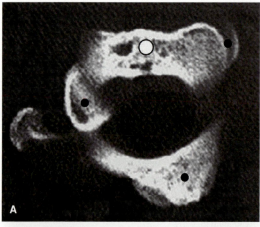

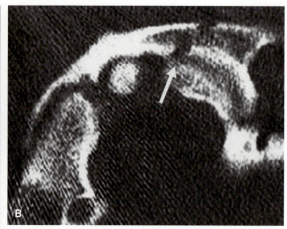

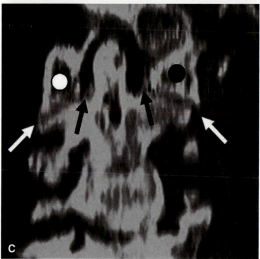

FIGURE 6-38. Atlantoaxial rotatory subluxation associated with left lateral mass of C1 fracture. **A:** Axial CT image at the level of the lateral masses and posterior arch of C1 (*black dots*) and body of C2 (*white dot*) shows rotation of C1 to the right. **B:** Axial CT image at the level of the anterior arch of C1 demonstrates a fracture of the left lateral mass of C1 (*white arrow*). **C:** Coronal CT multiplanar reformation shows asymmetry of the lateral atlanto-dental spaces (*black arrows*) and a difference in the atlantoaxial joint spaces (*white arrows*) secondary to rotational malalignment. Increased transverse diameter of the left lateral mass of C1 (*black dot*) and truncated appearance on the right (*white dot*) indicate rotation of C1 to the right.

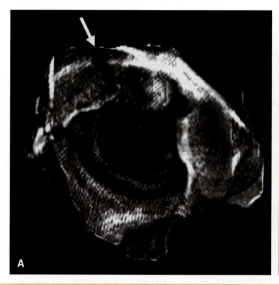

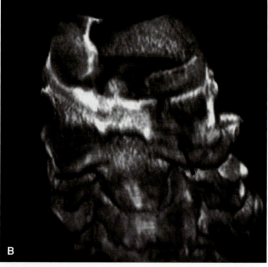

FIGURE 6-39. Atlanto-axial rotatory subluxation associated with left lateral mass of C1 fracture. **A:** Reformatted 3D volume rendered superior axial view shows rotation of C1 to the right without anterior displacement of C1. In addition, there is an oblique fracture of the left lateral mass of C1 (*white arrow*). **B:** Frontal-superior reformatted 3D CT volume rendered view shows rotation of C1 to the right and an oblique fracture of the left lateral mass of C1 (*black arrow*).

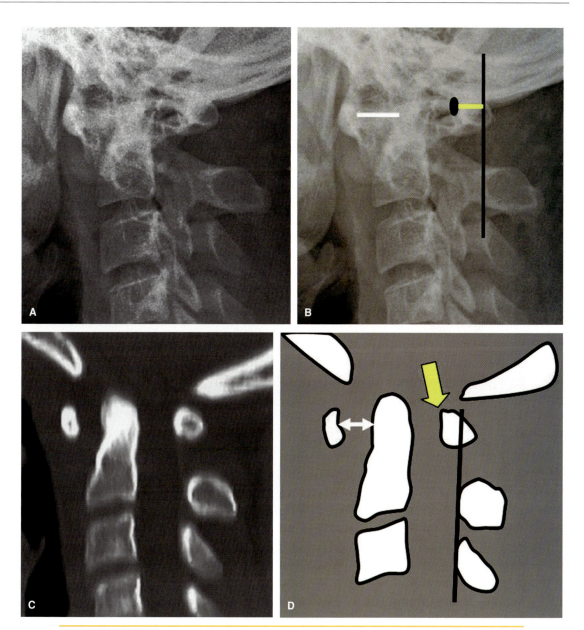

FIGURE 6-40. Acute traumatic rupture of the transverse atlantal ligament (TAL). **A,B:** Lateral radiographs show anterior translation of C1 evidenced by the abnormally wide (>5 mm) anterior atlanto-dental interval (AADI) (*white line in B*) and the anterior position of its spinolaminar line (*yellow line in B*) with respect to that of C2-3 spinolaminar lines (*black line*). The abnormal cervico-cranial prevertebral soft tissue contour reflects a retropharyngeal hematoma. **C:** Sagittal CT multiplanar reformation and **(D)** TAL injury illustration show anterior translation of C1 evidenced by the abnormally wide (>5 mm) anterior atlanto-dental interval (AADI) (*white arrow in D*) and the anterior position of its spinolaminar line (*yellow arrow in D*) with respect to that of C2-3 spinolaminar lines (*black line in D*). The abnormal cervico-cranial prevertebral soft tissue contour reflects a retropharyngeal hematoma **(C)**. *(continued)*

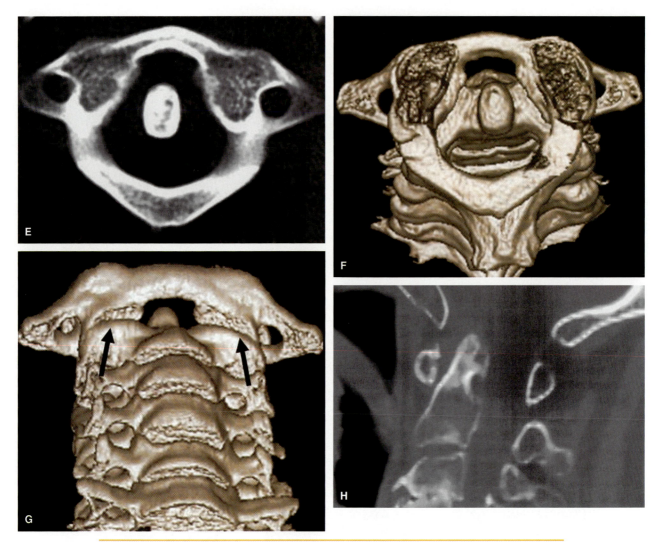

FIGURE 6-40. *(CONTINUED)* **E:** Axial CT image confirms the anterior displacement of C1 with widening of the AADI. **F:** Reformatted 3D CT surface rendered superior axial view shows anterior displacement of C1 (AADI >5 mm) with no significant associated rotation. Note moderate involvement of the spinal canal with narrowing of its AP diameter. **G:** Anterior-inferior oblique coronal reformatted 3D CT surface rendered view shows the anterior displacement of the C1 lateral masses (*arrows*). **H:** Sagittal CT multiplanar reformation in a patient with rheumatoid arthritis also shows anterior translation of C1 with widening of the AADI and anterior position of its spinolaminar line. Note the characteristic dens erosions, as well as narrowing and endplate erosions at C3-4.

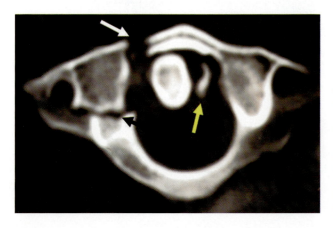

FIGURE 6-41. Atypical Jefferson fracture associated with avulsion fracture at the left transverse atlantal ligament (TAL) insertion. Axial CT image shows a displaced single fracture of the right anterior arch of C1 (*white arrow*) and right lateral fracture of the posterior atlas ring (*black arrow*). Avulsed fragment from the medial surface of the left lateral mass of C1 by the transverse atlantal ligament is noted (*yellow arrow*). This atypical Jefferson fracture two-part pattern often is associated with a TAL tear and instability.

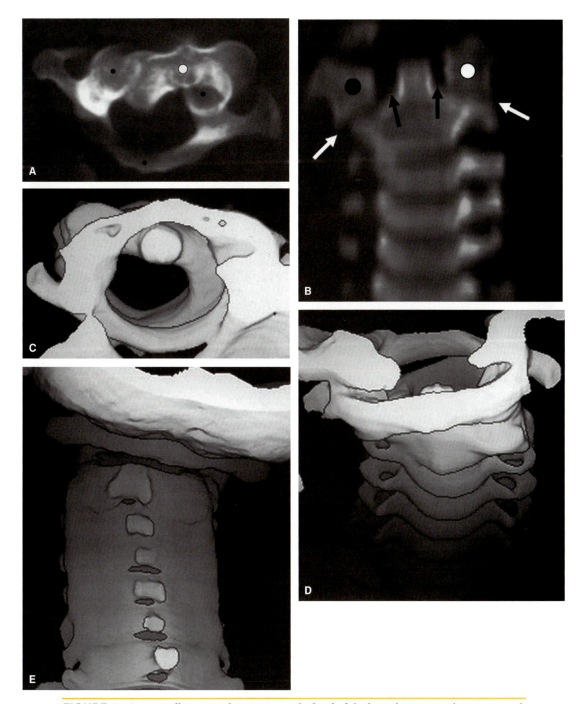

FIGURE 6-42. Torticollis. **A:** Axial CT image at the level of the lateral masses and posterior arch of C1 (*black dots*) and vertebral body of C2 (*white dot*) shows rotation of C1 to the left. **B:** Coronal CT multiplanar reformation shows asymmetry of the lateral atlanto-dental spaces (*black arrows*) and a difference in the atlanto-axial joint spaces (*white arrows*) secondary to rotational malalignment. Increase in the transverse diameter of the right lateral mass of C1 (*black dot*) and the truncated appearance of that on the left (*white dot*) indicate rotation of C1 to the left. **C:** Reformatted 3D CT surface rendered axial view clearly shows rotation of C1 to the left and a normal spinal canal. Anterior (**D**) and posterior (**E**) coronal reformatted 3D surface rendered views show rotation of C1 to the left (**D**) and lateral tilt of the head to the right (**E**).

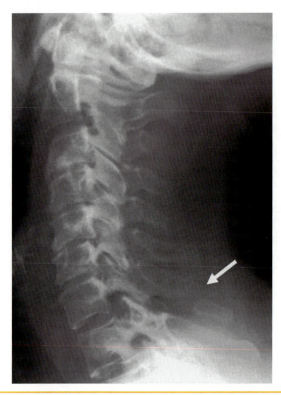

FIGURE 6-43. Typical clay-shoveler fracture of the spinous process of C7 (*white arrow*).

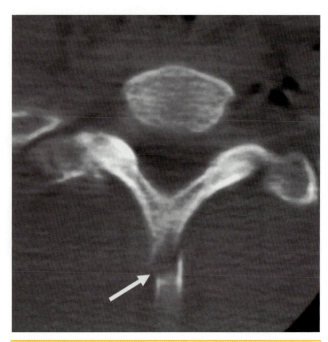

FIGURE 6-44. Axial CT image shows a typical clay-shoveler fracture of the spinous process of T1 (*white arrow*).

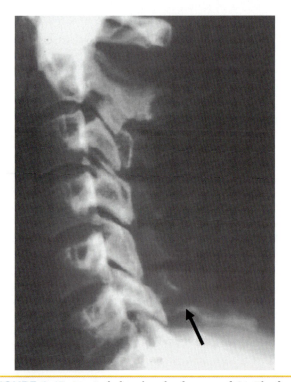

FIGURE 6-45. Atypical clay-shoveler fracture of C6. The fracture line extends beyond the spinous process into the lamina (*black arrow*). Spinal cord injury is possible with this fracture.

ligament remains intact. No associated bony injury is seen. Anterior subluxation is caused by a combination of flexion and distraction. Anterior subluxation is considered clinically significant because of the morbidity associated with the 20% to 50% incidence of failure of ligamentous healing (65,66), or "delayed instability." The radiographic manifestation of AS may be subtle and easy overlooked, despite the severity of the injury and its resultant instability.

Simple Wedge Compression Fracture

A simple wedge fracture occurs as a result of compression of the anterior aspect of the vertebral body. There is loss of vertebral body height, predominantly anteriorly. The typical compression fractures are the result of a flexion injury with no >25% compression of the anterior column and no injury to the posterior longitudinal ligament. Generally, this occurs in the mid and lower cervical segments. The simple wedge fracture is characterized radiographically by an impaction fracture of the superior endplate of the involved vertebral body while the inferior endplate remains intact. This injury commonly occurs in association with hyperflexion sprain and signs of posterior ligamentous injury. Assessment of posterior longitudinal ligament and posterior ligamentous complex injury can be made on lateral radiographs taken with the spine in flexion and extension. MRI can also be used for diagnosis. The simple wedge fracture is considered mechanically stable.

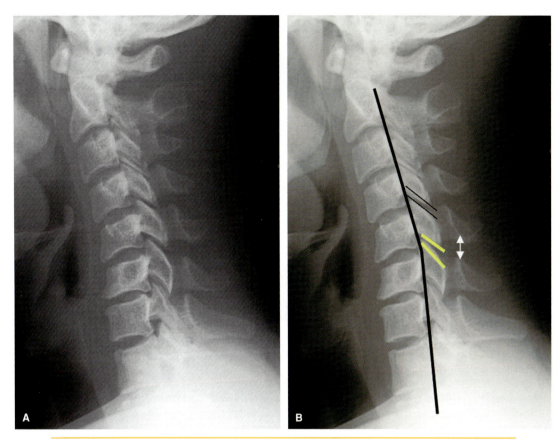

FIGURE 6-46. Anterior subluxation of C5. **A,B:** Lateral radiographs of the cervical spine show mild incongruity and lack of parallelism of the C5-6 facets (*yellow lines in B*) as compared to C4-5 facets (*thin black lines in B*) as well as widening of the interspinous distance at C5-6 ("fanning") (*white arrow in B*). Note the subtle localized hyperkyphotic angulation at C5-6 (*thick black lines in B*).

Bilateral Facet Dislocation

Bilateral facet dislocation (BFD) is an extreme form of anterior subluxation that occurs when a significant degree of flexion, distraction, and anterior subluxation causes ligamentous disruption and significant anterior displacement of the spine at the level of injury (Table 6-10, Figs. 6-49, 6-50, 6-51, 6-52, 6-53, 6-54, 6-55). Both inferior articular facets from one vertebral body can dislocate anterior to the superior facets of the subjacent vertebra, implying disruption or stripping of all major support ligaments of the anterior, middle, and posterior columns and facet capsules between levels. This injury may occur at any level from C2-3 (Fig. 6-52) through C7-T1, however, it usually occurs in the lower cervical spine. The more superior vertebra subluxes forward by 50% or more of the AP diameter of the vertebral body below (Figs. 6-49, 6-50). The spinal canal is severely compromised by this displacement, and spinal cord injuries are frequent. There are typically no facet fractures because the posterior column is distracted. However, it is common for small impaction fractures to occur at the margins of the articular masses involved in BFD, and these fractures are commonly not visible radiographically. Uncommonly, when the causative force is of sufficient magnitude, a major posterior column fracture may occur with BFD. There may also be compression deformities of the subjacent vertebra. A significant number of bilateral facet dislocations are accompanied by disc herniation (67) and in patients who have such an injury, catastrophic compression of the spinal cord can result from an uncontrolled facet reduction. Therefore, a careful neurologic examination should accompany closed reduction in these patients. BFD is unstable and is associated with extensive soft tissue damage and a high incidence of cord damage (67–69). "Perched" facets occur when the tips of the articular facets of adjacent vertebrae levels are in apposition (Fig. 6-53). In some cases, one facet may dislocate while the other perches atop the subjacent facet tip, leading to subtle signs of rotation on the lateral radiograph or AP radiograph. MRI is the modality indicated for subsequent imaging of patients with BFD as it best assesses the nature and extent of spinal cord injury as well as any associated disc and ligamentous injury (Fig. 6-50).

(text continues on page 132)

▶ **TABLE 6-10** Bilateral Facet Dislocation

Plain film findings: Radiographic findings are usually obvious given the marked degree of anterior displacement of the vertebral body.

Lateral view:
- Displacement of >50% of the anteroposterior diameter of the vertebral body (Figs. 6-49 and 6-50).
- Dislocation of articular facets (Fig. 6-50).
- There may be fractures of superior or inferior articular facets.
- Narrowing of the disc space at the injured level indicates possible extrusion of a disc fragment.
- Dislocation may be incomplete (perched facets), with varying degrees of anterolisthesis of facets of one body relative to another. Radiographically, the perched vertebra may be subtle on the lateral projection, evidenced primarily by "fanning" and anterior translation of the involved segment. The perched vertebra is mechanically unstable but may not be associated with a neurologic deficit.
- Increased thickness of the prevertebral soft tissues secondary to hematoma formation.
- There may be compression deformities of the subjacent vertebra.

AP view:
- Increased interspinous distance at the level of dislocation.

UNSTABLE:
- BFD is unstable and is associated with extensive soft tissue damage.
- CT findings: CT is valuable for detection of radiographically occult fractures of the posterior arch or articular facets.

Axial images:
- Fractures undetectable at plain radiography may be revealed.
- A cautious search for contiguous fractures is critical.
- The superior facet is rounded anteriorly and straight posteriorly at the joint surface, while the opposite is true of the inferior facet, which is flat anteriorly at the joint surface and rounded posteriorly. When the joints are normal, the flattened joint surfaces face each other. When they are dislocated, the rounded surfaces face each other. The "hamburger bun" sign of normal facet joints and the "reverse hamburger bun" sign is useful in establishing a diagnosis of facet dislocation: normal facet joints are oriented on CT examination so that they resemble the sides of a hamburger bun. Facet dislocation upsets this relationship and reverses the orientation of the "bun" halves to each other (112) (Figs. 6-51 and 6-52, and Figs. 5-25 and 5-26).

Naked facet sign: Anterior subluxation of vertebral bodies usually occurs as a result of an excessive flexion force that causes disruption of the ligamentous complex that stabilizes the facet joint. Consequently, the superior vertebra undergoes forward subluxation, with anterior displacement of its inferior articulating facet on the superior articulating facet of the vertebra below. In perched facets there is complete uncovering of the articulating facet surfaces. The naked facet sign refers to the CT appearance of uncovered articulating processes. On axial CT images, there are bilateral solitary nonarticulating facets with loss of the joint space (3) (Fig. 6-53).

Sagittal reconstruction: Sagittal MPR images clearly show the facet, the articular pillar, and vertebral body relationships.
- Displacement of >50% of the anteroposterior diameter of the vertebral body (Figs. 6-52 and 6-54).
- There may be compression deformities of the subjacent vertebra.
- Dislocation of articular facets (Fig. 6-54).
- There may be fractures of superior or inferior articular facets.
- Narrowing of the disc space at the injured level indicates possible extrusion of a disc fragment.
- Dislocation may be incomplete (perched facets), with varying degrees of anterolisthesis of facets of one body relative to another (Fig. 6-53).
- Increase in thickness of the prevertebral soft tissues as a result of hematoma formation.

Coronal reconstruction:
- Lateral dislocation, also called lateral translation, may occur.

3D reconstructions:
- The BFD and associated articular fractures are clearly demonstrated by surface or volume rendered 3D CT reconstructions (Figs. 6-54 and 6-55).

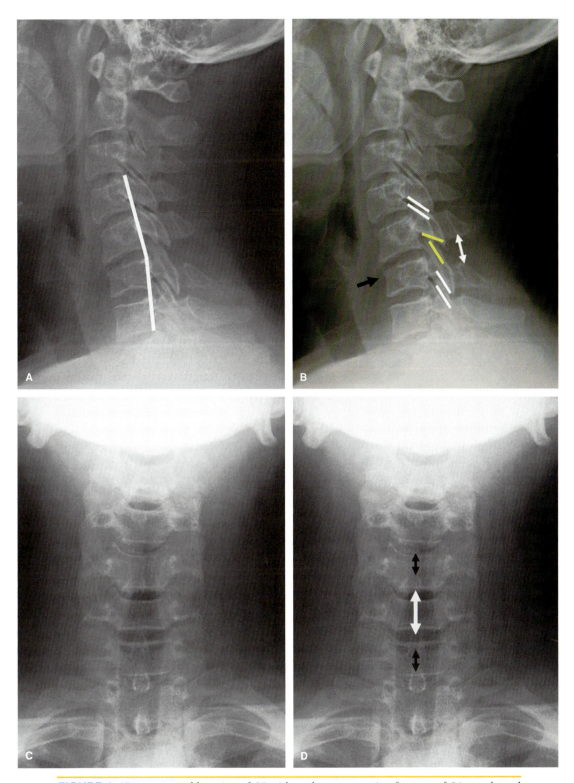

FIGURE 6-47. Anterior subluxation of C5 with wedge compression fracture of C6. **A,B:** lateral radiographs of the cervical spine show incongruity and lack of parallelism of the C5-6 facets (*yellow lines in B*), exposure of the superior facet joint surface of C6, and widening of the interspinous distance at C5-6 ("fanning") (*white arrow in B*) relative to adjacent levels. Note the subtle localized hyperkyphotic angulation at C5-6 (*white lines in A*). There is loss of anterior stature of the body of C6 secondary to the compression fracture involving its superior end plate (*black line in B*). **C,D:** AP radiographs of the cervical spine. On the frontal projection the C5-6 interspinous space is abnormally wide (*white arrow in D*). This represents the "fanning" seen on the lateral radiograph.

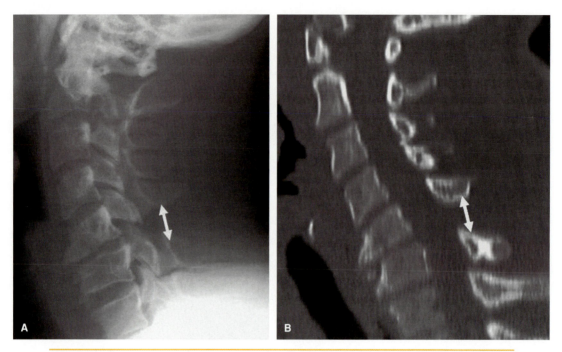

FIGURE 6-48. Anterior subluxation of C5. Lateral radiograph of the cervical spine **(A)** and sagittal multiplanar reformation **(B)** show widening of the interspinous distance at C5-6 ("fanning") (*white arrows*) and subtle localized hyperkyphotic angulation at C5-6.

Flexion Teardrop Fracture

The flexion teardrop fracture (FTF) represents the most severe injury of the cervical spine and is a highly unstable injury (Table 6-11). This occurs with severe flexion and axial compression loading forces, resulting in a fracture dislocation of a cervical vertebra (70), typically involving the lower cervical spine (especially C5). This injury shares the posterior ligamentous disruption of the other hyperflexion injuries, but there is also complete disruption of all soft tissues at the level of injury, including the posterior longitudinal ligament, intervertebral disc, and anterior longitudinal ligament. There is a typical large triangular fracture fragment of the anteroinferior margin of the upper vertebral body (teardrop fragment) (Figs. 6-56, 6-57, 6-58). There are two fracture patterns associated with the anteroinferior corner (teardrop) fracture fragment. The first is the isolated fracture, which is usually not associated with permanent neurologic sequelae. The second is the three-part, two-plane fracture in which there is an associated sagittal vertebral body fracture and a fracture of the posterior neural arch. This latter pattern is almost always associated with permanent neurologic sequelae (71). The spinal cord injury can be due to the severe narrowing of the spinal canal by retropulsed bone fragments and hyperkyphotic angulation at the level of the fracture dislocation. Patients frequently have acute anterior cervical cord syndrome: instant, complete quad-riplegia with loss of pain, touch, and temperature sensations but retention of posterior column sensations (position, motion, and vibration). The flexion teardrop fracture can be distinguished from the similarly named hyperextension teardrop fracture by the larger size of the triangular fragment and by distraction of the posterior elements (indicating the flexion mechanism).

FLEXION-ROTATION INJURIES

Flexion-rotation injuries result from simultaneous flexion and rotation of the cervical spine, and, in the subaxial spine, this mechanism can result in unilateral facet dislocation (UFD).

Unilateral Facet Dislocation

Flexion and rotation may result in dislocation of one facet. The inferior articular process of the dislocated facet lies in front of the superior articular process of the subjacent vertebra, and the posterior ligaments (including the capsule and annulus) are torn on the side of the dislocation (Table 6-12, Figs. 6-49, 6-59, 6-60, 6-61, 6-62). The dislocation occurs on the side opposite the direction of rotation. In many cases (73%), fractures of the articular facets and pillars occur (72). In most patients with unilateral facet

▶ **TABLE 6-11** **Flexion Teardrop Fracture**

Plain film findings:

Lateral view:
- Comminuted fracture of the vertebral body with an anteriorly displaced triangular fracture fragment ("teardrop") of the antero-inferior aspect of the vertebral body (Fig. 6-56, 6-57, 6-58). The teardrop fragment maintains alignment with the cervical spine below the level of injury.
- Displacement of the involved posterior vertebral body fragment into the spinal canal. The posterior vertebral body fragment and the cervical spine above the injury level move as a unit (Figs. 6-56, 5-57, 6-58).
- Abrupt kyphotic angulation at the level of the injury (Fig. 6-58).
- Widening of the interspinous distance at one level ("fanning") relative to adjacent levels (Fig. 6-56).
- Exposure of the superior facet joint surface of the subjacent vertebra.
- Increase in the thickness of the prevertebral soft tissues secondary to hematoma formation.

AP view:
- Sagittal fracture of the involved vertebral body (71,113) (Fig. 6-57).
- Increased interspinous distance at the level of dislocation.
- Disruption of the lateral columns.
- Loss of definition of endplates and disc spaces.
- Distorted Luschka joints.

UNSTABLE:
- FTF is the most unstable lower cervical spine injury.

CT findings: With CT, it is possible to determine the extent of fracture of the involved vertebra and the extent of fragment displacement into the spinal canal; adjacent vertebrae can also be assessed.

Axial images:
- Comminuted fracture of the vertebral body with an anteriorly displaced triangular fracture fragment ("tear-drop") of the anterior-inferior aspect of the vertebral body (Figs. 57 and 58).
- The teardrop fragment may be split sagitally.
- Sagittal fracture of the involved vertebral body in 87% of patients (70,71,113) (Figs. 6-57, 6-58).
- Displacement of involved posterior vertebral body fragment into the spinal canal.
- Fracture of the posterior arch (Figs. 6-57, 6-58)

Sagittal reformation:
- Triangular fracture fragment ("teardrop") of the anterior-inferior aspect of the vertebral body (Figs. 6-57, 6-58).
- Displacement of the involved posterior vertebral body fragment into the spinal canal.
- Abrupt kyphotic angulation at the level of injury.
- Widening of the interspinous distance at one level ("fanning") relative to adjacent levels.
- Exposure of the superior facet joint surface of the subjacent vertebra (Fig. 6-58).
- Increase in the thickness of the prevertebral soft tissues secondary to hematoma formation.

Coronal reformation:
- Sagittal fracture of the involved vertebral body (71,113) (Fig. 6-57).

fracture subluxation, the fracture has a vertical orientation through the articular pillar (72,73). Other isolated fractures, or extension of articular pillar fractures into the ipsilateral lamina and pedicle, can occur. Fractures can also involve the contralateral facets. Braakman and Vinken (74) noted that the capsule of the nondislocated (contralateral) interfacetal joint is frequently disrupted. According to Argenson et al. (75), 25% of all cases of UFD are associated with another traumatic lesion of the lower or upper cervical spine, and there is a 30% rate of radicular complications clinically. Shapiro et al. (76), in a study of 51 cases of UFD, reported a 73% incidence of radiculopathy, a 16% incidence of neck pain only, and a 12% incidence of cord injury. MRI may be warranted in patients with UFD who manifest neurologic symptoms to assess for cord injury or epidural cord compression from herniated disc material or hematoma. MRI can also evaluate flow in the vertebral arteries, which are prone to injury in patients with rotational lesions (77,78).

EXTENSION INJURY

Cervical spine injuries caused by hyperextension are characterized by distraction of the anterior and middle columns and by compression of the posterior column (Table 6-13, Figs. 6-63, 6-64, 6-65). Therefore, avulsion injuries are seen anteriorly while impaction injuries are seen posteriorly. Hyperextension injuries represent 7% to 26% of all cervical spine injuries (79). In general, hyperextension injuries tend to occur at the lower cervical levels. Hyperextension injuries are more common in patients with ankylosing spondylitis, diffuse idiopathic skeletal hyperostosis (DISH or Forestier disease), cervical spondylosis, congenital spinal stenosis, or severe degenerative disease (79–83). Cervical spondylosis narrows the central canal and makes the spinal cord more susceptible to compression by the bulging ligamentum flavum during hyperextension (80). The diagnosis of hyperextension injury to the cervical spine after a fall is easily overlooked in the elderly. This is because the pattern of neurologic deficit, usually that of the central cord syndrome, is complex and because radiologic signs of trauma are subtle (81). In these patients with pre-existing disease, injuries tend to occur as a result of low-impact trauma (e.g., a fall from standing).

Hyperextension Sprain, Dislocation, and Fracture Dislocation

Hyperextension sprain (HS) and hyperextension dislocation (HD) are soft tissue injuries caused by a force delivered to the face, which drives the head and neck into

▶ **TABLE 6-12** Unilateral Facet Dislocation

Plain film findings:

Lateral view:
- Anterior translation of the dislocated vertebra 25% to 50% of the AP diameter of the vertebral body, a distance greater than occurs with anterior subluxation (<25%), but less than occurs with bilateral facet dislocation (>50%) (Fig. 6-49).
- Offset of the articular pillars at the level of injury due to rotation. At one level they appear superimposed, and at the adjacent level there is an abrupt offset. This appearance has been referred to as the "bowtie sign" (Fig. 6-59 and 6-62).
- Abrupt alteration of the laminar space between two adjacent levels. Young et al. (114) have described use of the "laminar space" to indicate rotational injuries of the cervical spine (Fig. 6-59). The laminar space is the distance between the spinolaminar line and the posterior surface of the articular pillars (Fig. 5-7). Head turning, with physiologic rotation between adjacent levels, will produce a gradual transition in the laminar space on the lateral cervical radiograph.
- Abrupt kyphotic angulation at the level of the UFD.
- Widening of the interspinous distance at one level ("fanning") relative to adjacent levels.
- The disc space is widened posteriorly and narrowed anteriorly.
- Increase in the thickness of the prevertebral soft tissues secondary to hematoma formation.

AP view:
- Displacement of the spinous process off the midline in the direction of the side of the dislocated facet joint from the level of the dislocation upward. The displaced spinous processes point to the side of dislocation (Fig. 6-60).
- Widened interspinous space at level of injury.

UNSTABLE:
- In pure UFD the dislocated articular mass and accompanying soft tissues are stuck in the intervertebral foramen. The injury has been referred as the "locked" vertebra. Because of the common association of UFD with major cervical ligament tears, rotational facet injuries should be regarded as mechanically unstable.
- Unilateral facet fracture dislocation refers to a UFD associated with a fracture at the base of either the inferior articular process of the dislocated articular mass or the base of the superior articular process of the subjacent articular mass. The integrity of the facet joint is not restored following reduction since one of its components is a separate fracture fragment. This fracture-dislocation injury is unstable.

CT findings: CT is valuable in the diagnosis of radiographically occult fractures of the posterior arch or articular facets.

Axial images: (Figs. 5-25 and 5-26)
- Fractures undetectable at plain radiography may be revealed.
- A cautious search for contiguous fractures is critical.
- The superior facet is rounded anteriorly and straight posteriorly at the joint surface, while the opposite is true of the inferior facet, which is flat anteriorly at the joint surface and rounded posteriorly. When the joints are normal, the flattened joint surfaces facet each other. When they are dislocated, the rounded surfaces face each other. The "hamburger bun" sign of normal facet joints and the "reverse hamburger bun" sign is useful in establishing a diagnosis of facet dislocation. Normal facet joints are oriented on CT examination so that they resemble the sides of a hamburger bun. Facet dislocation upsets this relationship and reverses the orientation of the "bun" halves to each other (112). When fractures accompany UFD the images are more complex.
- In 10% of cases of UFD there is an avulsion fracture of the posterior cortex of the involved vertebra (72). The posterior longitudinal ligament avulses a posterior cortical fragment with the rotational torque applied to the vertebral body.

Sagittal reconstruction: Sagittal MPR images clearly show the facet, the articular pillar, and vertebral body relationships.
- Anterior translation of the dislocated vertebra 25% to 50% of the AP diameter of the vertebral body. This is a distance greater than occurs with anterior subluxation (<25%), but less than occurs with bilateral facet dislocation (>50%).
- Unilateral dislocation of articular facets/pillars (Fig. 6-62).
- CT frequently demonstrates diastasis of the contralateral facet joint.
- There may be fractures of superior or inferior articular facets/pillars.
- Narrowing of the disc space at the injured level indicates possible extrusion of a disc fragment.
- Increase in the thickness of the prevertebral soft tissues secondary to hematoma formation.
- In 10% of cases of UFD there is an avulsion fracture of the posterior cortex of the involved vertebra (72). The posterior longitudinal ligament avulses a posterior cortical fragment with the rotational torque applied to the vertebral body.

3D reconstructions:
- The UFD and associated articular fractures are clearly demonstrated by surface or volume rendered 3D CT reconstructions (Figs. 6-61, 6-62).

▶ **TABLE 6-13 Hyperextension Injuries**

Plain film findings: Cervical hyperextension injuries often show minimal radiographic abnormalities, even with severe or unstable lesions. The momentary posterior displacement of the involved vertebra is usually completely reduced when the causative force disappears.

Lateral view: The hallmarks are normal vertebral alignment with extensive prevertebral soft tissue swelling. According to Edeiken-Monroe et al. (84), this combination of findings was the only radiographic sign in 30% of patients.

- Increase in the thickness of the prevertebral soft tissues secondary to hematoma formation (evidence of disc, longus colli and longus capitis muscle, or ligament damage).
- Avulsion fracture fragment from the anterior aspect of the inferior endplate of the superior vertebra. The transverse dimension of the avulsed fragment exceeds its vertical height.
- Normally aligned vertebrae.
- Vacuum defect in the intervertebral disc subjacent to the dislocated vertebra (Fig. 6-63).
- Anteriorly widened disc space.
- Less commonly, fractures of posterior elements (particularly spinous processes) are encountered.

AP view:
- No value.

UNSTABLE:
- Hyperextension dislocation is mechanically unstable.

CT findings: Patients with underlying ankylosing spondylitis, diffuse idiopathic skeletal hyperostosis (Forestier disease), spondylosis, congenital spinal stenosis, or severe degenerative disease who have neck pain following trauma should undergo helical CT of the cervical spine with sagittal and coronal reconstructions. CT is valuable for detecting radiographically occult fractures that involve the posterior arch or articular facets.

Axial images:
- Fractures undetectable at plain radiography may be revealed. Fractures of the posterior elements, particularly the spinous processes, are encountered (Fig. 6-63).
- A cautious search for contiguous fractures is critical.

Sagittal reformation:
- Increase in the thickness of the prevertebral soft tissues secondary to hematoma formation (evidence of disc, longus colli and longus capitis muscle, or ligament damage).
- Avulsion fracture fragment from the anterior aspect of the inferior endplate of the superior vertebra. The transverse dimension of the avulsed fragment exceeds its vertical height.
- Normally aligned vertebrae.
- Vacuum defect in the intervertebral disc space subjacent to the dislocated vertebra.
- Anteriorly widened disc space.

severe hyperextension. Acute angulation of the spine can result in tearing of the longus colli and longus capitis muscles, disruption of the anterior longitudinal ligament and annulus, avulsion of the intervertebral disc from the superior vertebral body at the level of the injury, stripping of the posterior longitudinal ligament from the dorsal surface of the inferiorly situated vertebrae, and disruption of the ligamentum flavum. Posterior displacement of the involved vertebral body compresses the spinal cord against the ligamentum flavum and lamina of the subjacent vertebrae, producing a central cord syndrome (upper extremity deficit greater than lower extremity). The dislocation frequently is momentary and reduces spontaneously. Part of the clinical picture of HS/HD is evidence of facial trauma. In hyperextension sprain, the middle and posterior columns of the spine remain intact. Hyper-

extension sprain generally occurs in younger individuals as a result of high-impact trauma (84). Hyperextension dislocation injury results from a force of sufficient magnitude to disrupt the anterior and middle ligament supports of the cervical spine. MRI is useful to investigate ligamentous integrity following these hyperextension injuries (85–88).

Hyperextension fracture dislocation is an injury most often encountered in elderly patients with severe spondylosis or with spinal ankylosis from other etiologies. Hyperextension fracture dislocation occasionally occurs in younger individuals with severe HS/HD. In hyperextension fracture dislocation the posterior spinal elements experience impaction forces, producing loading fractures

(text continues on page 139)

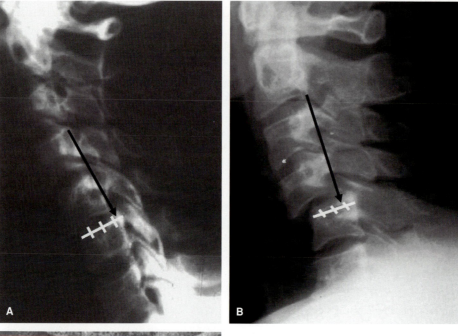

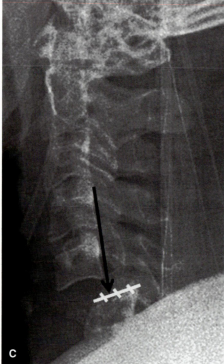

FIGURE 6-49. Anterior vertebral translation in different flexion injuries. The amount of anterior translation with unilateral dislocation (**B**) is less than occurs with bilateral facet dislocation (**C**) but greater than that of anterior subluxation (**A**). **A:** In anterior subluxation the involved vertebra may be displaced slightly anteriorly (1 to 3 mm), <25% of the AP diameter of the subjacent vertebral body. **B:** Unilateral facet dislocation demonstrating anterior translation of the dislocated vertebra 25% to 50% of the AP diameter of the subjacent vertebral body. **C:** Bilateral facet dislocation with anterior displacement of the involved vertebra >50% of the anteroposterior diameter of the subjacent vertebral body.

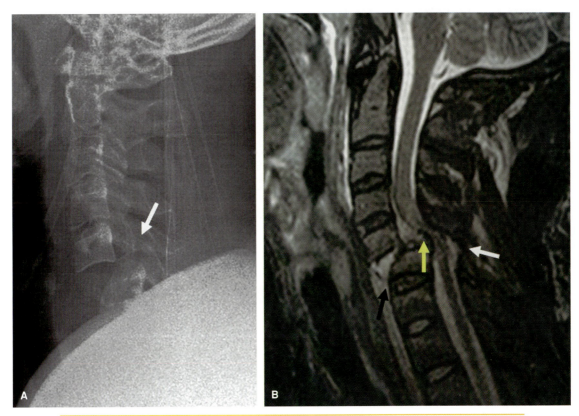

FIGURE 6-50. Bilateral facet dislocation. **A:** Lateral cervical radiograph demonstrates C5-6 bilateral facet dislocation (*white arrow*), with >50% anterolisthesis. **B:** Midsagittal T2-weighted MR image shows disruption of the anterior longitudinal ligament (*black arrow*) and posterior longitudinal ligament (*yellow arrow*), and stripping or tearing of the ligamentum flavum (*white arrow*). There is marked narrowing of the spinal canal at the level of dislocation with extensive cord contusion and central hemorrhage from C5 to C6.

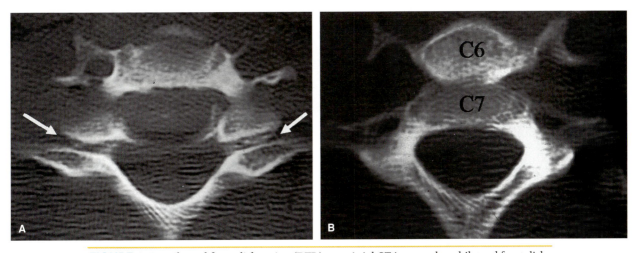

FIGURE 6-51. Bilateral facet dislocation (BFD). **A,B:** Axial CT images show bilateral facet dislocation (*white arrows in A*) and the "double vertebral body" sign **(B)**.

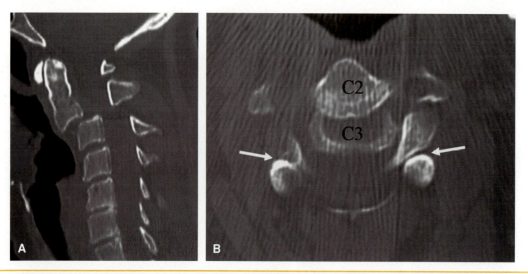

FIGURE 6-52. Bilateral facet dislocation of C2-3. **A:** Sagittal multiplanar reformation and **(B)** axial CT image show C2-3 bilateral facet dislocation (*white arrows in B*) with >50% anterolisthesis of C2 **(A)**. Note the "double vertebral body" sign **(B)**.

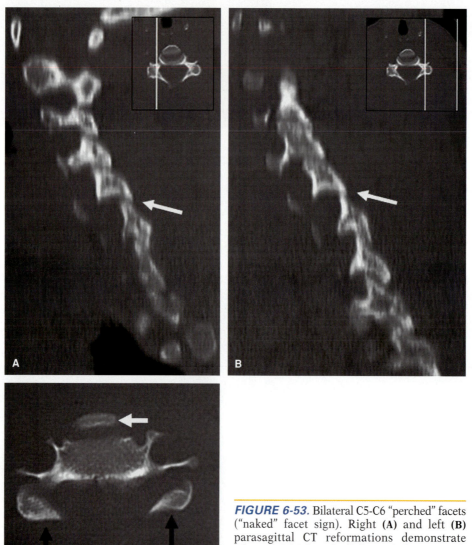

FIGURE 6-53. Bilateral C5-C6 "perched" facets ("naked" facet sign). Right **(A)** and left **(B)** parasagittal CT reformations demonstrate bilateral C5-6 "perched" facets (*white arrows*). **C:** Axial CT image at the level of the upper body of C6 reveals uncovered ("naked") C6 superior articulating processes (*black arrows*) and C5 anterior subluxation (*white arrow*).

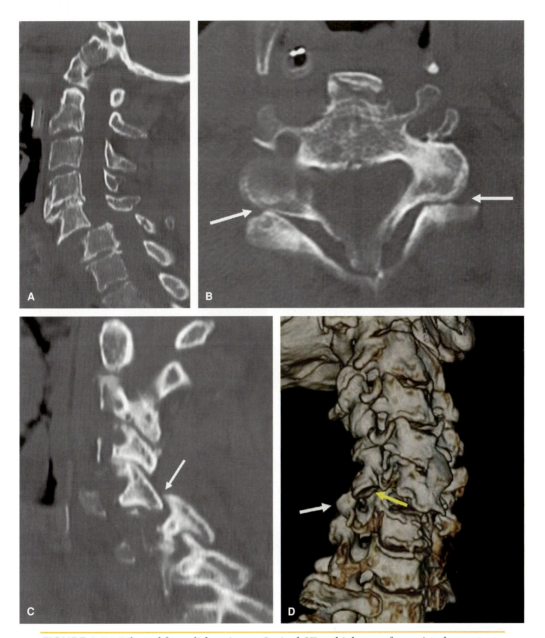

FIGURE 6-54. Bilateral facet dislocation. **A:** Sagittal CT multiplanar reformation demonstrates C5-6 bilateral facet dislocation with >50% anterolisthesis. **B:** Axial CT image show bilateral facet dislocation (*white arrows*). **C:** Right para-sagittal CT multiplanar reformation demonstrates C5-6 facet dislocation (*white arrow*). **D:** Reformatted 3D CT volume rendered anterior oblique view shows the right C5-6 facet dislocation. Inferior facet of C5 is indicated (*yellow arrow*) and superior facet of C6 is indicated (*white arrow*).

of the articular pillars, posterior vertebral body, laminae, spinous process, or pedicles (Fig. 6-63). Characteristically, the spine above the level of injury is posteriorly displaced (retrolisthesis), the intervertebral disc space is widened anteriorly and narrowed posteriorly (Fig. 6-64), and the facet joints are disrupted. Hyperextension fractures occurring in patients with ankylosing spondylitis or diffuse idiopathic skeletal hyperostosis (Forestier disease) are fractures of the anterior calcification that extend either obliquely through the disc into the subjacent verte-

bral body or extend posteriorly through the disc space itself (Fig. 6-65).

Extension Teardrop Fracture

The extension teardrop fracture (ETDF) is an avulsion fracture at the site of attachment of the anterior longitudinal ligament (Figs. 6-66, 6-67, 6-68). It involves the anteroinferior aspect of the vertebral body. Typically, it occurs in elderly osteoporotic patients and is associated

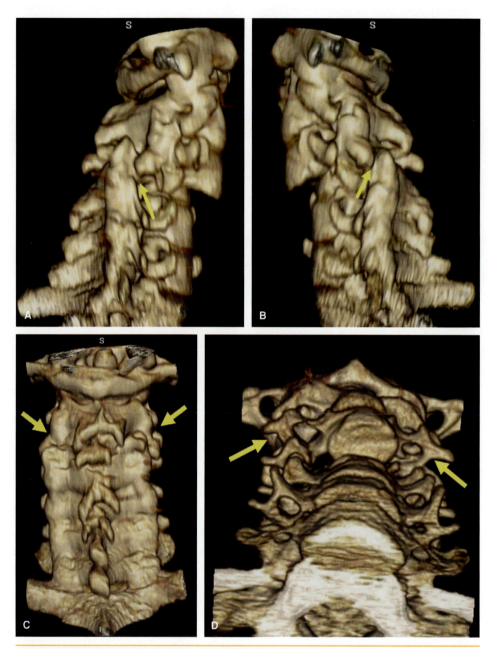

FIGURE 6-55. Bilateral facet dislocation. Right lateral **(A)**, left lateral **(B)**, posterior **(C)**, and anterior-inferior **(D)** reformatted 3D CT volume rendered views show bilateral C3-4 facet dislocation (*arrows in A, B, and C*) from different perspectives. The anterior-inferior view **(D)** demonstrates the anterior translation of C3 (*arrows*).

with little or no prevertebral hematoma. The "typical" ETDF fractures most commonly affect C2 (89). As opposed to the avulsed fragment seen in hyperextension dislocation, the vertical height of the ETDF fragment is equal or exceeds its transverse dimension. There is a high incidence of coexisting lesions at the same or at more distal levels (90). The "typical" C2 ETDF is usually mechanically and neurologically stable. In young adults, a variant of ETDF may occur in the lower cervical spine. When this

ETDF variant is associated with massive prevertebral soft tissue swelling, 80% of patients have an acute central cervical cord syndrome (91). This ETDF variant is stable in flexion but highly unstable in extension.

Laminar Fractures

Laminar fractures are usually components of complex injuries of the cervical spine, such as burst fractures of

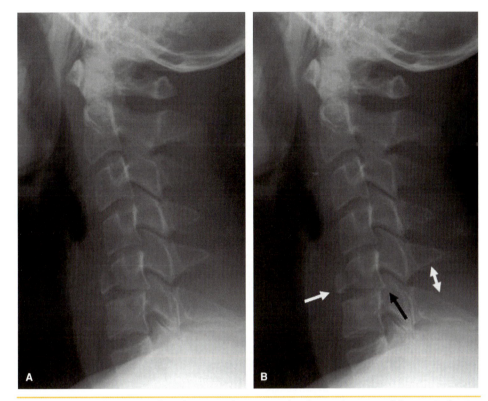

FIGURE 6-56. Flexion teardrop fracture of C5. Lateral radiographs **(A,B)** of the cervical spine show typical flexion teardrop fracture with anteriorly displaced triangular fracture fragment ("teardrop") of the anterior-inferior aspect of vertebral body of C5 (*white arrow in B*) and retropulsion of its posterior vertebral body fragment into spinal canal (*black arrow in B*). Note a subtle localized kyphotic angulation at C5-6 and widening of the interspinous distance at C5-6 ("fanning") (*white double arrow in B*).

the lower cervical spine, pedico-laminar fracture separation, and FTF. Isolated fractures confined to the laminae secondary to blunt trauma are rare (92) but, when seen, are commonly caused by hyperextension. Laminar fractures may be associated with fractures of the adjacent spinous process. The radiographic features may be quite subtle, and, therefore, isolated laminar fractures are often missed. In the plain-film examination of the cervical spine, the laminar fracture is best seen on the lateral projection. CT may reveal fractures undetectable at plain radiography and is also important in establishing the relation of laminar fragments with respect to the spinal canal. It is unusual for these injuries to cause neurologic compromise. The isolated laminar fracture is usually mechanically stable since the anterior column and the interfacetal joints are intact. Neurologic stability depends upon location of fragments within the spinal canal.

EXTENSION-ROTATION INJURY

Pillar Fracture

The pillar fracture (PF) is a vertical or oblique fracture limited to one articular mass caused by impaction by the ipsilateral suprajacent articular mass during hyperextension and rotation (93) or lateral bending. These fractures are frequently difficult to visualize (94). On the AP projection the fracture line may be visible or there may be a focal disruption of the smooth, undulating margin of the lateral column secondary to lateral displacement of a fracture fragment (Fig. 6-69). On the lateral projection, posterior displacement of a separate fragment causes the "double outline" sign, where the distance between the posterior cortex of the posteriorly displaced fragment and the cortex of the contralateral mass is greater than at any other level

(text continues on page 146)

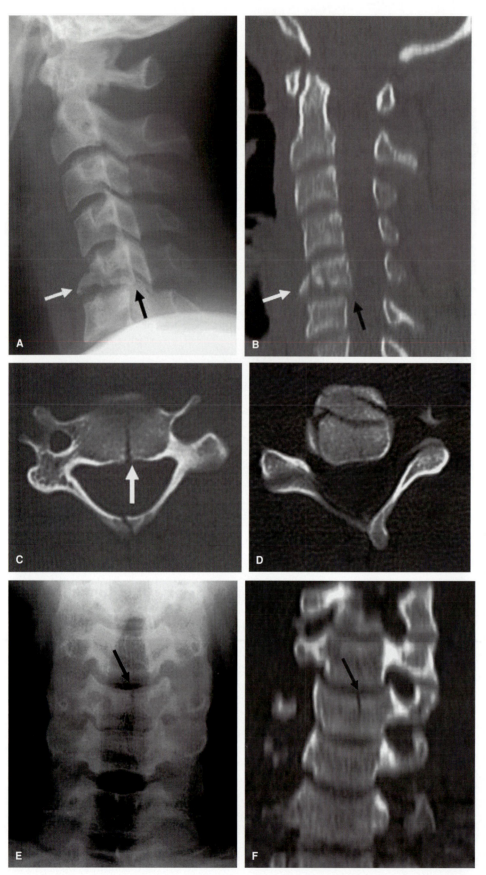

FIGURE 6-57. Flexion teardrop fracture of C5. Lateral radiograph of cervical spine **(A)** and sagittal multiplanar CT reformation **(B)** show compression of the body of C5 associated with a mild posterior subluxation of C5 upon C6 (*black arrows in A,B*). The fragment from the anterior inferior surface of C5 (*white arrow*) is the "teardrop." **C:** Axial CT image through the top of C5 demonstrates a sagittal fracture of the vertebral body (*white line*) and sagittal fracture of the spinous process. **D:** Axial CT image through the lower half of C5 shows a comminuted fracture of the anteroinferior end plate. Anteroposterior radiograph **(E)** and coronal multiplanar CT reformation **(F)** show a vertical fracture of the body of C5 oriented in the sagittal plane (*black arrows*).

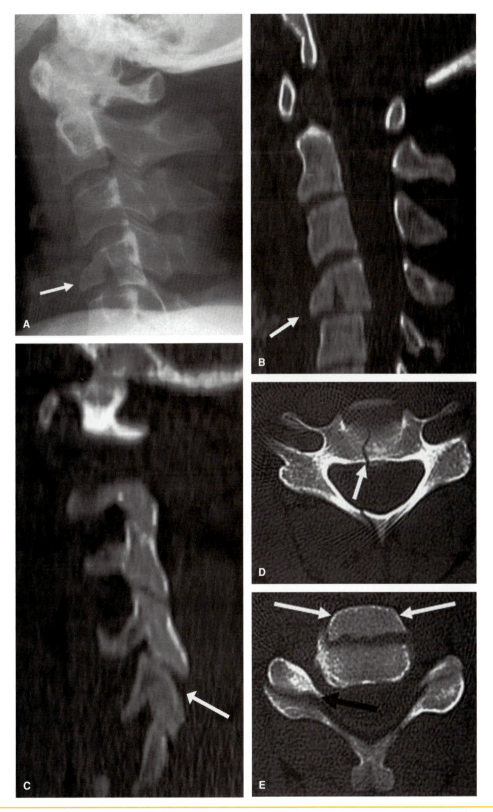

FIGURE 6-58. Flexion teardrop fracture of C4. Lateral radiograph of cervical spine **(A)** and midsagittal multiplanar CT reformation **(B)** show anterior triangular fracture fragment ("teardrop") of the anteroinferior aspect of the vertebral body of C4 (*white arrows*). Note localized kyphotic angulation at C4-5. **C:** Right parasagittal multiplanar CT reformation shows mild facet joint diastasis (*white arrow*). **D:** Axial CT image through the top of C4 demonstrates a sagittal fracture of the vertebral body (*white line*) and an associated right laminar fracture. **E:** Axial CT image through the lower half of C4 shows the anterior "teardrop" fracture fragment (*white arrows*). Note mild right C4-5 facet joint diastasis (*black arrow*).

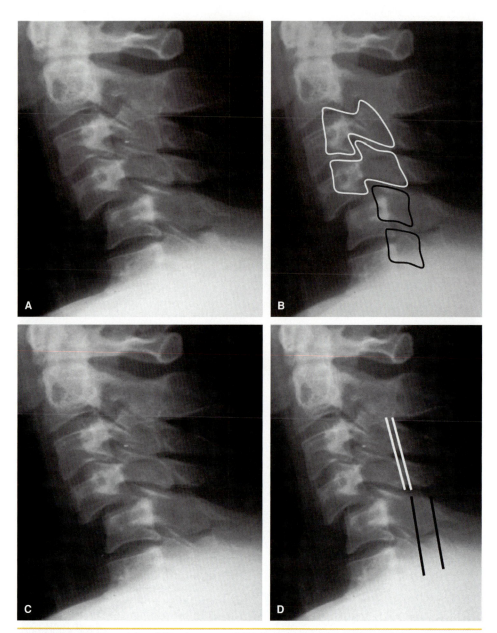

FIGURE 6-59. "Bowtie" and "laminar space" (114) signs in unilateral facet dislocation of C4-5. **A,B:** Lateral cervical spine radiographs show anterolisthesis of C4-5 with about 25% displacement. The articular pillars are offset from C4 above (*white lines in B*) and are seen in oblique profile giving the "bowtie" appearance; the "bowtie" sign indicates rotation. The articular pillars are superimposed at C5 and below and are seen in lateral profile (*black lines in B*). **C,D:** Lateral cervical spine radiographs. The laminar space is the distance between the spinolaminar line and the posterior surface of the articular pillars. The laminar space changes abruptly between C4 and C5, with the laminar space reduced above the C5 level (compare the black lines and white lines in **D** indicating sudden rotation).

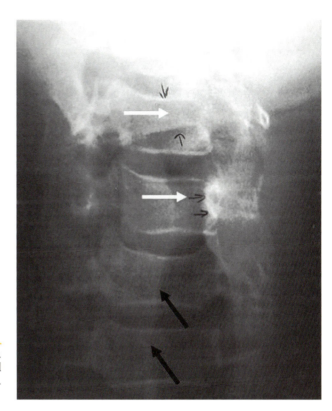

FIGURE 6-60. Unilateral facet dislocation. Anteroposterior view. The spinous process from C4 (*white arrows*) upward are deviated to the left while those of C5 and C6 remain midline (*black arrows*). The displaced spinous processes point to the side of dislocation.

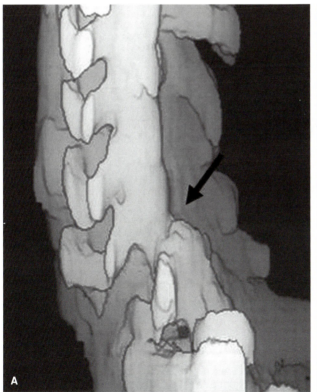

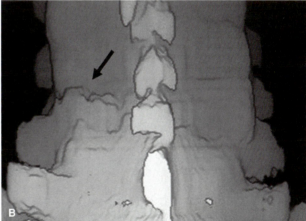

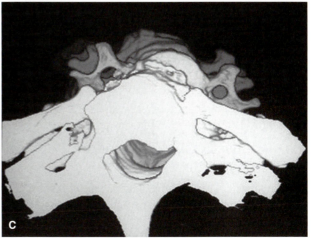

FIGURE 6-61. Unilateral facet dislocation. Lateral (**A**), posterior (**B**), and inferior (**C**) reformatted 3D CT surface rendered views show left C6-7 unilateral facet dislocation (*arrows in A and B*) from different perspectives. The inferior view (**C**) demonstrates the rotational component of the lesion to the right.

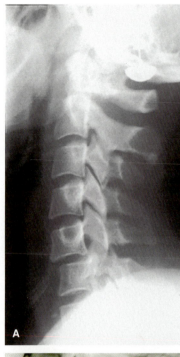

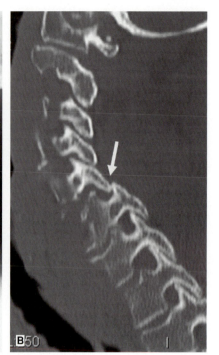

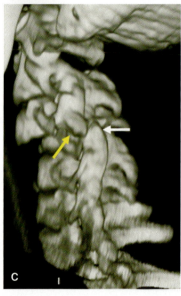

FIGURE 6-62. Unilateral facet dislocation. **A:** Lateral cervical spine radiograph shows anterolisthesis of C5-6. The articular pillars are offset from C5 above and are seen in oblique profile giving the "bowtie" appearance. The "bowtie" sign indicates rotation. **B:** Left parasagittal CT multiplanar reformation shows the left C5-6 facet dislocation (*arrow*). **C:** Reformatted 3D CT volume rendered left lateral view shows the C5-6 facet dislocation. Inferior facet of C5 (*yellow arrow*) and superior facet of C6 (*white arrow*).

(95). The PF usually extends into the transverse process or into the lamina. In patients with cervical spine trauma and a cervical radiculopathy, CT should be performed to evaluate the articular processes (94). The PF is usually considered mechanically and neurologically stable.

Pedicolaminar Fracture/Separation (Isolated Articular Pillar)

The isolated articular pillar (IAP) can occur with simultaneous fracture through the lamina and ipsilateral pedicle (96,97) (Figs. 6-70, 6-71, see Fig. 5-1). In this injury disrup-

tion of the superior and inferior facet joints occurs, permitting the pillar to rotate freely (97). Some studies (98–100) have suggested that injury is the result of combined rotation and compressive hyperextension. Shanmuganathan et al. (97) suggest that IAP is the result of either hyperflexion and rotation (17 out of 21 cases, 81%), or hyperextension and rotation. Fuentes et al. (101) classified the pediculolaminar fracture separation into four types based upon degree of ligamentous and osseous injury:

Type I: Pedicle and laminar fractures without displacement (disc intact).

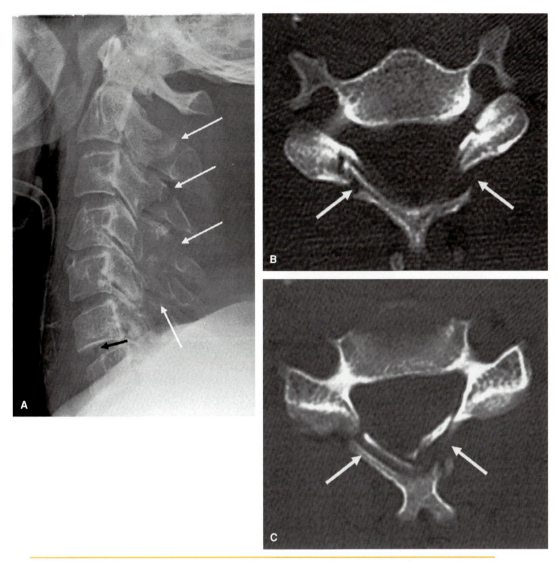

FIGURE 6-63. Hyperextension comminuted laminar and spinous processes fractures. Cervical spine injuries caused by hyperextension are characterized by distraction of the anterior and middle columns and compression of the posterior column **(A)**. Lateral radiograph demonstrates posterior impaction with multiple comminuted laminar and spinous processes fractures from C2 to C6 (*white arrows*). The acute vacuum disc (*black arrow*) with abnormal widening of the anterior C6-7 disc space is a sign of anterior and middle column distraction. **B,C:** Axial CT images demonstrate displacement of the spinous processes and bilateral comminuted laminar fractures (*white arrows*).

Type II: Type I features and disrupted capsule with articular mass rotation, displacement, or both (with rupture of the disc and ALL) (Fig. 6-70).

Type III: Type II features and disc narrowing plus vertebral anterolisthesis by ~3 mm (Fig. 6-71).

Type IV: Type III features and body and articular mass displacement (with disruption of the disc above and below the involved vertebra). In type IV injury there are ipsilateral pedicle–laminar fractures and contralateral apophyseal joint disruption.

The radiographic signs of the pediculolaminar fracture vary with the type of injury. On the AP projection there is lateral displacement of the articular mass fragment and the laminar fracture line is frequently visible (Figs. 6-70, 6-71). In types II to IV, rotation of the articular mass fragment results in the "bow-tie" sign (Figs. 6-70, 6-71). On the lateral projection, the separate articular mass fragment is rotated anteriorly and posteriorly

(text continues on page 152)

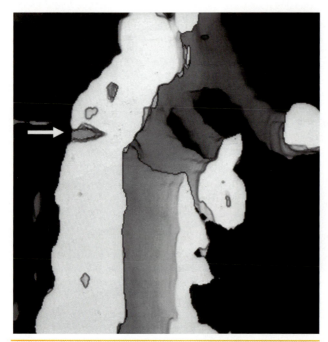

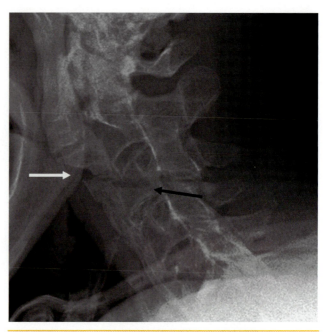

FIGURE 6-64. Hyperextension dislocation. Reformatted 3D CT surface rendered cutaway lateral view show widening of the disc space at C2-3 (*white arrow*) with posterior displacement and angulation of C2.

FIGURE 6-65. Hyperextension fracture. Lateral cervical radiograph shows an extension fracture traversing the C3 vertebral body (*black arrow*) and anterior syndesmophyte (*white arrow*) in a patient with diffuse idiopathic skeletal hyperostosis.

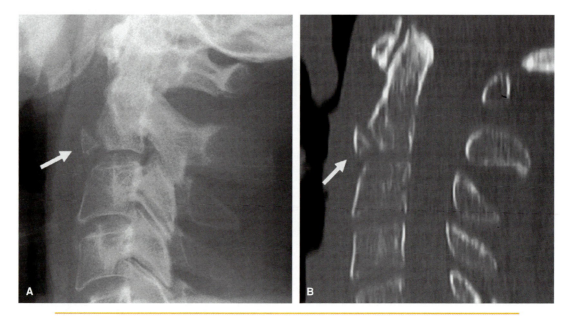

FIGURE 6-66. Hyperextension teardrop fracture of C2. **A:** Lateral cervical radiograph and (**B**) sagittal multiplanar CT reformation show a triangular fragment arising from the anterior inferior margin of C2 (*white arrows*).

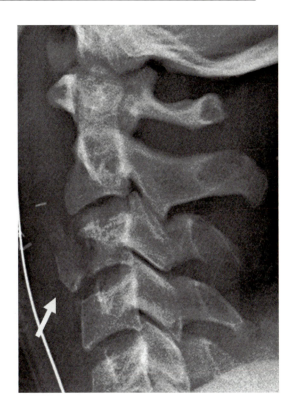

FIGURE 6-67. Hyperextension teardrop fracture of C3. Lateral cervical radiograph shows a large triangular bone fragment avulsed from the anterior inferior margin of C3, representing a teardrop fragment (*white arrow*). The C3-4 disc space appears intact. Note that the vertical dimension of this fracture fragment is greater than the transverse dimension.

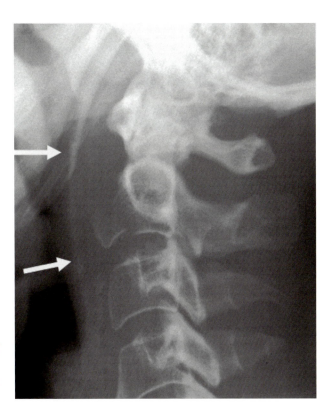

FIGURE 6-68. Hyperextension teardrop fracture of C2. Lateral cervical radiograph shows a triangular fragment arising from the anterior inferior margin of C2. Note associated prevertebral soft tissue swelling (*white arrows*).

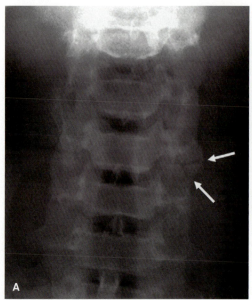

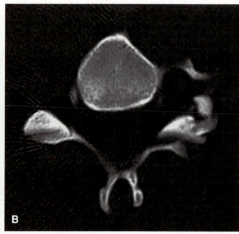

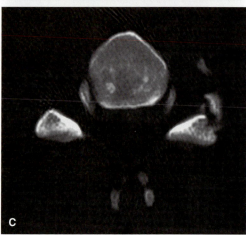

FIGURE 6-69. Pillar fracture. **A:** On the AP radiograph, fractures of the lateral column (*white arrows*) are seen, including the left articular mass of C5. **B,C:** Axial CT images show a comminuted left pillar fracture with extension into the transverse process.

▶ **TABLE 6-14** Burst Fracture (Dispersion, Axial Loading)

Plain film findings:

Lateral view (Fig. 6-72):
- Biconcave vertebral body due to endplate fracture.
- Fragments displaced anteriorly and posteriorly.
- Prevertebral soft tissue swelling.
- Cervical spine normally aligned without signs of hyperflexion or hyperextension.
- Disruption of the vertebral body posterior cortical line.
- Loss of height of the involved vertebral body.

AP view:
- Vertical fracture line extending through the midportion of the vertebral body.
- Fracture of each endplate.
- Widening of suprajacent and narrowing of subjacent uncovertebral joints secondary to lateral displacement of hemivertebral fragments. For the hemivertebral fragments to disperse laterally there must be at least one posterior arch fracture; the posterior arch fracture is typically a minimally displaced laminar fracture that is usually not visible on the lateral projection.

UNSTABLE:
- Burst fractures are mechanically unstable.

CT findings: Laminar fractures are clearly shown on axial CT images.

Axial images: (Fig. 6-72)
- Comminuted fracture of the vertebral body.
- Assess relationship of retropulsed fragment(s) to spinal cord.
- Confirm posterior arch fracture (laminar fracture).
- Cautious search for contiguous fractures is critical.

Sagittal reconstruction: (Fig. 6-72)
- Biconcave vertebral body secondary to endplate fractures.
- Fragments displaced anteriorly and posteriorly.
- Prevertebral soft tissue swelling.
- Cervical spine is normally aligned without signs of hyperflexion or hyperextension.
- Coronal reconstruction: (Fig. 6-72).
- A vertical fracture line extending through the midportion of the vertebral body.
- Fracture of each endplate.
- Widening of suprajacent and narrowing of subjacent uncovertebral joints secondary to lateral displacement of hemivertebral fragments.

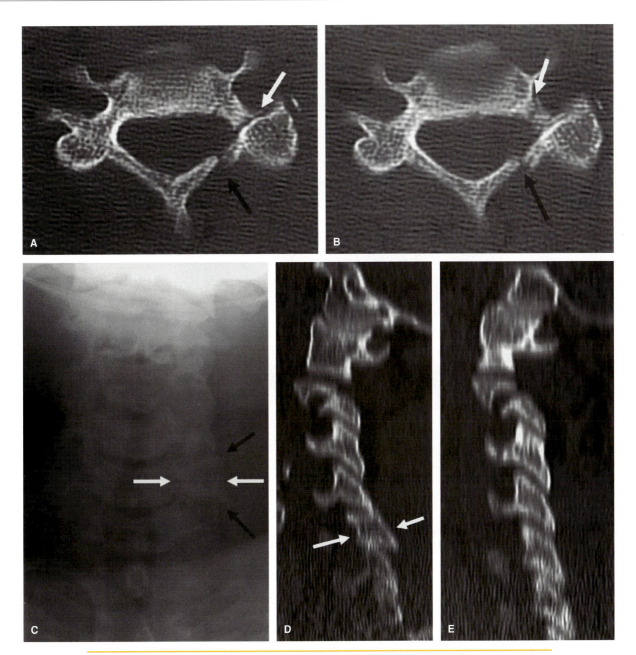

FIGURE 6-70. Type II pedicolaminar fracture of C5. **A,B:** Axial CT images demonstrate a fracture of the left pedicle that extends into the posterior aspect of the transverse process (*white arrow*) and a fracture of the left lamina (*black arrows*). **C:** On the AP radiograph the left articular mass of C5 is rotated (*white arrows*). The rotated articular mass appears as one half of a bowtie ("bowtie" sign). Additionally, the adjacent facet joint spaces are visible in the lateral column (*black arrows*). Left **(D)** and right **(E)** parasagittal multiplanar reformations. The left parasagittal reformation **(D)** clearly delineates rotation of the left C5 articular mass (*white arrows*).

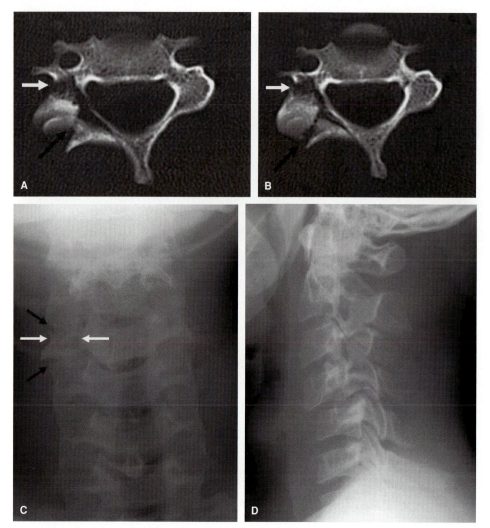

FIGURE 6-71. Type III pedico-laminar fracture of C4. **A,B:** Axial CT images demonstrate a comminuted fracture of the right pedicle that extends into the posterior aspect of the transverse process (*white arrow*) and a comminuted fracture of the right lamina (*black arrows*). **C:** On the AP radiograph the right articular mass of C4 is rotated (*white arrows*). The rotated articular mass appears as one half of a bowtie ("bowtie" sign). Additionally, the adjacent facet joint spaces are visible in the lateral column (*black arrows*). **D:** Lateral radiograph shows anterior translation of C4 with narrowing of the C4-5 disc space.

displaced. There is anterior translation of the vertebral body in type III (Fig. 6-71). Subluxation or frank dislocation of the contralateral facet joint is characteristic of type IV injury. CT and 3D CT can identify the unilateral pedicle and laminar fractures.

VERTICAL COMPRESSION (AXIAL LOADING) INJURY

Burst Fracture (Dispersion, Axial Loading)

The cervical burst fracture is a relatively uncommon injury (Table 6-14, Fig. 6-72). When axial compression forces are transmitted to the intervertebral disc, the liquid nucleus pulposus is imploded through the inferior endplate into the center of the vertebral body. The abrupt increase in pressure results in the vertebral body explod-

ing from the inside out, driving fragments in all directions (102). Retropulsed fragments may impinge on the spinal canal. The primary determinant of neurologic outcome is the extent of posterior bone fragment displacement into the thecal sac with concomitant spinal cord compression. Neurologic signs may vary from minor transient paresthesias to complete quadriplegia.

CONCLUSION

In this chapter we reviewed the common patterns of traumatic lesions that result from traumatic mechanisms that exceed the normal range of motion of the cervical spine. CT, with the use of high-resolution multiplanar and 3D reformations, has resulted in improved fracture pattern classification with better differentiation between stable or unstable injuries.

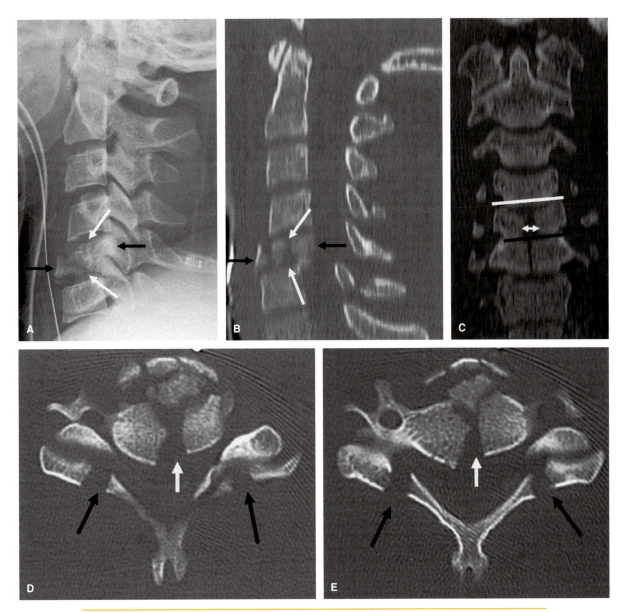

FIGURE 6-72. Burst (dispersion, axial loading) fracture of C5. Lateral radiograph **(A)** and sagittal multiplanar reformation **(B)** demonstrate fractures of each end plate (*white arrows*) with both anterior and posterior displacement of fracture fragments (*black arrows*), the latter into the central spinal canal. Note the typical straight alignment of the cervical spine in patients with burst fractures. **C:** Coronal multiplanar CT reformation shows vertical fracture lines extending through the midportion of the vertebral bodies of C5 and C6 with widening of suprajacent (*white line*) and narrowing of subjacent uncovertebral joints (*black line*) secondary to lateral displacement of hemivertebral fracture fragments (*white double-headed arrow*). **D,E:** Axial CT images demonstrate a comminuted fracture of the vertebral body with fragment dispersion; there is a vertical body fracture (*white arrows*), fragment retropulsion into the spinal canal, and bilateral fractures at the junctions of the laminae and articular masses (*black arrows*).

REFERENCES

1. Harris JH Jr. Mechanistic classification of acute cervical spine injuries. In: Harris JH Jr, Mirvis SE, eds. *The Radiology of Acute Cervical Spine Trauma*, 3rd ed. Baltimore: Williams and Wilkins; 1996:213–244.
2. Fielding JW. Cineroentgenography of the normal cervical spine. *J Bone Joint Surg*. 1957;39(A):1280–1288.
3. White AA III, Panjabi MM. *Clinical Biomechanics of the Spine*. 2nd ed. Philadelphia: JB Lippincott; 1991.
4. Denis F. Spinal instability as defined by the three-column spine concept in a acute spinal trauma. *Clin Orthop*. 1984;189:65–76.
5. Burke JT, Harris JH Jr. Acute injuries of the axis vertebra. *Skeletal Radiol*. 1989;18:335–346.
6. Leone A, Cerase A, Colosimo C, et al. Occipital condylar fractures: a review. *Radiology*. 2000;216:635–644.
7. Clayman DA, Sykes CH, Vines FS. Occipital condyle fractures: clinical presentation and radiologic detection. *AJNR Am J Neuroradiol*. 1994;15:1309–1315.
8. Stroobants J, Fidlers L, Storm JL, et al. High cervical pain and impairment of skull mobility as the only symptoms of an occipital condyle fracture. Case report. *J Neurosurg*. 1994;81:137–138.
9. Bloom AI, Neeman Z, Slasky BS, et al. Fractures of the occipital condyles and associated craneocervical ligament injury:incidence, CT imaging and implications. *Clin Radiol*. 1997;52:198–202.
10. Young WF, Rosenwasser RH, Getch C, et al. Diagnosis and management of occipital condyle fractures. *Neurosurgery*. 1994;34:257–260.
11. Anderson PA, Montesano PX. Morphology and treatment of occipital condyle fractures. *Spine*. 1988;13:731–736.
12. Przybylski GJ, Clyde BL, Fitz CR. Craniocervical junction subarachnoid hemorrhage associated with atlanto-occipital dislocation. *Spine*. 1996;21:1761–1768.
13. Fisher CG, Sun JCL, Dvorak M. Recognition and management of atlanto-occipital dislocation: improving survival from an often fatal condition. *Can J Surg*. 2001;44:412–420.
14. Shamoun JM, Riddick L, Powell RW. Atlanto-occipital subluxation/dislocation: a "survivable" injury in children. *Am Surgeon*. 1999;65:317–320.
15. Bucholz RW, Burkhead WZ. The pathologic anatomy of fatal atlanto-occipital dislocation. *J Bone Joint Surg Am*. 1979;61:248–250.
16. Traynelis VC, Marano GD, Dunker RO, et al. Traumatic atlanta-occipital dislocation. Case report. *J Neurosurg*. 1986;65:863–870.
17. Harris JH, Carson GC, Wagner LK. Radiologic diagnosis of traumatic occipitovertebral dissociation: 1. Normal occipitovertebral relationships on lateral radiographs of supine subjects. *AJR*. 1994;162:881–886.
18. Harris JH, Carson GC, Wagner LK, et al. Radiologic diagnosis of traumatic occipitovertebral dissociation: 2. Comparison of three methods of detecting occipitovertebral relationships on lateral radiographs of supine subjects. *AJR*. 1994;162:887–892.
19. Powers B, Miller MD, Kramer RS, et al. Traumatic anterior atlantooccipital dislocations. *Neurosurgery*. 1979;4:12–17.
20. Ferrera PC, Bartfield JM. Traumatic atlanto-occipital dislocation: a potentially survivable injury. *Am J Emerg Med*. 1996;14:291–296.
21. Lee C, Woodring JH, Goldstein SJ, et al. Evaluation of traumatic atlantooccipital dislocations. *AJNR*. 1987;8:19–26.
22. Brinkman W, Cohen W, Manning T. Posterior fossa subarachnoid hemorrhage due to an atlanto-occipital dislocation. *AJR*. 2003;180 (5):1476.
23. Jefferson G. Fracture of the atlas vertebra: report of four cases, and a review of those previously recorded. *Br J Surg*. 1920;7:407–422.
24. Harris JH. Jr, Mirvis SE. Vertical compression injuries. In Harris JH Jr, Mirvis SE, eds. *The Radiology of Acute Cervical Spine Trauma*, 3rd ed. Baltimore: Williams & Wilkins; 1996:340–365.
25. Landells CD, Van Pethegem PK. Fractures of the atlas: classification, treatment and morbidity. *Spine*. 1988;13:450–452.
26. Lee C, Woodring JH. Unstable Jefferson variant atlas fractures: an unrecognized cervical injury. *AJNR Am J Neuroradiol*. 1991;12:1105–1110.
27. Mirvis SE, Shanmuganathan K, eds. Imaging of Cervical Spine Trauma. *Imaging in Trauma and Critical Care: Imaging of Cervical Spine Trauma*, 2nd ed. Philadelphia: Saunders; 2003:185–296.
28. Suss RA, Zimmerman RD, Leeds NE. Pseudospread of the atlas: false sign of Jefferson fracture in young children. *AJR Am J Roentgenol*. June 1983;140(6):1079–1082.
29. Wirth RL, Zatz LM, Parker BR. CT detection of a Jefferson fracture in a child. *AJR*. 1987;149:1001–1002.
30. Shapiro R, Youngberg AS, Rothman SL. The differential diagnosis of traumatic lesions of the occipito-atlanto-axial segment. *Radiol Clin North Am*. 1973;11:505–526.
31. Sherk HH, Nicholson JT. Fractures of the atlas. *J Bone Joint Surg*. 1970;52:1017–1024.
32. Hadley MN, Dickman CA, Browner CM, et al. Acute traumatic atlas fractures: management and long term outcome. *Neurosurgery*. 1988;23:31–35.
33. Landells CD, Van Peteghem PK. Fractures of the atlas: classification, treatment and morbidity. *Spine*. 1988;13:450–452.
34. Stewart GC Jr. Gehweiler JA, Laib RH, et al. Horizontal fracture of the anterior arch of the atlas. *Radiology*. 1977;122:349–352.
35. Jevtich V. Horizontal fractures of the anterior arch of the atlas. *J Bone Joint Surg*. 1986;68:1094–1095.
36. Pepin JW, Hawkins RJ. Traumatic spondylolisthesis of the axis: hangman's fracture. *Clin Orthop*. 1981;157:133–138.
37. Cybulski GR, Stone JL, Arnold PM, et al. Multiple fractures of the cervical and upper thoracic spine without neurological deficit: case report. *Neurosurgery*. 1989;24:768–771.
38. Shacked I, Rappaport ZH, Barzilay Z, et al. Two-level fracture of the cervical spine in young child. *J Bone Joint Surg*. 1983;65:119–122.
39. Shear P, Hugenholtz H, Tichard MT, et al. Multiple noncontiguous fractures of the cervical spine. *J Trauma*. 1988;28:655–659.
40. Ersmark H, Kalen R. Injuries of the atlas and axis. A follow-up study of 85 axis and 10 atlas fractures. *Clin Orthop*. 1987;217:257–260.
41. Hadley MN, Sonntag VKH, Grahm TW, et al. Axis fractures resulting from motor vehicle accidents. The need for occupant restraints. *Spine*. 1986;11:861–864.
42. Schneider RD, Livingstone KE, Cove AJE, et al. "Hangman's fracture" of the cervical spine. *J Neurosurg*. 1965;22:141–154.
43. Lachman E. Anatomy of the judicial hanging. *Resident Staff Phys*. 1972;46:54.
44. Wood-Jones F. The ideal lesion produced by judicial hanging. *Lancet*. 1913;1:53–54.
45. Elliot JM, Rogers LF, Wissinger JP, et al. The hangman's fracture. *Radiology*. 1972;104:303–307.
46. Mollan RAB, Watt PCH. Hangman's fracture. *Injury*. 1982;14:265.
47. Effendi B, Roy D, Cornish B, et al. Fractures of the ring of the axis: a classification based on the analysis of 131 cases. *J Bone Joint Surg*. 1981;63B:319–327.
48. Levine Am, Edwards CC. The management of traumatic spondylolisthesis of the axis. *J Bone Joint Surg Am*. 1985;67:217–226.
49. Anderson LD, D'Alonzo RT. Fractures of the odontoid process of the axis. *J Bone Joint Surg*. 1974;56A:1663–1674.
50. Scott EW, Haid RW Jr, Peace D. Type I fractures of the odontoid process: implications for atlanto-occipital instability. Case report. *J Neurosurg*. 1990;72:488–492.
51. Gehweiler JA, Osborne RL, Becker RF. *The Radiology of Vertebral Trauma*. Vol. 16. Saunders Monographs in Clinical Radiology. Philadelphia: WB Saunders; 1980.
52. Alexander E Jr, Forsyth HF, Davis CH, et al. Dislocation of the atlas on the axis: the value of early fusion of C1, C2, and C3. *Neurosurgery*. 1958;15:353–371.

53. Hadley MN, Browner CM, Liu SS, et al. New subtype of acute odontoid fractures (type IIA). *Neurosurgery*. January 1988;22(1 Pt 1):67–71.

54. Koivikko MP, Kiuru MJ, Koskinen SK. Occurrence of comminution (type IIA) in type II odontoid process fractures: a multi-slice CT study. *Emerg Radiol*. October 2003;10(2):84–86.

55. Greene KA, Dickman CA, Marciano FF, et al. Acute axis fractures: analysis of management and outcome in 340 consecutive cases. *Spine*. 1997;22:1843–1852.

56. Weisskopf M, Reindl R, Schroder R, et al. CT scans versus conventional tomography in acute fractures of the odontoid process. *Eur Spine J*. June 2001;10(3):250–256.

57. Fielding JW Hawkins RJ. Atlantoaxial rotatory fixation. *J Bone Joint Surg*. 1977;59A:37–44.

58. Maheshwaran S, Sgouros S, Jeyapalan K, et al. Imaging of childhood torticollis due to atlanto-axial rotatory fixation. *Childs Nerv Syst*. 1995;11:667–671.

59. Kowalski HM, Cohen WA, Cooper P, et al. Pitfalls in the CT diagnosis of atlantoaxial rotatory subluxation. *Am J Neuroradiol*. 1987;8:697–702.

60. Philips WA, Hensinger RN. The management of rotatory atlantoaxial subluxation in children. *J Bone Joint Surg*. 1987;71A:664–668.

61. Roche CJ, O'Malley M, Dorgan JC, et al. A pictorial review of atlanto-axial rotatory fixation: key points for the radiologist. *Clin Radiol*. 2001;56:947–958.

62. Parke WW, Rothman RH, Brown MD. The pharyngovertebral veins: an anatomical rationale for Grisel's syndrome. *J Bone Joint Surg Am*. April 1984;66(4):568–574.

63. Wortzman G, Dewar F. Rotatory fixation of the atlanto-axial joint: rotational atlantoaxial subluxation. *Radiology*. 1968;90:479–487.

64. Cancelmo JJ Jr. Clay shoveler's fracture. A helpful diagnostic sign. *Am J Roentgenol Radium Ther Nucl Med*. July 1972;115(3):540–543.

65. Cheshire DJ. The stability of the cervical spine following the conservative treatment of fractures and fracture-dislocations. *Paraplegia*. 1969;7:193–203.

66. Bohlman HH. Acute fractures and dislocations of the cervical spine—an analysis of three hundred hospitalized patients and review of the literature. *J Bone Joint Surg Am*. 1979;61:1119–1142.

67. Doran SE, Papadopoulos SM, Ducker TB, et al. Magnetic resonant imaging documentation of co-existent traumatic locked facets of the cervical spine and disc herniation. *J Neurosurg*. 1993;79:341–345.

68. Sonntag VK. Management of bilateral locked facets of the cervical spine. *Neurosurgery*. 1981;8:150–152.

69. Wolf A, Levi L, Mirvis SE. Operative management of bilateral facet dislocation. *J Neurosurg*. 1991;75:883–890.

70. Kahn EA, Schneider RC. Chronic neurological sequelae of acute trauma to the spine and spinal cord. I. The significance of the acute-flexion or tear-drop fracture-dislocation of the cervical spine. *J Bone Joint Surg Am*. October 1956;38A(5):985–997.

71. Torg JS, Pavlov H, O'Neill MJ, et al. The axial load teardrop fracture. A biomechanical, clinical and roentgenographic analysis. *Am J Sports Med*. July–August 1991;19(4):355–364.

72. Shanmuganathan K, Mirvis SE, Levine AM. Rotational injury of cervical facets: CT analysis of fracture patterns with implications for management and neurologic outcome. *AJR Am J Roentgenol*. November 1994;163(5):1165–1169.

73. Sim E. Vertical facet splitting: a special variant of rotary dislocations of the cervical spine. *J Neurosurg*. February 1995;82(2):239–243.

74. Braakman R, Vinken PJ. Unilateral facet interlocking in the lower cervical spine. *J Bone Joint Surg Br*. May 1967;49(2):249–257.

75. Argenson C, Lovet J, Sanouiller JL, et al. Traumatic rotatory displacement of the lower cervical spine. *Spine*. July 1988;13(7):767–773.

76. Shapiro S, Snyder W, Kaufman K, et al. Outcome of 51 cases of unilateral locked cervical facets: interspinous braided cable for lateral mass plate fusion compared with interspinous wire and facet wiring with iliac crest. *J Neurosurg Spine*. July 1999;91(1):19–24.

77. Louw JA, Mafoyane NA, Small B, et al. Occlusion of the vertebral artery in cervical spine dislocations. *J Bone Joint Surg Br*. July 1990;72(4):679–781.

78. Willis BK, Greiner F, Orrison WW, et al. The incidence of vertebral artery injury after midcervical spine fracture or subluxation. *Neurosurgery*. March 1994;34(3):435–441; discussion 441–442.

79. Kiwerski J. Extension injuries of the cervical spine. *Chir Narzadow Ruchu Ortop Pol*. 1976;41(3):233–237.

80. Regenbogen VS, Rogers LF, Atlas SW, et al. Cervical spinal cord injuries in patients with cervical spondylosis. *AJR Am J Roentgenol*. February 1986;146(2):277–284.

81. Scher AT. Hyperextension trauma in the elderly: an easily overlooked spinal injury. *J Trauma*. December 1983;23(12):1066–1068.

82. Murray GC, Persellin RH. Cervical fracture complicating ankylosing spondylitis: a report of eight cases and review of the literature. *Am J Med*. May 1981;70(5):1033–1041.

83. Taylor AR. The mechanism of injury to the spinal cord in the neck without damage to vertebral column. *J Bone Joint Surg Br*. November 1951;33B(4):543–547.

84. Edeiken-Monroe B, Wagner LK, Harris JH Jr. Hyperextension dislocation of the cervical spine. *AJR Am J Roentgenol*. April 1986;146(4):803–808.

85. Warner J, Shanmuganathan K, Mirvis SE, et al. Magnetic resonance imaging of ligamentous injury of the cervical spine. *Emerg Radiol*. 1996;3:9–15.

86. Davis SJ, Teresi LM, Bradley WG Jr, et al. Cervical spine hyperextension injuries: MR findings. *Radiology*. July 1991;180(1):245–251.

87. Schweighofer F, Ranner G, Schleifer P, et al. Hyperextension injury of the lower cervical spine and diagnosis of dorsal unstable motion segments. *Langenbecks Arch Chir*. 1995;380(3):162–165.

88. Harris JH, Yeakley JW. Hyperextension-dislocation of the cervical spine. Ligament injuries demonstrated by magnetic resonance imaging. *J Bone Joint Surg Br*. July 1992;74(4):567–570.

89. Lee C, Kim KS, Rogers LF. Triangular cervical vertebral body fractures: diagnostic significance. *AJR*. June 1982;138(6):1123–1132.

90. Korres DS, Zoubos AB, Kavadias K, et al. The "tear drop" (or avulsed) fracture of the anterior inferior angle of the axis. *Eur Spine J*. 1994;3(3):151–154.

91. Lee JS, Harris JH Jr, Mueller CF. The significance of prevertebral soft tissue swelling in extension teardrop fracture of the cervical spine. *Emerg Radiol*. 1997;4(3):132–139.

92. Cimmino CV, Scott DW. Laminar avulsion in a cervical vertebra. *AJR*. July 1977;129(1):57–60.

93. Babcock JL. Cervical spine injuries: diagnosis and classification. *Arch Surg*. June 1976;111(6):646–651.

94. Woodring JH, Goldstein SJ. Fractures of the articular processes of the cervical spine. *AJR*. 1982;139(2):341–344.

95. Smith GR, Beckly DE, Abel MS. Articular mass fracture: a neglected cause of post-traumatic neck pain? *Clin Radiol*. July 1976;27(3):335–340.

96. Judet J, Roy-Camille R, Zerah JC, et al. Fractures of the cervical spine: fracture-separation of the articular column. *Rev Chir Orthop Reparatrice Appar Mot*. March 1970;56(2):155–164.

97. Shanmuganathan K, Mirvis SE, Dowe M, Levine AM. Traumatic isolation of the cervical articular pillar: imaging observations in 21 patients. *AJR Am J Roentgenol*. April 1996;166(4):897–902.

98. Forsyth Hf E. extension injuries of the cervical spine. *J Bone Joint Surg Am*. December 1964;46:1792–1797.

99. Scher AT. Radiological assessment of lateral flexion injuries of the cervical spine. *S Afr Med J*. December 26, 1981;60(26):983–985.

100. Allen BL Jr, Ferguson RL, Lehmann TR, et al. A mechanistic classification of closed, indirect fractures and dislocations of the lower cervical spine. *Spine*. January–February 1982;7(1):1–27.

101. Fuentes JM, Benezech J, Lussiez B, et al. Fracture-separation of the articular process of the lower cervical spine. Its relation to fracture-dislocation in hyperextension. *Rev Chir Orthop Reparatrice Appar Mot*. 1986;72(6):435–440.

102. Roaf RA. A study of the mechanics of spinal injuries. *J Bone Joint Surg Br*. 1960;42:810–823.

103. Schlicke LH, Callahan RA. A rational approach to burst fractures of the atlas. *Clin Orthop*. 1981;154:18–21.

104. Segal LS, Grimm JO, Stauffer ES. Non-union of fractures of the atlas. *J Bone Joint Surg Am*. December 1987;69(9): 1423–1434.

105. Harris JH, Burker JT, Ray RD, et al. Low (type III) odontoid fracture: a new radiographic sign. *Radiology*. 1984;153: 353–356.

106. Smoker WR, Dolan KD. The "fat" C2: a sign of fracture. *AJR*. 1987;148:609–614.

107. Fielding WJ, Hensinger RN, Hawkins RJ. Os odontoideum. *J Bone Joint Surg*. 1980;62:376–383.

108. Kathol MH. Cervical spine trauma. What is new? *Radiol Clin North Am*. 1997;35:507–532.

109. Green JD, Harle TS, Harris JH. Anterior subluxation of the cervical spine: hyperflexion sprain. *AJNR*. 1981;2:243–250.

110. Abel MS. *Occult Traumatic Lesions of the Cervical and Thoraco-lumbar Vertebrae*. 2nd ed. St. Louis: Warren Green; 1982.

111. Lingawi SS. The naked facet sign. *Radiology*. 2001;219: 366–367.

112. Daffner SD, Daffner RH. Computed tomography diagnosis of facet dislocations: the "hamburger bun" and "reverse hamburger bun" signs. *J Emerg Med*. November 2002;23(4): 387–394.

113. Kim KS, Chen HH, Russell EJ, et al. Flexion teardrop fracture of the cervical spine: radiographic characteristics. *AJR Am J Roentgenol*. February 1989;152(2):319–326.

114. Young JW, Resnik CS, DeCandido P, et al. The laminar space in the diagnosis of rotational flexion injuries of the cervical spine. *AJR Am J Roentgenol*. January 1989;152(1):103–107.

C h a p t e r   7

Imaging of Thoracolumbar Spinal Injury

George Koulouris, Amy Y. I. Ting, and William B. Morrison

Spinal trauma affects a variety of osteoligamentous supports that make up the vertebral column. The pattern of injury serves as a diagnostic clue as to the mechanism of injury, the latter being critically dependent on the degree of force involved and the force vectors on the portion of the spine affected. The potential for significant mechanical disruption exists, and, therefore, devastating neurologic deficits can occur with irreversible morbidity or even death. The goals of therapy primarily are to stabilize the patient in order to preserve life and to maintain and maximize neurologic function by providing a painless and stable vertebral column.

The imaging evaluation of the traumatized patient with possible spinal injury depends on many variables, including the nature of the injury, whether the patient is conscious, local imaging protocols, and the preference of trauma physicians/surgeons. In addition, institutions, particularly trauma centers, have adopted individual protocols based on what their clinicians feel is best practice given their patient population and imaging facilities available. To date, no standard uniform imaging algorithm is in widespread use; reflecting the complexity of possible spinal injuries, but also on the evolving nature and advances made in the field of diagnostic radiology and trauma. Indeed, controversy exists not only with issues pertaining to diagnosis, but with respect to the selection of surgical candidates, the preferred operative approach, and timing of surgery.

Despite the controversies, certain basic principles exist. Imaging assessment usually commences with radiographs, which are useful in screening the entire spine, without exposure to significant amounts of radiation. Most institutions will radiograph the entire spine as a minimum in the presence of one spinal fracture in order to exclude at least a noncontiguous fracture. The reported time to diagnosis for missed fractures has been recorded as high as 53 days (1). The second injury may be adjacent to the primary fracture (contiguous) or distant (noncontiguous) (2) with almost three quarters of noncontiguous fractures occurring at the cervicothoracic and lumbosacral transition zones (3). Computed tomography (CT), in particular with the advent of multidetector CT (MDCT), allows for excellent depiction of bone detail (particularly the cortex) and superbly demonstrates on multiplanar reformatted views vertebral alignment without osseous and soft tissue superimposition; a significant inherent limitation of radiographs. Even the most subtle-subtlest disruption can be visualized in all three planes, providing improved three-dimensional (3D) appreciation by allowing accurate depiction of osseous displacement. As spinal trauma patients often have coexisting visceral trauma requiring CT evaluation, images obtained from a MDCT study of the abdomen and pelvis can be used to create secondary reconstructions targeted to the spine. Overlapping thin slice multiplanar reformatted images (4,5) and 3D surface reconstructions (6) are of sufficient quality to obviate the need for standard radiographic assessment (7–10). The latter may be performed at the physician's request as required (11).

Magnetic resonance imaging (MRI) is a complementary examination to CT, often assisting in diagnosing subtle fractures as well as assisting in cases where a possible fracture is identified with CT, but cannot be confidently excluded. Also, minor alterations in alignment, possibly indicative of severe soft tissue injury, may be further evaluated with MRI. The main strength of MRI lies in its exquisite depiction of normal and pathologically affected soft tissue structures. This includes accurate visualization of the intervertebral discs, supporting ligaments, and of most importance, the status of the spinal cord and nerves. Extra- and intra-axial lesions can also be visualized, such as a hematoma, which may be seen in the context of trauma.

THORACOLUMBAR ANATOMY

The vertebral column consists of 32 vertebral segments, each of these segments is further subdivided into the weight-bearing vertebral body and the neural (dorsal) arch, the latter protecting the spinal cord, which occupies the spinal canal. The morphology of the vertebral bodies reflects their function. The vertebral bodies progressively increase in size in the thoracic and lumbar spine, consistent with an increased weight-bearing role (Fig. 7-1). Unique to the thoracic spine are facets for the costal articulations and characteristically long inferiorly directed overlapping spinous processes (Fig. 7-2A). The lumbar vertebral bodies are broad and flat, with large pedicles and facet joints orientated in the sagittal plane (Fig. 7-2B).

Intervening intervertebral discs represent symphyseal articulations, the disc consisting of the tough outer annulus fibrosus and the inner notochordal remnant, the nucleus pulposus. The annulus fibrosus consists of laminated type-I and type-II collagen fibers, which are orientated in an oblique direction (Fig. 7-3). Fibers on either side then run in an opposite direction, a feature designed to resist tensile forces in all directions. The nucleus pulposus is somewhat posteriorly located within the intervertebral disc complex and consists of large macromolecules that trap water molecules, giving this structure its gelatinous and mucoid consistency. Interposed between the disc and vertebral body cortical endplates is a layer of hyaline (articular) cartilage.

Dorsal (spinous process) and lateral (transverse) processes project from the neural arches and serve as levers upon which powerful muscles attach, conferring both mobility as well as dynamic stability when undergoing eccentric contraction (Fig. 7-4). The erector spinae muscle complex lies deep to the thoracolumbar fascia and is divided into three major subgroups, the spinalis

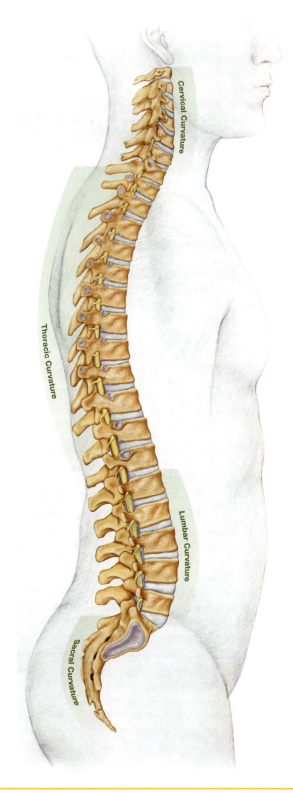

FIGURE 7-1. Vertebral column. Schematic image for the entire spine, demonstrating progressive enlargement of the vertebral bodies from the superior aspect of the thoracic spine to the lower lumbar spine. Also note the transition from kyphosis to lordosis at the thoracolumbar junction. Asset provided by Anatomical Chart Co.

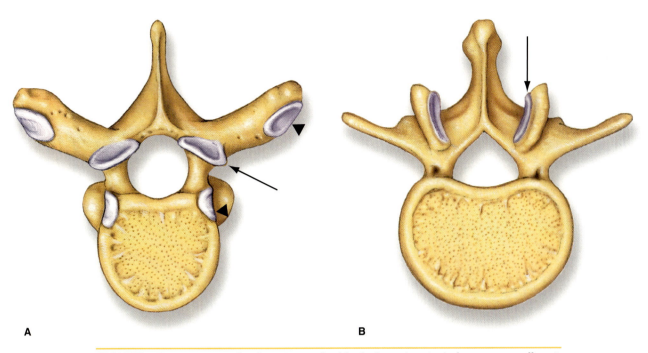

A   B

FIGURE 7-2. **A:** Diagram of a thoracic vertebral body (superior view) shows a coronally oriented facet joint (*black arrow*), as well as the costovertebral articulations (*black arrowheads*). Asset provided by Anatomical Chart Co. **B:** Diagram of a lumbar vertebral body (*superior view*) shows a sagittally oriented facet joint (*black arrow*). Asset provided by Anatomical Chart Co.

(medial), iliocostalis (intermediate), and longissimus (lateral). These muscles attach to the spinous processes. The thicker multifidus group arises from the sacrum and mammillary processes of the lumbar spine and attaches to the posterior aspect of the laminae and spinous processes. The muscles anterior to the thoracolumbar fascia are the quadratus lumborum, psoas major, and the variably present psoas minor. The psoas major gains its origin from anteromedial aspect of the transverse processes, and annulus and adjacent vertebral bodies

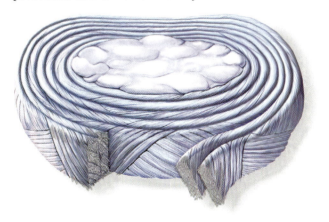

FIGURE 7-3. Diagram of intervertebral disc shows central nucleus pulposus surrounded by the annulus fibrosus, which consists of obliquely oriented collagen fibers. Asset provided by Anatomical Chart Co.

from the T12 to first sacral segments. The quadratus lumborum originates from the anterolateral portion of the transverse processes from L1 to L4. Further osseous projections, superiorly and inferiorly, consist of inferior and superior articular processes respectively (with the intervening pars interarticularis), which when interlock with their counterparts above and below and form the synovial facet joints. The orientation of the facet joints is critical with respect to the range and orientation of movement that is permitted in that region of the vertebral column.

The ligamentous constraints of the thoracolumbar spine are extensive, functioning to confer stability while allowing motion, and are best demonstrated with MRI (12,13) (Fig. 7-5). The principal ligaments include the anterior and posterior longitudinal ligaments (ALL and PLL) (14), which share a reciprocal relationship with respect to size, with the ALL thinner cranially and thicker caudally. The ALL gains its origin from the basiocciput and inferiorly is broader, terminating anteriorly on the sacrum. Its primary role is to resist extension. At the level of C1 and above, the ALL is continuous as the anterior atlanto-occipital membrane. The PLL is broad in the cervical spine (15) and possesses a serrated appearance throughout its course, being widest at the intervertebral disc level, to which it is adherent though loosely attached to the vertebral bodies. It terminates on the posterior aspect of the sacrum and acts to resist flexion. Both longitudinal ligaments are composed of fibers deep and superficial

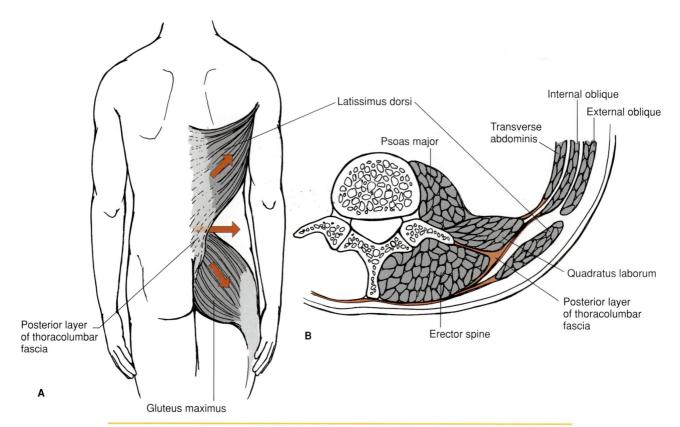

FIGURE 7-4. **A:** Diagram shows the attachments of the major muscle groups of the back and relationship to the vertebral bodies. (From Oatis CA. *Kinesiology—The Mechanics and Pathomechanics of Human Movement*. Baltimore: Lippincott Williams & Wilkins; 2004, with permission.) **B:** Diagram shows the three major columns of the erector spinae musculature. (From Hendrickson T. *Massage for Orthopedic Conditions*. Baltimore: Lippincott Williams & Wilkins; 2002, with permission.)

relative to the vertebral bodies, the former coursing only over one vertebral body and the latter crossing three to four levels. Superiorly, the PLL continues as the tectorial membrane, attaching to the anterior aspect of the foramen magnum to insert and become inseparable from the dura mater.

The posteriorly positioned ligamentum flavum is composed of elastic fibers (16), giving this ligament its characteristic yellow color. It connects the laminae between vertebral bodies and prevents separation of the posterior structures by acting as a dynamic restraint against excessive flexion. The interspinous ligaments are composed of short fascicles connecting the spinous processes together to adjacent spinous process and arise from the origin of the process to its tip. At the tip, the ligament fuses with the supraspinous ligament, which forms a continuous superficial longitudinal ligament, extending from the sacrum to the C7 vertebral body (and continues to the occiput as the ligamentum nuchae). Both these ligaments act as further restraints of hyperflexion.

The thoracic spine from T1 to T8 is positioned in kyphosis and is less mobile than the cervical and lumbar spine because of the rib cage, smaller intervertebral discs, and the significant overlap provided by the articular facets and associated musculoligamentous supports. The sternum and ribs limit the thoracic spine's inherent tendency to hyperflex when subjected to axial forces. To an extent, this relative rigidity protects the thoracic spine from injury and accounts for the relative decreased incidence of fractures. The weight-bearing axis of the body is anterior to the thoracic spine, so that the anterior vertebral structures undergo physiologic compression, whereas the posterior aspect is under tension. This anatomy results in a flexion force during axial load injuries with the result of characteristic anterior flexion wedge-type fracture patterns. However, with a greater amount of force, fractures may involve the posterior vertebral body and posterior elements, as well as the ribs.

Several key anatomic points account for the increased susceptibility of the thoracolumbar region to injury. The

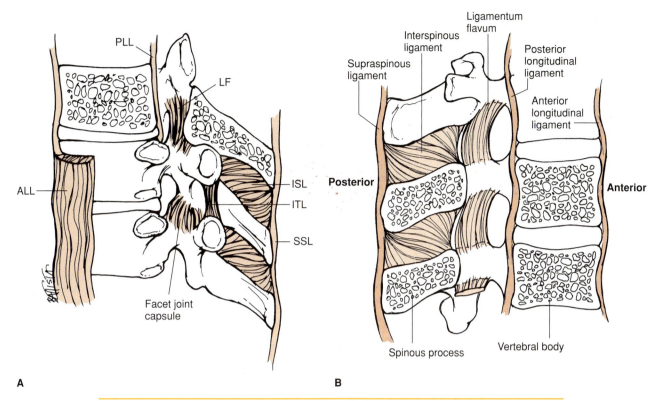

FIGURE 7-5. Diagrams of the thoracic spine **(A)** and lumbar **(B)** demonstrate the major ligamentous structures. ALL, anterior longitudinal ligament; PLL, posterior longitudinal ligament; LF, ligamentum flavum; ITL, intertransverse ligament; ISL, interspinous ligament; SSL, supraspinous ligament. (From Oatis CA. *Kinesiology—The Mechanics and Pathomechanics of Human Movement*. Baltimore: Lippincott Williams & Wilkins; 2004, with permission.)

thoracolumbar junction is a region of transition (17), the junction of the relatively fixed thoracic spine and the highly mobile lumbar spine and simultaneous transition from a posture of kyphosis to lordosis (Fig. 7-1). The lower two thoracic vertebral bodies possess short ribs, which, unlike at higher levels, possess no sternal articulation and hence offer no additional protection. Furthermore, a sudden alteration in the plane of orientation of the facet joints from coronal (thoracic) to sagittal (lumbar) also accounts for a greater propensity for injuries in this region (18). The orientation of the facet joints is felt to be important with respect to injury mechanism; for example, sagittal-orientated facets, as seen in the lumbar spine (relative to the thoracic facets) allow for a greater range in motion with respect to hyperflexion, and thus such injuries are common (Fig. 7-2). Conversely, injuries secondary to a rotational force are less common. These factors make the thoracolumbar junction (T9 to L3) particularly susceptible to injury; two thirds of all thoracolumbar fractures occur at T12, L1, or L2, and an estimated 90% occur between T11 and L4. Axial load injuries to this region are common, with additional rotation, lateral bending, and shearing vectors demonstrated in this biomechanical transition zone. Also concentrated in this

area are flexion/distraction injuries resulting from restraint by automobile lap belts.

The lumbar spine is positioned in lordosis and is very mobile, making it susceptible to varying force vectors. Because of the lordotic curve, the center of gravity is shifted more posteriorly; flexion injuries often straighten the spine and result in an axial load type burst injury, with little or no anterior wedging. The thoracolumbar spine has a higher incidence for visceral trauma when compared to the cervical spine (19). The radiologist must have a high index of suspicion for associated chest injuries, which may be seen in up to 26% of cases (19), as well as being aware of a 6% to 10% (20,21) incidence of abdominal and pelvic visceral trauma. Particular fractures that have extremely high associations with visceral injury require extremely careful abdominal scrutiny, such as the classic Chance fracture, resulting from a flexion-distraction force, which has had a previously reported incidence as high as 89% (22).

Neurologic injury depends partly on type and severity of injury, but is also related to the configuration of the spinal canal and cord. The spinal cord typically terminates at approximately L1 (L2 or L3 in children). The spinal canal size in the thoracic region averages 16 (anteroposterior) by

16 mm (transverse), whereas in the lumbar spine the canal averages 17 (anteroposterior) by 26 mm (transverse). Therefore, relatively minor thoracic trauma can result in significant neurologic compromise, which is also contributed to in part by the close approximation of the cord to the posterior cortex of the vertebral body. In contrast, the lumbar spine is more capacious and has the advantage of the cord terminating as the conus medullaris at the L1 level. Moreover, the nerve roots of the cauda equina, unlike the spinal cord, are relatively resistant to blunt trauma. Hence, a significant burst injury with retropulsed fragments has potential for relatively minimal effect on neurologic status in this region.

The spinal cord commences at the level of the foramen magnum as a continuation of the medulla oblongata and extends inferiorly to the level of the L1-2 intervertebral disc (L2-3 level in the newborn), where it terminates as the conus medullaris and its distal cordlike extension, the filum terminale. The latter inserts to the posterior aspect of the coccyx. Surrounding the cord are the typical coverings of the central nervous system, the dura mater (itself surrounded by epidural fat and venous plexus and terminating at the S2 level), the arachnoid and pia mater. Cerebrospinal fluid is present in the subarachnoid space, with the subdural space only being a potential space. The epidural space is a true space, principally composed of fat. Cervical and lumbar enlargement of the cord is secondary to the brachial and lumbar plexus.

Emanating from the spinal cord are tiny rootlets that coalesce to form spinal roots, the ventral (motor) and dorsal (sensory). As the cord terminates at the level of the L1-2 intervertebral disc, the spinal nerves inferior to this level must traverse a long segment of the spinal canal to finally reach their respective neural exit foramen, hence forming the characteristic cauda equina. The exiting nerves in the thoracolumbar spine are numbered from the vertebral body pedicle they pass under; hence, the L1 nerve root emanates from the L1-2 level, under the pedicle of L1.

FRACTURE CLASSIFICATION AND STABILITY

Vertebral fractures, like fractures in the peripheral skeleton, occur in a predictable and reproducible manner, related to the kind of force applied to the bone. The purpose of a classification scheme is to act as a tool to assist the clinician in determining whether instability (mechanical or neurologic) is present. Classification schemes also allow for research to be reproduced, such that accurate comparison and conclusions are made possible. However, in some instances, classification schemes force stratification of processes that can be better characterized as a continuous spectrum. As such, the different magnitude

and complex vectors of force applied to variably mobile vertebral segments, in any of the three regions of the spine, compounded by individual variability and possible concomitant disease processes, allow for an extremely wide variability of injury patterns, which may not fall neatly into a specific class of injury. Thus, if a scheme is relatively simplified, it is considered too broad and not specific enough; one that is comprehensive becomes cumbersome and unwieldy (23) with low interobserver agreement. Introduction of novel classification schemes, which evolve continuously, particularly with emerging imaging technology such as with MRI (24), only adds to the lack of consistency. Nevertheless, knowledge of basic traumatic force vectors, anatomy, and biomechanics allows for a reasonable understanding of injury patterns and hence, a comprehension of the etiology of vertebral column fractures.

As mentioned above, the more comprehensive the classification system, the lower the interobserver agreement. This creates a dilemma for the radiologist who wants to communicate with the referring clinician using relevant terminology. Therefore, as in many other instances of radiologic standard practice, it is prudent and best practice to be descriptive when reporting fractures as opposed to simply subcategorizing an injury into a classification scheme. This allows accurate communication between clinicians and other radiologists and will still remain a historically correct interpretation despite the emergence of further differing classification schemes. However, the radiologist needs to be aware of the relevant findings to report, for example, if there is an anterior wedge fracture indicated on an MRI, or if the integrity of the posterior longitudinal ligament should be described. Essentially, it is not so important to be aware of the classification as it is to understand the concepts of stability and the mechanism of injury. This approach enables accurate communication of the most important information and aids in detection of associated injuries, including any unusual injuries that might change management.

Fractures of the vertebral column are divided traditionally into those affecting the thoracolumbar region (as the fracture pattern and mechanism share many similarities) and the cervical spine. Many theories and classification schemes have been proposed for cervical and thoracolumbar fractures; some deal primarily with mechanism of injury, others with the pattern of fracture (25), still others with stability or neurologic compromise. These systems are still not optimal for the evaluation of stability, prognosis, and management options and are perhaps simplified as two key concepts: mechanical and neurologic stability (either stable or unstable) with each having potential for being acute or chronic. A full discussion of the various classification schemes is beyond the scope of this discussion (Table 7-1). Denis (26) in 1983 reviewed the radiographs, pathology results, and surgical and operative

▶ **TABLE 7-1 Evolution of Thoracolumbar Fracture Classification Schemes**

Watson-Jones 1938 (92)
Wedge fracture
Comminuted fracture
Fracture-dislocation

Holdsworth 1963 (93)
Two-column theory:
   Flexion
   Flexion-rotation
   Extension
   Extension-compression
   Shear

Denis 1983 (26)
Three-column theory:
   Demarcation between anterior and middle columns *midway* of
     vertebral body

Compression
 Type A: Both endplates fractured
 Type B: Superior endplate fracture
 Type C: Inferior endplate fracture
 Type D: Lateral wedging

Burst
 Type A: Both endplates fractured
 Type B: Superior endplate fracture
 Type C: Inferior endplate fracture
 Type D: Burst fracture with rotatory component
 Type E: Burst fracture with lateral flexion

Flexion-distraction
 Type A: Single level, classic Chance fracture with bone disruption only
 Type B: Single level, soft tissue/ligamentous disruption
 Type C: Two level disruption through bone at middle column
 Type D: Two level disruption through soft tissues at middle column

Fracture-dislocation
 Type A: Flexion rotations through body
 Type B: Flexion rotation through disc

Type C: Posteroanterior shear injury
Type D: Posteroanterior shear injury with floating lamina
Type E: Anteroposterior shear injury
Type F: Flexion distraction

McAfee et al. 1983 (33)
Wedge compression
Stable burst
Unstable burst
Chance fracture
Flexion distraction
Translational

Ferguson and Allen 1984 (94)
Demarcation between anterior and middle columns at junction of
anterior two thirds and posterior one third of vertebral body
Compressive flexion
Distractive flexion
Lateral flexion
Translational
Torsional flexion
Vertical compression
Distractive flexion

Magerl et al. 1994 (25)
Type A: Compression: resulting in fracture due to axial load $\pm$ flexion
Type B: Distraction: disrupted anterior and posterior soft tissues in
   the transverse plane
Type C: Rotation: anterior and posterior element injuries
Further subdivided into groups and subgroups utilizing the
   AO 3-3-3 grid

McCormack et al. 1994 (95)
Load-sharing classification
   Used as a predictor of implant failure
   Grading of fracture on:
     Degree of comminution: 1, little; 2, more; 3, gross
     Fragment displacement: 1, little; 2, more; 3, gross
     Corrected traumatic kyphosis: 1, little; 2, more; 3, gross

notes in 412 thoracolumbar injuries and modified the Holdsworth two-column concept to devise the "three-column spine concept" in acute spinal trauma (Fig. 7-6). This classification scheme forms the basis of the contents discussed in this chapter owing to its widespread use and relative simplicity. Though real-life vectors are a complex combination of forces, usually one force predominates to result in a main pattern of injury. Force vectors applied to certain areas of the spine result in predictable patterns of fracture, which essentially serve as a "fingerprint" (27). Force vectors can therefore be divided into two groups; *rotational* (flexion, extension, lateral bending, and torsion) and *linear* (compression, distraction, and translation) (28). Thoracolumbar fractures commonly result from falls (29,30) or motor vehicle accidents (31). By applying basic assessment of alignment, bone integrity, joint space, and ligamentous supports, in conjunction with appreciating

the mechanism of injury, a highly accurate and clinically relevant radiologic interpretation can be communicated to the referring physician.

Mechanical Stability

Essentially, the mechanically unstable spine is one that undergoes deleterious deformation when subjected to the normal physiologic force vectors and normal ranges of motion; this can be acute or delayed. Denis (26,32) proposed the three-column theory to help predict instability associated with different patterns of injury of the thoracolumbar spine.

The three-column theory of Denis consists of subdividing the spinal column into three anatomical zones: the anterior, middle, and posterior columns (Fig. 7-6). The *anterior column* consists of the anterior vertebral body,

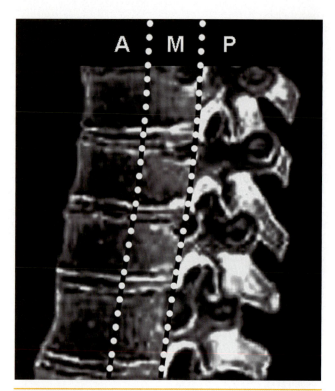

FIGURE 7-6. Three-column theory of spinal stability. The anterior column (*labeled "A"*) includes the ALL (anterior longitudinal ligament), anterior disc annulus, and anterior vertebral body. The middle column (*labeled "M"*) consists of the posterior vertebral body, the posterior disc annulus, and PLL (posterior longitudinal ligament). The posterior column (*labeled "P"*) consists of the posterior elements (pedicles, facets, lamina, spinous processes), the posterior interspinous ligament, and the ligamentum flavum. Disruption of two or three columns indicates mechanical instability.

the anterior longitudinal ligament, and the anterior annulus. The *middle column* consists of the posterior vertebral body, the posterior longitudinal ligament, and the posterior annulus. The *posterior column* is comprised of the posterior elements (pedicles, lamina, facets, and spinous processes) and associated ligaments (ligamentum flavum, interspinous, and supraspinous ligaments), as well as the associated facet joint capsule. When only one column is disrupted, the injury is considered mechanically stable. For example, most thoracolumbar spine fractures have a hyperflexion component (27), such as the anterior wedge compression fracture (anterior column involvement only) with intact posterior ligaments. With increasing degree of flexion secondary to greater forces, a second column may be disrupted, hence resulting in mechanical instability. Using the above example, an anterior wedge compression fracture with posterior ligament disruption on MRI (or exceeding 50% loss in vertical vertebral body height anteriorly, considered to have disrupted the posterior ligamentous supports) represents a two-column injury and, therefore, is deemed mechanically unstable. Another typical

example is that of a burst fracture, which by definition is a two- or three-column injury. Overall, of the three columns, more importance has been placed on the integrity of the middle column (33,34). The integrity of the middle column has been demonstrated on biomechanical testing to have a higher correlation with mechanical instability when compared to the anterior or posterior columns. In addition, assessment of the integrity of the posterior ligamentous complex is an important determinate for surgical stabilization.

Despite the numerous classification schemes for fractures, it is perhaps more important to be familiar with the signs of instability, as this affects functional and neurologic outcome and is at least uniform in its description of the significance of a fracture despite its morphology (Table 7-2) (35).

White and Punjabi (36) proposed a point-scoring checklist for instability, combining clinical and radiologic parameters, with five or more points equating to instability. Disruption of either the anterior or posterior columns is assigned two points each. Cauda equina damage is designated three points, and "dangerous loading anticipated" a further one point. Radiographic signs satisfying criteria for instability are listed and valued at two points (Table 7-3).

Neurologic Stability

Denis (32) further classified injuries as neurologically stable or unstable based on neurologic deficit at presentation, or impending neurologic deterioration secondary to impingement upon the spinal cord or nerve roots. Injuries therefore can be classified as having mechanical or neurologic instability, which can be helpful to guide management options. The greater the degree of canal compromise, the greater the probability of neurologic injury, however, the degree of spinal canal compromise is not indicative of the degree of neurologic deficit (37–39). Considering that the spinal cord terminates in the upper lumbar region, injury at the level of the lower lumbar spine does not result in

▶ TABLE 7-2 Radiologic Hallmarks of Instability

1. Displacement/translation >2 mm, indicative of disruption to the main ligamentous supports.
2. Widening of the interspinous space, widening of facet joints and/or widening of the interpedicular distance.
3. Disruption of the posterior vertebral body line equates to a disrupted anterior and posterior column or articular process fractures.
4. Widened intervertebral canal, indicative of sagittally orientated vertebral body trauma.
5. Vertebral body height loss >50%.
6. Kyphosis >20 degrees.

Source: Daffner et al. (35).

▶ **TABLE 7-3** Radiographic Criteria for Clinical Instability

Flexion and Extension Views:

1. Sagittal plane translation >4.5 mm or 15%	2 points
2. Sagittal plane rotation:	
>15 degrees (L1-2 to L3-4 levels)	2 points
>20 degrees (L4-5 level)	2 points
>25 degrees (L5-S1 level)	2 points

OR

Static Radiographs:

1. Sagittal plane displacement >4.5 mm or 15%	2 points
2. Relative sagittal plane angulation >22 degrees	2 points

Source: White and Punjabi (36).

cord compression, however, the possibility exists for a conus medullaris or cauda equina syndrome with severe canal compression (40,41).

Awareness of neurologic and mechanical stability therefore allows the clinician to choose the appropriate treatment strategy, which may be either conservative or surgical. Basic treatment principles include conservative treatment for mechanically and neurologically stable patients. Similarly, mechanically stable patients, though with irreversible neurologic deficit, may also be managed conservatively. Patients with reversible neurologic deficit (regardless of mechanical stability) are treated emergently in the hope of partial, if not complete, recovery. The patient with a complete neurologic deficit but mechanically unstable spine may be surgically stabilized on an elective basis in order to prevent future kyphotic deformity in order to improve functional activities of daily living.

THORACOLUMBAR SPINE FRACTURES: FORCE VECTORS

Flexion/Compression Injury

As previously discussed, flexion/compression (or hyperflexion/compression) injuries predominate in the thoracic spine. The most basic form of this type of injury is the typical anterior wedge compression fracture (Fig. 7-7) and accounts for nearly half of all thoracolumbar fractures (26,32). The axis of flexion of the lumbar spine occurs through the midportion of the nucleus pulposus. Since the distance of the anterior vertebral body is closer to this axis when compared to the posterior elements, concentration of compressive forces anteriorly is possible in comparison to the posterior distractive forces (42). This relative anterior positioning of the nucleus pulposus accounts for greater injury anteriorly. Radiographically, cortical end-

plate buckling almost always involves the anterosuperior endplate. Associated paraspinal soft tissue swelling may be apparent. Disruption of the anterior column alone is generally stable, although some patients (especially those with osteoporosis) may experience progressive loss of height. Neurologic instability is rare in this fracture and when present, is associated with a favorable outcome. Radiologic stability in these patients is best facilitated by CT, as this is more sensitive than radiographs in identifying the presence of subtle two-column injury, which alters the treatment outcome and prognosis (43). Flexion/compression fractures may occur at multiple levels, be contiguous, or noncontiguous. The depression usually involves only the superior endplate (rarely the inferior) and may be cup shaped or angular. It is distinguished from Scheuermann disease (Fig. 7-8) and physiologic anterior vertebral wedging; the latter two usually involve both superior and inferior endplates. Overall, this injury has a bimodal distribution, occurring in the young (in the context of high-speed trauma) and in the elderly (osteoporosis). As the middle column is preserved, there is no compromise of the spinal canal and a lack of neurologic deficits. A potential pitfall exists in differentiating a subtle fracture from the gentle anatomical anterior wedging. In the latter, the wedging of the vertebral bodies is slight and uniform and not isolated to one vertebral body.

Sagittal reformatted CT images or a lateral radiograph can provide morphologic information about the injury; there is preservation of the vertical height of the posterior vertebral body, in contradistinction to the axial/burst fractures, where the reduction in height of the anterior and posterior vertebral margins is relatively symmetrical. However, radiography for signs of middle-column injury can sometimes be unreliable, with imaging findings of middle-column instability present in only one third of patients (44,45). In some instances, MRI may have value, as this might show the disrupted PLL in middle-column injuries (13).

With increased force, anterior wedging becomes more pronounced. It is thus essential to exclude posterior ligamentous injury (and hence multicolumn trauma), which results in a mechanically unstable spine and can cause progressive loss of anterior vertebral height with kyphotic deformity and persistent pain. Increasing loss of vertebral body height anteriorly results in increased tensile forces on the posterior structures, with progressive anterior kyphosis increasing the likelihood of an associated posterior ligament tear. With 50% or greater loss of anterior vertebral body height (43), disruption of the posterior ligaments (and hence posterior column) can be assumed, rendering the fracture mechanically unstable. Posterior ligamentous disruption may also be apparent radiographically, as indicated by posterior interspinous distance widening at the level of injury, focal kyphosis and spondylolisthesis greater than 2 mm. If not suspected at the time

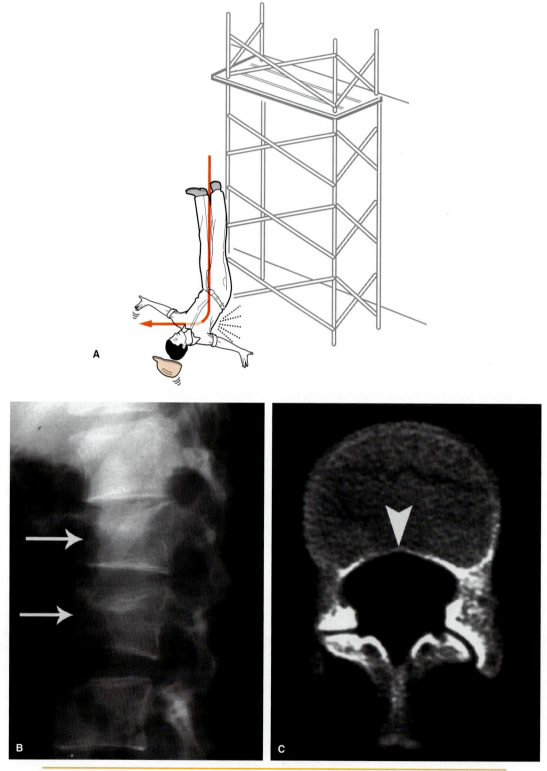

FIGURE 7-7. Flexion compression mechanism of injury. **A:** This type of injury often results from a fall, with flexion of the spine along with an axial load mechanism. Anterior wedge fractures occur with more major force resulting in burst fracture. **B:** Lateral radiograph of the L1 and L2 vertebral body demonstrates loss of vertebral body height anteriorly with cortical buckling of the superior endplates (*arrows*), consistent with flexion compression (*wedge*) fractures. The posterior cortical margins of the vertebral bodies are intact. **C:** Axial CT through the same region images the fracture and confirms an intact middle column, or posterior vertebral body at this level (*arrowhead*).

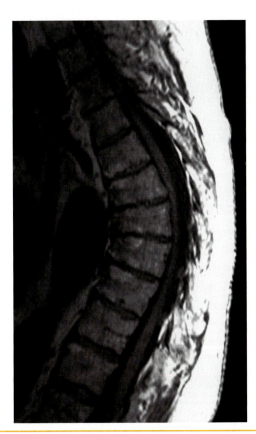

FIGURE 7-8. Sagittal T1 weighted image shows kyphotic deformity in the thoracic spine due to Scheuermann disease. As opposed to flexion compression injuries, note the deformity in both the superior and inferior endplates.

of injury, posterior ligamentous disruption should be presumed if there is progressive kyphotic deformity on follow-up imaging. MRI is very useful for identification of posterior soft tissue edema associated with posterior ligamentous injury, but care should be taken to obtain *fat-suppressed* T2-weighted fast spin echo sequences (46), or alternatively, to obtain short tau inversion recovery (STIR) images in order to optimally evaluate the edema pattern.

Axial Load Injury

Axial force (vertical compression) is most commonly associated with burst fractures of the thoracolumbar junction and lumbar spine, in contradistinction to the flexion/compression injury produced in the upper and midthoracic spine due to the kyphotic curvature. This type of injury is common, accounting for 14% of spinal injuries (26,32) and classically occurs after landing on both feet or buttocks following a fall from a height (*lover's fractures* when associated with bilateral calcaneal fractures). Rarely, the injury may be due to seizure (47) or electrocution (48).

Axial loading results in shear and tensile forces highest at the base of pedicle and superior margin of the vertebral body (49), where the microstructure of the trabecular pattern demonstrates changes consistent with this region being a focus of stress concentration (50). The forces transmitted to the pedicle base result in an anterior shear force (51). This is combined with the simultaneous axial compression of the vertebral body from above by the nucleus pulposus (52), which explodes into the superior vertebral endplate to result in centripetal displacement of the body and its fracture fragments. The tip of the fragment arises from the level of the basivertebral foramen (53). A varying degree of rotation and comminution of the fracture fragments may occur (usually vertically orientated) (54). The retropulsion of the posterior aspect of the vertebral body (middle column) into the spinal canal (or posterior bowing of the posterior vertebral body margin) is pathognomonic of a burst fracture (55) (Figs. 7-9, 7-10, 7-11, 7-12, 7-13, 7-14, 7-15). Despite the disruption of the posterior vertebral cortex and the inherent associated instability, the PLL is uncommonly injured and remains in contact with the displaced fragment. As the PLL is often intact, spinal traction can reduce this displaced fragment by tightening the PLL. Interestingly, a deficient nucleus pulposus, as seen in intervertebral disc degeneration, is thought to account for a decrease in the incidence of burst fractures in this subset of patients, despite the presence often of concomitant osteoporosis. In the intact nucleus pulposus, the concentration of forces occurs at the endplate overlying the nucleus. In the case of intervertebral degeneration, no such concentration of forces is able to occur (56). The high incidence of burst fractures at the thoracolumbar junction can be partially attributed to the orientation of the facet joint. The sagittal orientation of the facet joints increases significantly from T12 to L1 (57) and thus allows for an increase in load transmission (51).

Applying the three-column principle, there is as a minimum two-column disruption (the anterior and middle) in a burst fracture. Evaluation of the posterior column is paramount to this determination, as debate exists over whether a two-column burst fracture is unstable (58). For example, a burst fracture is diagnosed by the presence of the characteristic retropulsion pattern; however, only minimal disruption to other elements may be otherwise demonstrated to support findings associated with instability (44) (Table 7-4). The integrity of the posterior column thus critically alters clinical decision making and outcome.

▶ **TABLE 7-4** **Determinants of Burst Fracture Instability**

Widened interspinous and interlaminar distance
Kyphosis >20 degrees
Dislocation
Vertebral body height loss greater than 50%
Articular process fractures

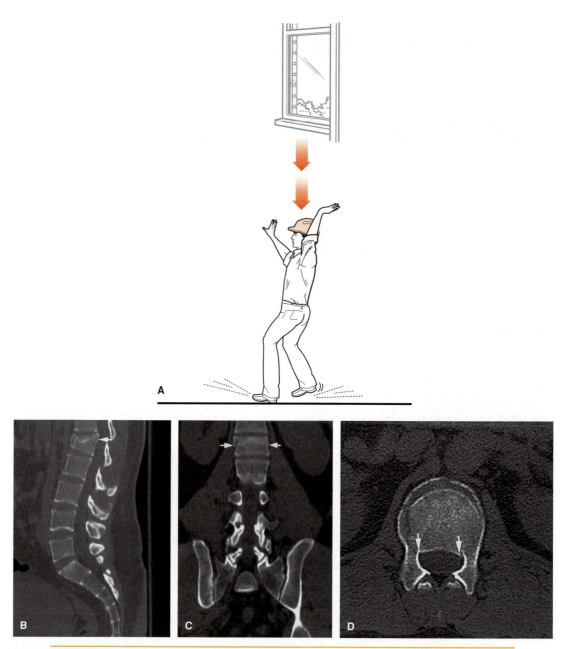

FIGURE 7-9. Axial load mechanism of injury. **A:** This mechanism is also generally related to a fall from a height, often resulting in burst fractures. Multiple levels are often involved, which may not be contiguous. Sagittal **(B)** and **(C)** coronal reformatted MDCT images demonstrate a subtle vertical-compression (burst) fracture of L1, which on plain radiographs was initially thought to represent a simple flexion-compression fracture. However, the convexity of the upper margin of the posterior vertebral cortex (*arrow Fig. 7-3B, 7-3D*), best visualized on the axial image, is a finding that precludes the diagnosis of a flexion-compression fracture and hence the diagnosis of a burst fracture.

Burst fractures most commonly occur at the thoracolumbar junction, especially T12 and L1; in this region, retropulsion of fragments can cause significant neurologic compromise and surgical decompression and fixation is usually performed. However, burst fractures of the lower lumbar spine can be treated conservatively when there is no associated neurologic deficit, in the context where the injury is considered stable given the absence of the findings elucidated above (Table 7-3) (59). The probability of neurologic deficit may be determined by the percentage of the cross-sectional area that the retropulsed fragment occupies of the estimated original

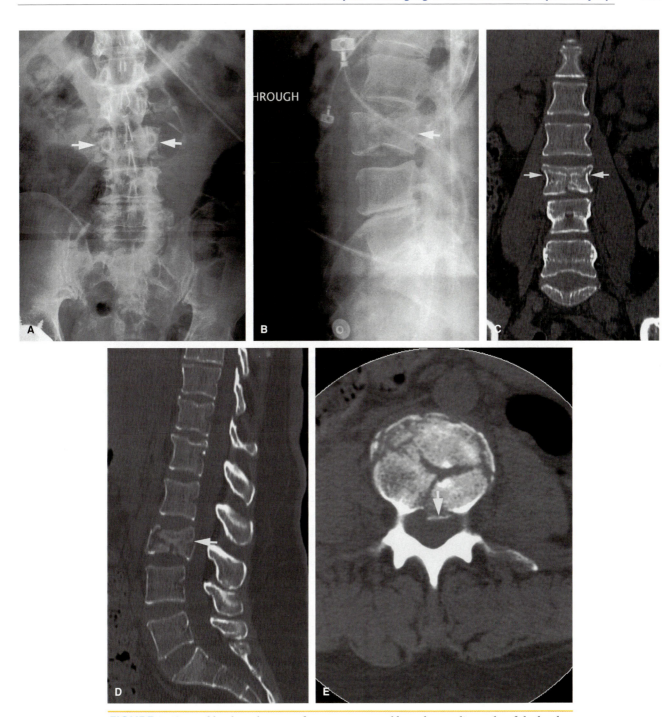

FIGURE 7-10. Axial load mechanism of injury. AP **(A)** and lateral **(B)** radiographs of the lumbar spine demonstrate a decrease in vertebral body height of L3 due to transverse and anteroposterior widening (*arrows*). Posterior bowing of the vertebral body margin is diagnostic of an axial-compression (burst) fracture. The posterior elements are intact, with no widening of the interpediculate distance. Coronal **(C)** and sagittal **(D)** reformatted MDCT correspond to the findings depicted on the radiographs (*arrows*). Single axial image **(E)** through this level allows for accurate evaluation of the degree of canal compromise caused by the retropulsed fragment (*arrow*), which in this instance is <50%. (*continued*)

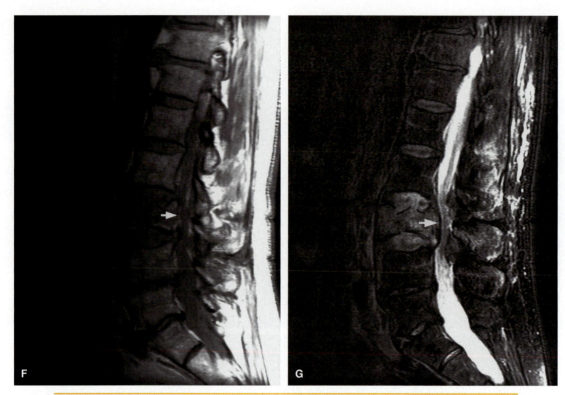

FIGURE 7-10. *(CONTINUED)* Sagittal T1 **(F)** and fat-saturated T2 **(G)** weighted MRI also reveal the buckled and retropulsed posterior cortex (arrows).

spinal canal area, with a significant risk of neurologic sequelae naturally occurring at higher levels with greater degrees of stenosis (60). Conversely, a greater degree of stenosis may be tolerated at lower levels without event due to the relative resistance of the cauda equina to direct trauma. Measurement of the anteroposterior (AP) dimension is compared to the average of the levels above and below to assess the degree of canal compromise (assuming the absence of contiguous fracture involvement).

A burst fracture is characterized on imaging by loss of height of the anterior and posterior vertebral body cortex, with posterior bowing or retropulsion of the posterior wall. Often, extension of the fracture occurs posteriorly to result in fracture of the posterior elements and the neural arch (vertebral body/pedicle) junction. This causes widening of the interpedicular distance on the AP radiograph (Fig. 7-10). CT is helpful to detect subtle posterior wall disruption. As many as 15% of burst fractures are missed on routine radiographic assessment (61). Careful attention should be paid to the morphology of the posterior vertebral body margin, which should be concave on the axial and sagittal reformatted images. Any flattening or posterior bowing present confirms the diagnosis (Fig. 7-9). CT precisely quantifies the degree of canal compromise due to the fragment(s) and identifies any potential posterior

element fractures, evaluating the latter more accurately than MRI.

It is further essential to alert the clinician to the presence of a laminar split fracture, which can critically alter management and surgical approach (Fig. 7-11, 7-14). The significance of the sagittal split fracture through lamina is the high association with posterior dural laceration. Impaction of the thecal sac with the vertical fracture results in this characteristic laceration. When combined with compression anteriorly from the retropulsed fragment, neural extrusion, entrapment, and neurologic instability are possible (62). The laminar split fracture almost exclusively occurs with the burst fracture, with an incidence of 7.7% of such fractures having a dural tear, which in turn has an 86% association with neurologic deficit (63). The presence of a dural tear requires detection prior to surgery, as reduction of the neural extrusion and closure of the dural laceration requires a posterior approach and should be performed prior to any spinal reduction maneuver (64), which would worsen compression of the extruded neural contents. The fracture may only involve the cortex of the lamina closer to the thecal sac (greenstick fracture). Burst fractures with a posterior column fracture have a higher association with neurologic deficit on initial examination (65). The 3D configuration of the fracture (Fig. 7-16) and the retropulsed fragment, as well

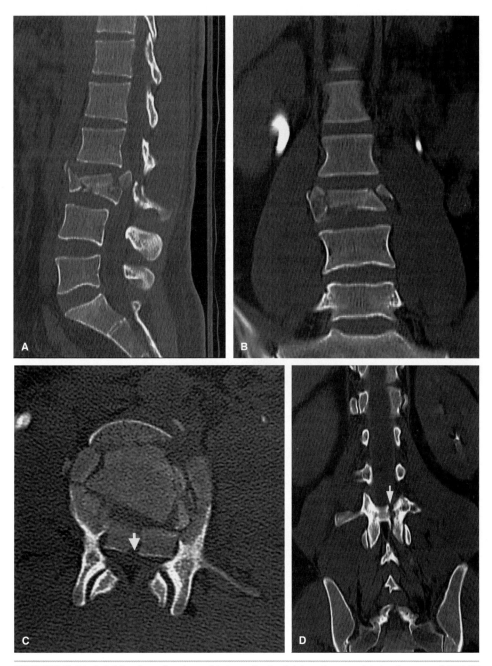

FIGURE 7-11. Axial load mechanism of injury. Sagittal **(A)** and coronal **(B)** reformatted MDCT images demonstrate an axial-compression (burst) fracture with at least 50% loss of height of the L3 vertebral body, as well as ~50% canal narrowing, best evaluated on the axial **(C)** images (*arrow*). Further, the more posterior coronal images **(D)** confirm the presence of a laminar split fracture (*arrow*), for which preoperative detection is mandatory.

as concomitant posterior column injury, are also best assessed with CT, as osseous superimposition clearly remains a limitation of standard radiographs.

Once a burst fracture is diagnosed, as with many vertebral fractures, radiographic survey of the entire spine is recommended as noncontiguous level involvement may occur in as many as 6.4% to 34% (3,66) of patients with burst fractures. There is also an increased incidence of associated sacral (26%) and pelvic (7.7%) fractures.

Features of *mechanical* instability include a widened interspinous and interlaminar distance, greater than 2 mm of translation, kyphosis >20 degrees, dislocation, height loss >50%, and articular process fractures (Table 7-4) (44). Neurologic instability (actual or impending) has

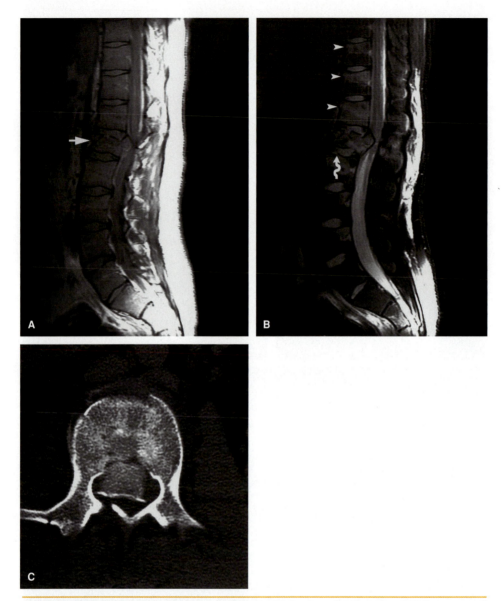

FIGURE 7-12. Axial load mechanism of injury. Sagittal proton density **(A)** and T2 fat-saturated **(B)** MRI demonstrate an axial compression (burst) fracture of the L1 vertebral body (*arrow*), with retropulsion resulting in near total occlusion of the canal, best assessed on the axial CT **(C)**. A minimally displaced fracture of the L2 superior endplate (*curved arrow*) is also likely the result of an axial compression injury, with the finding in these two vertebrae likely representing a spectrum of injury. Note further flexion-compression fractures of T10, T11, and T12 (*arrowheads*), resulting in buckling of the anterior vertebral cortex and without disruption of the posterior column. Contusions also of the posterosuperior margins of the L3 and L4 vertebral bodies are probably due to local hyperextension forces given the greater lordosis at this level.

been defined as spinal canal stenosis >50% of normal (44,67,68).

Treatment of burst fractures without neurologic sequelae has been particularly controversial, with many authors advocating a conservative approach, reserving surgical intervention only in cases of delayed (chronic) instability or pain (69). This has ranged from complete bed rest to mobilization (early [70] or delayed) with or

without casting/bracing (71). No additional benefit has been demonstrated for anatomical reduction of displaced osseous fragments in the canal in patients without neurologic deficit. Indeed, studies have shown that retropulsed fragments will spontaneously remodel over time, presumably due to disuse and the effects of normal cerebrospinal fluid (CSF) pulsation on the adjacent bone fragments, ultimately decreasing the degree of posttraumatic canal

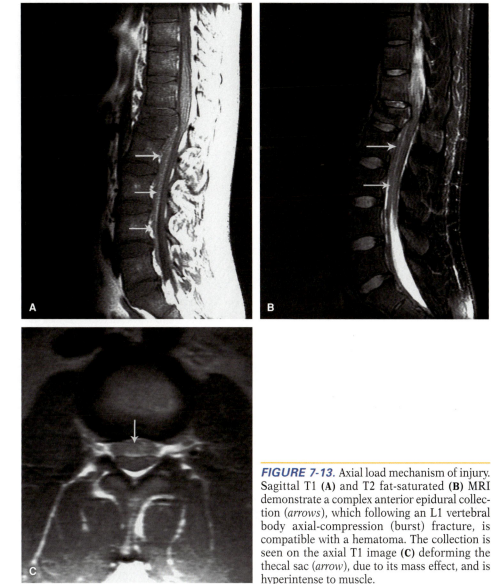

FIGURE 7-13. Axial load mechanism of injury. Sagittal T1 **(A)** and T2 fat-saturated **(B)** MRI demonstrate a complex anterior epidural collection (*arrows*), which following an L1 vertebral body axial-compression (burst) fracture, is compatible with a hematoma. The collection is seen on the axial T1 image **(C)** deforming the thecal sac (*arrow*), due to its mass effect, and is hyperintense to muscle.

stenosis in both nonoperative and surgical patients. The notion that displaced fragments may be a source of ongoing cord or neural impingement has been questioned; burst fractures, like other traumatic incidents, represent a momentary event (72), when maximal canal occlusion, cord compression, and, hence, neurologic damage occurs dynamically and instantly at the time of injury (73), with the final resting place of the centripetally displaced fragments (including the retropulsed posterosuperior vertebral margin) thought by some to have no correlation with the presence or degree of neurologic deficit.

Alternatively, recent data have demonstrated that 25%, 50%, and 75% narrowing of the thoracolumbar canal is correlated with a 12%, 41%, and 78% incidence respectively with neurologic deficits (74). Moreover, a positive correlation was made with the degree of *incomplete* neurologic deficit and the percentage of canal stenosis. However, investigators also found a lack of correlation with the degree of canal stenosis and *complete* neurologic deficit (34.3%), which occurred at a comparable rate to those *without* neurologic deficit (35.7%) (74). As an absolute percentage of area involved, burst fractures considered at increased risk for neurologic sequelae have been shown to be those at the T11 and T12 level with 35% canal compromise, 45% compromise at L1, and 55% at L2 and below (75). Ultimately, the decision as to whether decompression is performed rests with the spinal surgeon based on local practice and experience, patient comorbidities, and overall prognosis.

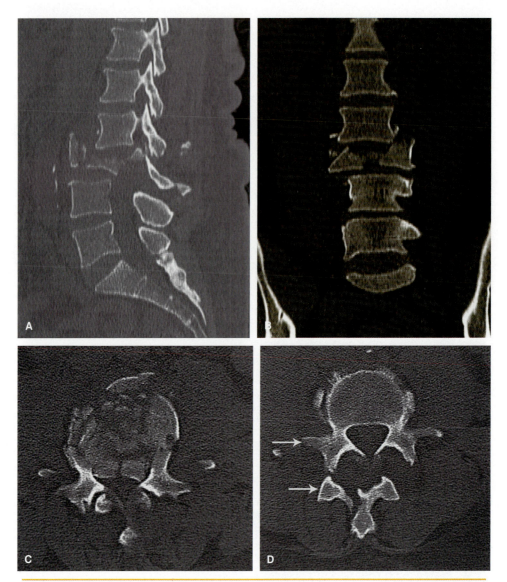

FIGURE 7-14. Axial load mechanism of injury. Sagittal **(A)** and coronal **(B)** reformatted MDCT images demonstrate a severe L3 vertebral body axial-compression (burst) fracture with concomitant dislocation of the vertebral column at this level. Axial image **(C)** at the level of injury, demonstrates the degree of canal compromise, and above this, the inferior displacement and anterolisthesis (*arrows*) of L2 relative to L3 is appreciated **(D)**, with the two bodies visualized on a single axial image. Note the laminar split fracture on the right L3 lamina.

Current long-term surgical data and follow-up for simple burst fractures is lacking. This situation is made more difficult due to the multitude of surgical approaches and devices over time that make standardization for effective comparison difficult. There are a small number of clinical series that report successful use of percutaneous vertebroplasty alone, or in combination with short segment pedicle screw fixation to treat burst fractures (76–78). Large series are yet to be reported, with data from only small numbers and carefully selected patients. Patient selection included those without neurologic deficit, contraindications to surgery, and failure of conservative treatment (orthoses),

such as intractable pain. In the context of incomplete neurologic deficit, surgery with decompression is indicated and has a demonstrated benefit (79) as well as in those demonstrating radiologic criteria of severe instability (68). In the setting of complete neurologic deficit, the role of surgery is not to improve neurologic function but to preserve alignment in order to prevent further mechanical instability and ongoing progressive kyphotic deformity. The choice of whether a patient undergoes conservative therapy or surgery should be considered with the inherent surgical complication and revision rate (the latter reported up to 41%) in mind (80). Other than a more prolonged

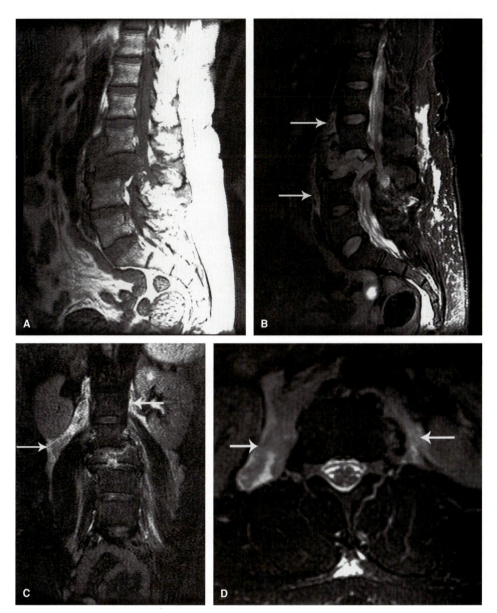

FIGURE 7-15. Axial load mechanism of injury. Sagittal T1 (**A**), sagittal (**B**), coronal (**C**), and axial (**D**) T2 fat-saturated MRI demonstrate near complete obliteration of the L3 vertebral body, which is associated with a large retroperitoneal hematoma (*arrows*). The hematoma extends superiorly to at least the level of L1 (*arrow, D*).

hospital stay and later return to rehabilitation and employment, no significant increase in immobility related complications prescribed in conservative therapy occurs when compared with postoperative immobility.

Flexion/Rotation Injury

In combined flexion/rotation injuries, the flexion component results in anterior wedge compression or burst fracture. The addition of a rotational force vector can cause significant injury to the posterior ligaments or fractures of the facets (Fig. 7-17). As such, this injury tends to be unstable. Residual offset, or *subluxation* of the facet joints is compatible with this mechanism. With more extreme flexion/rota-

tion injuries, complete offset, or *dislocation,* of the facets may occur, and, hence, a greater degree of traumatic spondylolisthesis. This can occur secondary to disruption of either the intervertebral disc at the level below or due to a fracture extending through the superior portion of the vertebral body above and displacement of the spine superior to this cleft. This injury pattern is seen most commonly at the thoracolumbar junction because of the transition between relatively immobile and mobile segments, particularly of the facet joints. Soft tissue trauma is a common finding, and as such, MRI assessment is useful. Along with involvement of the anterior column, coexistent avulsion of the ALL may occur. Not surprisingly, given the forces involved and the degree of displacement, neurologic impairment is common.

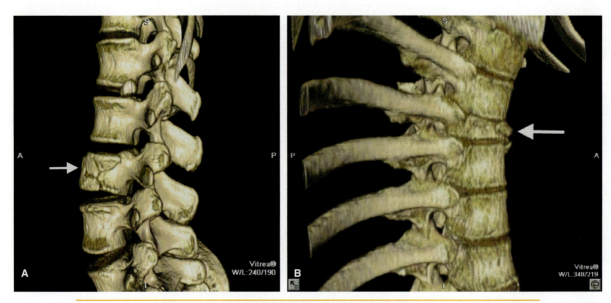

FIGURE 7-16. Axial load mechanism of injury. CT 3D volume rendered images of a lumbar burst fracture (*arrow*, **A**) and thoracic burst fracture (*arrow*, **B**).

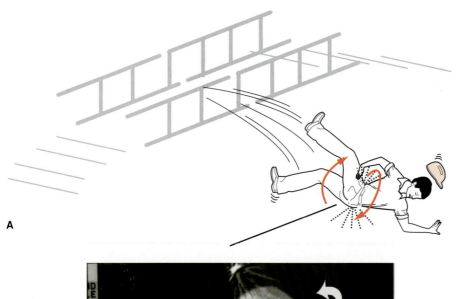

A

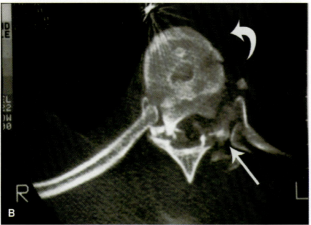

B

FIGURE 7-17. Flexion rotation mechanism of injury. **A:** This mechanism often occurs from motor vehicle accidents, in which a flexion force is applied as the upper body turns relative to the pelvis and lower body. The spinal column fails at a certain point and results in a complex pattern of injury with disruption of the three columns, facet fractures, and rib fractures (if thoracic); severe neurologic compromise results. **B:** Axial CT demonstrates a complex and comminuted thoracic vertebral body fracture, with rotation to the patient's right side (*curved arrow*), resulting in canal compromise. The disruption of the posterior elements (*arrow*) makes rotation possible.

Flexion/Distraction Injury

Flexion/distraction injuries are also most common at the thoracolumbar junction, though are infrequent when compared with other forms of thoracolumbar fractures. *Distraction* occurs with complete vertebral step-off combined with separation in a cranial-caudal direction. This mechanism is a result of a flexion force applied to the spine with an axis of rotation anterior to the spine (81) to result in hyperflexion of the upper thoracic spine while the lower spine remains relatively fixed. The consequence of these force vectors is posterior and middle-column disruption under severe tension (82) with concomitant distraction (Figs. 7-18, 7-19, 7-20). This injury is classically caused by a deceleration-type motor vehicle accident in which the

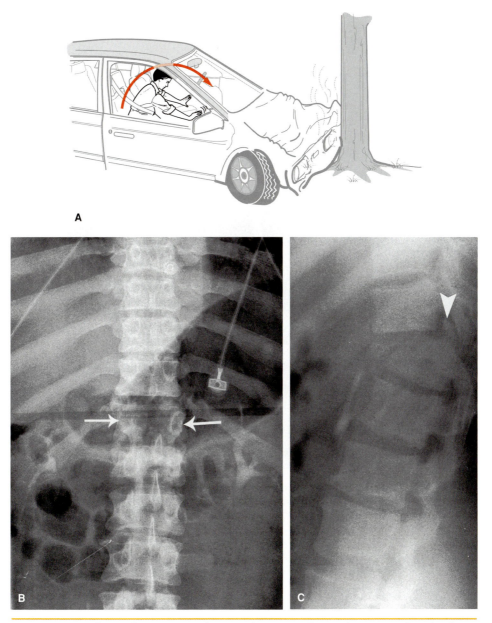

FIGURE 7-18. Flexion distraction mechanism of injury. **A:** This mechanism involves the classic "lap belt" injury. The flexion force is centered anterior to the spine, resulting in distraction extending through the posterior elements to the anterior column. The distractive nature of injury often leaves patients neurologically intact, although there may be significant abdominal organ injury. This leads to the classic Chance fracture (purely osseous) and Chance variants (soft tissue or combined osseous/soft tissue). AP **(B)** radiograph demonstrates widening of the interpediculate (*arrows*) and interspinous distance of T12, findings consistent with a flexion-distraction fracture. Acute hyperflexion deformity is appreciated on the lateral radiograph **(C)** with decrease in vertebral body height anteriorly, characteristic of the flexion vector. (*continued*)

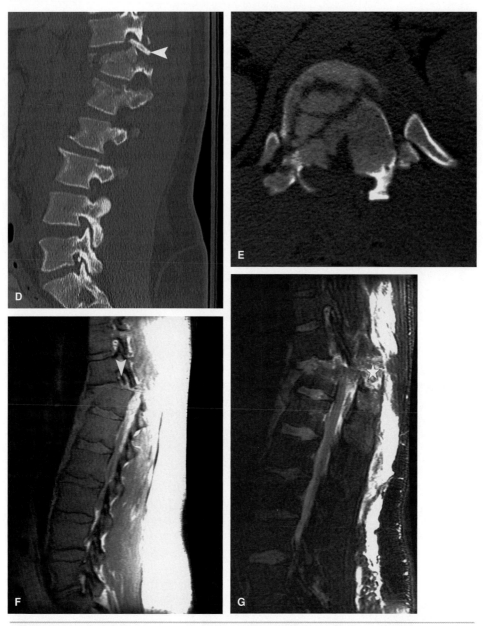

FIGURE 7-18. (*CONTINUED*) In this specific case, the injury is similar to bilateral interfacetal dislocation seen in the cervical spine, given the manner that the facet joints of T11 are perched on T12 **(D)**. A small osseous fragment, consistent with a displaced rib fracture is present within the neural exit foramen (*Figs. 7-18C, 7-18D, and 7-18F, arrowhead*). The horizontal orientation of a portion of the fracture through the vertebral body is best appreciated on the sagittal reformatted MDCT (D), which also demonstrates the fracture continuing posteriorly into the posterior elements. The status of the canal is assessed on the on the axial image **(E)**. Disruption of the posterior soft tissues (*asterisk*) can be seen on the midline sagittal MR images **(F and G)**. Compression of the thecal sac is also visualized.

occupant is restrained only by a lap belt (also known as a lap-belt injury), though it has been reported in other activities with similar hyperflexion mechanisms. The resultant fracture has been classically described as the "Chance fracture," this first described in 1948, but variations to this have since been described such that the term Chance-type fractures is commonly used to encompass similar injuries. With the routine use of conventional three-point restraint (shoulder harness and lap belt), the incidence of the classic Chance fracture has decreased and burst fractures are now more prevalent (83). The classic Chance fracture, with a two-point restraint system, has traditionally been associated

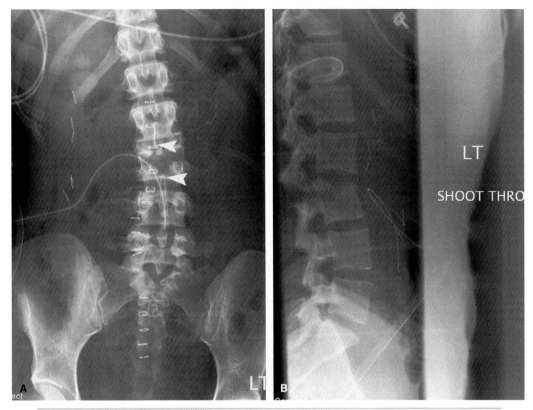

FIGURE 7-19. Flexion distraction mechanism of injury. AP **(A)** and lateral **(B)** radiographs demonstrate a flexion-distraction (Chance) fracture of the L3 vertebral body, with interspinous process widening (*arrowheads, A*) and a horizontal fracture extending through the vertebral body posteriorly, with compression anteriorly.

with an extremely high rate of solid abdominal visceral trauma, up to 89% (22); however, the true incidence of abdominal injury more recently has been reported to be lower, closer to 25% (22). With the three-point restraint system, the incidence of abdominal injuries is significantly lower, having been decreased by roughly 50% in one series (26.7% compared to 57.1%) (83).

A "classic" Chance fracture consists of a pure osseous injury in which there is a horizontal split through the spinous process, lamina, pedicles, and the extends through the intervertebral disc space, resulting in a small anteroinferior corner fracture of the lower vertebral body. The classic Chance fracture accounts for approximately 50% of Chance-type injuries and is usually isolated to one vertebral body (L1, L2, or L3). It is acutely unstable, however, as it is purely an osseous disruption; it also has excellent healing potential with good prognosis for long-term stability. Incidence of neurologic deficit is low, estimated at 10%. A lateral projection/sagittal reformatted image (MDCT) demonstrates a horizontally orientated fracture extending across the posterior elements, continuing into the vertebral body with more separation of the fragments posteriorly. Depiction of the involvement of the posterior elements on the lateral radi-

ograph is often unreliable due to overlap. This may be visualized on the AP radiographs as a "double" spinous process, interspinous distance widening, and horizontal fractures through the pedicles. Retropulsion of bone into the spinal canal is typically absent, and the decompressive effects of this type of injury on the spinal canal help to explain the relative absence of neurologic deficits with this type of injury.

Chance variants are either a combined osseous/soft tissue injury or pure soft tissue disruption. The fracture may extend through the posterior elements as for the classic Chance fracture, but continues anteriorly through the disc or it may involve the posterior ligaments and vertebral body. In the pure soft tissue Chance variant, anteriorly the intervertebral disc is disrupted with posterior extension through the interspinous and supraspinous ligaments without osseous involvement. This can result in "naked facets" on axial imaging and an imaging pattern similar to bilateral interfacetal dislocation (BID) of the cervical spine. The degree of osseous involvement is important as the osseous structures have better regenerative potential in contrast to the soft tissue supports.

On plain radiography, the features of a Chance variant can be subtle, with posterior element distraction and disc

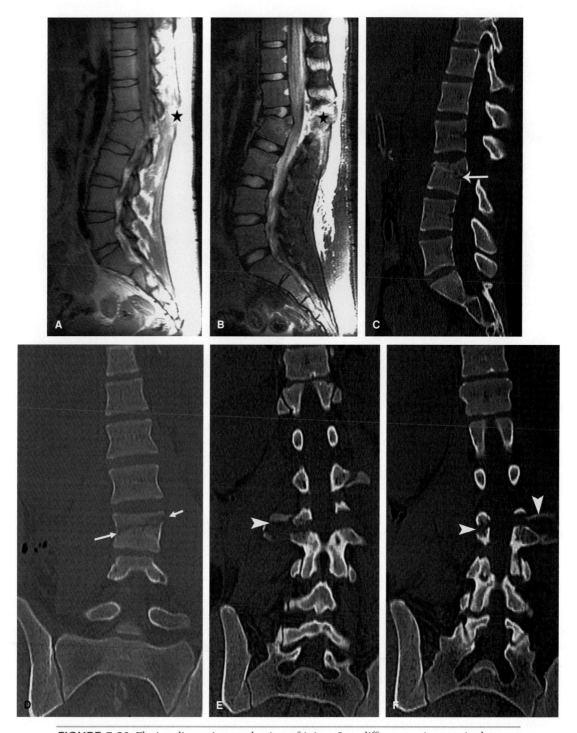

FIGURE 7-20. Flexion distraction mechanism of injury. In a different patient, sagittal proton density **(A)** and T2 fat-saturated **(B)** MRI and sagittal **(C)** reformatted MDCT of the lumbar spine demonstrate a flexion-distraction (Chance) fracture also of L3, with disruption of the interspinous ligaments (*asterisk*) and a horizontally oriented fracture through the vertebral body (*arrow*), the latter finding also appreciated on the anterior coronal reformatted image (*arrows*) **(D)**. Further posteriorly, the coronal reformatted images also demonstrate transverse fractures through the right **(E)** and left **(F)** transverse processes and pedicles (*arrowheads*).

widening, or a horizontally or obliquely oriented fracture plane through a portion of the vertebra as the only finding. In more severe injuries, the ALL can be stripped off the vertebral bodies or torn, permitting a translational component to the injury as is seen with associated features of jumped facets or vertebral dislocation (84,85). Chance fractures are uncommon in children due to the differences in mechanical properties of the vertebrae, ligaments, and ring in children compared to adults. Instability in the adult is defined as >13 degrees (partial) or 19 degrees (complete) kyphosis and/or >20 mm (partial) or 33 mm (complete) (86) on AP radiographs.

Lateral Compression Injury

Lateral compression injury is similar to the previously described flexion/compression injury, except that the flexion force is applied laterally, as opposed to symmetrical application of the force through the spinal column. This results in compressive forces to one side, resulting in fracture, with distraction forces on the contralateral side of the vertebral column (Fig. 7-21). Hence, the radiographic pattern is similar to flexion-compression injuries except that the vertebral body height loss is laterally located (as opposed to anterior) and best appreciated on the AP radiograph, where a scoliotic deformity will be appreciated. As with anterior-flexion injuries, a simple lateral vertebral body compression is usually stable; however, it is considered to be mechanically unstable with additional column involvement.

Shear Injury

A shearing mechanism, either pure or in association with other force vectors, typically results in a severe and unstable three-column injury, with anterior, posterior, or lateral subluxation, as well as posterior element fracture or ligamentous disruption (Fig. 7-22). The force vectors in this type of injury are both enormous and complex. The shear mechanism results in severe anatomic disruption of all tissue planes, and neurologic impairment is frequent. In

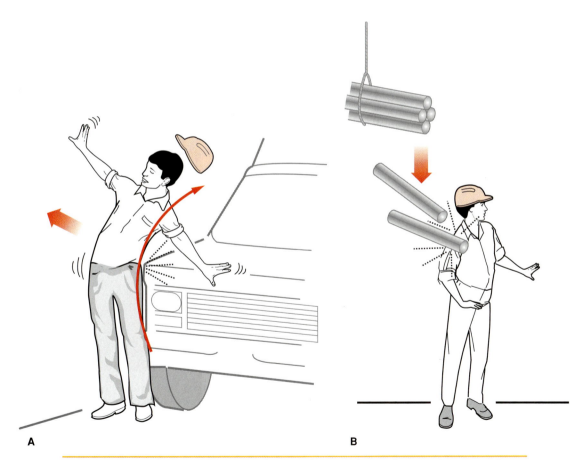

A   **B**

FIGURE 7-21. Lateral compression mechanism of injury. This mechanism often occurs from a laterally applied load to the body **(A)** but may also occur from an axial load directed eccentrically across the spinal column **(B)**. The lateral aspect of the vertebral body and posterior elements are compressed asymmetrically. (*continued*)

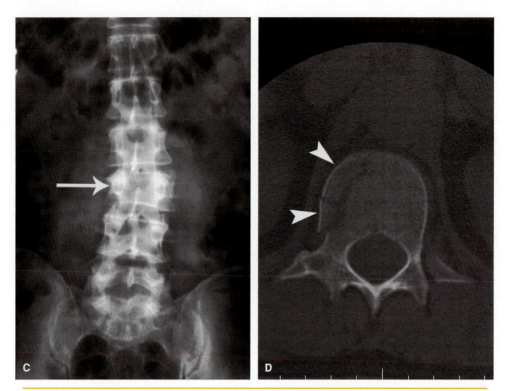

FIGURE 7-21. (*CONTINUED*) **C:** AP radiograph of the lumbar spine demonstrates loss of L3 vertebral body height (*arrow*) on the right side, consistent with an ipsilateral compression injury. **D:** Axial CT of the T12 vertebral body again demonstrates asymmetric compression (*arrowheads*) of the right side of the vertebral body.

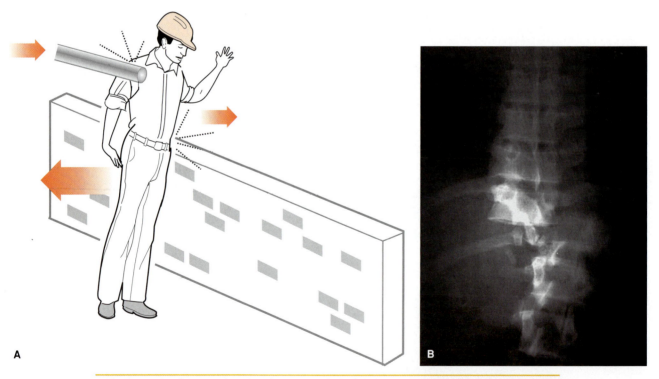

FIGURE 7-22. Shear mechanism of injury. **A:** This injury occurs as a horizontal force is applied to one end of the body as the other end is fixed or moving in a different direction. Severe neurologic compromise is the rule, and dislocation may occur. **B:** Lateral dislocation at the lower thoracic spine is evident on this AP view.

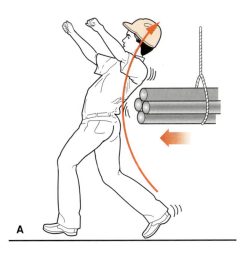

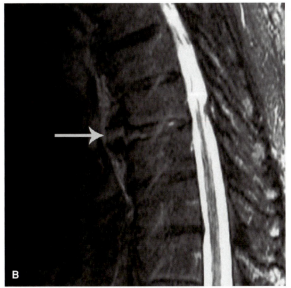

FIGURE 7-23. Extension mechanism of injury. **A:** This mechanism typically occurs from a strike on the back (the classic "lumberjack injury") or from a fall with landing on the face or chest and extension of the spinal column. Radiographs are often negative; occasionally subtle anterior disc widening or focal lordosis may be seen. However, a T2-weighted MRI **(B)** shows the typical findings of disruption of the anterior longitudinal ligament (*arrow*) and prevertebral soft tissue swelling. Widening of the intervertebral disc space anteriorly implies a hyperextension force.

fact, it is unusual for this type of injury to be without neurologic sequelae. This injury has a high association with thoracic and abdominal injury.

Extension Injury

An extension injury pattern is produced when the upper trunk is thrust backward, or when there is a direct blow to the back. The resultant radiographic pattern is characterized by posterior element impaction, with fractures (often comminuted) of the spinous process, lamina, or facets, in association with anterior disc widening or avulsion fracture of the anterior endplate (Fig. 7-23). Instability results when there is disruption of the anterior ligaments that results in the converse of hyperflexion injuries, that being anterior intervertebral disc widening and retrolisthesis. If severe enough, the injury may result in the "lumberjack fracture-dislocation" in which there is complete loss of continuity of the upper and lower spinal segment associated with an extremely high rate of paraplegia and dural tear (Fig. 7-24) (62). Compression fractures of the posterior elements may coexist. As seen in the cervical spine, patient with ankylosing spondylitis are at higher risk of extension-type injuries (Fig. 7-25). Imaging findings of extension injury in the setting of ankylosing spondylitis include acute lordosis, anterior intervertebral disc space widening, anterior soft tissue swelling, and posterior element fracture. Ligamentous ossification in ankylosing spondylitis results in complete loss of spinal flexibility; therefore, a minimal amount of trauma can produce severe disruption of the spinal axis. In many cases, the imaging findings can be subtle. MRI can be helpful to identify the associated soft tissue component of injuries in this subset of patients (12–14, 87).

Transverse Process Fractures

Lumbar transverse process fractures commonly occur at multiple adjacent levels and can be relatively insignificant if the mechanism is an avulsion-type force from the surrounding paraspinal musculature (Figs. 7-26, 7-27). The injury should serve as a sentinel sign, alerting one to the possibility of other injury, including the presence of another lumbar spine fracture (up to 11%) *not* involving the transverse processes (88) and abdominal visceral injury (89,90) in up to 50%. Hence, strong consideration should be given to performing a CT. Importantly, the fracture is often missed on plain radiography (91), and its significance when detected is frequently underestimated. For example, an isolated L5 transverse process fracture is commonly seen in association with a vertically oriented sacral fracture (Malgaigne fracture/dislocation) on the same side, indicating a vertical shearing force; this injury is commonly associated with nerve root injury.

SUMMARY

Imaging plays a pivotal role in assessing the mechanical and neurologic stability of the traumatized thoraco-lumbar spine. By correlating the clinical findings with the radiologic features and with a thorough knowledge of spinal anatomy and biomechanics, the original pattern of injury can be elucidated. Furthermore, this essential understanding allows one to examine for associated noncontiguous

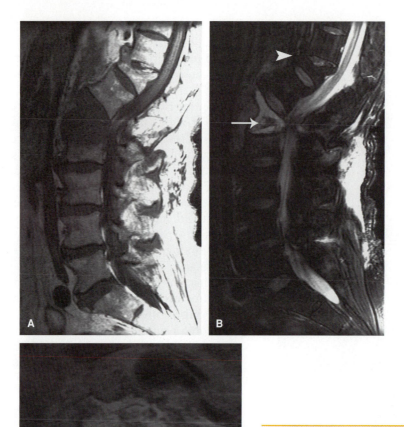

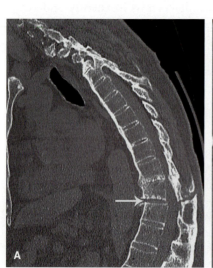

FIGURE 7-24. Extension mechanism of injury. Sagittal T1 **(A)** and T2 fat-saturated **(B)** MRI demonstrate a severe hyperextension injury at the L1-2 level, resulting in complete disruption of the anterior longitudinal ligament and a disrupted intervertebral disc (*arrow*). A hyperflexion-compression injury of the T12 vertebral body is also present (*arrowhead*), though without edema, and thus is a sequela of prior injury. The degree of canal compromise (*arrow*) can be assessed on the T1 axial image **(C)** through this level.

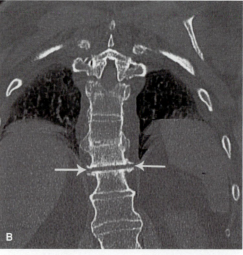

FIGURE 7-25. Ankylosing spondylitis with extension mechanism of injury. Sagittal **(A)** and coronal **(B)** reformatted MDCT images demonstrate a complete horizontally oriented fracture (*arrows*), through the thoracic spine, consistent with a "chalk-stick" fracture in a patient with ankylosing spondylitis following a hyperextension injury mechanism.

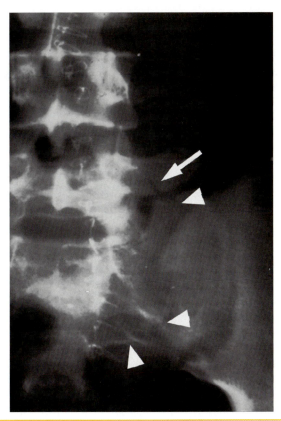

FIGURE 7-26. Transverse process fracture. AP radiograph of the lumbar spine demonstrates an acute left transverse process fracture of L5 (*arrow*). This injury is often associated with a sacral fracture, here seen as a fracture line and interruption of the sacral foramina (*arrowheads*).

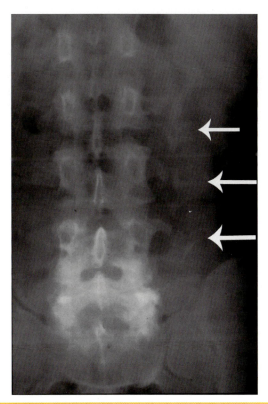

FIGURE 7-27. Transverse process fracture. AP radiograph shows healed left sided transverse process fractures of L2, L3, and L4 (*arrows*).

vertebral and other nonosseous injuries, providing greater assistance to the clinician and ultimately improved patient management and optimal outcome.

REFERENCES

1. Kewalramani LS, Taylor RG. Multiple non-contiguous injuries to the spine. *Acta Orthop Scand*. 1976;47:52–58.
2. Tearse DS, Keene JS, Drummond DS. Management of non-contiguous vertebral fractures. *Paraplegia*. 1987;25:100–105.
3. Keenen TL, Antony J, Benson DR. Non-contiguous spinal fractures. *J Trauma*. April 1990;30(4):489–491.
4. Herzog C, Ahle H, Mack MG, et al. Traumatic injuries of the pelvis and thoracic and lumbar spine: does thin-slice multidetector-row CT increase diagnostic accuracy? *Eur Radiol*. 2004;14:1751–1760.
5. Begemann PG, Kemper J, Gatzka C, et al. Value of multiplanar reformations (MPR) in multidetector CT (MDCT) of acute vertebral fractures: do we still have to read the transverse images? *J Comput Assist Tomogr*. 2004;28:572–580.
6. Kosling S, Dietrich K, Steinecke R, et al. Diagnostic value of 3D CT surface reconstruction in spinal fractures. *Eur Radiol*. 1997;7:61–64.
7. Roos JE, Hilfiker P, Platz A, et al. MDCT in emergency radiology: is a standardized chest or abdominal protocol sufficient for evaluation of thoracic and lumbar spine trauma? *AJR*. 2004;183:959–968.
8. Hauser CJ, Visvikis G, Hinrichs C, et al. Prospective validation of computed tomographic screening of the thoracolumbar spine in trauma. *J Trauma*. 2003;55:228–234; discussion 234–235.
9. Wintermark M, Mouhsine E, Theumann N, et al. Thoracolumbar spine fractures in patients who have sustained severe trauma: depiction with multi-detector row CT. *Radiology*. 2003;227:681–689.
10. Sheridan R, Peralta R, Rhea J, et al. Reformatted visceral protocol helical computed tomographic scanning allows conventional radiographs of the thoracic and lumbar spine to be eliminated in the evaluation of blunt trauma patients. *J Trauma*. 2003;55:665–669.
11. Brandt MM, Wahl WL, Yeom K, et al. Computed tomographic scanning reduces cost and time of complete spine evaluation. *J Trauma*. 2004;56:1022–1026; discussion 1026–1028.
12. Haba H, Taneichi H, Kotani Y, et al. Diagnostic accuracy of magnetic resonance imaging for detecting posterior ligamentous complex injury associated with thoracic and lumbar fractures. *J Neurosurg Spine*. 2003;99:20–26.
13. Terk MR, Hume-Neal M, Fraipont M, et al. Injury of the posterior ligament complex in patients with acute spinal trauma: evaluation by MR imaging. *AJR*. 1997;168:1481–1486.
14. Brightman RP, Miller CA, Rea GL, et al. Magnetic resonance imaging of trauma to the thoracic and lumbar spine. The importance of the posterior longitudinal ligament. *Spine*. 1992;17:541–550.
15. Bertram C, Prescher A, Furderer S, et al. Attachment points of the posterior longitudinal ligament and their importance

for thoracic and lumbar spine fractures. *Orthopade*. 2003; 32:848–851.

16. Yahia LH, Garzon S, Strykowski H, et al. Ultrastructure of the human interspinous ligament and ligamentum flavum. A preliminary study. *Spine*. 1990;15:262–268.

17. Vaccaro AR, Kim DH, Brodke DS, et al. Diagnosis and management of thoracolumbar spine fractures. *Instr Course Lect*. 2004;53:359–373.

18. Singer KP, Willen J, Breidahl PD, et al. Radiologic study of the influence of zygapophyseal joint orientation on spinal injuries at the thoracolumbar junction. *Surg Radiol Anat*. 1989;11:233–239.

19. Saboe LA, Reid DC, Davis LA, et al. Spine trauma and associated injuries. *J Trauma*. 1991;31:43–48.

20. Jeanneret B, Holdener HJ. Vertebral fractures and abdominal trauma. A retrospective study based on 415 documented vertebral fractures. *Unfallchirurg*. 1992;95:603–607.

21. Rabinovici R, Ovadia P, Mathiak G, et al. Abdominal injuries associated with lumbar spine fractures in blunt trauma. *Injury*. 1999;30:471–474.

22. Tyroch AH, McGuire EL, McLean SF, et al. The association between Chance fractures and intra-abdominal injuries revisited: a multicenter review. *Am Surg*. May 2005;71(5): 434–438.

23. Mirza SK, Mirza AJ, Chapman JR, et al. Classifications of thoracic and lumbar fractures: rationale and supporting data. *J Am Acad Orthop Surg*. 2002;10:364–377.

24. Oner FC, van Gils AP, Dhert WJ, et al. MRI findings of thoracolumbar spine fractures: a categorisation based on MRI examinations of 100 fractures. *Skeletal Radiol*. 1999;28: 433–443.

25. Magerl F, Aebi M, Gertzbein SD, et al. A comprehensive classification of thoracic and lumbar injuries. *Eur Spine J*. 1994;3:184–201.

26. Denis F. The three column spine and its significance in the classification of acute thoracolumbar spinal injuries. *Spine*. 1983;8:817–831.

27. Daffner RH. Thoracic and lumbar vertebral trauma. *Orthop Clin North Am*. 1990;21:463–482.

28. Vollmer DG, Gegg C. Classification and acute management of thoracolumbar fractures. *Neurosurg Clin North Am*. 1997;8:499–507.

29. Stubbs SN, Pasque CB, Brown S, et al. Spinal cord injuries due to falls from hunting tree stands in Oklahoma, 1988–1999. *J Okla State Med Assoc*. 2004;97:156–159.

30. Belmont PJ Jr, Taylor KF, Mason KT, et al. Incidence, epidemiology, and occupational outcomes of thoracolumbar fractures among U.S. Army aviators. *J Trauma*. 2001;50:855–861.

31. Dai LY, Yao WF, Cui YM, et al. Thoracolumbar fractures in patients with multiple injuries: diagnosis and treatment—a review of 147 cases. *J Trauma*. 2004;56(2):348–355.

32. Denis F. Spinal instability as defined by the three-column spine concept in acute spinal trauma. *Clin Orthop*. 1984;189:65–76.

33. McAfee PC, Yuan HA, Fredrickson BE, et al. The value of computed tomography in thoracolumbar fractures. An analysis of one hundred consecutive cases and a new classification. *J Bone Joint Surg Am*. 1983;65:461–473.

34. Panjabi MM, Oxland TR, Kifune M, et al. Validity of the three-column theory of thoracolumbar fractures. A biomechanic investigation. *Spine*. 1995;20:1122–1127.

35. Daffner RH, Deeb ZL, Goldberg AL, et al. The radiologic assessment of post-traumatic vertebral stability. *Skeletal Radiol*. 1990;19(2):103–108.

36. White AA III, Panjabi MM. The problem of clinical instability in the human spine: a systematic approach. In: *Clinical Biomechanics of the Spine*. 2nd ed. Baltimore: Lippincott Williams & Wilkins; 1990:352.

37. Fontijne WP, de Klerk LW, Braakman R, et al. CT scan prediction of neurological deficit in thoracolumbar burst fractures. *Bone Joint Surg Br*. 1992;74:683–685.

38. Eberl R, Kaminski A, Muller EJ, et al. Importance of the cross-sectional area of the spinal canal in thoracolumbar and lumbar fractures. Is there any correlation between the

39. Braakman R, Fontijne WP, Zeegers R, et al. Neurological deficit in injuries of the thoracic and lumbar spine. A consecutive series of 70 patients. *Acta Neurochir (Wien)*. 1991;111:11–17.

40. Thongtrangan I, Le H, Park J, et al. Cauda equina syndrome in patients with low lumbar fractures. *Neurosurg Focus*. 2004;16:E6.

41. Harrop JS, Hunt GE Jr, Vaccaro AR. Conus medullaris and cauda equina syndrome as a result of traumatic injuries: management principles. *Neurosurg Focus*. 2004;16:E4.

42. Angtuaco EJC, Binet EF. Radiology of thoracic and lumbar fractures. *Clin Ortho Rel Res*. 1984;189:43–57.

43. Campbell SE, Phillips CD, Dubovsky E, et al. The value of CT in determining potential instability of simple wedge-compression fractures of the lumbar spine. *AJNR*. 1995;16:1385–1392.

44. Petersilge CA, Emery SE. Thoracolumbar burst fracture: evaluating stability. *Semin Ultrasound CT MR*. 1996;17:105–113.

45. Petersilge CA, Pathria MN, Emery SE, et al. Thoracolumbar burst fractures: evaluation with MR imaging. *Radiology*. 1995;194:49–54.

46. Lee HM, Kim HS, Kim DJ, et al. Reliability of magnetic resonance imaging in detecting posterior ligament complex injury in thoracolumbar spinal fractures. *Spine*. 2000;25:2079–2084.

47. Youssef JA, McCullen GM, Brown CC. Seizure-induced lumbar burst fracture. *Spine*. 1995;20:1301–1303.

48. van den Brink WA, van Leeuwen O. Lumbar burst fracture due to low voltage shock. A case report. *Acta Orthop Scand*. 1995;66:374–375.

49. Hongo M, Abe E, Shimada Y, et al. Surface strain distribution on thoracic and lumbar vertebrae under axial compression. The role in burst fractures. *Spine*. 1999;24:1197–1202.

50. Heggeness MH, Doherty BJ. The trabecular anatomy of thoracolumbar vertebrae: implications for burst fractures. *Spine*. 1988;13:1268–1272.

51. Sharma M, Langrana NA, Rodriguez J. Modeling of facet articulation as a nonlinear moving contact problem: sensitive study on lumbar facet response. *J Biomech Eng*. 1998;120:118–125.

52. Ochia RS, Ching RP. Internal pressure measurements during burst fracture formation in human lumbar vertebrae. *Spine*. 2002;27:1160–1167.

53. Jelsma RK, Kirsch PT, Rice JF, et al. The radiographic description of thoracolumbar fractures. *Surg Neurol*. 1982;18:230–236.

54. Guerra J Jr, Garfin SR, Resnick D. Vertebral burst fractures: CT analysis of the retropulsed fragment. *Radiology*. 1984; 153:769–772.

55. Daffner RH, Deeb ZL, Rothfus WE. The posterior vertebral body line: importance in the detection of burst fractures. *AJR Am J Roentgenol*. 1987;148(1):93–96.

56. Shirado O, Kaneda K, Tadano S, et al. Influence of disc degeneration on mechanism of thoracolumbar burst fractures. *Spine*. 1992;17:286–292.

57. Panjabi MM, Oxland T, Takata K, et al. Articular facets of the human spine. Quantitative three-dimensional anatomy. *Spine*. 1993:18:1298–1310.

58. James KS, Wenger KH, Schlegel JD, et al. Biomechanical evaluation of the stability of thoracolumbar burst fractures. *Spine*. 1994;19:1731–1740.

59. Kinoshita H, Nagata Y, Ueda H, et al. Conservative treatment of burst fractures of the thoracolumbar and lumbar spine. *Paraplegia*. 1993;31:58–67.

60. Sapkas G, Korres D, Babis GC, et al. Correlation of spinal canal post-traumatic encroachment and neurological deficit in burst fractures of the lower cervical spine (C3-7). *Eur Spine J*. 1995;4:39–44.

61. Ballock RT, Mackersie R, Abitbol JJ, et al. Can burst fractures be predicted from plain radiographs? *J Bone Joint Surg Br*. 1992;74:147–150.

62. Denis F, Burkus JK. Shear fracture-dislocations of the thoracic and lumbar spine associated with forceful hyperextension (lumberjack paraplegia). *Spine*. 1992;17(2):156–161.

63. Keenen TL, Antony J, Benson DR. Dural tears associated with lumbar burst fractures. *J Orthop Trauma*. 1990;4(3):243–245.

64. Kahamba JF, Rath SA, Antoniades O, et al. Laminar and arch fracture with dural tear and nerve root entrapment in patients operated upon for thoracic and lumbar spine injuries. *Acta Neurochir (Wien)*. 1998;140:114–119.

65. Kim NH, Lee HM, Chun IM. Neurological injury and recovery in patients with burst fracture of the thoracolumbar spine. *Spine*. 1999;24(3):290–294.

66. Greene KA, Dickman CA, Marciano FF, et al. Acute axis fractures. Analysis of management and outcome in 340 consecutive cases. *Spine*. 1997;22:1843–1852.

67. Hitchon PW, Torner JC. Recumbency in thoracolumbar fractures. *Neurosurg Clin North Am*. 1997;8:509–517.

68. Hitchon PW, Torner JC, Haddad SF, et al. Management options in thoracolumbar burst fractures. *Surg Neurol*. 1998;49:619–626; discussion 626–627.

69. Celebi L, Muratli HH, Dogan O, et al. The efficacy of non-operative treatment of burst fractures of the thoracolumbar vertebrae. *Acta Orthop Traumatol Turc*. 2004;38:16–22.

70. Aligizakis A, Katonis P, Stergiopoulos K, et al. Functional outcome of burst fractures of the thoracolumbar spine managed non-operatively, with early ambulation, evaluated using the load sharing classification. *Acta Orthop Belg*. 2002; 68(3):279–287.

71. Tropiano P, Huang RC, Louis CA, et al. Functional and radiographic outcome of thoracolumbar and lumbar burst fractures managed by closed orthopaedic reduction and casting. *Spine*. 2003;28:2459–2465.

72. Wilcox RK, Boerger TO, Allen DJ, et al. A dynamic study of thoracolumbar burst fractures. *J Bone Joint Surg Am*. 2003;85A(11):2184–2189.

73. Limb D, Shaw DL, Dickson RA. Neurological injury in thoracolumbar burst fractures. *J Bone Joint Surg Br*. 1995;77: 774–777.

74. Meves R, Avanzi O. Correlation between neurological deficit and spinal canal compromise in 198 patients with thoracolumbar and lumbar fractures. *Spine*. April 1, 2005;30(7):787–791.

75. Hashimoto T, Kaneda K, Abumi K. Relationship between traumatic spinal canal stenosis and neurologic deficits in thoracolumbar burst fractures. *Spine*. 1988;13:1268–1272.

76. Chen JF, Wu CT, Lee ST. Percutaneous vertebroplasty for the treatment of burst fractures. Case report. *Neurosurg Spine*. 2004;1:228–231.

77. Chen JF, Lee ST. Percutaneous vertebroplasty for treatment of thoracolumbar spine bursting fracture. *Surg Neurol*. 2004;62(6):494–500.

78. Cho DY, Lee WY, Sheu PC. Treatment of thoracolumbar burst fractures with polymethyl methacrylate vertebroplasty and short-segment pedicle screw fixation. *Neurosurgery*. 2003;53:1354–1360; discussion 1360–1361.

79. Hu SS, Capen DA, Rimoldi RL, et al. The effect of surgical decompression on neurologic outcome after lumbar fractures. *Clin Orthop*. 1993;288:166–173.

80. Knop C, Bastian L, Lange U, et al. Complications in surgical treatment of thoracolumbar injuries. *Eur Spine J*. 2002; 11:214–226.

81. Hoshikawa T, Tanaka Y, Kokubun S, et al. Flexion-distraction injuries in the thoracolumbar spine: an in vitro study of the relation between flexion angle and the motion axis of fracture. *Spinal Disord Tech*. 2002;15:139–143.

82. Liu YJ, Chang MC, Wang ST, et al. Flexion-distraction injury of the thoracolumbar spine. *Injury*. 2003;34:920–923.

83. Ball ST, Vaccaro AR, Albert TJ, et al. Injuries of the thoracolumbar spine associated with restraint use in head-on motor vehicle accidents. *J Spinal Disord*. 2000;13:297–304.

84. Arnold PM, Malone DG, Han PP. Bilateral locked facets of the lumbosacral spine: treatment with open reduction and transpedicular fixation. *J Spinal Cord Med*. 2004;27: 269–272.

85. Stuart RM, Song SJ. Unilateral lumbosacral facet joint dislocation without associated fracture. *Australas Radiol*. 2004; 48:224–229.

86. Neumann P, Nordwall A, Osvalder AL. Traumatic instability of the lumbar spine. A dynamic in vitro study of flexion-distraction injury. *Spine*. 1995;20:1111–1121.

87. Wang YF, Teng MM, Chang CY, et al. Imaging manifestations of spinal fractures in ankylosing spondylitis. *Am J Neuroradiol*. 2005;26(8):2067–2076.

88. Krueger MA, Green DA, Hoyt D, et al. Overlooked spine injuries associated with lumbar transverse process fractures. *Clin Orthop*. 1996;327:191–195.

89. Shen FH, Crowl A, Shuler TE, et al. Delayed recognition of lumbosacral fracture dislocations in the multitrauma patient: the triad of transverse process fractures, unilateral renal contusion and lumbosacral fracture dislocation. *Trauma*. 2004;56:700–705.

90. Miller CD, Blyth P, Civil ID. Lumbar transverse process fractures—a sentinel marker of abdominal organ injuries. *Injury*. 2000;31:773–776.

91. Patten RM, Gunberg SR, Brandenburger DK. Frequency and importance of transverse process fractures in the lumbar vertebrae at helical abdominal CT in patients with trauma. *Radiology*. 2000;215:831–834.

92. Watson-Jones R. The results of postural reduction of fractures of the spine. *J Bone Joint Surg Am*. 1938;20:567–586.

93. Holdsworth FW. Fractures, dislocations and fracture-dislocations of the spine. *J Bone Joint Surg Br*. 1963;45:6–20.

94. Ferguson RL, Allen BL. A mechanistic classification of thoracolumbar spine fractures. *Clin Orthop*. 1984;189:77–88.

95. McCormack T, Karaikovic E, Gaines RW. The load sharing classification of spine fractures. *Spine*. 1994;19(15):1741–1744.

Magnetic Resonance Imaging of Acute Spinal Trauma

Adam E. Flanders

Prior to the development of magnetic resonance imaging (MRI), the extent of associated soft tissue injury to the intervertebral discs, ligaments, and spinal cord was determined primarily by inference from known biomechanical principles rather than by direct imaging of the affected tissues (1,2). Consequently, many of the established therapies for spinal cord injuries (SCI) are based on radiologic classifications of osseous injury to the spinal column. These traditional therapeutic interventions for SCI are directed primarily by radiographic findings such as re-establishment of normal anatomic alignment of the spinal canal and removal of bone fragments. Current management of SCI, however, has become more directed toward the correction of the associated soft tissue and spinal cord damage (3–6), and MRI has become increasingly important in the diagnostic evaluation of spinal injuries.

The greatest impact that MRI has made in the evaluation of SCI has been in assessment of the intracanalicular and paraspinal soft tissues (3–5,7–15). The integrity of the intervertebral discs and ligamentous complexes can be routinely evaluated with MRI. In addition, MRI permits direct visualization of the morphology of the injured cord parenchyma and the relationship of the surrounding structures to the spinal cord (2,16). No other imaging modality has been able to faithfully reproduce the internal architecture of the spinal cord, and it is this particular feature of MRI that promises to have the greatest impact on the management of the SCI patient in the future.

Although MRI is a powerful diagnostic tool, it has not supplanted conventional radiologic imaging in the initial evaluation of SCI (16). The conventional diagnostic algorithm of plain radiography supplemented by computed tomography (CT) is the most appropriate and cost-effective method to evaluate most cases of spinal trauma (7,10,16–18). MRI has replaced myelography and CT myelography (CTM), however, as the primary imaging option available to assess for residual soft tissue compression of the spinal cord (10,12,14,19,20) due to factors such as acute disc herniations and epidural hematomas. Identification of residual compression of the spinal cord has significant implications in regard to timing of subsequent surgery and the type of surgical approach that is required (8,12,20). MRI is also an essential diagnostic modality in cases of SCI without radiographic abnormality (SCIWORA) (11,17,20–25). An MRI examination in the acute period is warranted in any patient who has a persistent neurologic deficit after spinal trauma (10,11,17).

The focus of this chapter is the application of MRI in the evaluation of injuries of the spinal axis and spinal cord. For a comprehensive reference of the radiology of spine trauma, the reader is encouraged to pursue the reviews found in Chapters 5, 6, and 7.

DEMOGRAPHICS OF SPINAL CORD INJURY

SCI is a significant cause of disability in the United States. Although the number of individuals who sustain paralysis yearly is substantially less than the number of people who sustain moderate to severe traumatic brain injury (TBI) (11,000 SCI per year versus 70,000 to 90,000 TBI per year), the financial costs to society for SCI are significant. Since most patients survive the acute SCI, there are approximately 225,000 to 288,000 SCI patients with partial or complete paralysis currently being cared for in the United States. The total lifetime costs for medical treatment and rehabilitation range from $200,000 to $800,000 per affected individual. The lifetime direct costs may exceed $2.8 million, for a high tetraplegic patient injured at age 25 (26–27). Nearly 55% of all SCI occur in young adults between the ages of 16 to 30 years. Most SCI victims are white males (81.7%). The etiologies of SCI are vehicular (37.4%), acts of violence (25.9%), falls (21.5%), and sports injuries (7.1%) (27). Because SCI primarily affects employed (60.5%) young adults, there is a tremendous financial loss to society in terms of overall lifetime productivity.

Injuries to the spinal axis can be subdivided into *spinal injuries* (damage to the spinal axis without neurologic injury) and *SCI* (damage to the spinal cord with or without spinal axis abnormality). An accurate estimate of the total number of SCI is difficult to define because patients who expire in the field from a fatal SCI (i.e., high cervical cord) or from related injuries (e.g., cerebral trauma) are not included in the national statistics. Tetraplegia (quadriplegia) is defined as an injury to one of the eight cervical plegia) is defined as an injury to one of the eight cervical segments of the spinal cord with paralysis of all four limbs. Paraplegia usually results from injury to the thoracic, lumbar, or sacral segments of the spinal cord with dysfunction of both legs. A neurologically complete lesion is one in which there is no motor or sensory function three segments below the neurologic level of injury. Of those spinal cord–injured persons who survive to reach a medical facility, the most frequent neurologic deficit is incomplete tetraplegia (29.5%), followed by complete paraplegia (27.9%), incomplete paraplegia (21.3%), and complete tetraplegia (18.5%) (27). Less than 1% of SCI patients recover completely during the initial hospitalization.

MAGNETIC RESONANCE IMAGING TECHNIQUES

Imaging Considerations

The spinal cord–injured patient requires special consideration before MRI with regard to patient transfer, life support, monitoring of vital signs, fixation devices, choices of surface coils, and pulse sequences. The potential risks from transporting a medically and neurologically unstable patient must be carefully weighed against the potential benefits derived from the diagnostic information provided by MRI. Most SCI patients can be accommodated with minimal risk to the patient as long as appropriate precautions are adhered to. As with all critical care patients, myriad life-sustaining devices may need to accompany the SCI patient to the MRI suite. Many of these devices are incompatible with the MRI environment. Conventional ventilatory equipment is safe to use only in the fringe field of ultralow field strength units. For mid- and high-field strength MRI units, several manufacturers offer MRI-compatible ventilators. The unit itself is operated remotely, and the ventilator controls remain inside the control room. Similarly, MRI-compatible monitors are now available that can relay heart rate, respiration, blood pressure, and oxygenation information directly into the MRI control area. Indwelling central venous catheters with thermocouples and conventional intravenous medication pumps are prohibited in the MRI environment.

External spinal fixation devices warrant special attention because, if used improperly in the MRI suite, they can pose a significant safety hazard to both the patient and personnel (28). Moreover, fixation devices that are composed of ferromagnetic alloys may destroy the static magnetic field close to the region of interest, resulting in image degradation.

Most patients will arrive for an MRI examination following closed reduction of the spinal injury and fixation with the appropriate external spinal stabilization device (Fig. 8-1). Occasionally, traction will be applied using cranial tongs and a system of pulleys and weights (Fig. 8-1C). Although it is possible to maintain traction on the scanning

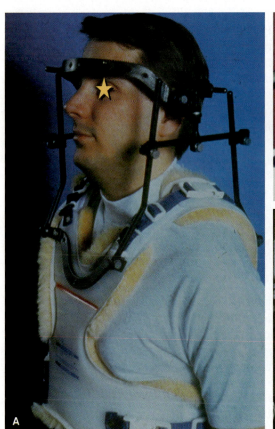
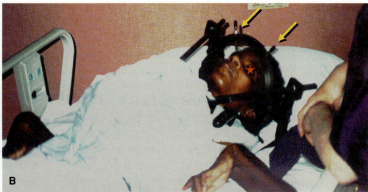
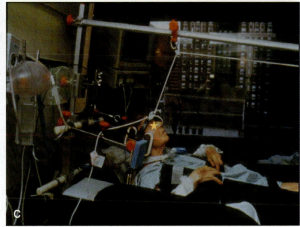

FIGURE 8-1. Various forms of spine stabilization. **A:** Detailed view of a standard halo vest applied to a normal volunteer. The fiberglass vest is fixed to a rigid frame made of a nonferrous graphite alloy composite. The frame connects to a ring that encircles the head. The head is transfixed to the ring through a series of four pins. **B:** Halo device applied to a patient. Note the pins that rigidly fix the skull to the ring (*arrows*). **C:** Traction device that applies constant distractive force between the head and lower body to maintain spinal alignment.

table, it is not advisable to do so for several reasons: (a) it is cumbersome to attach the weights and pulleys to the scanning table, (b) the traction device may interfere with table motion, and (c) conventional traction weights ("sandbags") contain metallic pellets that pose a significant projectile hazard to patient and personnel (Fig. 8-2) (28). Only MRI-compatible weights are permitted inside the scanning area (29).

Patients with cervical spine injuries are usually stabilized with a fiberglass cervical collar or, in more severe injuries, a halo and halo vest are used (30). For thoracic and lumbar injuries, the patient may be transported on a rigid spine board, a body cast, or in traction. MRI-compatible halo vests are often composed of a graphite composite, titanium, aluminum, and plastic, and are devoid of stainless steel components (31,32). If the fixation pins used for femoral traction are ferrous, they usually do not interfere to any noticeable degree with the images of the spine, although tissue heating can occur at the contact points with skin.

Only properly trained personnel should perform transfer of a patient with spine instability to and from the scanning table. Patient motion should be minimized, as there is potential risk for further neurologic deterioration from moving of a patient with an unstable spine.

Patient motion (voluntary or involuntary) can also be detrimental to the quality of any MRI study. Even a patient with acute tetraplegia can seriously degrade a cervical MRI examination either by movement of the head and neck or from irregular ventilation. Sedation may be necessary to complete an examination.

Choice of surface coil is determined by the location(s) of injury, access to the area of interest, and the types of coils available. The proximity of the surface coil to the area of interest is a key factor in determining image quality. Temporary removal of a cervical collar, for example, will permit the use of specially designed quadrature or anterior/posterior neck coils. Wherever possible, a dedicated spine-phased array coil system should be used to maximize coverage and optimize MRI signal.

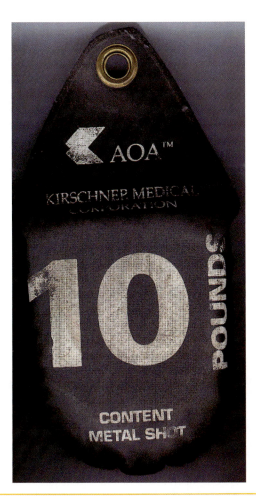

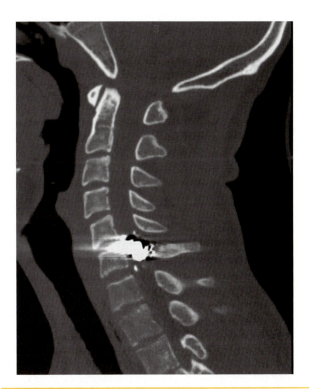

FIGURE 8-3. Sagittal CT reconstruction of the cervical spine showing a large bullet fragment lodged within the spinal canal. There is a potential risk of fragment migration in the MR environment, therefore, MRI evaluation is usually prohibited in these instances.

FIGURE 8-2. Traction weight (aka "sandbag"). Earlier versions were filled with sand or other dense inert material. In some cases, these bags are filled with metal pellets with ferromagnetic properties (see label on bag). This type of bag is prohibited in the MR environment because they can act as projectiles in high field systems.

When the neck is fixed in a halo vest (Fig. 8-1A,B), use of a phased-array coil system can be problematic as the distance between the coil surface is increased, which can diminish the returned signal strength. Instead, a pair of 5-inch circular surface coils closely applied to the back of the neck can be used effectively. A multicoil phased-array system can be accommodated in most thoracic and lumbar evaluations. Alternatively, the patient can be placed over a sliding surface coil tray, which permits repositioning of the coil without moving the patient. A conventional 5-inch by 11-inch "license plate" surface coil provides adequate coverage for sagittal fields of view up to 32 cm.

MRI evaluation of the spine following penetrating trauma requires special consideration for two reasons: (a) retained metallic fragments within the spinal canal may be regarded as a safety hazard to the patient, and (b) depending on their composition, these fragments can

produce significant local image degradation (Fig. 8-3). Most firearm projectiles are nonferrous and therefore will not move in the static magnetic field (33). A ferrous fragment in the spinal canal could theoretically migrate, dislodge, or produce thermal injury when exposed to the strong static magnetic field and radiofrequency energy, potentially producing further neurologic injury (34). Bullets encased in steel, copper, or copper-nickel exhibit significant deflection force in a high-field MRI unit (34). Although we are not aware of any reports of ascending paralysis from retained bullet fragments in the spinal canal, any MRI examination following penetrating trauma to the spine should be performed at the discretion of the radiologist after review of radiographs or CT of the area of interest. Additional consideration should be given to the length of time the fragment has been embedded in the tissue as the potential risk of movement is diminished in mature scar tissue. If there are sufficient safety concerns, then myelography or CTM should be used.

Imaging Methods

At a minimum, evaluation of the injured spine should be performed both in the axial and sagittal planes using a

▶ **TABLE 8-1** Proposed Trauma MR Scan Protocol

Imaging Plane	Sequence	Comments
Sagittal	T1	Anatomic images
Sagittal	Proton density or intermediate weighted (TSE or FSE)	Improves identification of epidural fluid collections and ligament disruption.
Sagittal	T2 weighted (TSE or FSE) with fat suppression	Best sequence for visualizing spinal cord injury, ligamentous edema/disruption, marrow edema and disc herniation.
Sagittal	Gradient echo	Useful to confirm presence and location of hemorrhage in spinal cord injury. Identify fractures.
Axial	Gradient echo	Useful to confirm existence and location of hemorrhage in spinal cord injury and to identify fractures.
Axial	T2 weighted (TSE or FSE)	Useful to confirm damage to spinal cord parenchyma.
Axial (cervical spine)	2D-Time-Of-Flight-MRA (cervical only)	Useful to identify posttraumatic vertebral occlusion.
Axial (cervical spine)	T1 with fat-suppression and superior/inferior spatial saturation (black blood technique)	Useful to identify vascular dissection.

combination of pulse sequences. At a minimum, T1- and T2-weighted information are both necessary to completely assess the spinal axis and the spinal cord. Additional sequences are performed as needed, depending on the portion of the spine that is injured, the degree of injury, and patient tolerance. Conventional fast spin-echo (FSE) or turbo spin-echo (TSE) and gradient-echo pulse sequences are used most often (Table 8-1).

An inherent property of the FSE pulse sequences is that the images exhibit less magnetic susceptibility artifact

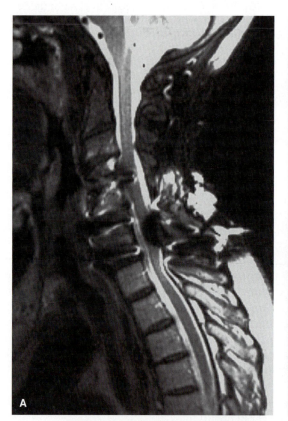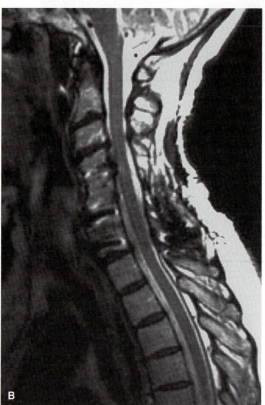

FIGURE 8-4. Effect of fat suppression and bandwidth in reducing artifact from hardware. **A:** Sagittal FSE T2-weighted, fat-suppressed image (2500/85Ef/4 NEX/ETL 8, RBW 32 kHz) shows significant distortion of the image and artifact over the spinal cord. **B:** Sagittal FSE T2-weighted image without fat-suppression (2500/85Ef/4 NEX/ETL 8, RBW 64 kHz) shows a dramatic reduction of the artifact and improved visibility of the spinal cord parenchyma. (From Flanders AE, Croul SE. Spinal trauma. In: Atlas SW. *Magnetic Resonance Imaging of the Brain and Spine*. 3rd ed. Philadelphia: Lippincott Williams & Wilkins; 2002:1772, with permission.)

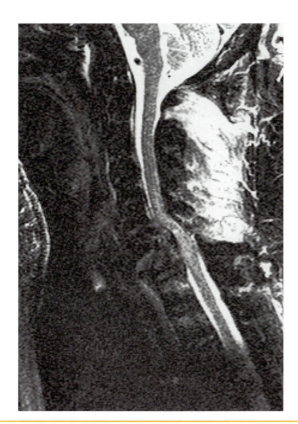

FIGURE 8-5. GRASE (gradient spin echo) sagittal image of a cervical injury. Note the increased amount of background noise associated with this technique.

as compared to conventional spin-echo and gradient-echo images (35). Although this property may seem theoretically disadvantageous when searching for small areas of acute spinal cord hemorrhage, FSE images have been shown to be comparably sensitive to conventional spin-echo images for detecting intramedullary hemorrhage (36). The decrease in magnetic susceptibility with FSE may be advantageous when imaging postoperative spines with instrumentation that otherwise would be obscured by artifacts (Fig. 8-4) (35). Use of hybrid techniques such as GRASE (gradient spin-echo) may provide improved visualization of intramedullary hemorrhage in SCI over FSE images; however, the increase in artifacts and noise may prohibit its routine use in this application (Fig. 8-5) (37). Manually increasing receiver bandwidth (RBW) decreases the read-out period, which has the added benefit of diminishing susceptibility effects (Fig. 8-4).

Imaging of the cervical, thoracic, or lumbar regions begins with a low-resolution gradient-echo localizer in the coronal plane. This image(s) can be obtained in less than 1 minute and can be used subsequently to prescribe the sagittal sequences. A maximum of nine to 12 sagittal images are usually required to interrogate the spine to

include the lateral elements. Sagittal images should be no more than 3 to 4 mm thick with a 0- to 1-mm slice gap. The field of view of the area of interest is adequate at 22 to 24 cm. In the thoracic spine, a large sagittal localizer is also needed (48 cm field-of-view) for accurate labeling of the involved levels.

Modern MRI equipment has the capacity to rapidly image multiple regions of the spine simultaneously without repositioning the patient. With the availability of combined head and spine array surface coils and moving MRI tables, the entire spine can be imaged without repositioning the patient. This "survey" method may be useful when multiple levels of the spinal axis need to be rapidly interrogated at one time (Fig. 8-6).

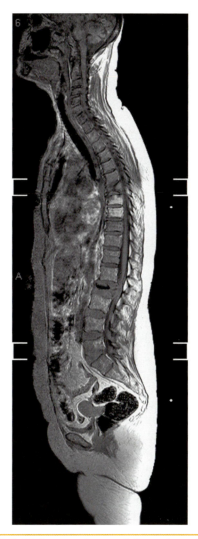

FIGURE 8-6. MRI survey image of the entire spine. Patient with metastatic disease who sustained a fall and presents with new lower extremity weakness. This technique combines separate image acquisitions from the cervical, thoracic, and lumbar region in one display for easier review. The patient has pathologic fractures in both the thoracic and lumbar regions.

The prescribed spatial resolution depends on the inherent limitations of the MR scanner, the type of sequence used and acquisition time limitations. T2-weighted information is obtained using a single FSE acquisition using a split echo train, resulting in an intermediate and T2-weighted image. Alternatively, two separate FSE acquisitions can be used with different echo train lengths. To produce a short effective echo time (TE_{ff}) image (intermediate weighted) an echo train of four with two excitations is suggested, whereas for the long TE_{ff} image an echo train of eight with four excitations is recommended. At a minimum, 256 steps are prescribed in both the frequency (x_{res}) and phase (y_{res}) axes. Unlike spin echo sequences, fat-containing structures remain bright on FSE/TSE images due to the effects of J-coupling. Therefore, fat suppression must be employed on the long repetition time (TR) sequences to improve visualization of edema in the posterior ligamentous complexes. Typically, a spectrally selective fat-saturation pulse is applied that is tuned to the resonance frequency of lipid on a T2-weighted image. Alternatively, a short tau inversion recovery (STIR) sequence can be employed to produce effective suppression of lipid signal in the soft tissues, thereby improving the conspicuity of edema. Increased signal-to-noise and shorter acquisition times can be achieved by applying driven equilibrium pulses (38). Fat saturation techniques can have a deleterious effect on image quality when ferromagnetic hardware is present (Fig. 8-4). When available, parallel imaging methods can be advantageous in spinal imaging by reducing imaging time, reducing blurring in FSE/TSE sequences, and by helping to reduce motion artifacts (39). The phase-encoding axis is oriented parallel to the spine so that phase ghosting is not propagated across the spinal canal. A form of gradient moment nulling (GMN) should also be employed in the cervical and thoracic regions to compensate for cerebrospinal fluid (CSF) flow artifacts. Cardiac gating is another option for correcting cerebrospinal flow artifacts on T2-weighted sequences. Anteriorly placed saturation pulses are helpful in reducing artifacts produced by swallowing, breathing, and cardiac motion. Respiratory compensation may be of benefit when imaging the thoracic and lumbar regions. Resolution can be maintained with reduced imaging times by implementing options that vary the number of phasing encoding steps and field of view.

Cross-sectional information on MRI is essential, especially when assessing the cervical and thoracic spinal cord. The choice of axial pulse sequence varies, depending on the part of the spine being evaluated, extent of injury, type of tissue contrast required, personal preferences, and time constraints. Usually, axial images that provide hyperintense CSF are preferred and are obtained using gradient-echo (GE) or FSE pulse sequences. In the cervical spine, a myelographic-like image is produced using an axial three-dimensional Fourier transform (3D

FT) GE pulse sequence to obtain 28 or 64 contiguous images, at 1.5 mm thickness. Technical parameters include 5-degree flip angle, minimum TR/TE, 256 by 192 matrix and two excitations. The TE should be <15 msec in order to minimize unwanted susceptibility effects that might exaggerate bony stenoses (40). To maximize detection of acute intramedullary hemorrhage, at least one GE sequence should be performed. High-resolution cross-sectional imaging of the spinal cord can be performed using FSE techniques in the study of the cervical and thoracic spine.

As a supplement to the cervical examination, a survey of the extracranial vasculature is useful to detect posttraumatic occlusion or dissection of the carotid and vertebral arteries. This may be achieved with routine two-dimensional (2D) time-of-flight (TOF) magnetic resonance angiography (MRA), 3D TOF MRA, or a contrast-enhanced MRA (CEMRA) using ellipticocentric reordering of k-space. An axial cross-sectional evaluation of the neck using a T1-weighted "black-blood" technique (employing superior/inferior spatial and fat saturation) is helpful to identify subtle arterial dissections of the extracranial vasculature.

Although there are reported cases in which gadolinium was useful in the evaluation of acute SCI, the justification for routine use is unsubstantiated (41–44). In humans, some degree of enhancement of the posttraumatic spinal cord lesion has been reported at 1 to 14 weeks after injury (43,44). The enhancement is postulated to represent breakdown of the blood-brain barrier in the acute phase and reparative granulation tissue late after injury (43,44). In our experience, contrast agents have no clinical utility in the routine MRI evaluation of acute spinal trauma.

CHARACTERIZATION OF SPINAL INJURY USING MAGNETIC RESONANCE IMAGING

Although the biomechanics and types of injuries to the spine vary by location, the observed soft tissue and osseous changes to the spinal axis and spinal cord on MRI are relatively similar. Any interpretation of an MRI examination performed for spinal injury should include a discussion of the integrity of the intervertebral discs, vertebral bodies, vertebral alignment, ligaments, and neural elements. Specifically, the types of changes that are observed with MRI in SCI can be grouped into osseous injuries, ligamentous and joint disruption, intervertebral disc injury, fluid collections, vascular injury, and SCI. The force of injury is often dissipated primarily at one level in the spine; therefore, injury to all of the tissues (e.g., bone, ligament, disc, and spinal cord) is usually anticipated at one to two isolated levels.

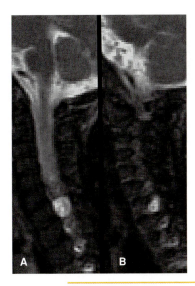
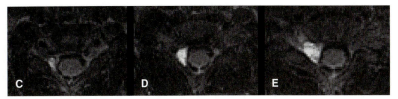

FIGURE 8-7. Dilated nerve-root sheath following root avulsion. **A,B:** Sagittal T2-weighted images show prominent intraforaminal CSF-filled space without characteristic hypointensity of exiting nerve root. **C,D,E:** Axial T2-weighted images confirm dilatation of exiting nerve-root sheath filled by CSF. (From Flanders AE, Croul SE. Spinal trauma. In: Atlas SW. *Magnetic Resonance Imaging of the Brain and Spine*. 3rd ed. Philadelphia: Lippincott Williams & Wilkins; 2002:1774, with permission.)

Identification of injury to one tissue type should prompt the observer to scrutinize the same level for injuries to other tissues.

Most of the diagnostic information in spinal cord injury is derived from the sagittal images. Axial images serve as a supplement (2). Sagittal T1-weighted images offer an excellent anatomic overview. Disc herniations, epidural fluid collections, subluxations, vertebral body fractures, cord swelling, and cord compression are also visualized (18). The fat-suppressed sagittal T2-weighted images are usually relied upon to depict most of the soft tissue abnormalities including spinal cord edema and hemorrhage, ligamentous injury, disc herniation, and epidural fluid collections (13). Axial and sagittal GE images aid in the identification of acute spinal cord hemorrhage, disc herniations, and fractures. MRI has not been successful in reliably demonstrating traumatic nerve root avulsions. Occasionally, posttraumatic root pouch cysts are identified. High-resolution T2-weighted cross-sectional images may reveal traumatized rootlets (Fig. 8-7). CT with intrathecal contrast remains the diagnostic method of choice for demonstrating the characteristic empty nerve root sheath and the periradicular cavities (45,46).

Osseous Injury

Currently, MRI does not offer any advantage over plain radiography or high-resolution multidetector CT (MDCT) in the evaluation of associated osseous injuries following spinal trauma (8,16,18,24). Moreover, even when MRI is available, it should only be performed *after* appropriate radiographic evaluation of the osseous injury.

The overall incidence of cervical spine injury from a multi-institutional survey of 615 US trauma centers was estimated to be 4.3%. The incidence of cervical spine injury *without* SCI was 3.0% and the incidence of cervical SCI *without* fracture was 0.7% (47).

The traumatic osseous changes to the spinal axis on MRI are divided into subluxations, fracture deformities, and compressive injuries. Relative loss of alignment at a specific level of the spinal axis is readily depicted on a mid-sagittal MRI image. The sensitivity of MRI in detecting anterior subluxation is probably better than conventional radiography or CT because the morphology of the thecal sac is also demonstrated and because portions of the spine obscured on plain radiography (e.g., cervical-thoracic junction) are clearly identified on MRI (16).

Nondisplaced fracture lines through the vertebral bodies and posterior elements are poorly demonstrated on MRI. The fracture line is sometimes visible on GE images as a thin hyperintense band that traverses the vertebral body. Depending on the mode of injury, this band may be oriented vertically, horizontally, or obliquely (Figs. 8-8–8-14) (2,10,12,16). A fracture line that extends through the cortex may interrupt the continuity of the characteristic hypointense peripheral margin of cortical bone (2,10). It may be difficult to distinguish cortical bone fragments

(text continues on page 198)

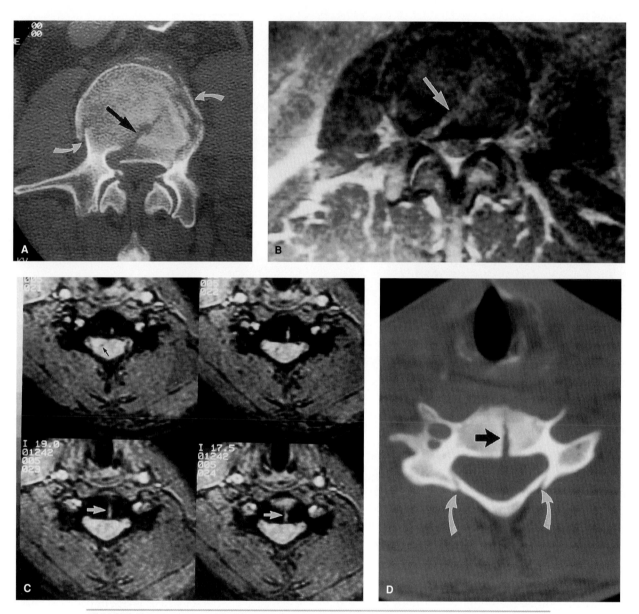

FIGURE 8-8. Depiction of fractures with MRI and CT. **A:** Axial CT image shows a comminuted fracture of L3. An oblique fracture line (*arrow*) demarcates a fragment of retropulsed bone. Fractures extend out to the peripheral cortical margin (*curved arrows*). **B:** Axial FSE intermediate-weighted image at the same level as (A). The fracture line (*arrow*) appears similar to the CT image; however, the additional fracture lines and fragments are poorly delineated. **C:** Axial GE images 3DFT in another patient show a vertically oriented fracture line that extends through the midportion of a cervical vertebral body (*white arrows*). There is a tiny focus of residual hemorrhage within the right ventral aspect of the cord (*black arrow*). **D:** Axial CT image obtained through the same level as (C) also demonstrates the vertical fracture line (*black arrow*). Additional fractures of the lamina are present bilaterally (*white arrows*). This finding is difficult to appreciate on the MRI. (From Flanders AE, Croul SE. Spinal trauma. In: Atlas SW. *Magnetic Resonance Imaging of the Brain and Spine*. 3rd ed. Philadelphia: Lippincott Williams & Wilkins; 2002:1775, with permission.)

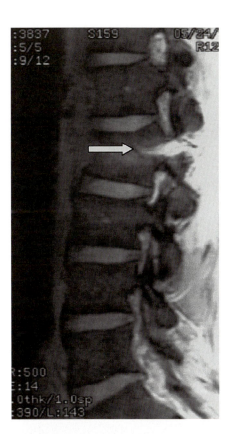

FIGURE 8-9. Chance fracture of L2. Sagittal gradient echo image shows depression of the superior endplate of the L2 vertebral body and a horizontal fracture line extending from the posterior cortex of L2 through the posterior elements (*arrow*). (From Flanders AE, Croul SE. Spinal trauma. In: Atlas SW. *Magnetic Resonance Imaging of the Brain and Spine*. 3rd ed. Philadelphia: Lippincott Williams & Wilkins; 2002:1776, with permission.)

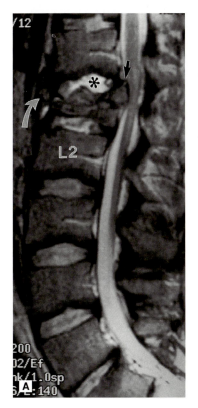

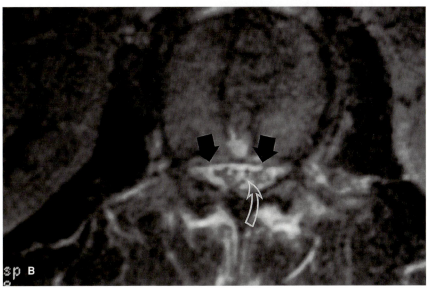

FIGURE 8-10. Burst fracture of L1. **A:** Sagittal FSE T2-weighted image shows changes of a burst fracture involving the L1 vertebra body. There is loss of height anteriorly with displacement of a fracture fragment, which is contained by the intact ALL (*curved arrow*). There is retropulsion of the posterior-superior corner of the L1 body into the spinal canal (*black arrow*). The T12-L1 intervertebral disc (*asterisk*) is hyperintense relative to the other levels secondary to injury. Note that the height of the posterior aspect of the body is maintained, suggesting column stability. Also note the absence of ligamentous injury. **B:** Axial FSE T2-weighted image at the level of the lower half of L1 shows the retropulsed bone (*arrows*) compressing the ventral theca and the roots of the cauda equina (*curved arrow*). (From Flanders AE, Croul SE. Spinal trauma. In: Atlas SW. *Magnetic Resonance Imaging of the Brain and Spine*. 3rd ed. Philadelphia: Lippincott Williams & Wilkins; 2002:1777, with permission.)

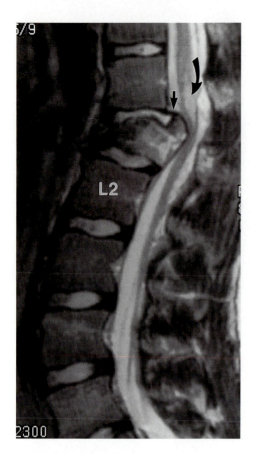

FIGURE 8-11. Burst fracture of L1. Sagittal FSE T2-weighted image shows a burst fracture of the L1 vertebral body with rotation of the posterior-superior corner of the vertebral body into the spinal canal. The PLL is stretched, but appears intact (*short arrow*). The marrow of the vertebral body is hyperintense relative to the other segments due to compressive injury. A focal region of cord edema is present in the conus medullaris (*curved arrow*). No other ligamentous injury is demonstrated. (From Flanders AE, Croul SE. Spinal trauma. In: Atlas SW. *Magnetic Resonance Imaging of the Brain and Spine*. 3rd ed. Philadelphia: Lippincott Williams & Wilkins; 2002:1778, with permission.)

from ligament on MRI because both structures exhibit low signal intensity on all pulse sequences (48). Displaced fractures produce concomitant deformity of the involved vertebral body and, if directed posteriorly, compress on the thecal sac. The latter is readily apparent on sagittal images (2). Although identification of a vertebral body or posterior element fracture is not predictive of a neurologic deficit, burst fractures do have a high propensity for associated neurologic deficit (8,16).

MRI is notoriously insensitive to all types of fractures involving the posterior elements (Fig. 8-8) (5,16,24,49–51). This decreased sensitivity is attributed to the smaller size, the complex geometry, and the lower proportion of medullary space of the posterior elements relative to the vertebral bodies. These characteristics are particularly true in the cervical spine (2). Comparison of axial CT and axial GE MRI images shows that MRI has low sensitivity and moderate specificity for posterior element fractures (8,49). Moreover, fractures of C1 and C2 are also extraordinarily difficult to demonstrate on MRI (Fig. 8-15). In an evaluation of 32 patients with cervical spine fractures, MRI was found to have a sensitivity of 36.7% in the detection of anterior column fractures and 11.5% sensitivity for posterior element fractures in comparison to CT (51). The improved sensitivity to anterior column injury was

attributed partly to marrow edema, which served as an indicator of deformity.

MRI is unique, however, in its ability to demonstrate compressive injury to the marrow elements even without evidence of fracture deformity or cortical failure. Compressive injury is manifested by hypointensity of the marrow space within the involved vertebral body on the short TR images and relative hyperintensity on the long TR images (Figs. 8-16, 8-17) (2,8,9,12,52). These signal alterations presumably are the result of microfractures within the medullary bone and resultant hemorrhage. As these signal changes are transient, they can be used as a secondary indicator of an acute osseous injury.

Ligamentous and Joint Disruption

MRI is the only imaging modality available that directly visualizes changes to the ligaments as a result of trauma. The ligamentous structures that are readily identified on routine sagittal MRI of the spine include the anterior longitudinal ligament (ALL), posterior longitudinal ligament (PLL), ligamentum flava (LF), and interspinous ligaments (ISP) (Fig. 8-18). They are relatively avascular structures composed primarily of strong fibroelastic tissue with very short T2 relaxation properties. Therefore, ligaments appear relatively hypointense to other structures on all

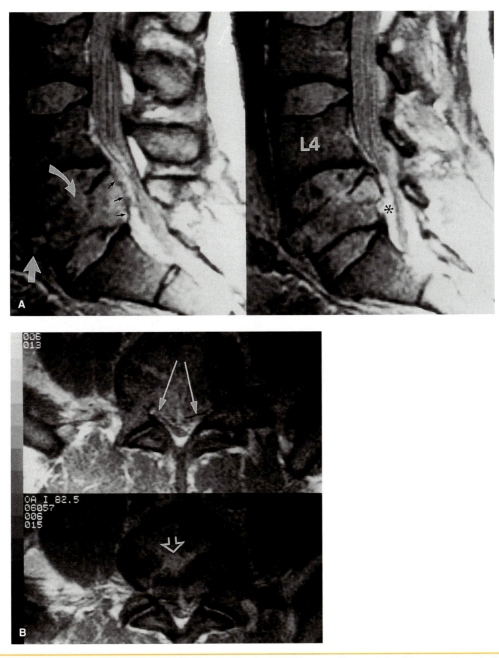

FIGURE 8-12. Cauda equina compression from L5 fracture. **A:** Sagittal FSE intermediate-weighted images. There is diminished height of the L5 vertebral body both anteriorly and posteriorly. Disc material from L4-5 has herniated into the centrum of the L5 vertebral body with interruption of the superior endplate of L5 (*curved arrow*). A fracture fragment is rotated into the prevertebral space (*white arrow*). The posterior cortex is retropulsed into the anterior epidural space (*black arrows*). A small epidural hematoma is incidentally noted (*asterisk*). **B:** Axial FSE intermediate-weighted at the L5 level shows the retropulsed bone fragments compressing the thecal sac. Disc material has herniated through the endplate (*open arrow*). (From Flanders AE, Croul SE. Spinal trauma. In: Atlas SW. *Magnetic Resonance Imaging of the Brain and Spine.* 3rd ed. Philadelphia: Lippincott Williams & Wilkins; 2002:1776–1777, with permission.)

MRI pulse sequences. When overstretched or ruptured, a gap in the ligament may be identified and the surrounding tissues may increase in signal intensity on T2-weighted or GE images because of an increase in free water content from extracellular fluid or adjacent hemorrhage (9,10,16). Because of the similarity in imaging characteristics, dis-

tinction between a ligament fragment and cortical bone fragment may prove difficult on MRI (16,48).

The longitudinal ligaments are solitary, continuous strips of fibroelastic tissue that extend from the skull base to the sacrum. They function to maintain vertebral body alignment and provide elasticity during flexion, extension,

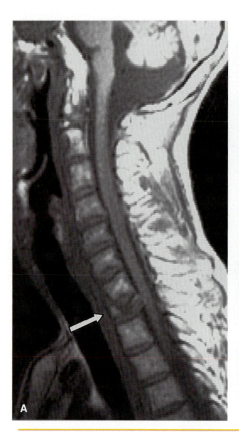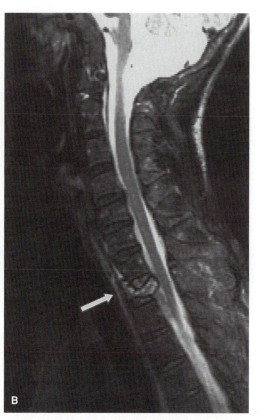

FIGURE 8-13. Burst fracture of T1 without spinal cord injury. **A:** Sagittal T1-weighted image shows collapse of the T1 vertebral body (*arrow*) and diminished signal intensity of the marrow elements. **B:** Sagittal T2-weighted FSE image shows the hyperintense vertebral marrow elements. Note that the posterior cortex encroaches upon the spinal canal; however, there is no damage to the spinal cord. (From Flanders AE, Croul SE. Spinal trauma. In: Atlas SW. *Magnetic Resonance Imaging of the Brain and Spine*. 3rd ed. Philadelphia: Lippincott Williams & Wilkins, 2002:1778, with permission.)

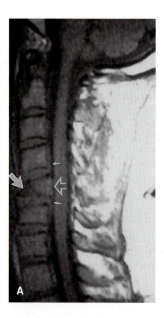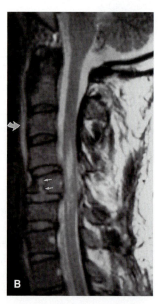

FIGURE 8-14. Flexion teardrop fracture of C5. **A:** Sagittal T1-weighted image shows loss of height of the C5 vertebral body anteriorly (*large arrow*). The marrow signal of the compressed segment is hypointense. The posterior aspect of the vertebral body is retropulsed into the spinal canal (*open arrow*). There is associated elevation of the PLL (*small arrows*) and there is mild swelling of the spinal cord. **B:** Sagittal FSE T2-weighted image depicts the hyperintense vertically oriented fracture line that interrupts the inferior endplate (*small arrows*). A small amount of prevertebral edema is also present (*curved arrow*). There is edema in the spinal cord without a discrete focus of hemorrhage. (Hypointense focus in brainstem is artifactual.) (From Flanders AE, Croul SE. Spinal trauma. In: Atlas SW. *Magnetic Resonance Imaging of the Brain and Spine*. 3rd ed. Philadelphia: Lippincott Williams & Wilkins; 2002:1776, with permission.)

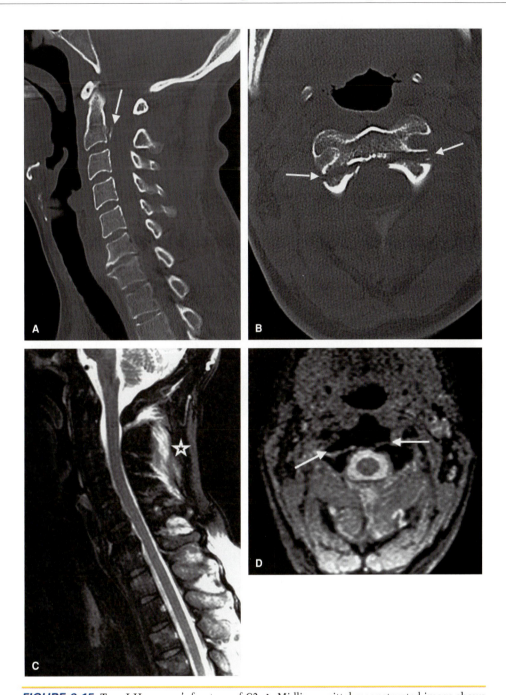

FIGURE 8-15. Type I Hangman's fracture of C2. **A:** Midline sagittal reconstructed image shows avulsion of a cortical fragment dorsal to the C2 vertebral body (*arrow*). **B:** Axial CT image shows a bilateral fracture line extending through the isthmus of C2 (*arrows*). **C:** Midline sagittal T2 weighted MRI shows some signal in the posterior ligamentous complex (*asterisk*) but the fracture fragment is not visible. **D:** Axial gradient echo image at the same level as (B) shows the distracted fracture line through C2 (*arrow*).

and rotation. Failure of either ligament at any spinal level is indicative of spinal instability (Figs. 8-19–8-32). On MRI the ALL is a thin, continuous band of low signal intensity that lies ventral to the anterior cortical surface of the vertebral bodies (53,54,55). The ALL is a critical component of the *anterior column*, which includes the anterior one half of the vertebral body and annulus fibro-

sis. Normally, the ALL may be indiscernible from the cortex or the outer annulus of the intervertebral disc; however, when elevated by fluid, disc, or bone, it may be more apparent (Figs. 8-20–8-22) (55). Portions of the ligament merge with Sharpey fibers at the vertebral endplate and

(text continues on page 204)

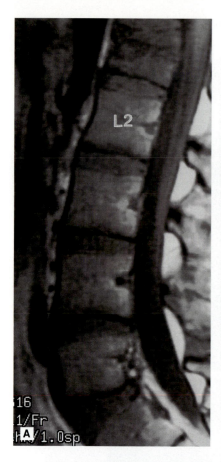
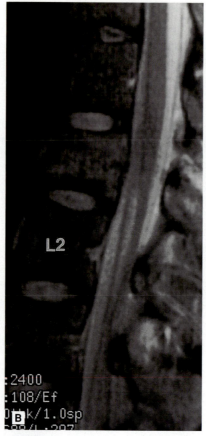

FIGURE 8-16. Compressive injury of the L1 vertebral body marrow. **A:** Sagittal T1-weighted image shows loss of height of the L1 vertebral body secondary to a burst fracture. The signal intensity of the marrow in the upper half of the involved vertebral body is hypointense relative to the other vertebral bodies. **B:** Sagittal FSE T2-weighted image shows that the marrow elements in L1 revert to hyperintensity secondary to compressive injury. Note that there is minimal retropulsion of the posterior aspect of the vertebral body; however, there is no significant compression of the theca. (From Flanders AE, Croul SE. Spinal trauma. In: Atlas SW. *Magnetic Resonance Imaging of the Brain and Spine*. 3rd ed. Philadelphia: Lippincott Williams & Wilkins; 2002:1779, with permission.)

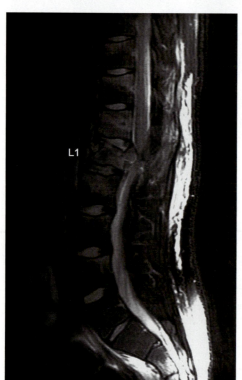

FIGURE 8-17. Burst fracture of L1 with multi-level axial loading injuries. Sagittal FSE T2-weighted image with fat-suppression shows loss of stature of the L1 vertebral body consistent with a burst type fracture. There is rotation of a fracture fragment that compromises the spinal canal. Note the increased signal in the endplates of the adjacent vertebral bodies of T10-12 and L2-4 indicative of compressive marrow injury.

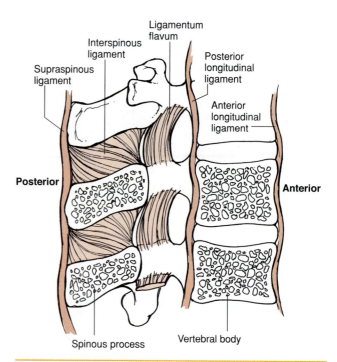

FIGURE 8-18. Diagrammatic representation of the ligamentous structures in the spine. (From Oatis CA. *Kinesiology—The Mechanics and Pathomechanics of Human Movement*. Baltimore: Lippincott Williams & Wilkins; 2004, with permission.)

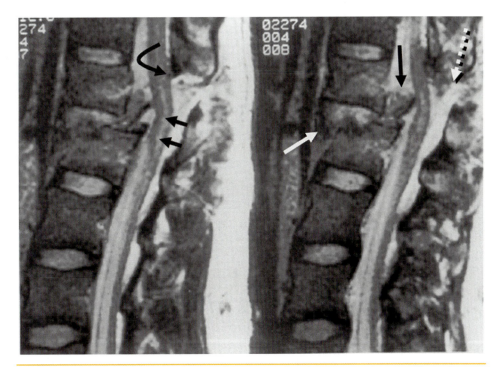

FIGURE 8-19. Fracture dislocation at T12-L1. Sagittal FSE T2-weighted images show the associated soft tissue components to this injury. The ALL is torn at the L1 level (*white arrow*). The free end of the ruptured LF is demonstrated (*curved black arrow*). The PLL is disrupted and a portion of the attached bone fragment that has rotated into the spinal canal (*black arrow*) is displacing the conus medullaris. A small region of edema is noted within the spinal cord (*small black arrows*). The interspinous and supraspinous ligaments are also disrupted (*dotted white arrow*).

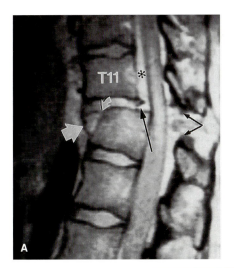
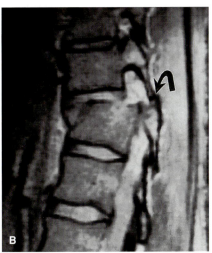
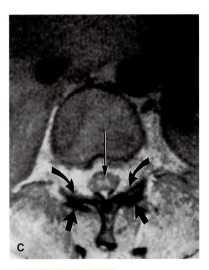

FIGURE 8-20. Fracture dislocation at T11-12 with locked facets. **A:** Sagittal intermediate weighted FSE image shows subluxation and angulation at T11-12. There is a fracture deformity of the T12 vertebral body. The disc at T11-12 is damaged with interruption of the annulus anteriorly (*curved white arrow*) and posteriorly (*long black arrow*). There is an anterior disc herniation that appears contained by the ALL (*large white arrow*). The LF is ruptured (*black arrows*). A hematoma is present in the ventral epidural space (*asterisk*) that extends cephalad from the disc injury. **B:** Parasagittal intermediate-weighted FSE image shows the right inferior facet of T11 dislocated anterior to the superior facet of T12 (*curved arrow*). The same finding was present on the left side. **C:** Axial intermediate-weighted FSE image of T11 demonstrates the abnormal relationship of the facet joints. The inferior facet surfaces (*curved arrows*) are displaced anterior to the superior facet surfaces (*arrows*). Note the edema in the central gray matter of the spinal cord (*long arrow*). (From Flanders AE, Croul SE. Spinal trauma. In: Atlas SW. *Magnetic Resonance Imaging of the Brain and Spine.* 3rd ed. Philadelphia: Lippincott Williams & Wilkins; 2002:1781, with permission.)

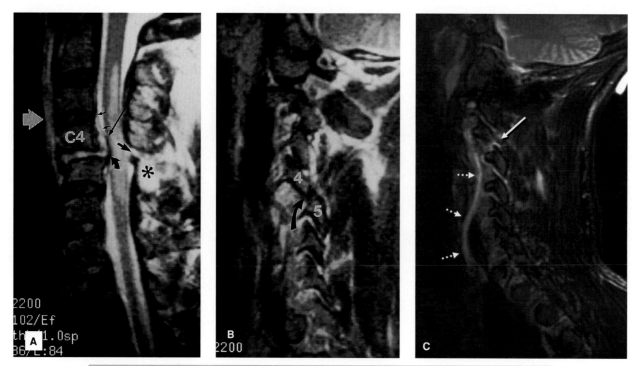

FIGURE 8-21. Flexion-rotation injury at C4-5. **A:** Sagittal FSE T2-weighted image. The body of C4 is subluxed relative to C5. A moderate-sized disc herniation (*curved black arrow*) has impacted on the swollen and edematous spinal cord. No blood products are identified in the spinal cord. Note the separation of the PLL from the midportion of the C4 body (*long black arrow*). The ventral dura margin is represented by a thin hypointense line (*small black arrows*). There is associated disruption of the ligamentum flavum (*black arrow*) and the interspinous ligaments (*asterisk*). Prevertebral edema is also present (*white arrow*). **B:** Right parasagittal image (same sequence as A). The right C4 inferior facet is jumped and locked in front of the C5 superior facet (*arrow*). **C:** Unilateral facet dislocation at C3-4 in another patient. There is increased fluid within the joint capsule in the subluxed facet joint (*white arrow*). Note the incidental thrombosed right vertebral artery (*dotted arrows*). (Figure 8-21A,B from Flanders AE, Croul SE. Spinal trauma. In: Atlas SW. *Magnetic Resonance Imaging of the Brain and Spine.* 3rd ed. Philadelphia: Lippincott Williams & Wilkins; 2002:1781, with permission.)

with the outer annular fibers. The ALL may rupture as the result of hyperextension injury (Figs. 8-27, 8-28) (17,53,56,57,58). This is seen on all pulse sequences as a focal discontinuity of the hypointense band that is adherent to the ventral aspect of the vertebral bodies (Figs. 8-22–8-24). This finding may be associated with an avulsion of the vertebral endplate (Figs. 8-22–8-24) or hemorrhage in the prevertebral musculature (17,53,57,58). The accumulation of hemorrhage and fluid in the prevertebral space is seen on T2-weighted or GE sequences as a crescent-shaped mass of high signal intensity centered over the segment of injured ligament (Figs. 8-21–8-25) (14,24,53).

Unlike the ALL, the PLL is much more variable in width. The PLL is widest at the level of the intervertebral disc and thinner as it passes behind the vertebral bodies (54). Therefore, the PLL may normally appear discontinuous on sagittal MRI images (14). The PLL is represented on MRI as a thin, hypointense band that is interposed between the ventral dural sac and the posterior margin of the vertebral bodies and intervertebral discs. The PLL is the principal ligament of the *middle column*, which includes the posterior one half of the vertebral body and the annulus fibrosis. The PLL is best visualized on T2-weighted and intermediate-weighted sagittal images; however, the PLL is often impossible to resolve as a separate structure from the ventral dura or annulus on midsagittal images. The PLL is better delineated when elevated away from the posterior cortex by a herniated disc or posttraumatic fluid collection (Figs. 8-19–8-22, 8-24–8-26, 8-29). As with the ALL, rupture of the PLL is identified as a focal region of discontinuity. Typically, rupture of the PLL occurs in hyperflexion and hyperextension type injuries.

The LF forms a continuous strip of fibroelastic tissue that bridges adjacent lamina. Along with the ISP, they act as check ligaments to oppose hyperflexion and distraction of the posterior elements and maintain alignment. They

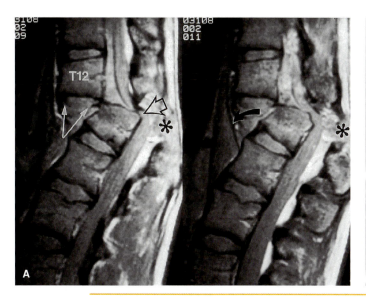
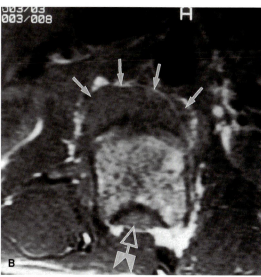

FIGURE 8-22. Complete dislocation at T12-L1. **A:** Sagittal intermediate-weighted FSE image. The body of T12 is dislocated relative to L1. The T12-L1 disc is avulsed and free edges of the annular fibers are demonstrated (*white arrows*). The PLL is discontinuous. The posterior ligamentous complex is disrupted (*asterisk*). The spinal cord is markedly distorted and compressed at the level of the dislocation (*open arrow*). Hematoma is present in the anterior epidural space. The ALL is stretched over the dislocated segments (*curved black arrow*). **B:** Axial T1-weighted image shows the avulsed disc (*arrows*) displaced anteriorly to the L1 vertebral body. The spinal cord (*open arrow*) is draped over the vertebral body. Note the absence of the posterior elements. (From Flanders AE, Croul SE. Spinal trauma. In: Atlas SW. *Magnetic Resonance Imaging of the Brain and Spine*. 3rd ed. Philadelphia: Lippincott Williams & Wilkins; 2002:1782, with permission.)

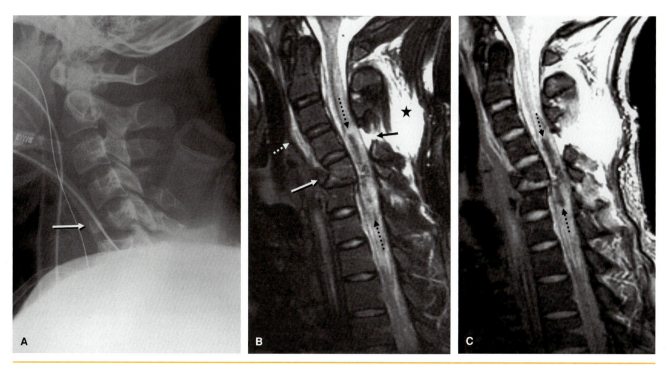

FIGURE 8-23. Flexion teardrop fracture of C5 with severe SCI. **A:** Lateral radiograph shows the typical teardrop configuration of the C5 vertebral body (*arrow*) in which a large anterior bone fragment is disassociated from the vertebral body from combined axial loading and flexion. **B:** Sagittal FSE T2-weighted image shows a flexion teardrop fracture of the C5 vertebral body with avulsion of a fragment ventrally (*white arrow*). There is prevertebral soft tissue swelling (*dotted white arrow*). The ligamentum flavum (LF) and posterior ligamentous complex is ruptured (*small black arrow*) and the posterior musculature is edematous (*asterisk*). An extensive intramedullary hemorrhage is present (*dotted black arrows*). **C:** Sagittal gradient echo image shows the extensive hypointense intramedullary hemorrhage (*dotted black arrows*).

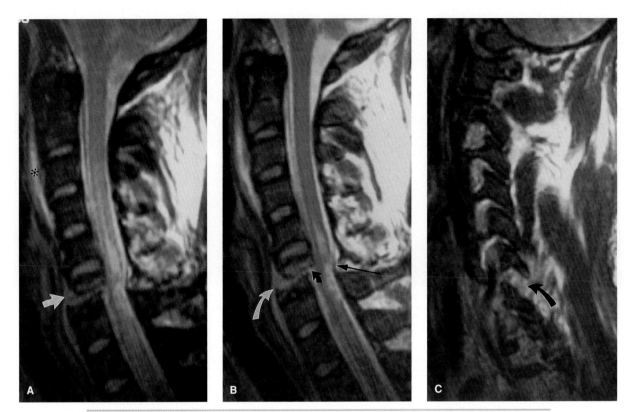

FIGURE 8-24. Fracture dislocation at C6 in a 29-year-old man. **A:** Sagittal T2-weighted image reveals a horizontal fracture line that extends through the C6 vertebral body (*arrow*). There is off-set of the upper segment relative to the lower segment. Spinal cord edema is present, extending the length of three vertebral segments. There is a mound of prevertebral soft tissue swelling/hemorrhage (*asterisk*). **B:** Sagittal FSE T2-weighted image shows the details of the injury with better clarity than the SE image. There is disruption of the ALL (*curved white arrow*), the PLL (*curved black arrow*), and the LF (*straight black arrow*). Note that the borders defining the spinal cord edema are better defined than in (A). **C:** Parasagittal FSE T2-weighted image shows distraction of the C6 and C7 facet joints on the right (*curved arrow*). (From Flanders AE, Croul SE. Spinal trauma. In: Atlas SW. *Magnetic Resonance Imaging of the Brain and Spine.* 3rd ed. Philadelphia: Lippincott Williams & Wilkins; 2002:1783, with permission.)

are the principal ligaments of the *posterior column*, which includes all of the posterior elements. Normally, the LF are small structures (especially in the cervical and thoracic regions), which are oriented parallel to the adjacent lamina. Focal discontinuity of the LF can be identified on the parasagittal MRI (Figs. 8-30–8-32). The LF may enlarge either on a degenerative basis or physiologically by bulging into the spinal canal in hyperextension. LF rupture is often associated with fractures of the posterior elements. The injured LF can be easier to visualize when the damaged segment projects into the spinal canal and distorts the posterolateral aspect of the thecal sac. This finding is best seen on parasagittal and axial images (Figs. 8-19–8-21, 8-23–8-26, 8-29–8-32).

Disruption of the ISP is best appreciated on the fat-suppressed midsagittal T2-weighted views. Fat suppression is essential for the detection of the typical high signal intensity in the tissues interposed between the widened spinous processes (Figs. 8-19, 8-21, 8-31, 8-33) (16). The

supraspinous ligament forms a long contiguous band connecting the tips of the adjacent spinous processes and also serves as a posterior tension band that resists hyperflexion. The ruptured free edge of this structure may be visible within the edematous posterior paraspinal soft tissues (Fig. 8-19).

The facet joint complexes are easily identified on sagittal and axial images, particularly in the cervical and lumbar region where the structures are somewhat larger in size and the joint plane is oriented in the sagittal direction. In the thoracic spine, the facet joints are small in size and the joint is oriented in the coronal plane.

The facet joint complex is a dynamic structure that permits limited compression and distraction of the posterior elements during extension and flexion while resisting rotation and translation. Although fractures that involve the facet surfaces are better detected with tomography and CT, subtle damage to the synovial capsule and cartilaginous surface of the joint is best appreciated

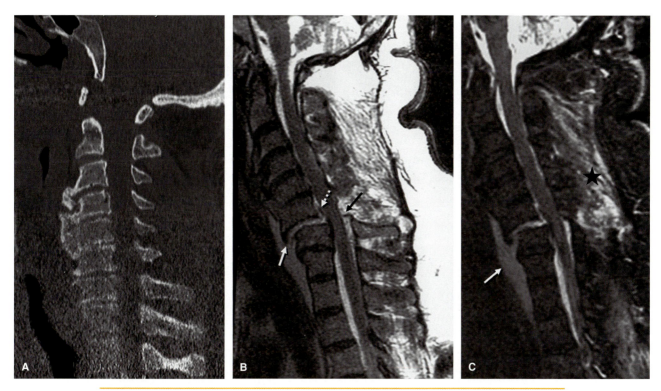

FIGURE 8-25. Multicolumn ligamentous disruptions and spinal instability. **A:** Sagittal reformatted image from multidetector CT study is limited by artifact. There are extensive degenerative changes noted but no gross evidence of malalignment. **B:** Sagittal T2-weighted image shows a previously unsuspected instability with anterior angulation deformity at C6-7 and subluxation. The ALL (*white arrow*), LF (*black arrow*), and PLL (*dotted arrow*) are disrupted. There is widening of the interspinous distance. Note that none of these findings are evident on the CT image. **C:** Sagittal STIR (fat-suppressed inversion recovery sequence) shows the edema in the posterior paraspinal soft tissues (*asterisk*), which is not clearly depicted in the nonfat-suppressed sequence in (B). Note that the damaged intervertebral disc is hyperintense. A prevertebral hematomas is also noted (*white arrow*). (Images courtesy of Eric D. Schwartz MD, Hospital of the University of Pennsylvania.)

with MRI. The facets are demonstrated on the far left and right parasagittal images of a well-centered sagittal sequence. The articular surface of the superior facet normally maintains close apposition to the inferior facet surface. Widening of this space is suggestive of a distraction injury (Fig. 8-24). The imaging criteria of altered facet alignment or subluxation are similar to the plain film appearance (Figs. 8-20, 8-21, 8-24, 8-29, 8-33, 8-34). Increased fluid within the joint space is suggested by a well-demarcated hyperintense focus interposed between the articular surfaces on T2-weighted and GE images (Fig. 8-21). The increased fluid is contained within the joint space and joint capsule.

Disc Injury

The identification and classification of a traumatic disc injury are important factors in determining the timing of and type of surgical decompression and stabilization

(59,60). Although posttraumatic disc herniation does not correlate with the degree of associated injuries or neurologic deficit, unrecognized disc herniation is a cause of neurologic deterioration after stabilization (8,59,61). Formerly, myelography, noncontrast CT, and CT myelography played an important role in determining whether extruded disc material compromised the epidural space and the thecal sac. Noncontrast CT is relatively insensitive to disc herniation as compared to MRI; however, the high resolution and isotropic data sets produced with MDCT often routinely depict disc herniations and the soft tissue contents of the spinal canal (8,10,49).

Although degenerative disc herniations are probably more common in the lumbar spine, posttraumatic disc herniations are encountered more frequently in the cervical and thoracic regions (17,53,59). In the cervical region, disc herniations most commonly occur at the C4-7 levels (8,62). The incidence of posttraumatic thoracic

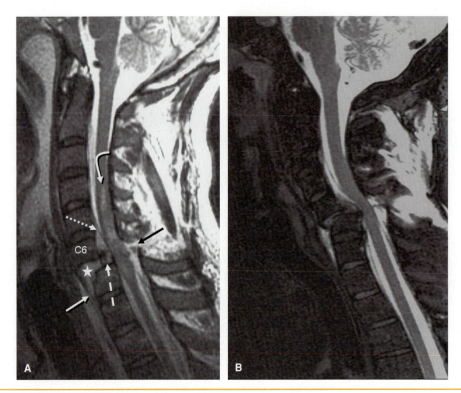

FIGURE 8-26. Multicolumn ligamentous disruption secondary to a bilateral interfacetal dislocation (BID) with and without SCI. **A:** Sagittal T2-weighted MRI shows the marked anterior subluxation of C6 relative to C7. The C6-7 intervertebral disc is macerated (*asterisk*) and a portion of it is herniated anteriorly likely intermixed with hemorrhage. A portion of the disc is herniated posteriorly (*dashed white arrow*). The anterior-superior corner of C7 is fragmented. The anterior longitudinal ligament (ALL) is distorted and stretched (*white arrow*) and is peeled off the anterior cortex. The posterior longitudinal ligament (PLL) is also stretched and pulled away from the posterior cortical margin (*dotted white arrow*). The ligamentum flavum (LF) is ruptured (*black arrow*). A sizable spinal cord injury is present spanning from C4 to C7 comprised primarily of swelling and edema (*curved white arrow*). **B:** Sagittal T2-weighted MRI using fat supression in another patient with a BID type injury and complete ligamentous disruption and the anterior and posterior columns. Note that the spinal cord shows no intrinsic signal abnormality and this patient was neurologically intact.

disc herniations are more common than previously estimated; they occur in up to 50% of thoracic injuries (59). When only single detector CT and CTM, were available, for the evaluation of spine trauma, cervical disc herniations were estimated to occur in only 3% to 9% of all cervical spine injuries. In addition, a large number of false-positive cervical disc herniations were reported using CT and myelography alone (59). With the routine use of MRI, the reported incidence of cervical disc herniation is reported as high as 54% (8,60–62). Cervical disc herniations were associated with 80% of bilateral facet dislocations, 60% of hyperextension injuries, 47% of central cord injuries, and all cases of anterior cord syndromes (60). Twenty-two percent of neurologically normal patients demonstrated disc herniations on MRI (62). Cervical disc herniation is reported to occur more frequently in flexion-distraction and flexion-compression–type injuries (63). The existence of thecal sac compression by herniated disc mate-

rial is a significant factor in determining whether a discectomy should be performed at the time of surgical stabilization (60,63). In addition, residual spinal cord compression from a posttraumatic disc herniation is associated with more severe neurologic injuries than disc herniation without cord compression (8,64,65). However, in a study by Dai and Jai (60), the authors found no significant relationship between neurologic deficit or neurologic recovery rate and severity of spinal cord compression by herniated disc material. Nevertheless, the authors concluded that surgical management is advised when residual spinal cord compression is demonstrated on MRI.

Posttraumatic disc changes on MRI can be classified as either disc injury or disc herniation. Normally, the well-hydrated intervertebral disc is hypointense relative to bone marrow on T1-weighted images and intermediate in signal on T2-weighted FSE images. The nondegenerated disc is uniform and symmetric in height, and

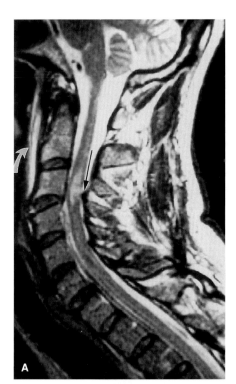
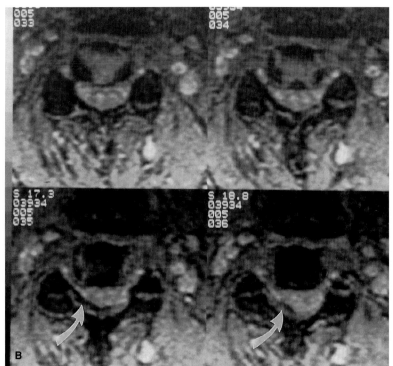

FIGURE 8-27. Hyperextension strain injury at C3-4. **A:** Sagittal FSE T2-weighted image shows anterior widening of the C3-4 disc space and an associated prevertebral hematoma (*curved arrow*). There is buckling of the LF (*arrow*). A discrete area of spinal cord edema is also present. **B:** Axial GE axial images show deformity of the right posterolateral aspect of the thecal sac by the buckled LF. The spinal cord was compressed between the vertebral body anteriorly and the LF posteriorly. (From Flanders AE, Croul SE. Spinal trauma. In: Atlas SW. *Magnetic Resonance Imaging of the Brain and Spine.* 3rd ed. Philadelphia: Lippincott Williams & Wilkins; 2002:1784, with permission.)

the peripheral fibers of the annulus fibrosus merge imperceptibly with the longitudinal ligaments. *Disc injury* is implied whenever there is asymmetric narrowing or widening of an isolated disc space on sagittal images and focal hyperintensity of the disc material on T2-weighted images. The injured disc is often higher in signal intensity than the adjacent discs on T2-weighted images, and the level of injury is usually contiguous with other damaged tissues (Figs. 8-21, 8-25, 8-28, 8-33). The observed signal changes in the disc may be the result of tearing of the disc substance during hyperflexion, hyperextension, or subluxation (8,14,53). As the adult intervertebral disc is an avascular structure, the observed, potentially hemorrhagic MR signal changes of a damaged disc may therefore be, in part, due to damage to the adjacent endplates. The signal changes of the injured disc may be easier to identify in patients with hypointense discs from pre-existing degenerative disc disease (Fig. 8-28).

An acute, posttraumatic disc herniation has a similar MRI appearance to nontraumatic disc herniation. The nucleus pulposus is forced under pressure to extrude into the peripheral annulus fibrosus and, in some instances, extend beyond the outer annulus into the anterior epidural space. The herniation may be broad-based or eccentric and may or may not be associated with a vertebral body fracture. On a sagittal MRI, the disc herniation is isointense and contiguous with the disc of origin (2,8,10,12,14,18). A small herniated disc fragment often appears as a focal area of expansion of the annulus beyond the border of the posterior cortical margin (Figs. 8-21, 8-29, 8-35, 8-36). Occasionally, a small rent in the annulus may appear that allows passage of nuclear material into the epidural space. On axial images, the herniated disc produces focal distortion of the ventral theca (Fig. 8-35). Depending on the size and location of the disc herniation, the fragment may be demonstrated on multiple sagittal and axial images.

The degree of compressive injury to the neural elements depends on the size of the herniated fragment, the width of the spinal canal at the level of injury, and the

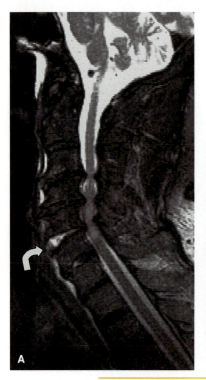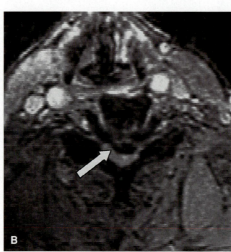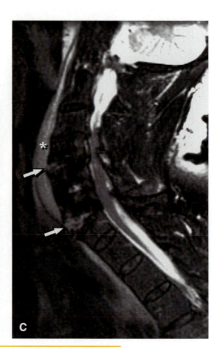

FIGURE 8-28. Extension mechanism injury at C5-6. **A:** Sagittal FSE T2-weighted image shows changes of multi-level degenerative cervical spondylosis and stenosis spanning C3-6. There is acute widening of the anterior aspect of the C5-6 disc space (*curved arrow*) and the disc material is hyperintense secondary to injury. Spinal cord edema is also present. **B:** Axial GE axial image obtained through the C5-6 interspace shows the retropulsed spondylotic disc fragment (*arrow*) compressing the thecal sac. **C:** Sagittal T2 weighted image in a different patient shows extension type injury at two distinct levels (C4-5 and C6-7). Note the anterior widening of the interspaces with increased signal in the damaged discs (*arrows*). There is a large prevertebral hematoma (*asterisk*). (Figure 8-28A,B from Flanders AE, Croul SE. Spinal trauma. In: Atlas SW. *Magnetic Resonance Imaging of the Brain and Spine*. 3rd ed. Philadelphia: Lippincott Williams & Wilkins; 2002:1784, with permission.)

diameter of the spinal cord. For example, a small disc herniation in the thoracic region may cause more neural impingement than an identical fragment would cause in the lumbar or cervical regions (66).

Identification of an acute disc herniation can be difficult in the setting of superimposed degenerative spondylotic changes (17). In such instances, multiple chronic spondylotic disc herniations associated with osteophytes may complicate the correct identification of an acute traumatic disc herniation (24). Imaging factors that may aid in the identification of an acute disc herniation with superimposed spondylosis include alteration in signal of the disc material at one level, asymmetric width of the intervertebral disc space, subluxation, and associated injuries at the same level (Fig. 8-28). In some circumstances, definitive identification may be impossible.

Epidural Hematoma

The incidence of asymptomatic posttraumatic spinal epidural hematomas is greater than was previously recognized (16). They have been reported to occur in up to 41% of spine injuries (16). Spinal epidural hematomas occur as the result of tearing of a portion of the epidural venous plexus with focal extravasation of blood into the anterior epidural space. Most epidural hematomas from closed trauma are found in association with other injuries, are relatively small in size, and are probably not clinically significant (14). Since the spinal dura is not firmly adherent to the vertebral canal, relatively large epidural hematomas may remain clinically silent because they extend over multiple levels and therefore do not result in substantial compromise to the thecal sac and contents. The imaging characteristics of epidural

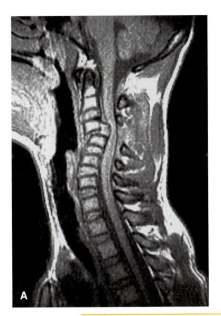 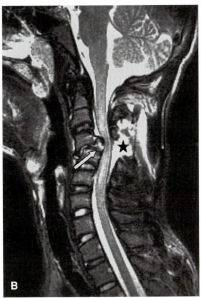 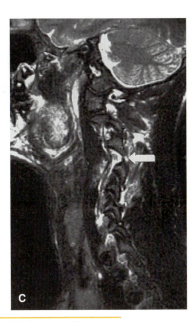

FIGURE 8-29. Hyperflexion mechanism injury at C3-4 in a 15-year-old male following a wrestling injury. **A:** Sagittal T1-weighted image shows acute angulation of C3 on C4 with spinal cord compression. **B:** Sagittal T2-weighted FSE image shows a large herniated disc fragment (*arrow*) compressing the spinal cord with the free edge of the ruptured PLL adjacent to the disc fragment. The posterior elements are splayed apart and there is rupture of the interspinous ligaments and ligamentum flavum (*asterisk*). Spinal cord edema is present from C2 to C5. **C:** Parasagittal T2-weighted FSE image shows a perched C3-4 facet complex (*arrow*). (From Flanders AE, Croul SE. Spinal trauma. In: Atlas SW. *Magnetic Resonance Imaging of the Brain and Spine*. 3rd ed. Philadelphia: Lippincott Williams & Wilkins; 2002:1780, with permission.)

FIGURE 8-30. Hyperflexion injury associated with ligamentum flavum and posterior ligamentous complex rupture. **A:** Sagittal intermediate weighted image shows discontinuity of the ligamentum flavum at the C6-7 level (*arrow*). **B:** Sagittal T2-weighted image with fat suppression shows the discontinuity of the LF (*arrow*) and edema in the posterior paraspinal musculature (*asterisk*).

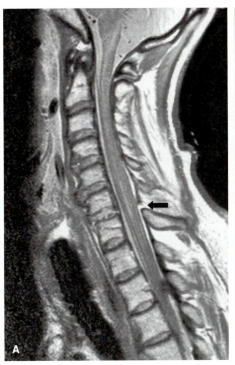 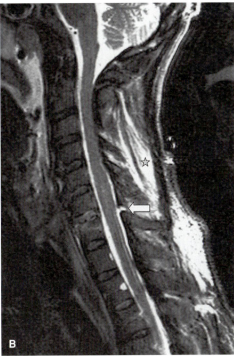

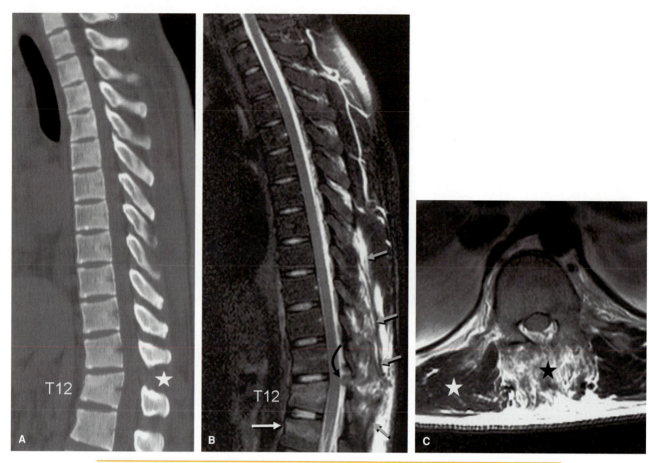

FIGURE 8-31. Isolated rupture of the posterior ligamentous complex (PLC) at the thoraco-lumbar junction. **A:** Sagittal MPR CT image of the thoracic spine shows a wedge deformity of the T12 vertebral body. There is widening of the interspinous distance at T11-12. Note that the posterior cortex of T12 is intact indicating no failure of the middle column. **B:** Sagittal T2-weighted image of the thoracic spine with fat suppression shows marrow edema in the T12 segment as well as in the adjacent L1 body (*white arrow*). The ligamentum flavum (LF) is disrupted (*curved black arrow*) and there is extensive soft tissue injury in the posterior paraspinal soft tissues (*gray arrows*). **C:** Axial T2-weighted image at the T12 level shows the high signal intensity in the posterior paraspinal soft tissue indicative of edema/hemorrhage (*black asterisk*) compared to the normal adjacent paraspinal muscles (*white asterisk*).

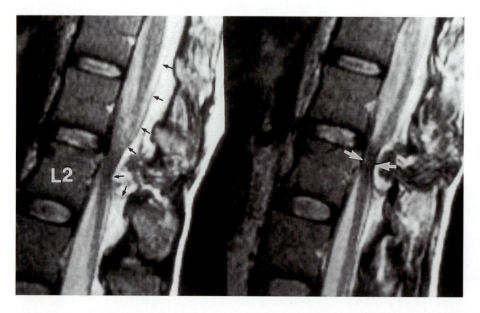

FIGURE 8-32. Dorsal epidural hematoma from ligamentum flavum rupture. Sagittal fast spin echo (FSE) T2-weighted images. A large dorsal epidural hematoma is displacing the posterior margin of the dura (*small black arrows*). The hematoma is heterogeneous with both hypointense and hyperintense components. The hematoma likely originates at the site of rupture of the ligamentum flavum at the L2 level. The roots of the cauda equina are compressed against the vertebral body by the hematoma (*white arrows*). (From Flanders AE, Croul SE. Spinal trauma. In: Atlas SW. *Magnetic Resonance Imaging of the Brain and Spine*. 3rd ed. Philadelphia: Lippincott Williams & Wilkins; 2002:1786, with permission.)

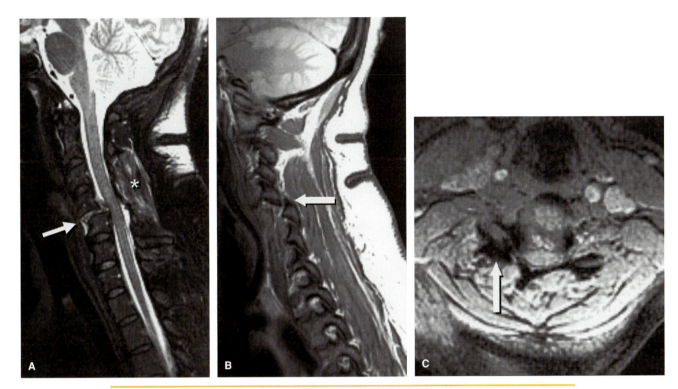

FIGURE 8-33. Unilateral interfacetal dislocation at C4-5. **A:** Sagittal T2-weighted FSE image with fat suppression shows anterior subluxation of C4 on C5 with disc disruption and anterior herniation of disc material (*arrow*). Note the edema in the posterior paraspinal musculature (*asterisk*) related to the rotational component of the injury. **B:** Right parasagittal intermediate weighted image shows the abnormal orientation of the C4 inferior articular process located anterior and inferior to the C5 superior articular process (*arrow*). **C:** Gradient echo axial image obtain through the C4-5 disc space shows the abnormal morphology of the right facet joint (*arrow*) compared to the left.

hematomas are variable as they depend on the oxidative state of the hemorrhage and the effects of clot retraction (Figs. 8-12, 8-20, 8-32, 8-35, 8-37–8-40) (50,67,68). In the acute phase, the epidural hematoma is isointense with spinal cord parenchyma on T1-weighted images and isointense with CSF on intermediate- and T2-weighted sequences (2). The epidural collection may be difficult to distinguish from the adjacent CSF in the subarachnoid space (Fig. 8-35). This distinction can often be made by the hypointense dura, which separates the two compartments (Figs. 8-35, 8-38, 8-40). The reported incidence of posttraumatic epidural hematoma in patients with ankylosing spondylitis (AS) is greater than in the general population, ranging from 10% to 50% (Fig. 8-40) (69). Traumatic epidural hematomas in the AS population are frequently larger and occur more often in the posterior epidural space compared to the general population.

Vascular Injury

The true incidence of associated posttraumatic dissection or thrombosis of the extracranial carotid and verte-bral arteries following cervical spine injury is unknown because the vascular injury often remains clinically occult. Prior investigations have suggested that damage to the vertebral arteries can be demonstrated angiographically in up to 40% of patients following cervical subluxation/dislocation (70). Dissection of the vertebral artery is more frequent than carotid artery dissection following fracture/subluxation because a portion of the cervical vertebral artery is contained within the foramen transversarium. A fracture that extends through the foramen transversarium may compress the ipsilateral vertebral artery. Because the artery is fixed within the foramen, it may also be subject to severe stretching and torsional forces from cervical subluxation (Figs. 8-21C, 8-41–8-43) (71–75).

Early recognition of vertebral artery injury remains important because of its potential to produce significant neurologic comorbidity and permanent neurologic damage. Moreover, the secondary injury is potentially preventable with early institution of therapy (e.g., anticoagulation, embolization, or surgical ligation) (72). The incidence of isolated vertebral artery injury in the setting of cervical

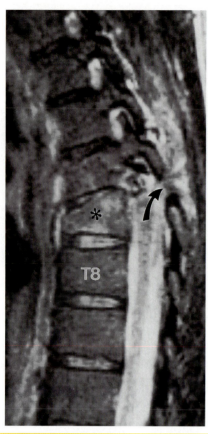

FIGURE 8-34. Interfacetal dislocation. Sagittal fast spin echo (FSE) T2-weighted image. There is fracture deformity of the T7 vertebral body with loss of height anteriorly. The marrow signal of T7 is hyperintense secondary to compressive injury (*asterisk*). The right T6-7 facet joint is disrupted (*curved arrow*). (From Flanders AE, Croul SE. Spinal trauma. In: Atlas SW. *Magnetic Resonance Imaging of the Brain and Spine*. 3rd ed. Philadelphia: Lippincott Williams & Wilkins; 2002:1786, with permission.)

spine trauma is not well known because the patient is frequently asymptomatic at the time of injury (73).

In a prospective study of 47 cervical spine trauma patients, Parbhoo et al. (73) reported that 26% (n = 12) of the patients showed vertebral artery damage on MRI/MRA; in nine patients (19%), the vertebral artery was thrombosed. Most of the patients with vertebral artery injury (n = 10) had an associated unilateral facet dislocation (73).

Willis et al. (74) prospectively selected 26 patients with bony injuries associated with vertebral artery injury and found vertebral artery thrombosis (VAT) in nine patients (35%), normal vertebral arteries in 14 patients (54%), and dissection in three patients (11%) by using angiography; SCI was present in half of the patients, and no neurologic sequelae were attributed to the arterial injuries.

In another prospective MRI/MRA study, Friedman et al. (75) identified VAT in 9 (24%) of 37 consecutive cervical SCI patients. VAT was significantly more common in the motor-complete SCI patients than in the motor-incomplete patients.

Using cerebral arteriography, Biffl et al. (76) found 47 vertebral artery injuries in 38 patients in a selected cohort derived from 7,205 consecutive patients (0.53%) admitted with blunt trauma to a single level-I trauma center; 350 patients were selected for cerebral arteriography on the basis of mechanism of injury or the existence of acute cerebrovascular symptoms. The most frequent related injuries associated with vertebral injury included spine fracture/dislocation (71%), followed by chest and extremity injury (45%). The actual frequency of VAT in the subgroup evaluated with angiography was 2.6%. These authors found no relationship between grade of vertebral artery injury, neurologic deficit, or neurologic outcome (76).

Other investigators have shown a higher incidence of vertebral artery thrombosis on cerebral arteriography when selecting for patients with specific types of cervical injuries, such as facet joint dislocations (75%; unilateral or bilateral) and foramen transversarium fractures (88%) (3,4). The frequency of VAT was lower overall for similar studies that used MRA as the imaging technique: 33% for patients with foramen transversarium fractures and as high as 24% for multiple contiguous cervical spinal injuries (4,12,16).

There is some disparity in the literature whether the severity of neurologic deficit has a relationship to the frequency of VAT. Giacobetti et al. (77) prospectively reviewed MRA examinations of 61 consecutive cervical spine injuries, finding VAT in 12 (19.7%). Twenty-eight of the 61 patients sustained some form of SCI. The frequency of VAT stratified by American Spinal Injury Association (ASIA) impairment scale included ASIA A (n = 3), ASIA B (n = 3), ASIA D (n = 2), and ASIA E (n = 4). This suggested that the severity of neurologic injury was not predictive of VAT. No permanent neurologic deficits related to the VAT were identified (77). Six of the patients were reimaged by MRA 12 to 26 months after injury. The vertebral arteries in five patients remained thrombosed on the subsequent MRA study (78).

In the largest retrospective review, which evaluated the association of VAT with severity of spinal cord injury, Torina et al. (79) assessed the vertebral arteries of 632 patients with nonpenetrating injuries using MRA/MRI. Eighty-three (13%) patients had VAT on the admission MRI/MRA. Fifty-nine percent (49/83) of VAT patients had an associated SCI. VAT was significantly more common in motor-complete patients (ASIA A and B, 20%) than in neurologically intact (ASIA E, 11%) cervical spine–injured patients (p = .019). VAT incidence was not significantly different between motor-incomplete (ASIA C and D, 10%) and neurologically intact (ASIA E, 11%) cervical spine–injured patients (p = .840). They concluded that the absence of neurologic symptoms from the SCI does not preclude VAT (Fig. 8-41). Therefore, MRA evaluation is warranted as part of the routine MRI evaluation of cervical injuries.

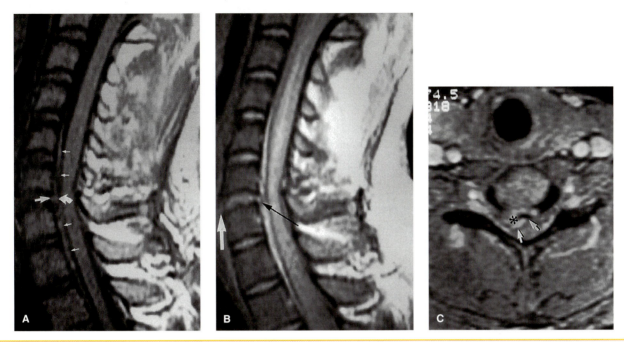

FIGURE 8-35. Traumatic disc herniation with epidural hematoma. **A:** Sagittal SE T1-weighted image shows interruption of the posterior annulus at the C6-7 level (*white arrow*). A mound of tissue projects behind and above the disc space (*curved arrow*) representing herniated material bounded by the elevated PLL. The associated epidural hematoma (*small arrows*) is minimally hyperintense. Also note the marked swelling of the spinal cord. **B:** Sagittal SE image shows that the epidural fluid collection is hyperintense. The margins around the herniated disc are better demonstrated (*black arrow*). Note the associated interruption of the ALL (*white arrow*). **C:** Axial 3DFT GE image in another patient shows a large extruded disc fragment (*asterisk*) that is compressing the right anterior margin of the thecal sac (*arrows*). (From Flanders AE, Croul SE. Spinal trauma. In: Atlas SW. *Magnetic Resonance Imaging of the Brain and Spine.* 3rd ed. Philadelphia: Lippincott Williams & Wilkins; 2002:1787, with permission.)

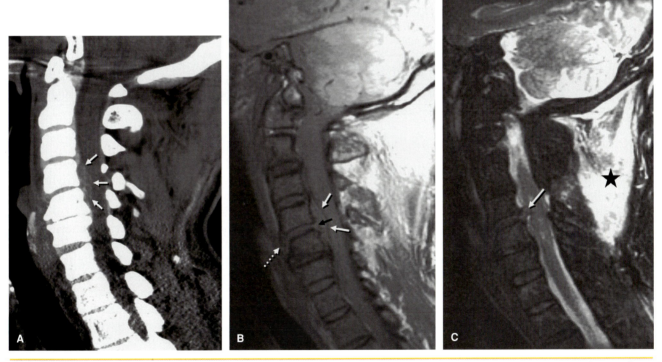

FIGURE 8-36. Large posttraumatic disc herniation with epidural hematoma. **A:** Sagittal CT MPR image shows a hyperdense soft tissue mound extending into the spinal canal and compromising the anterior epidural space (*arrows*). **B:** Sagittal intermediate weighted MRI shows discontinuity of the posterior annulus at C4-5 (*black arrow*) and a epidural tissue mound spanning the C4 and C5 vertebral bodies which compromises the spinal canal (*white arrows*). Note that disc material cannot be distinguished from hematoma. **C:** Off-midline sagittal T2 weighted MRI with fat suppression shows the herniated disc fragment that is not discernable on the other images. The remainder of the mound of tissue represents a combination of epidural hemorrhage and congested epidural venous plexus. Also note the complete disruption of the posterior paraspinal soft tissues (*asterisk*).

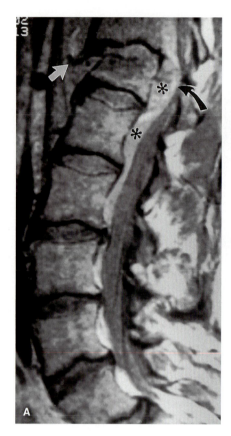

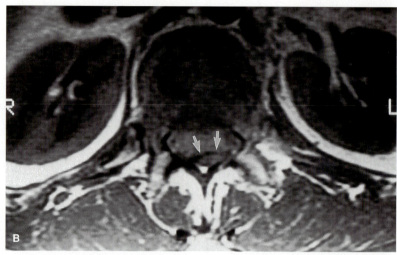

FIGURE 8-37. Large epidural hematoma. **A:** Sagittal FSE intermediate weighted image. There is a fracture of the T12 vertebral body with resultant kyphosis deformity of the spine. The ALL is ruptured at the T12 level (*white arrow*). A large hyperintense fluid collection is present in the ventral epidural space that extends caudally to approximately the L3 level (*asterisks*). There is marked compression of the thecal sac (*curved arrow*). **B:** Axial T1-weighted image. The epidural hemorrhage is forcing the thecal sac dorsally and causing severe compression of the conus medullaris (*arrows*). (From Flanders AE, Croul SE. Spinal trauma. In: Atlas SW. *Magnetic Resonance Imaging of the Brain and Spine*. 3rd ed. Philadelphia: Lippincott Williams & Wilkins; 2002:1785, with permission.)

The clinical significance of occult vertebral artery injury is not known; however, in some series the stroke rate has been as high as 54% for untreated vertebral artery injury (80). Biffl et al. (76) reported a posterior circulation stroke rate of 25% in his series of blunt vertebral artery injuries. It is noteworthy that no other published studies report a stroke rate of this magnitude.

Both Biffl et al. (76) and Miller et al. (80) advocate angiographic evaluation of selective patients at risk of vascular injury and aggressive management of VAI with anticoagulation, reporting significant protection from cerebral ischemia and improved neurologic outcomes. Although their reported incidence of vertebral artery injury and secondary cerebral ischemia is substantial, other reports would suggest that the incidence is much lower and that secondary neurologic complications are unusual, particularly with VAT (79). There is empirical evidence that a 6-month course of anticoagulation offers some protective

effect against thromboembolic events and cerebral ischemia from spontaneous carotid or vertebral dissection; however, no well-controlled studies have been performed to support routine use of anticoagulation in this setting (81).

Since the proportion of patients with clinically symptomatic posttraumatic vascular injury is small, conventional angiography cannot be justified to evaluate all patients with cervical trauma for occult vascular injury. However, MRA is an appropriate screening test to identify patients who may require subsequent catheter angiography. A 2D TOF sequence used in conjunction with a walking superior saturation pulse used to suppress venous inflow is effective in screening the extracranial vasculature for occlusion. This technique is adequate to evaluate vascular occlusion or significant narrowing; however, resolution limits the effectiveness of detecting subtle intimal injuries associated with dissection (Fig. 8-43). In cases of vertebral artery occlusion, axial GE images

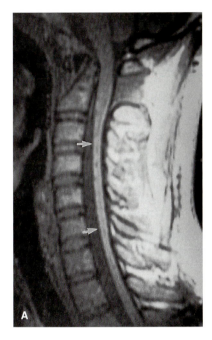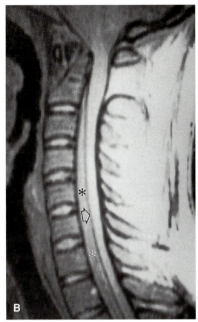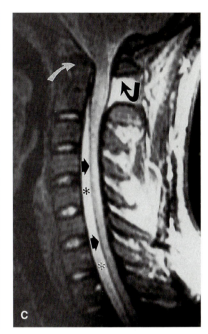

FIGURE 8-38. Large epidural collection following C2 fracture. **A:** Sagittal T1-weighted image shows a markedly widened ventral subarachnoid space. The spinal cord is displaced posteriorly (*arrows*). **B:** Sagittal intermediate-weighted image shows that the widened epidural space (*asterisks*) contains fluid that is somewhat hyperintense relative to CSF. The hypointense band (*arrow*) represents the ventral dura. **C:** Sagittal T2-weighted image shows a large epidural fluid collection (*asterisks*) separate from normal CSF that is displacing the spinal cord dorsally (*arrows*). The collection is bounded by dura as the PLL appears intact. There is diffuse high signal intensity within the spinal cord parenchyma from edema. Note that the deformity of the odontoid process is very difficult to appreciate (*curved white arrow*). There is associated rupture of the interspinous ligaments between C1 and C2 (*curved black arrow*). (From Flanders AE, Croul SE. Spinal trauma. In: Atlas SW. *Magnetic Resonance Imaging of the Brain and Spine*. 3rd ed. Philadelphia: Lippincott Williams & Wilkins; 2002:1779, with permission.)

reveal replacement of normal flow-related enhancement in the foramen transversarium by a hypointense clot (deoxyhemoglobin) (Figs. 8-41, 8-43). In contrast, the acute clot appears hyperintense on routine T2-weighted cross-sectional images compared to the normal flow-void in the normal artery (Figs. 8-41, 8-42). Use of black-blood techniques is also advocated to improve detection of subintimal dissections without occlusion. This technique suppresses signal from flowing blood and the surrounding tissues through the use of multiple spatial and chemical saturation pulses that render flowing blood hypointense and subintimal clot as hyperintense (75,79).

Biomechanics and Distribution of Injuries

Most SCI reported in any given year result in tetraparesis due to damage to the cervical spinal cord. The majority of victims of thoracic and lumbar spine trauma suffer no neurologic sequelae (66,82). The type of injuries that occur in the cervical, thoracic, and lumbar regions differ because of regional structural differences, biomechanical variations, and mechanisms of injury. Factors that may predispose to SCI include developmental or acquired spinal stenosis, degenerative spondylosis, and ankylosing spondylitis (53,58,69,83,84).

The pathophysiology of spinal injury can be better understood in a biomechanical framework (85). The spine is made up of relatively rigid components (vertebral bodies and posterior elements) and flexible components (intervertebral discs and ligaments). All the spinal segments work in concert with the adjacent segments to allow for reasonable amounts of flexion, extension, and rotation. The response of any substance to stretching or compression by an external force is defined by its *elastic modulus*. The application of too great a force over a short period of time results in tissue stress and eventual failure. Bone and ligament have different failure characteristics

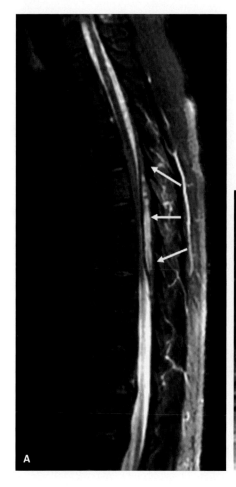

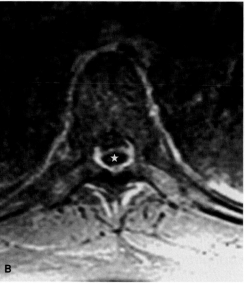

FIGURE 8-39. Unusual dorsal thoracic epidural hematoma not associated with a fracture in a 32-year-old woman after a fall. **A:** Sagittal FSE T2-weighted image shows a dorsal hyperintense epidural fluid collection that spans multiple segments of the thoracic spine (*arrows*). **B:** Contrast enhanced axial T1-weighted image shows the low signal intensity hematoma (*asterisk*) compressing the thecal sac. (From Flanders AE, Croul SE. Spinal trauma. In: Atlas SW. *Magnetic Resonance Imaging of the Brain and Spine.* 3rd ed. Philadelphia: Lippincott Williams & Wilkins; 2002:1789, with permission.)

(1). The dissipation of a force applied to the spine is well tolerated under the following circumstances: (a) the force is applied gradually over a prolonged period, and (b) the resultant motion of the spine by the force does not exceed the design specifications in terms of length of travel. If either of these rules is violated, then the elastic modulus of the tissues may be exceeded and tissue failure results. This phenomenon is well illustrated in the cervical region: the cervical spine supports a large free weight (the head) that allows for a full range of motion (flexion, extension, and rotation). During periods of rapid acceleration/deceleration, the head develops large amounts of kinetic energy that must be completely dissipated by the cervical spine. In this setting, a lower segment of the cervical spine may behave as a fulcrum against the relatively fixed thoracic spine, resulting in tissue failure. Tissue failure allows for focal dissipation of this kinetic energy; therefore, the osseous, ligamentous, and spinal cord damage tend to be in anatomic proximity (8,53,58).

Classification systems have been developed to help simplify the description of spinal injuries as an aid in

diagnosis, prognosis, and treatment (86,87). These systems are used to infer the amount of "invisible" soft tissue damage based on radiographic appearance. Some of these schemata are based on mechanisms of injury (i.e., hyperflexion, hyperextension, rotation, flexion-rotation, extension-rotation, axial loading, or lateral translation) (85). A major limitation of this method of analysis is that few injuries can be explained by "pure" mechanisms. Moreover, the biomechanics of the spine differ drastically by location and therefore the types of injuries produced by the same force vectors differ by location. A classification based on mechanism alone does not directly relate either to treatment or prognosis.

Other classification schemes of spinal injury are based solely on the presence of stability or instability of an injury. Potential instability is an important determining factor in the use and type of surgical stabilization. Instability is defined as the loss of ability of the spine to maintain normal anatomic alignment under normal physiologic loads (66,88). The properties of spinal instability are based on the three-column model of thoracolumbar spine trauma suggested by Holdsworth (89) and

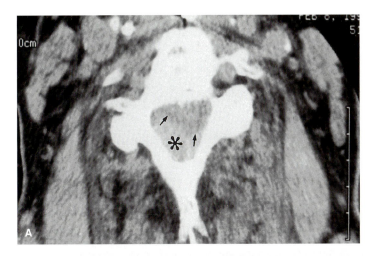
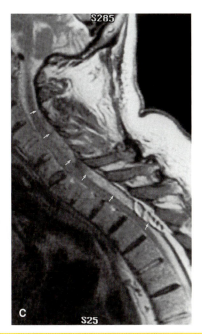
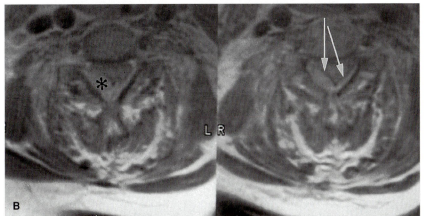

FIGURE 8-40. Dorsal epidural hematoma in patient with ankylosing spondylitis. **A:** Oblique axial CT image through lower cervical spine shows a large biconvex hyperdense collection (*asterisk*) dorsal to the thecal sac. The theca is displaced anteriorly (*arrows*). **B:** Axial FSE MRI confirms the presence of the epidural hematoma (*asterisk*) and the compression of the posterior dura (*arrows*). **C:** Sagittal FSE T2-weighted image shows the broad extent of the hemorrhage through the entire cervical region (*arrows*). The heterogeneous signal characteristics are secondary to heme in various stages of evolution. The accentuated configuration of the cervical spine is secondary to ankylosing spondylitis. (From Flanders AE, Croul SE. Spinal trauma. In: Atlas SW. *Magnetic Resonance Imaging of the Brain and Spine.* 3rd ed. Philadelphia: Lippincott Williams & Wilkins; 2002:1790, with permission.)

revised by Denis (87), and applied to the thoracic and lumbar spine. This model was devised so that inferences could be made about the status of soft tissue injury based solely on radiologic changes. In this model, the spine is represented by three columns: the *anterior column*, which is made up of the anterior one half of the vertebral body, the anterior annulus fibrosus, and the ALL; the *middle column*, composed of the posterior half of the vertebral body and the PLL; and the *posterior column*, which contains the posterior bony arch, ligamentum flavum, facets, and interspinous ligaments. Isolated disruption of the posterior column does not constitute instability; the structures of the middle column must also be involved to invoke instability in the thoracic and lumbar spine (87).

This type of classification offers information that aids in the diagnosis and treatment of specific injuries, yet it is an oversimplification that is probably not valid biomechanically (66). Tears of the posterior longitudinal ligament, ligamentum flavum, intraspinous and supraspinous ligaments, and facet joint disruption are potentially unstable (89). Some fractures that would be classified as stable can still harbor components that would render the injury unstable if not adequately treated (90). Furthermore, since MRI provides direct visualization of the integrity of the ligamentous complexes, MRI evaluation may supersede standard classification methods when MRI demonstrates unexpected soft tissue injuries.

(text continues on page 223)

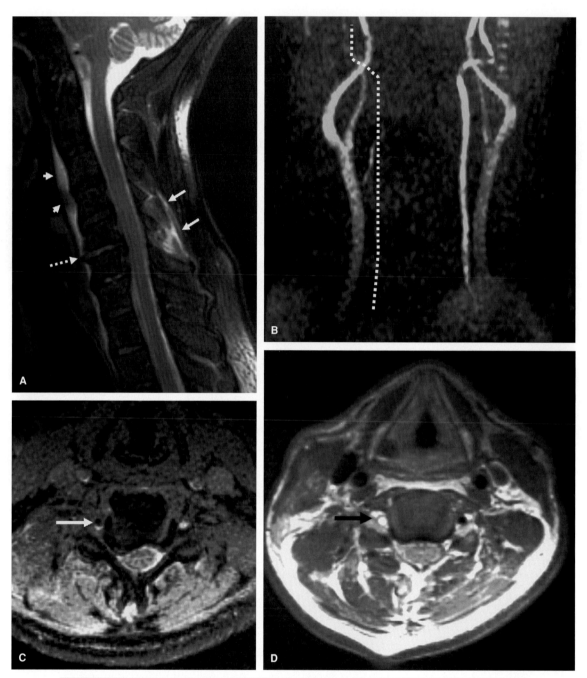

FIGURE 8-41. Clinically occult vertebral artery thrombosis after unilateral facet dislocation (UFD) at C5-6 without spinal cord injury at C5-6 without SCI. **A:** Sagittal T2-weighted fast spin-echo (FSE) image shows an injured disk at C5-6 with increased signal intensity in the disc and probably avulsion of the anterior longitudinal ligament (*dashed arrow*). Prevertebral edema (*arrowheads*) and edema in the posterior paraspinal musculature (*white arrows*) are present. **B:** Nonvisualization of the right vertebral artery. MIP image (*anterior view*) from a 2D TOF MRA acquisition shows absence of signal intensity in the expected course of the right vertebral artery (*dotted line*). **C:** Thrombus in the right foramen transversarium. Axial image from a 3D GRE acquisition shows an oval area of low signal intensity in the right foramen transversarium corresponding to thrombus in the right vertebral artery. Note the normal flow related enhancement in the left foramen transversarium. **D:** Thombus in the right vertebral artery. Axial FSE image obtained at a similar level to image in panel (C) shows a high-signal-intensity thrombus (*arrow*) in the right foramen transversarium indicative of a thrombosed vertebral artery. Note the normal flow void of the left vertebral artery. (From Torina PJ, Flanders AE, Carrino JA, et al. Incidence of vertebral artery thrombosis in cervical spine trauma: correlation with severity of spinal cord injury. *AJNR.* 2005;26:2645–2651, copyright © by American Society of Neuroradiology, with permission.)

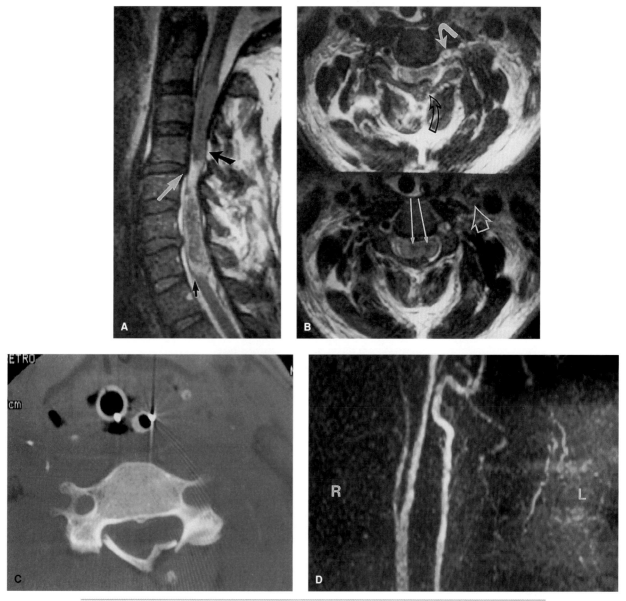

FIGURE 8-42. Crush injury from forklift in a 49-year-old man. **A:** Sagittal fast spin echo (FSE) T2-weighted image shows a massive hemorrhagic injury of the cervical spinal cord. The edema extends up to the level of the foramen magnum. A disc herniation is present at C4-5 (*white arrow*) and there is offset of the cervical segments at that level. The ligamentum flavum is disrupted at the C4 level (*black arrow*). Note the sharp change in caliber of the spinal cord caudally (*small black arrow*). **B:** Axial FSE T2-weighted images at the C3-4 level shows buckling of the lamina with encroachment on the posterior epidural space (*open black arrow*). The spinal cord is enlarged, deformed, and devoid of all normal internal anatomic features. Portions of the central gray matter are hypointense secondary to hemorrhage (*long white arrows*). Note the absence of normal flow void in the left vertebral artery (*curved white arrow*) and left internal carotid artery (*open white arrow*) suggestive of slow flow or occlusion (compare with normal right side). **C:** Axial computed tomographic image at the C4 level shows comminuted fractures of the lamina bilaterally with resultant narrowing of the spinal canal. **D:** Maximum intensity projection image from axial 2D TOF MRA acquisition reveals normal flow-related enhancement of the right carotid artery and right vertebral artery with absence of the left carotid and vertebral arteries. (*continued*)

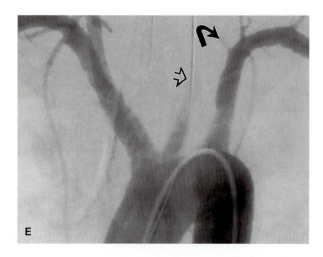

FIGURE 8-42 (*CONTINUED*) **E:** Right posterior oblique view from arch arteriography confirms the traumatic occlusion of the left common carotid artery (*open arrow*) and left vertebral artery (*curved arrow*). (From Flanders AE, Croul SE. Spinal trauma. In: Atlas SW. *Magnetic Resonance Imaging of the Brain and Spine*. 3rd ed. Philadelphia: Lippincott Williams & Wilkins; 2002:1791–1792, with permission.)

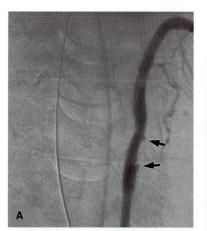

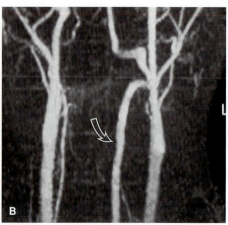

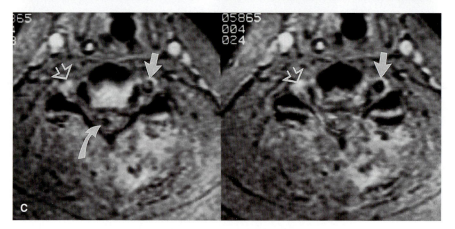

FIGURE 8-43. Traumatic intimal injury of vertebral artery. **A:** AP radiograph from a left vertebral arteriogram shows irregularity of the lateral wall (*arrows*) of the contrast column secondary to distractive injury at C3-4. (No associated fracture at this level.) **B:** Single projection from a 2D TOF MRA shows normal flow-related enhancement in all vessels. There is minimal irregularity of the left vertebral artery (*arrow*) but the intimal damage is not apparent. **C:** Axial 3DFT GE images in another patient with traumatic occlusion of the left vertebral artery. Hypointense acute clot is demonstrated within the lumen of the left vertebral artery (*arrows*). Compare with normal flow-related enhancement in the right vertebral artery (*open arrows*). Also note the massive hemorrhage in the spinal cord (*curved arrow*). (From Flanders AE, Croul SE. Spinal trauma. In: Atlas SW. *Magnetic Resonance Imaging of the Brain and Spine*. 3rd ed. Philadelphia: Lippincott Williams & Wilkins; 2002: 1793, with permission.)

Assessment of Spinal Instability

The integrity of the spinal ligamentous complexes is paramount to the assessment of spinal instability. The occurrence of radiographically occult unstable cervical spine injuries, while rare, (estimated at 0.04% to 0.6% in some series) underscores the need for improved detection of soft tissue injuries (91). Although MRI offers an unprecedented assessment of the ligamentous structures of the spine, MRI's role in predicting mechanical instability remains in question. Clearly, a ligament does not need to be torn or disrupted in order to be mechanically incompetent. Any ligament that has been stretched or distorted beyond its normal elastic tolerance will no longer provide effective resistance to abnormal translation of adjacent vertebral segments *even if it remains intact*. Therefore, controlled physiologic testing of spinal mechanical stability has been the primary means of assessment of ligamentous incompetence and mechanical instability.

Prior to the advent of MRI, the accepted method for testing spinal instability has been through the evaluation of lateral radiographs during controlled flexion and extension of the spine. Detection of abnormal translation or angulation between two adjacent vertebral segments (>3 mm or 11 degrees angulation) is considered an indication of mechanical instability, even in the absence of a fracture (92).

When a patient has an altered level of consciousness, immobilization of the spine may be necessary until the patient is alert enough to provide an adequate clinical examination. Alternatively, operator-controlled passive flexion and extension of the patient's cervical spine is sometimes advocated in conjunction with radiography; however, this technique has important limitations including significant operator dependency and diminished sensitivity to injury unless adequate motion is achieved. Many studies report an unacceptable false positive and false negative rates (93). In one study, 30% of the flexion-extension radiographs were evaluated as inadequate due to limited motion and a 12.5% false-negative rate (94). Dynamic flexion (DF) radiography was completely normal for 276 patients who required cervical spine clearance as a result of traumatic brain injury. Flexion-extension radiography did not offer any additional diagnostic value beyond that available with standard radiography and high resolution CT (95). Moreover, the method is potentially dangerous to perform in the unconscious patient who may harbor an unstable injury (93–96).

Because MRI offers a noninvasive method to visualize the spinal ligaments, it has been suggested that MRI can provide an objective assessment of ligament integrity (93–109). However, studies that rigorously assess the validity of MRI in this application are lacking (104). In a study that assessed the reliability of identifying intact ligaments on cervical MRIs in nontraumatic patients, Saifuddin et al. (55) found that complete ligaments were absent in a substantial proportion of normal subjects. Moreover, there was marked interobserver variation and identification varied by ligament type. The identification rate for a complete, intact ALL ranged from 74% to 79%, for an intact PLL the range was 36% to 74% and for the ligamentum flavum the rate of identification range was poor at 63% to 65%. Moreover, the prevalence of normal discontinuous longitudinal ligaments was greater in patients with cervical spondylosis. The authors concluded that the ALL, PLL, and LF are commonly not visualized, therefore, discontinuity of the ligament alone cannot be used as a reliable measure of ligament integrity especially in the setting of superimposed spondylosis.

A surprisingly high incidence of cervical soft tissue injuries were reported in a postmortem study of ten cadaver spines who died from multisystem trauma. In this study, a comparison was made of cervical specimen radiographs, anatomic dissection, and MRI of the specimens. Twenty-eight distinct injuries were found in eight of the ten specimens; the majority of the injuries consisted of soft tissue processes including facet joint capsule lesions, ligament and disc injury, and spinal cord injury. Observers were only able to identify 11 of the 28 pathologic findings prospectively on MRI, and 17 abnormalities were ultimately found retrospectively. The authors concluded that occult soft tissue lesions of the cervical spine are common in trauma victims and that MRI is limited in its ability to depict these injuries. An important limitation of this study was the absence of fat-suppressed T2-weighted MRI, which may have diminished the detection of associated soft tissue injury. This study does suggest that even in the best imaging conditions (i.e., motionless subject) the sensitivity of MRI in identifying traumatic soft tissue injuries may be limited (102).

In order to define the role of MRI in the preoperative evaluation of the spinal ligaments, Lee et al. (99) prospectively evaluated 34 thoracolumbar fracture patients with fat-suppressed T2-weighted MRI and assessed the posterior ligamentous complexes (PLC) by palpation and direct inspection during surgery. The authors found that the accuracy of palpation for posterior ligamentous complex injury was 53.6% and for plain radiography it was 66.7%. The performance of MRI was substantially better; the accuracy in the detection of injury to the supraspinous ligament (SSL) was 90.9%, the intraspinous ligament (ISL) was 97.0%, and for the ligamentum flavum (LF), 87.9%. The authors concluded that a fat-suppressed T2-weighted sagittal sequence was highly sensitive, specific, and accurate in the detection of PLC injuries.

A similar study by Haba et al. (98) determined the diagnostic accuracy of MRI in detecting injury to the SSL and ISL was 90.5% and 94.3% respectively. T1-weighted images had a significantly great specificity than T2-weighted images for detecting SSL injury. The kappa interrator values were 0.803 for PLC injury, 0.915 for ISL, and 0.69 for SSL injury. These authors concluded that MRI can reliably differentiate an inherently unstable three-column injury from a potentially stable two-column injury.

Other studies have examined the reproducibility of soft tissue damage in identical types of injuries. In a retrospective review of 48 MRI studies performed on unilateral (UID) and bilateral (BID) cervical facet dislocations (without controls), Vaccaro et al. (100) found disruption to the posterior ligamentous complex (PLC: 68.2%), facet capsule, ligamentum flavum (LF), posterior (PLL: 56.5%), and anterior longitudinal ligaments (ALL: 65.2%) in a statistically significant number of patients with BID. Disruption of these structures was also found in UID patients with the exception of the PLL. Disruption of the ALL, PLL, and the left facet capsule were significantly more common in BID compared to UID. Intervertebral disc injury was associated with both UID and BID, but was more common in BID.

A follow-up study evaluated ligamentous integrity in 30 BID patients with MRI and found a lower incidence of ligamentous disruption: ALL, 26.7%; PLL, 40%; PLC, 96.7% (101). The authors noted that the PLL was rated as intact in the majority of these BID patients, which contradicts accepted theory for the mechanism of this type of injury. The discrepancy in results between the two studies can be partially explained by dissimilar classification methods used for the two studies and the use of a separate category for mechanically compromised but intact ligaments (i.e., intact but elevated). The differences underscore the fact that ambiguities exist in classifying damage to the supporting spinal structures.

Although most trauma centers typically employ radiography and CT as their main diagnostic tools in the evaluation of spinal injury, the indication for use of MRI in the clearance of spinal injury (without neurologic injury) remains controversial. Several trauma centers have employed protocols that use MRI in conjunction with radiography and high resolution CT. In one such study, 97 cervical injury patients were evaluated with MRI after CT. In 83 cases, the MRI study confirmed the findings of CT yet did not offer any additional information. MRI reclassified fractures as degenerative changes in 12 cases, and MRI identified a new injury that was not depicted on CT in only two instances. The overall negative predictive value of CT was 98%, positive predictive value was 78%, and the sensitivity and specificity was 94% and 91% respectively. The findings suggested that routine use of MRI as part of a standard trauma protocol is not warranted unless under certain circumstances such as patient obtundation or confounding physical/clinical findings (97). This conclusion was also supported by Hogan and Mirvis (105) who assessed the added value of MRI in detecting occult cervical soft tissue injuries in 366 obtunded patients who also received high-resolution MDCT evaluation. The negative predictive value of MDCT was 98.9% for ligament injury and 100% for unstable cervical injury. Only four of the 366 patients with a negative MDCT study were subsequently found to have a ligament injury with MRI; none of these injuries were judged to be unstable. The authors concluded that a normal MDCT study alone will exclude unstable cervical injuries.

Sliker and Mirvis (106) reviewed the body of literature that addresses cervical spine stability in obtunded blunt trauma patients who were evaluated with MRI or dynamic fluoroscopy. The aggregate MR data from numerous studies yielded a frequency of ligamentous injury detected by MRI for the blunt trauma population at 22.7%; 80.8% of these injuries warranted treatment, with 5.6% requiring immobilization. For the subset of patients that were obtunded, MRI diagnosed ligament injuries at a lower frequency (19.5%), with 69.2% of these injuries requiring treatment, 12.8% needing surgery, and 2.5% receiving surgical stabilization. It is noteworthy that the MRI criteria for ligamentous injury and surgical indications were very inconsistent between studies.

The occipital-cervical junction and the atlanto-axial junction contain a complex of multiple nonparallel ligaments that confer stability to this area. Imaging assessment for rotatory instability has also traditionally been accomplished with rotational dynamic radiography or fluoroscopy. Today, MRI is often relied upon to exclude ligamentous strain or disruption of this area, despite the relative paucity of data that validates MRI for this application (Figs. 8-44, 8-45).

Wilmink and Patijn (107) evaluated the alar ligaments at the atlanto-axial junction of patients with whiplash-associated disorders (WAD) using 0.5 Tesla MRI. They were unable to identify a reliable set of imaging criteria that differentiated WAD patients from control subjects. Moreover, the level of agreement between observers in grading the ligaments was poor.

Kaale et al. (108) applied a MRI grading system to the alar and transverse ligaments as well as the tectorial and posterior atlanto-occipital membranes for 92 symptomatic WAD patients and 30 control subjects. The authors demonstrated a significant relationship between pain-disability scores and the grade of ligamentous damage; the highest association was found with alar ligament damage and the number of structures showing changes on MRI. One principal shortcoming of this study was the use of only a single observer to grade the ligaments; therefore, the validity and reproducibility of the grading system cannot be evaluated.

Although MRI is significantly more costly than radiography or CT, judicious use of MRI in the appropriate circumstances can be cost effective. At one pediatric center, incorporation of routine MRI into their pediatric spinal clearance protocol for obtunded patients resulted in a significant decrease in time-to-clearance

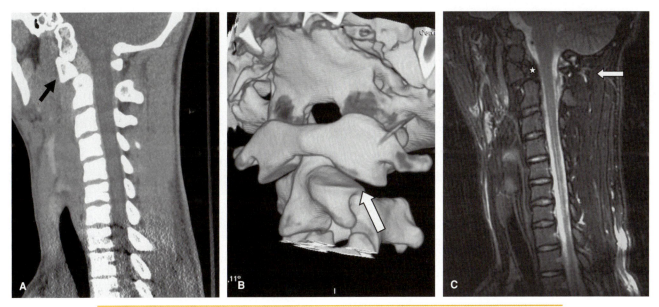

FIGURE 8-44. Absence of expected ligamentous injury in a rotatory subluxation of C1-2 in a 16-year-old who presented with the head fixed in rotation after trauma. **A:** Sagittal MPR reformatted CT image shows abnormal configuration and orientation of the skull base and atlas (C1) relative to the axis (C2) (*arrow*). **B:** Surface-rendered CT reformatted image of the C1-2 articulation shows the rotational malalignment of the lateral mass of C1 and C2 (*arrow*). **C:** Sagittal T2-weighted MRI with fat suppression obtained at the midline shows absence of any significant soft tissue damage including the transverse/alar ligaments (*asterisk*) and posterior ligamentous complex (*arrow*).

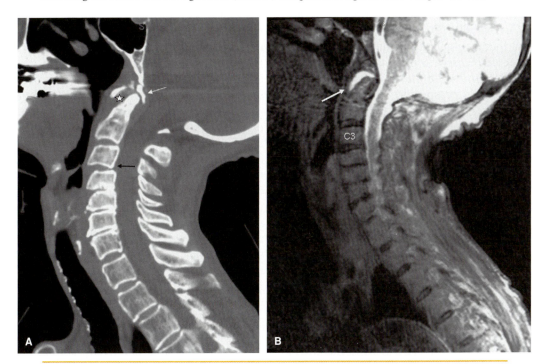

FIGURE 8-45. Use of MRI to assess ligamentous instability; C1-2 instability in an elderly female after a fall. **A:** Midsagittal MPR image of the cervical spine shows thinning of the anterior arch of C1 and dystrophic bone formation between the apex of the odontoid process and the anterior margin of the foramen magnum (*white arrow*) from a prior occult injury. There is abnormal increased distance between the odontoid process and the anterior arch of the atlas (*asterisk*). There is also anterior subluxation of the C3 vertebral body relative to C4 (*black arrow*). **B:** Sagittal T2-weighted MRI with fat suppression show fluid in the predental space (*arrow*) indicative of instability. Note that the subluxation at C3-4 has reduced and there are no associated signal changes of ligamentous injury at this area. This represents a degenerative subluxation rather than an acute traumatic episode.

(5.1 days to 3.2 days), average stay in the intensive care unit (9.2 days to 7.3 days), and an overall decrease in hospital stay. Taking these factors into account, they realized an average cost savings of $7,700 per patient by using MRI as an integral part of their spinal clearance protocol (103).

Although there is a body of evidence that suggests that MRI can be used as a reliable measure of spinal ligamentous instability from blunt trauma, there are several key shortcomings in the current literature that emphasize the need for critical reassessment of MRI in this application. These issues include a general lack of consistency in grading of ligament injury in studies without validation of the schema. While the MR findings in some of the studies have been confirmed at surgery, most have not. Moreover, routine surgical assessment of the longitudinal ligaments is not possible in many cases due to the surgical approach chosen and limited visualization of these structures. Although true discontinuity or avulsion of a ligament is likely an indicator of ligamentous failure, the significance of the MR signal changes seen in intact ligaments or surrounding soft tissues remains unclear; differentiation between a simple strain from a mechanically incompetent but *intact* ligament is unproven. Moreover, the absence of a signal change in a ligament on MRI may not always be predictive of mechanical stability (Fig. 8-44). Finally, with minimal exception, there are no studies that gauge the ligament soft tissue changes with physical disability and loss in range of motion. All of these factors underscore the need for controlled prospective trials to prove the complementary value of MRI in assessing soft tissue injury in blunt spinal trauma.

There is also a need to image the ligaments of the spine more reliably and to develop new MRI techniques that augment signal from the ligaments. One method that has received some interest is ultrashort TE (UTE) imaging, which has the capability of extracting signals from structures that normally elicit little to no signal using conventional pulse sequences. Standard MR pulse sequences are typically capable of receiving signals from tissues that have T2 relaxation properties greater than 10 milliseconds. However, the intrinsic T2 relaxation of ligaments is typically <1 millisecond. This is why ligaments are of low signal on conventional MRI. The typical echo times of the UTE sequence are on the order of 0.08 millisecond and are therefore capable of capturing signal from less conspicuous structures (Fig. 8-46).

Degenerative spondylosis alters the biomechanical properties of the spine by decreasing elasticity, thereby diminishing the ability of the tissues to uniformly dissipate applied force (Fig. 8-47) (58). The loss of spinal elasticity in AS is so severe that even minor trauma can result in a fracture dislocation (84). In AS, lower cervical spine fractures

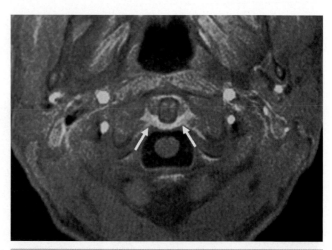

FIGURE 8-46. Ultrashort TE imaging of the transverse ligament of C1. Axial UTE image obtained at the level of C1 depicts the entire transverse ligament as a high signal intensity structure (*arrows*). The transverse ligament is usually difficult to identify using standard clinical MR sequences. (Image courtesy of Graham Bydder, PhD of the University of California in San Diego.)

predominate (75%) and hyperextension is the most frequent mechanism of injury. The loss of spinal elasticity associated with the disease augments fractures through both the anterior and posterior columns as well as the intervertebral disc space (Fig. 8-48) (84). As a result, spinal fractures in patients with AS are highly unstable and difficult to manage, with a high incidence of morbidity and secondary mortality, ranging from 35% to 50% (69,84).

Because of biomechanical differences, the pathophysiology of upper cervical spine injuries (C1-2) (Figs. 8-15, 8-49) differs from lower cervical spine injuries (C3-7) (21,82). Upper cervical spinal cord injuries are more common in children than adults because the head size for children is proportionally larger than for adults (21). Furthermore, in adults, the probability of developing a permanent neurologic deficit is much higher in the lower cervical spine injuries.

The classification system devised by Allen et al. (1) is the most widely used classification scheme for lower cervical injuries. Injuries are classified by major and minor injury force vectors and then are subclassified into degree of severity. The common classification groups are compressive flexion, vertical compression, distraction flexion, compressive extension, distraction extension, and lateral flexion (1). Most injuries to the cervical spine, however, are the result of hyperflexion mechanisms (79%) (67).

Although fractures of the thoracic spine are not unusual, they comprise only a small proportion of all fractures of the spinal column (16%) (66,110). The biomechanics of the upper thoracic spine (T1-10) differ from the cervical spine as well as from the lower thoracic

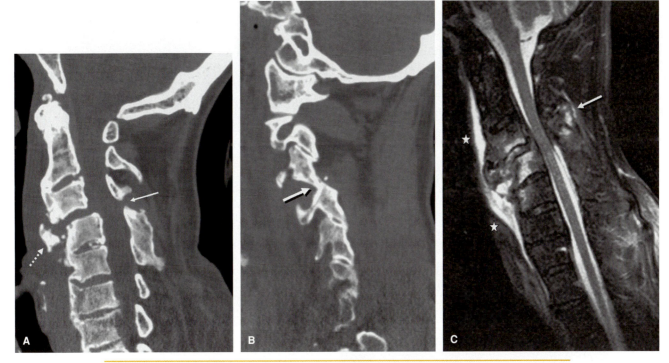

FIGURE 8-47. Severe fracture from minor trauma in a 50-year-old with pre-existing diffuse idiopathic skeletal hyperostosis (DISH). **A:** Sagittal MPR CT image shows posttraumatic sublux-ation of the C3 segment on C4 with widening of the interspinous distance (*arrow*) and a large fragmented osteophyte anteriorly (*dashed line*). Note the extensive bony bridging elsewhere. **B:** Sagittal MPR CT image shows the associated unilateral interfacetal dislocation. **C:** Sagittal T2-weighted MRI shows extensive prevertebral edema (*asterisk*) as well as marrow edema within the C3 and C4 vertebral bodies. There has been damage to the posterior ligamentous complex as well (*arrow*). There is a small associated posterior epidural fluid collection. Note the absence of injury to the spinal cord.

FIGURE 8-48. Classic exten-sion type injury in ankylosing spondylitis. **A:** Midsagittal MPR CT image shows widening of the anterior aspect of the C5-6 inter-space (*thick arrow*). Note the bony ankylosis of the skull base to the upper cervical spine (*thin arrow*) and the ossification of the ligamentum flavum (*dashed arrow*). **B:** T2-weighted fat sup-pressed sagittal MRI shows the disrupted intervertebral disc (*arrow*) and the extensive pre-vertebral edema (*asterisk*).

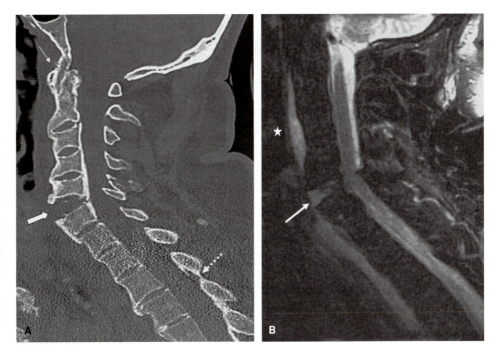

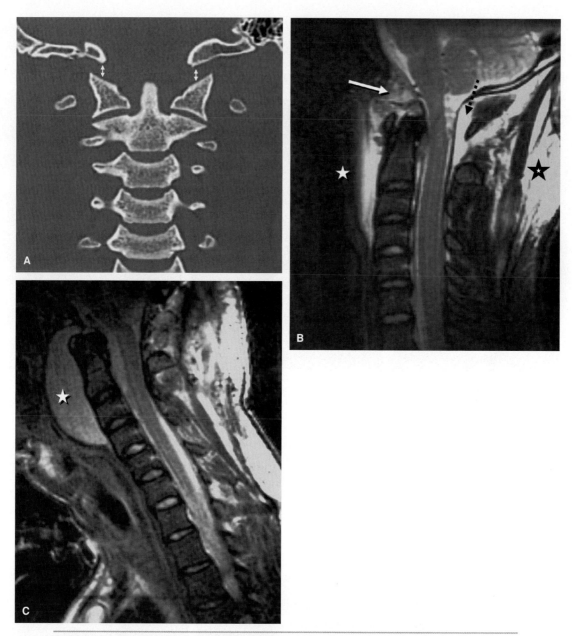

FIGURE 8-49. Atlanto-occipital dislocation. **A:** Coronal CT reformat image shows markedly increased distance between the superior articular process of C1 and the occipital condyles (*arrows*) without evidence of fracture. **B:** Midsagittal T2-weighted MRI with fat suppression shows distraction of the skull base and upper cervical spine with complete disruption of the ligamentous support structures between the apex of the dens and the foramen magnum (*white arrow*) with hematoma/fluid in the gap and prevertebral hematoma in the upper cervical spine (*white asterisk*). There is complete disruption of the posterior ligamentous complex with epidural hemorrhage interposed between the dura and the posterior ring of C1 (*dashed black arrow*). The posterior musculature is also edematous (*black asterisk*). **C:** Midsagittal T2-weighted MRI with fat suppression after surgery shows a massive prevertebral fluid collection from dural laceration that compromises the airway (*asterisk*).

spine (T10-12) and thoracolumbar junction. Most thoracic fractures occur at the thoracolumbar junction and remain neurologically intact (Fig. 8-50) (82). The thoracic cage offers a protective effect to the upper thoracic spine by adding stiffness and providing additional energy-absorbing capacity. The rib cage alters the moment of inertia of the spine and therefore imparts resistance to rotational forces. In addition, the facet joints have a coronal orientation in the upper thoracic spine that resists anterior translational forces. Considerable

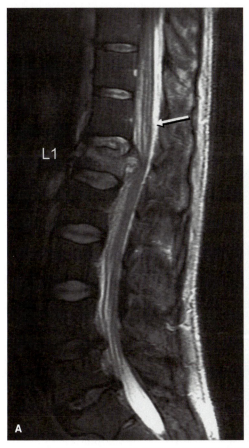

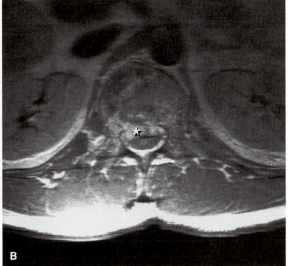

FIGURE 8-50. L1 burst fracture with failure of the middle column and compression of the thecal sac. **A:** Midsagittal T2-weighted MRI with fat suppression shows loss of height of the L1 vertebral body with disruption of the superior endplate. There is retropulsion of the posterior cortex into the anterior epidural space resulting in approximately 50% compromise of the spinal canal. Note that the conus medullaris (*arrow*) is above the level of injury. **B:** Axial proton-density MRI through the L1 level shows epidural hemorrhage compressing the thecal sac (*asterisk*).

force is therefore necessary to fracture or dislocate the thoracic spine. It is estimated that these anatomic features increase the compression tolerance of the thoracic spine by a factor of four (66). These factors contribute to the lower overall incidence of fracture dislocations in the upper thoracic spine compared to other areas (66).

Since the thoracic spinal canal is relatively narrow in dimension, there is a high association of complete SCI (63%) with fractures of the upper thoracic spine (Fig. 8-51) (110). Most of these injuries occur via hyperflexion mechanisms (66,110). When there are associated bilateral fractures of the posterior elements with resultant autodecompression of the spinal canal, the spinal cord sometimes escapes injury (66).

In adults, SCI without radiographic abnormality (SCIWORA) is a well-recognized syndrome of the cervical spine that is thought to occur secondary to hyperex-

tension dislocations or hyperextension sprain associated with cervical spondylosis (Fig. 8-52) (25,53,57,58,111, 112). This type of mechanism is reproduced in rear-end motor vehicle collisions and direct anterior craniofacial trauma (53). In one report, 96% of patients over the age of 40 years with SCIWORA had severe cervical spondylosis (58). Common to this type of injury is momentary compression of the thecal sac between the edge of the dorsally displaced vertebral body or disc and the buckled LF (24,25,53,57,58). Minimal changes that may be appreciated on radiographs include prevertebral swelling, focal widening of the disc space anteriorly, or avulsion of a small portion of the vertebral endplate. MRI is of particular diagnostic value in this type of injury because it depicts abnormalities that are invisible on conventional radiographs, including separation of the intervertebral disc, rupture of the ALL and annulus, prevertebral hemorrhage, and parenchymal SCI (Figs.

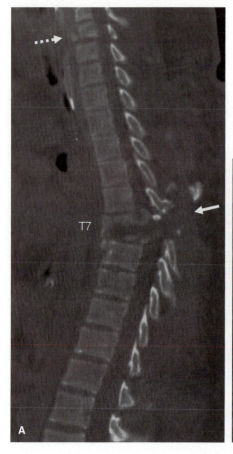
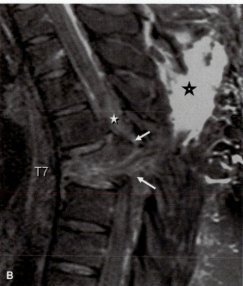

FIGURE 8-51. T7 fracture dislocation from high-speed motor vehicle accident. **A:** Midsagittal CT MPR image shows severe comminution of the T7 vertebral body with multiple retropulsed fragments that obliterate the spinal canal and complete disruption of the posterior ligamentous complex (*arrow*) resulting in acute angulation. There is a noncontiguous fracture at C6 (*dashed arrow*). **B:** Sagittal T2-weighted MRI with fat suppression reveals the extent of soft tissue disruption which has occurred at this level. The retropulsed cortical fragments from T7 have obliterated the entire spinal canal (*white arrows*). The entire posterior ligamentous complex has been disrupted (*black star*). The thoracic spinal cord is distorted and edematous (*white star*).

8-27, 8-28, 8-52) (24,53). Since SCIWORA was first described over 20 years ago, MRI has been central to improving our understanding the mechanisms of this syndrome, particularly in the pediatric population (112).

SPINAL CORD INJURY

Magnetic Resonance Imaging Findings of Spinal Cord Injury

MRI has had a greater impact on our understanding of SCI than any other diagnostic modality developed in the past decade. The clarity with which MRI is able to depict the internal architecture of the spinal cord is unmatched by any other imaging modality. Moreover, the depiction of parenchymal SCI on MRI not only correlates well with the degree of neurologic deficit, but it also bears significant implications in regard to prognosis and potential for neurologic recovery (4,8,9,42,44,61,64, 113–120).

Although the spinal cord can be reliably visualized with conventional MRI, it is often difficult to distinguish spinal gray matter from white matter as readily as the brain. This is particularly true in the sagittal plane, in

which the spinal cord is uniform in signal intensity on all pulse sequences. Spinal gray and white matter have very similar T1 and T2 relaxation characteristics, and therefore, the cord parenchyma appears relatively uniform in signal intensity (121–123). In vitro imaging of spinal cord specimens shows that the central gray matter is uniformly hyperintense relative to white matter on all pulse sequences. This is attributed to the higher spin density of gray matter (121–123) (Fig. 8-53). The gray-white matter interface is often best demonstrated in cross section on long TR SE and GE axial images. The tissue imaging characteristics are usually lost after SCI due to accumulation of edema and hemorrhage within the substance of the cord parenchyma. Despite these limitations, the basic MRI features of SCI that correlate with the pathologic changes of SCI are reliably demonstrated (Fig. 8-53) (124).

The foundation for understanding MRI patterns of SCI were developed initially in animal models (3,4,42,68,125). It has been shown in a rat model of SCI that the areas of low and high signal intensity in the cord on T2-weighted images were confirmed histologically as foci of intramedullary hemorrhage and edema, respectively (3,68,122,126).

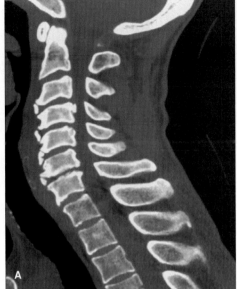

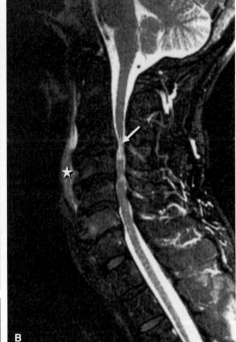

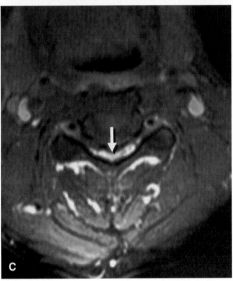

FIGURE 8-52. Spinal cord injury without radiographic abnormality (SCIWORA) in a 48-year-old male who experienced hand weakness (central cord syndrome) following a motor vehicle accident. **A:** Midsagittal CT MPR image shows multilevel cervical spondylosis with pre-existing developmental stenosis. Note the absence of an obvious fracture or subluxation. **B:** Sagittal T2-weighted MRI with fat suppression shows the markedly stenotic spinal canal with effacement of the subarachnoid space. There is edema within the spinal cord at the C3-4 level (*arrow*) and prevertebral edema (*star*) suggestive of an extension type injury. **C:** Axial T2-weighted MRI with fat suppression obtained at the C3-4 level shows the compression of the spinal cord and intrinsic edema (*arrow*).

Several investigators have been successful in quantifying the volume of injured parenchyma and the spatial/temporal evolution of the injury in experimental SCI (113,121,123,127,128). Decreased motor function was associated with lesions that had greater longitudinal and cross-sectional involvement of the spinal cord and evidence of central hemorrhage (42,121,123). In experimentally induced injuries, the typical MRI abnormalities were readily identifiable shortly after injury and were clearly manifest one day postinjury. The abnormal signal pattern reached maximum intensity within three days postinjury. Histologic preparations revealed the presence of hemorrhage, necrosis, and macrophages dispersed in the gray matter. The initial changes were attributed to the primary mechanical and vascular injury mechanism, whereas the prolonged growth in lesion size and intensity were related to the superimposed secondary or biochemical cascade that continued to expand the lesion for several days after

the actual injury (130). Since the complete MRI correlate of tissue injury becomes manifest as early as 72 hours after injury, the inherent value of serial MRI studies is questioned. For a detailed discussion of the pathophysiology of spinal cord injury, the reader is encouraged to review Chapter 1.

MRI provides excellent definition of intramedullary hemorrhage and edema in animal models (3,41,68,121, 128,129). The combination of MRI lesion length, cord caliber, and degree of preservation of white matter in MRI cross section have a significant relationship to functional status in animals and the pathologic findings at autopsy (121,123,130). The MRI appearance of experimentally induced SCI has been used to explain the variability in functional deficit among animals subjected to identical injuries (121). A significant shortcoming of MRI is its limited capability in demonstrating functionally preserved white matter tracts at the level of injury; this observation

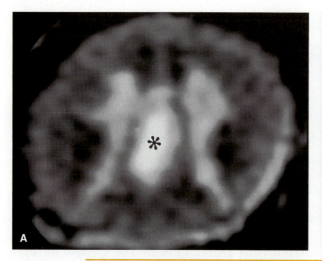

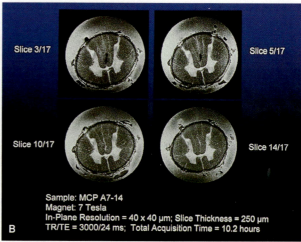

FIGURE 8-53. Cervical spinal cord specimen with hemorrhage in the posterior columns. **A:** Axial T1-weighted image at 1.5 Tesla shows a large focus of hemorrhage (*asterisk*) that involves the posterior columns bilaterally, with greater involvement on the right. **B:** The same lesion imaged in a 7 Tesla magnet shows far greater resolution of gray matter, white matter, and the hemorrhage in the posterior columns. (7 Tesla image courtesy of E. Wirth, MD, PhD, University of Florida School of Medicine.) (From Flanders AE, Croul SE. Spinal trauma. In: Atlas SW. *Magnetic Resonance Imaging of the Brain and Spine*. 3rd ed. Philadelphia: Lippincott Williams & Wilkins; 2002:1801, with permission.)

becomes significant in estimating preserved functional capacity (123,127,130). With the advent of diffusion techniques and tractography algorithms based upon diffusion parameters, MRI now has the capacity to assess the integrity of spinal white matter (see Chapter 13).

Several MRI classification schemes of human SCI have been proposed by prior investigators (4,5,9). Kulkarni et al. (9) first described three basic patterns of acute SCI with MRI. Schaeffer et al. (61) and Bondurant et al. (7) described a four-tiered classification system. Common to these schemes are three imaging observations: spinal cord hemorrhage, spinal cord edema, and spinal cord swelling (4,5,8–10,18,61,119). Each of these characteristics can be further defined by their rostral-caudal location in the spinal cord and the length or span of parenchyma that is involved. The typical SCI lesion on MRI is spindle-shaped, containing an epicenter of hemorrhage surrounded by a halo of edema; the latter has a greater rostral-caudal extent than the central hemorrhage (Fig. 8-54). These MRI findings have a direct relationship to the degree of neurologic deficit.

SPINAL CORD HEMORRHAGE

Posttraumatic spinal cord hemorrhage (i.e., hemorrhagic contusion) is defined as the presence of a discrete focus of hemorrhage within the substance of the spinal cord after an injury. The most common location is within the central

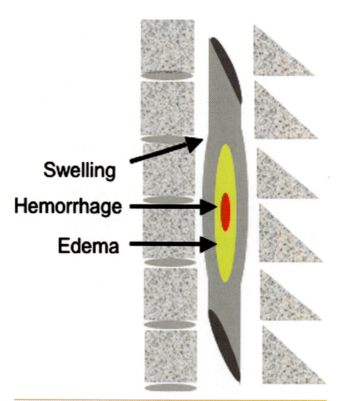

FIGURE 8-54. Graphic representation of spinal cord injury. A central focus of hemorrhage (*red oval*) is identified at the epicenter of the injury with a longer segment of edema (*yellow oval*) that spans the cord for a variable length.

gray matter of the spinal cord, and it is centered at the point of mechanical impact (Figs. 8-55–8-59) (3,7–9,131). Drawing from experimental and autopsy pathologic studies, the underlying lesion most often will be hemorrhagic necrosis of the spinal cord. True hematomyelia will rarely be found (42).

In the acute phase following injury, deoxyhemoglobin is the most common species generated (3,7,8,10,42,68, 132). Thus, the hemorrhagic component of the SCI on high field strength scanners is depicted as a discrete area of hypointensity on the T2-weighted and GE images (Figs. 8-55–8-59) (4,5,7–9,12,17,61,131,132). This represents the imaging manifestations of hemorrhagic necrosis of the spinal cord (Fig. 8-60) (8,9,18,133). The oxidative process in which deoxyhemoglobin evolves to methemoglobin is prolonged in the injured spinal cord. Methemoglobin appears approximately 3 to 5 days after an initial hemorrhage in the brain; however, conversion to intracellular methemoglobin may be delayed for 8 days or more in the spinal cord following injury (Figs. 8-57, 8-58) because degradation of deoxyhemoglobin is delayed due to local hypoxia/hypoperfusion of the injured segment (7–9,68). Early investigations in animal and human SCI suggested that identification of acute hemorrhage was unusual and that methemoglobin was the most prevalent species (7–9, 42). The low overall incidence of detecting deoxyhemoglobin in these early reports was a technical limitation rather than a direct contradiction of known pathologic evidence. Variable results in early studies are most likely due to the use of low static field strength magnets (4,7,8,12,42).

Parenchymal hemorrhage develops rapidly in the spinal cord after injury. In experimentally induced SCI models, hemorrhage was found in 12.5% of the cross-sectional area of the lesion epicenter initially, increasing exponentially to approximately 25% of the epicenter cross section within hours of injury. The rate of change in volume of hemorrhage is initially 0.15% per minute, with a maximal rate of 45% per minute within 5 hours after injury (129).

The MRI identification of hemorrhage in the spinal cord following trauma has significant clinical implications. It was originally thought that detection of intramedullary hemorrhage was predictive of a complete injury. However, the increased sensitivity and spatial resolution of current MRI techniques has shown that even small amounts of hemorrhage are identifiable in incomplete lesions. Therefore, the basic construct has been altered such that the detection of a sizable focus of blood (>10 mm in length on sagittal images) in the spinal cord is often indicative of a complete neurologic injury (119). The anatomic location of the hemorrhage closely corresponds to the neurologic level of injury, and the presence of frank hemorrhage implies a poor potential for neurologic recovery (7–9,64,115,131,133).

SPINAL CORD EDEMA

Spinal cord edema is defined on MRI as a focus of abnormal high signal intensity on T2-weighted images (17). This signal abnormality presumably reflects a focal accumulation of intracellular and interstitial fluid in response to injury (3–5,7–10,12,17,42,61,68). Edema is usually well defined on the midsagittal long TR image (Figs. 8-5, 8-11, 8-14, 8-19, 8-21, 8-24, 8-26–8-29, 8-42, 8-56, 8-58). Axial T2-weighted images offer supplemental information in regard to involvement of structures in cross section. Edema involves a variable length of spinal cord above and below the level of injury, with discrete boundaries adjacent to uninvolved parenchyma. Spinal cord edema is invariably associated with some degree of spinal cord swelling; however, it can occur without MRI evidence of intramedullary hemorrhage. Simple edema within the spinal cord in the setting of trauma has been referred to as a contusion by some investigators or as a hemorrhagic contusion when blood products are identified on MRI (18,61,68,119,131). The length of spinal cord affected by edema is directly proportional to the degree of initial neurologic deficit (8,61). Posttraumatic spinal cord hemorrhage always coexists with spinal cord edema; however, the converse is not always true, that is, edema alone can be produced following an injury. Cord edema alone connotes a more favorable prognosis than cord hemorrhage (9,67,115,119,131).

SPINAL CORD SWELLING

Spinal cord swelling is the most nondescriptive imaging finding associated with SCI. It is defined as a focal increase in caliber of the spinal cord centered at the level of an injury. By itself, swelling does not specifically describe any signal changes in the spinal cord. Spinal cord swelling is best demonstrated on the T1-weighted sagittal images (8,9,18,61); the parenchyma may be normal to slightly hypointense (8,61).

The normal spinal cord is relatively uniform in caliber, although it increases slightly in diameter at the lower cervical and lower thoracic areas. This normal enlargement may be difficult to discern on MRI. The change in caliber of the injured spinal cord is usually maximal at the level of trauma and tapers gradually cranially and caudally from the epicenter of the injury (Figs. 8-14, 8-21, 8-23, 8-24, 8-26, 8-27, 8-29, 8-42, 8-56, 8-58). In some instances, the swelling abruptly begins at the level of impact and progresses cranially only. Spinal cord swelling may be difficult to appreciate at a level of acute compression or when superimposed spinal canal stenosis is present. In this instance, the surrounding subarachnoid space is completely effaced, obscuring the upper and lower borders of the swelling. Although identification of spinal cord swelling alone is an

(text continues on page 236)

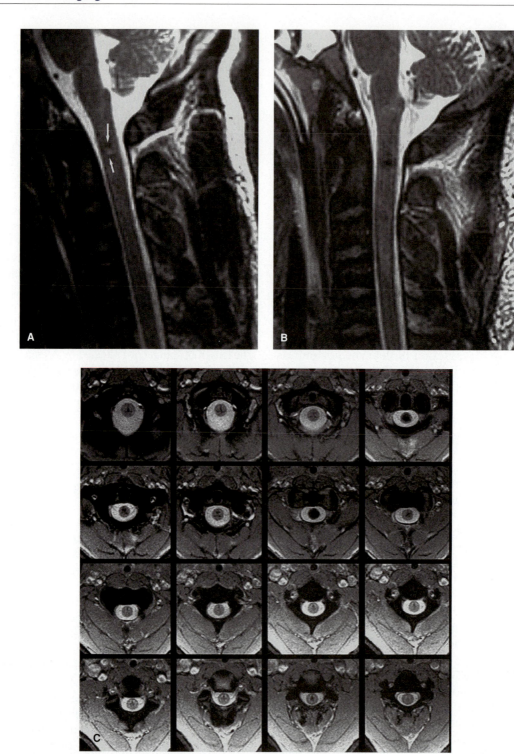

FIGURE 8-55. Hyperacute hemorrhage in high cervical cord trauma. **A:** Sagittal T2-weighted MR on admission. **B:** Sagittal T2-weighted MR 2 days later. **C:** Axial gradient echo images from cervicomedullary junction to midcervical spine. Initial MR (A) of cervical cord injury in football player showed small focus of hyperacute hemorrhage at C1-2 (*arrow*) and very subtle high-intensity edema. Two days later (B), more obvious edema extending down to C4 and clear hemorrhage in deoxyhemoglobin state is seen, particularly on axial GRE (C), where hemorrhage is noted within central portion of spinal cord. (From Flanders AE, Croul SE. Spinal trauma. In: Atlas SW. *Magnetic Resonance Imaging of the Brain and Spine*. 3rd ed. Philadelphia: Lippincott Williams & Wilkins; 2002:1805–1806, with permission.)

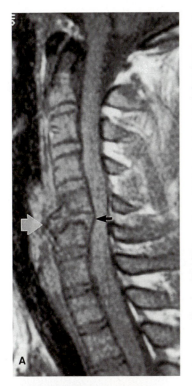
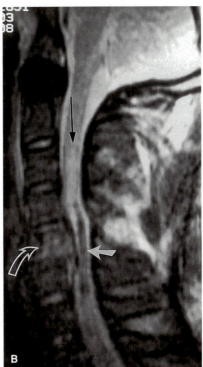
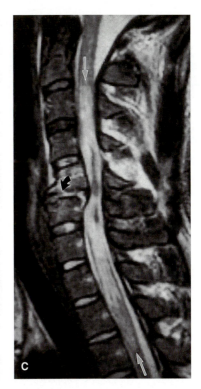

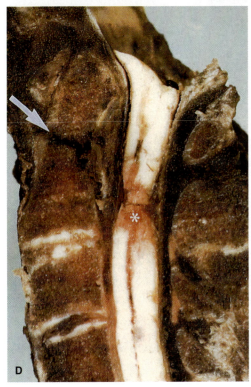

FIGURE 8-56. Hemorrhagic spinal cord injury. **A:** Sagittal SE T1-weighted image shows a flexion deformity centered at the C5-6 interspace (*white arrow*). There are fractures that extend through the inferior endplate of C5 and superior endplate of C6. Disc material is retropulsed into the anterior epidural space (*black arrow*). **B:** Sagittal SE T2-weighted image shows that the compressed marrow space of C5 reverts to hyperintensity (*open arrow*). A large hypointense focus of spinal cord hemorrhage (deoxyhemoglobin) is present extending from C4 to T1 (*white arrow*). The upper margin of spinal cord edema is indistinct (*black arrow*). **C:** Sagittal FSE T2-weighted image shows the injury with improved clarity due to increased matrix size and improved signal. This image shows interruption of the inferior endplate at C5 (*black arrow*). The upper and lower boundaries of the spinal cord edema are very distinct (*white arrows*). Note that the spinal cord hemorrhage is not as hypointense as it is in the SE image because of decreased magnetic susceptibility effects. **D:** This sagittal section of the cervical spine and cord was taken from a patient who died 3 hours after trauma. The odontoid process is fractured and displaced posteriorly (*arrow*). The cord is transected just caudal to the fracture with obvious tissue distortion and fresh hemorrhage (*asterisks*). Additional blood can be seen tracking centrally for several centimeters rostral and caudal to the transection. (Material courtesy of RO Weller MD, University of Southampton, UK, and Harvey Miller Publishers.) (From Flanders AE, Croul SE. Spinal trauma. In: Atlas SW. *Magnetic Resonance Imaging of the Brain and Spine*. 3rd ed. Philadelphia: Lippincott Williams & Wilkins; 2002:1788, with permission.)

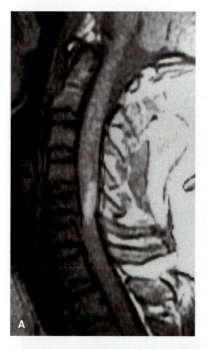
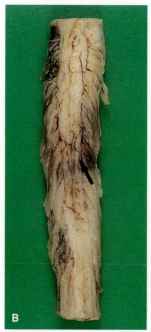
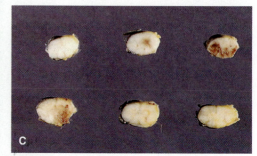
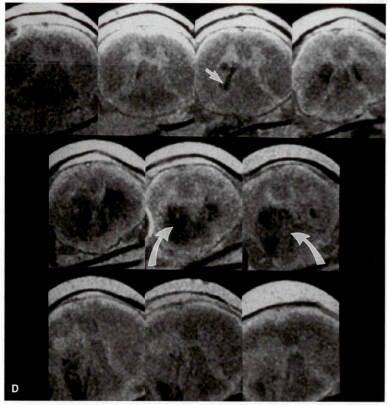

FIGURE 8-57. Methemoglobin in a 9-day-old spinal cord injury. **A:** Sagittal SE T1-weighted image demonstrates a markedly swollen spinal cord that effaces the surrounding subarachnoid space. There is associated herniation of disc material at C5-6. The large hyperintense focus within the spinal cord at the level of injury is methemoglobin. **B:** Cervical spinal cord from another patient who sustained a C6 lesion 1 week before demise. Dorsal view of the cord reveals a hematoma (*arrow*). **C:** Cross sections of the cord shown in (B) demonstrate extension of the contusion into the dorsal spinal white and gray. **D:** Serial axial T2-weighted SE images at 1.5 Tesla of specimen in (B) and (C) show well-demarcated areas of hypointense hemorrhage involving the central gray matter (*arrow*) as well as the surrounding white matter (*curved arrows*). (From Flanders AE, Croul SE. Spinal trauma. In: Atlas SW. *Magnetic Resonance Imaging of the Brain and Spine*. 3rd ed. Philadelphia: Lippincott Williams & Wilkins; 2002:1797, with permission.)

indicator of spinal cord dysfunction, it does not predict the extent of the parenchymal injury (8,64).

Clinical Measures of Spinal Cord Injury

The ASIA has devised standards for both neurologic and functional classification of spinal injuries (134). A standardized set of examination procedures allows the determination of sensory/motor deficits and a spinal level for the lesion. From these, a clinical spinal cord syndrome and an impairment scale are derived, including a measure of functional independence. The ASIA impairment scale is modified from Frankel (135,136) and is used to grade

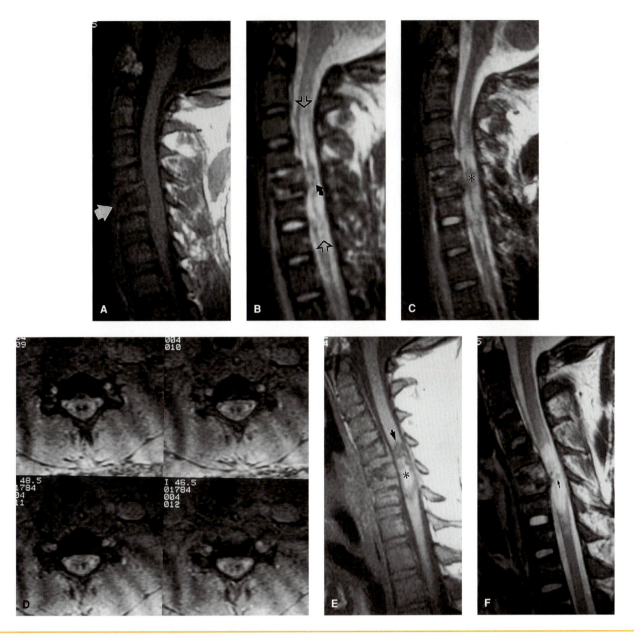

FIGURE 8-58. Evolution of intramedullary hemorrhage (18-year-old man). **A:** Sagittal T1-weighted image shows fracture deformity of C5 (*arrow*) with loss of height anteriorly. Extensive spinal cord swelling is present with effacement of the subarachnoid space. Note the lack of cord signal abnormality. **B:** Sagittal T2-weighted image shows a long segment of signal abnormality in the spinal cord. The hyperintensity that extends from C2 to T1 represents spinal cord edema (*open arrows*). The central focus of hypointensity centered at the C5 level is intramedullary hemorrhage (deoxyhemoglobin) (*curved arrow*). **C:** Sagittal FSE T2-weighted image also depicts the spinal cord signal abnormalities. Note that the intramedullary hemorrhage (*asterisk*) is not as hypointense as it is in (B). Acquisition time was half that of (B). **D:** Four 1.5-mm thick continuous axial images from a 3DFT GE sequence through the epicenter of the injury show discrete hypointense foci of hemorrhage within the central gray matter of the spinal cord. **E:** Sagittal T1-weighted image obtained 2 months after injury shows a well-defined area of cavitation within the still swollen spinal cord. The central portion of the cavity is now hyperintense (*asterisk*) from retained hemorrhagic breakdown products. The cavity is surrounded by a rind of myelo-malacia/gliosis (*arrow*). **F:** Sagittal FSE T2-weighted image shows the persistent swelling of the spinal cord. The necrotic cavity and malacic tissue are all hyperintense. Several discrete foci of low signal intensity are noted within the cavity (*arrow*) from hemorrhagic residue. (*continued*)

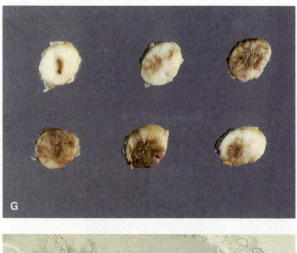
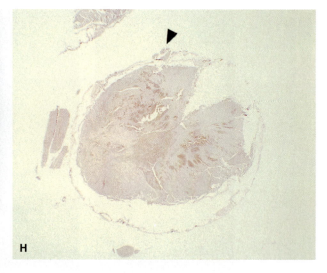
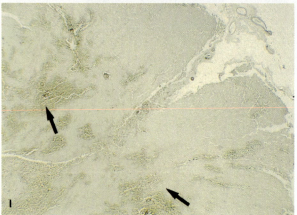

FIGURE 8-58. *(CONTINUED)* **G:** Sections of cervical spinal cord taken from a patient who died 6 days following a neurologically complete C6-7 anterior dislocation that did not come to medical attention immediately. Note that the hemorrhage occupies the complete extent of gray and white matter over several centimeters of spinal cord. **H:** Micrograph of spinal cord from case illustrated in (G). Even in this histologic preparation, the hemorrhage has distorted the spinal cord anatomy almost beyond recognition. For orientation, note preserved anterior spinal artery (*arrowhead*) (H and E). **I:** Impregnation for axons (Bodian stain). The axonal profiles (*arrows*) have been destroyed by the mechanical force of the cervical dislocation. Axonal profiles that would normally stain as black dots in white matter are not seen. Hemorrhage stains green in this preparation. (From Flanders AE, Croul SE. Spinal trauma. In: Atlas SW. *Magnetic Resonance Imaging of the Brain and Spine*. 3rd ed. Philadelphia: Lippincott Williams & Wilkins; 2002:1792,1803, with permission.)

the patient's overall degree of neurologic impairment due to the spinal lesion. Thus, complete (grade A) impairment connotes paralysis in the lower extremities and the absence of both sensation and motor function in the sacral segments S4-5. Incomplete impairment (grades B,C,D) ranges from preserved sensation without motor function below the level of the lesion (grade B) to preserved sensation with motor function approximating normal below the level of the lesion (grade D). Normal sensory and motor function is graded E. (For more detailed discussion, see Chapter 2.)

Lesions of the spinal cord have been classically divided into five classic neuroanatomic syndromes: anterior cord, central cord, Brown-Séquard, conus medullaris, and cauda equina.

Anterior cord syndrome most commonly results from occlusion of the anterior spinal artery (Fig. 8-60) (137–140). In the setting of trauma, processes that collapse a vertebral body with resultant canal compromise and compression of the cord may also result in this syndrome, probably on the basis of vascular insufficiency either from interruption of the arterial supply or from intrinsic changes to the vascular supply due to secondary injury. Patients experience profound loss of motor function and interruption of pain and temperature sensation below the level of lesion. There is relative preservation of vibration and position sense. Since the anterior two thirds of the spinal cord is supplied by the anterior spinal artery, this syndrome correlates anatomically with damage to the corticospinal and lateral spinothalamic tracts with relative sparing of the posterior columns.

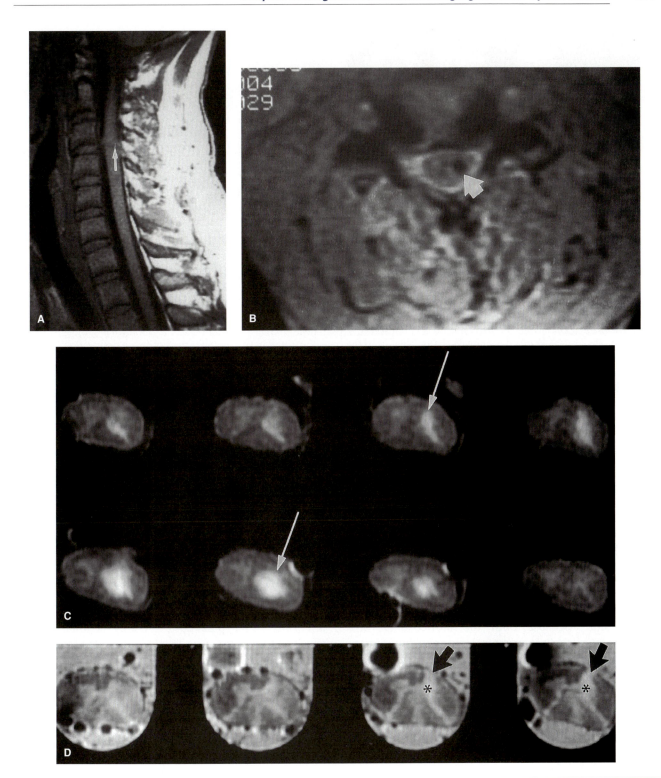

FIGURE 8-59. Brown-Séquard syndrome. **A:** Sagittal T1-weighted image shows an obliquely oriented hypointense band that traverses the width of the spinal cord between C3 and C4 (*arrow*), which represents the path of a knife blade. There is a mild degree of cord swelling at this level. **B:** Axial GE 3DFT in another patient shows a discrete hypointense focus in the central gray matter of the spinal cord on the left side (*arrow*) representing deoxyhemoglobin. **C:** Serial axial T1-weighted images of a human spinal cord specimen at 1.5 Tesla with a Brown-Séquard lesion. A focal area of hyperintensity is noted within the central gray matter on the left side secondary to hemorrhage (methemoglobin). **D:** Serial axial intermediate-weighted FSE images show abnormal morphology of the central gray matter on the left (*asterisks*). Tissue damage extends into the ventral white matter approximating the spinothalamic tracts (*arrow*). (Multiple magnetic susceptibility artifacts are present surrounding the specimen presumably from air bubbles in solution during preparation.) (*continued*)

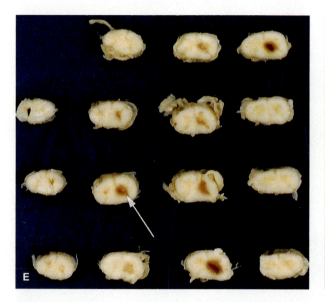 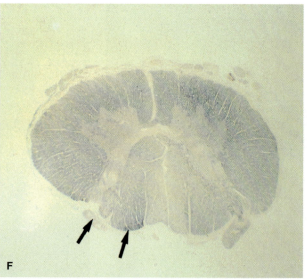

FIGURE 8-59. *(CONTINUED)* **E:** Gross specimen of (C) and (D). Note the asymmetrical hemorrhagic lesion involving the gray matter (*arrow*). **F:** Photomicrograph of a stained section taken from the case illustrated in (E). Note the area of tissue destruction in the left dorsal horn and dorsal columns (*arrows*). Although the lesion was hemorrhagic, the blood pigments fail to show with this method (Luxol fast blue). (From Flanders AE, Croul SE. Spinal trauma. In: Atlas SW. *Magnetic Resonance Imaging of the Brain and Spine.* 3rd ed. Philadelphia: Lippincott Williams & Wilkins; 2002:1804–1805, with permission.)

The *central cord syndrome* (141–143) is characterized by greater weakness in the arms than the legs, with sparing of sacral sensation. Patients with cervical spondylosis/stenosis are predisposed to central cord injuries (Figs. 8-27, 8-28, 8-52) (24). The proposed mechanism of injury suggests that the spinal cord is pinched between a dorsally displaced vertebral body and a buckled ligamentum flavum during hyperextension (144). Other authors describe central cord syndrome in association with disc herniations (60). The underlying pathology consists of contusion, hemorrhage, or necrosis of the central cervical gray matter. Because both the corticospinal and spinothalamic tracts in primates, and probably in man, are laminated such that the most rostral projections are most medial, central damage in the cervical cord would predict injury to the cervical laminations with sparing of the sacral laminations, resulting in the characteristic pattern of deficit. Recent work questions this traditional view. One study described 11 cases of acute central cord syndrome, nine of which had MRI correlation and three of which had pathologic examination (145). Blood or blood products were not found by imaging or pathology in any of these cases. In all cases, the most severe changes occurred in the white matter and included demyelination with or without axonal loss. No necrotic lesions were reported in the central gray matter. Since these findings are at variance with what has been previously accepted, they challenge other investigators to attempt independent confirmation.

The *Brown-Séquard syndrome* is due to a purely unilateral transverse lesion above midlumbar spinal cord levels. Probably the most common type of trauma associated with this syndrome is penetrating injury to the spinal cord (146,147) (Figs. 8-59, 8-61). The resultant loss of proprioception and motor control ipsilateral to the lesion reflects damage to the corticospinal tract and posterior columns on the side of the lesion, whereas contralateral loss of sensitivity to pain and temperature is due to damage to the crossing spinothalamic tracts.

Traumatic lesions of the lower spinal canal rarely affect the sacral spinal cord or conus medullaris exclusively, but they may also damage the surrounding cauda equina (148,149). Damage to the sacral spinal segments alone produces a pure *conus medullaris syndrome* resulting in an areflexic bladder, fecal incontinence, and saddle anesthesia (Fig. 8-62). Additional cauda equina injury may result in a variable degree of flaccid paralysis in the legs with accompanying multimodal sensory loss. Lesions that occur higher in the sacral cord may effectively isolate the distal-most cord, and thus these injuries exhibit preservation of bowel, bladder, and genital reflexes with loss of motor function in the lower extremities.

Injuries below the level of the sacral segments cause a pure *cauda equina syndrome* (Fig. 8-63). Damage to lumbosacral nerve roots results in flaccid paralysis of the bowel, bladder, and legs. All forms of sensory input are also affected. The cauda equina is said to be more resistant to trauma than the spinal cord and certainly shows a

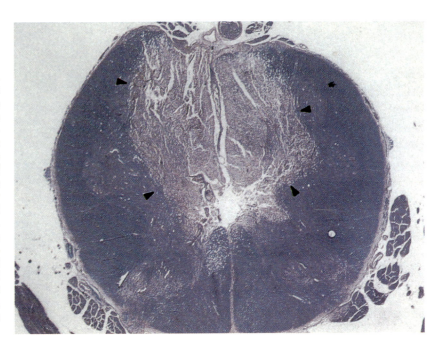

FIGURE 8-60. Anterior cord syndrome. The ventral aspect of the spinal cord shows infarction with necrosis (*arrowheads*). In this case, the most medial portions of the anterior horns bear the brunt of the injury with relative preservation of the remainder of the anterior circulation. Quite often, the area of damage spreads more laterally to involve the entire anterior horn and the white matter comprising spinothalamic and corticospinal tracts. (Luxol fast blue–periodic acid Schiff. Material courtesy of A Hirano, MD, Division of Neuropathology Montefiore Medical Center, Bronx, NY and Igaku-Shoin Publishers.) (From Flanders AE, Croul SE. Spinal trauma. In: Atlas SW. *Magnetic Resonance Imaging of the Brain and Spine*. 3rd ed. Philadelphia: Lippincott Williams & Wilkins; 2002:1807, with permission.)

greater propensity for recovery. The fact that it is composed of peripheral nerve roots rather than central nervous system tissue may account for its resistance to injury. Nerve roots are ensheathed by a substrate that includes fibrous tissue; this covering renders them more resistant to trauma than the spinal cord. The fact that peripheral axons are myelinated by Schwann cells rather than the oligodendrocytes found in the spinal white matter is a major factor that accounts for the unique ability of peripheral nerves to regenerate following trauma. Following injury to the cauda equina, Schwann cells provide a substrate for axonal elongation, thus setting the stage for restitution of the peripheral nerves and neurologic recovery.

Atypical mechanisms of SCI produce different patterns of MRI including penetrating trauma (e.g., knife wounds or gun shot injuries) (Figs. 8-59, 8-61, 8-64). Although physiologic transection of the spinal cord is typical of severe blunt injury, complete mechanical transection (i.e., separation of the spinal cord into two or more pieces) is uncommon and is usually secondary to a high-velocity motor vehicle accidents that produce marked translocation at a segmental level. Aside from the mechanical separation of the spinal cord fragments, the degree of injury to the preserved adjacent parenchyma is often less than that observed with injuries associated with intact spinal cords (Fig. 8-65).

The functional independence measure (FIM) (150–152) more fully defines the impact of SCI on the daily activities of the individual and serves as a benchmark against which to evaluate spontaneous or treatment-associated changes in overall function. By focusing on 18 items in six areas of function (self-care, sphincter control, mobility, locomotion, communication, and social cognition) a 7-point scale is constructed ranging from complete independence [7] to total assistance [1] for each item. The total score summed across all items gives a more complete estimate of total disability (see Chapter 2).

Clinical Significance of the Spinal Cord Magnetic Resonance Imaging Findings

Many clinical investigations have reported that the MRI patterns of SCI correlate with the neurologic deficit at presentation (7–9,61,64,67,119,131). Kulkarni et al. (9) initially proposed three MRI injury patterns for SCI and correlated these with the five-part ASIA impairment scale and total motor scores. Intramedullary hemorrhage (type I pattern of injury) equated with a severe neurologic deficit and a poor prognosis. Cord edema alone (type II pattern of injury) was found in patients with mild to moderate initial neurologic deficits who subsequently showed neurologic improvement (7,9,67,119,131).

Schaefer et al. (61) refined the MRI patterns of SCI by including the size of the injured segment. Cord edema that extended for more than the span of one vertebral segment was associated with a more severe initial deficit than smaller areas of edema. Cord hemorrhage was associated with the most severe neurologic abnormalities.

Flanders et al. (8) demonstrated that spinal cord hemorrhage in the cervical region was a strong predictive finding for a complete neurologic injury. The location of the hemorrhage corresponded anatomically to the level of neurologic injury. Although the location of spinal cord edema related imprecisely to the neurologic level, the

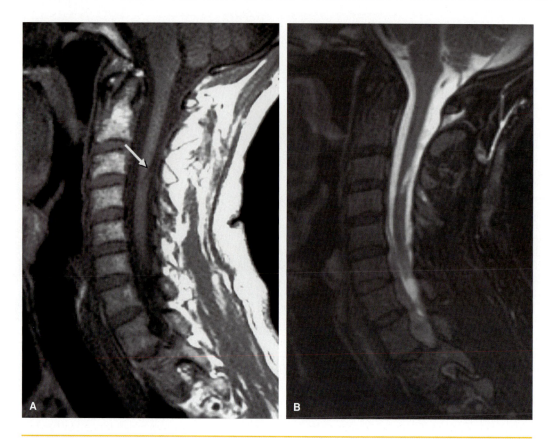

FIGURE 8-61. Chronic brown-sequard injury from stab wound to neck 32 years prior. **A:** Sagittal T1-weighted MRI shows a well-defined, low signal intensity cleft that obliquely traverses the left half of the spinal cord (*arrow*). **B:** Lesion reverts to hyperintensity on this corresponding T2-weighted, fat-suppressed image.

proportion of spinal cord affected by edema was directly related to the severity of initial neurologic injury. The presence of vertebral body fractures, disc herniation, and ligamentous injury was not predictive of the neurologic deficit; however, the presence of residual spinal cord compression by bone, disc, or fluid was predictive of a hemorrhagic spinal cord lesion located at the level of the compression. This latter finding supports the controversial concept of early decompressive surgery for SCI patients (8,12,63).

The imaging changes observed in the spinal cord parenchyma with MRI show a close correlation with the initial neurologic deficit. Furthermore, substantial evidence suggests that these MRI changes offer prognostic information regarding neurologic recovery (7,9,20,44, 64,67,113,115,118,119,131,132,142,153,154). Yamashita et al. (153,154) showed that poor recovery from SCI was associated with severe cord compression, cord swelling, and abnormal signal on T1-weighted and T2-weighted images. Moreover, patients with persistent signal changes in the spinal cord on follow-up MRI examinations demonstrated little or no clinical improvement, whereas prognosis was improved for patients who demonstrated resolu-

tion of signal abnormalities. The authors categorized MRI spinal cord injury patterns into five types. Signal patterns that correlate with the best prognosis include normal spinal cord signal or hyperintensity on T2-weighted images (intramedullary edema). Hypo- or hyperintensity on T1-weighted images with hyperintense parenchyma on T2-weighted images is a poor prognostic indicator (44,64,113,119,153,154). In two very similar studies, Shimada et al. (44,113) showed that persistent signal changes in the spinal cord on serial MRI studies were associated with no significant clinical improvement, whereas marked improvement in neurologic status was found in the subset of patients whose MRI studies became normal.

In an experimental model of SCI that included serial MRI studies, Ohta et al. (114) demonstrated results that validate similar results reported in clinical studies. Two types of paralysis were induced in rats using a weight-drop model (20 and 35 gm respectively) resulting in a transient and persistent motor paralysis. The animals were imaged and motor strength was tested two and 28 days after induction of the injury. The animals with the milder injury showed significant improvement in motor function after 28 days. Spinal cord edema was identified

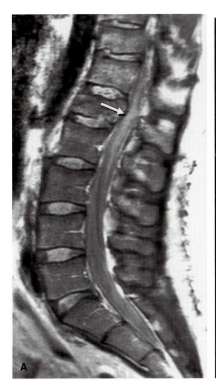
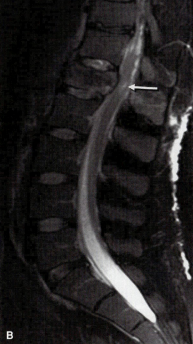
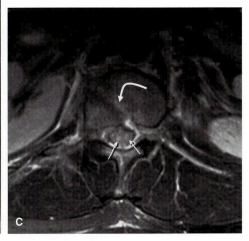

FIGURE 8-62. A 33-year-old male presenting with a conus medullaris syndrome from a L1 burst fracture. **A:** Sagittal intermediate-weighted image shows loss of stature of the L1 vertebral body secondary to a burst fracture. There is failure of the middle column and buckling of the posterior cortex into the spinal canal (*arrow*). **B:** Sagittal T2-weighted, fat-suppressed image shows a subtle focus of signal abnormality in the distal thoracic spinal cord (*arrow*) representing subacute, posttraumatic edema. **C:** Axial T2-weighted, fat-suppressed image obtained at the L1 level shows the oblique fracture line (*curved arrow*). There is a subtle increased signal intensity originating from the central gray matter of the conus medullaris (*paired white arrows*) indicative of posttraumatic edema.

on the initial and final MRI studies that corresponded histologically to edema and reactive gliosis. The subset of animals with the severe injury featured a central focus of hemorrhage surrounded by edema on the T2-weighted images on the initial MRI study. Low signal was observed on the T1-weighted images on the final study suggesting cavitation. Histologically, this injury resulted in hemorrhages, cavitation, and reactive gliosis. This supports the contention that identification of hemorrhage on MRI after SCI is an indicator of poor recovery.

Silberstein et al. (64) found that the presence of associated spinal fractures, subluxation, ligamentous injury, prevertebral swelling, and epidural hematoma was associated with a more severe clinical deficit at presentation and a poorer prognosis. All these associated imaging features suggested that residual spinal cord compression may be an important factor in determining poor neurologic recovery. Other investigators have not found a relationship between residual spinal cord compression and initial neurologic deficit or neurologic recovery (60).

Schaefer et al. (117) correlated the MRI appearance of the spinal cord on admission to the change in total motor index score (MIS) in 57 patients. Patients with hemor-

rhagic spinal cord lesions showed no statistical improvement in motor index score at follow-up. The group of patients with small areas of edema (less than one vertebral segment in length) demonstrated the largest improvement in MIS (72% recovery), whereas larger areas of edema showed intermediate recovery of MIS (42%).

In a similar study, Marciello et al. (115) compared the presence or absence of intramedullary hemorrhage to change in individual motor scores for the upper and lower extremities in 24 subjects. For patients with spinal cord hemorrhage, only 16% of muscles in the upper extremities and 3% of muscles in the lower extremities improved to a useful grade (>3/5) at follow-up and only 7% improved one or more motor levels. For patients without MRI evidence of spinal cord hemorrhage, 73% of upper extremity and 74% of lower extremity muscles improved to useful grade and 78% of subjects improved one or more motor levels.

In a subsequent comprehensive study, Flanders et al. (116) assessed the prognostic capabilities of MRI in forecasting motor recovery in 104 cervical SCI patients. Individual manual muscle test scores were compiled for the upper and lower extremities both at the time of admission

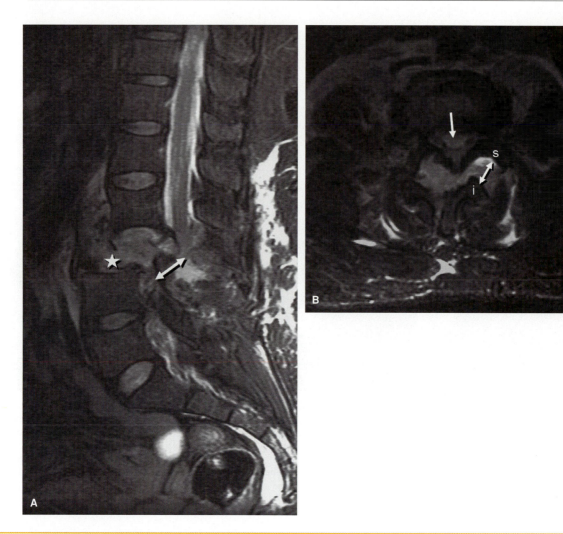

FIGURE 8-63. Cauda equina syndrome from translocation at the L3 level resulting from a high-speed motor vehicle accident. **A:** Sagittal T2-weighted, fat-suppressed image shows complete disruption of the L3 vertebral body and adjacent interspaces (*asterisk*) with translocation of the L3 and L4 vertebral segments. There is complete loss of continuity of the spinal canal (*double arrow*). **B:** Axial T2-weighted, fat-suppressed image obtained at the L3-4 level shows the markedly distracted left L4 superior articular process (*s*) and the inferior articular process of L3 (*i*). A large amount of hemorrhage fills the potential space. No recognizable components of the cauda equine are visible in the canal (*arrow*).

and 12 months after injury. A motor recovery rate for the upper and lower extremities was also determined. The injured spinal cord segment on MRI was measured using a unique method that quantified spinal cord hemorrhage and edema by length and location relative to known anatomic landmarks. Lesion length was directly proportional to neurologic impairment at the time of injury ($p <.001$). In addition, spinal cord hemorrhage was associated with the most severe injuries ($p <.001$). Although improvement in motor function after one year was observed in all patients, subjects with spinal cord hemorrhage on MRI had lower initial motor scores and had less improvement than those without hemorrhage. Nonhemorrhagic MRI lesions were associated with significantly higher motor recovery rates in the lower and upper extremities and had a higher proportion of useful muscle

function. Multiple regression analysis was used to determine the contribution of MRI in predicting the outcome parameters of motor function independent of the initial clinical evaluation. Initial motor scores, the presence of hemorrhage, and the length of edema were independent predictors of final motor score and the proportion of muscles with useful function at one year. The addition of the MRI parameters to the initial clinical information improved the statistical power of the SCI model by 16% for the upper extremities and 34% for the lower extremities.

In a similar study of 55 cervical SCI patients, Selden et al. (154) identified four MRI characteristics that were significant negative prognosticators of neurological recovery as measured by the ASIA grade that were independent from the initial clinical examination: presence of spinal cord hemorrhage, length of spinal cord

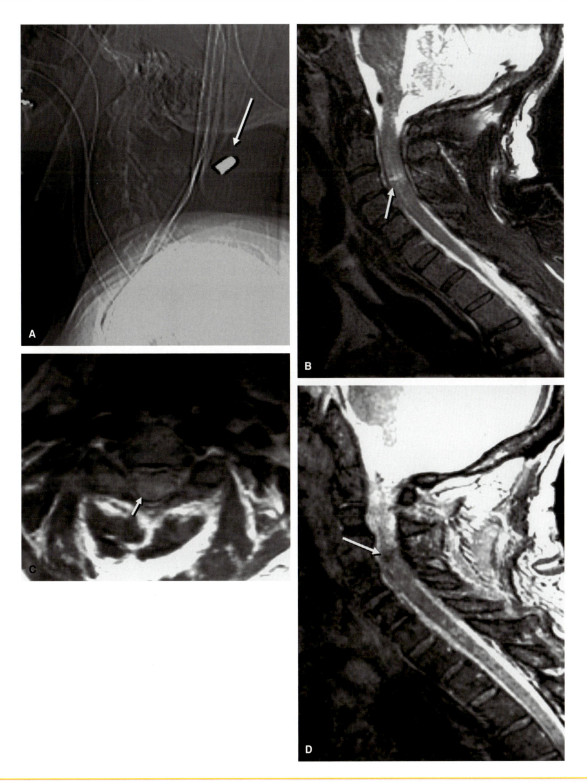

FIGURE 8-64. High cervical SCI secondary to gunshot wound that has traversed the spinal canal. **A:** Lateral digital radiograph shows an intact bullet fragment lodged in the posterior cervical soft tissues whose trajectory has passed through the upper cervical canal. **B:** Sagittal T2-weighted MRI with fat suppression shows a linear focus of signal abnormality traversing the cervical spinal cord at the C3 level (*arrow*). **C:** Axial intermediate weighted MRI obtained at the C3 level shows a markedly enlarged spinal cord with loss of internal features related to diffuse edema (*arrow*). **D:** Sagittal gradient echo MRI reveals a focus of low signal intensity at the injured level (*arrow*) as a result of the paramagnetic effects of hemorrhage. Note the relative absence of artifact from the bullet fragment on all imaging sequences. Also recognize that the severity of the injury on MRI is disproportionately small in spite of the amount of direct trauma to the spinal cord.

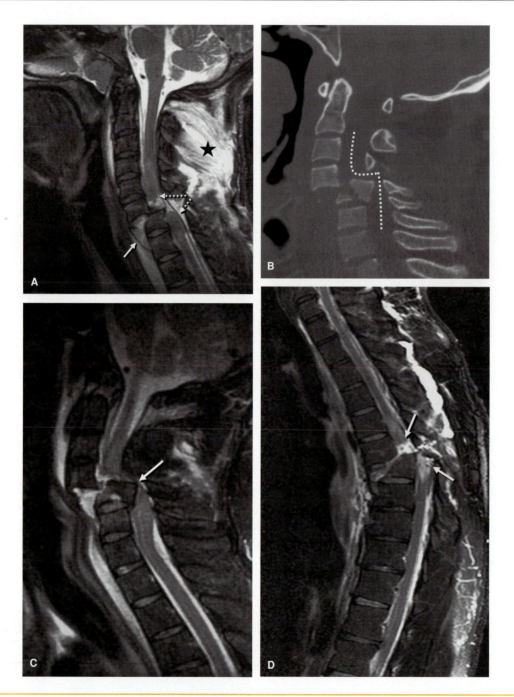

FIGURE 8-65. Mechanical transection of the spinal cord. **A:** Sagittal T2-weighted MRI of the cervical spine shows a complete disassociation of the C6 and C7 segments with disruption of the intervertebral disc and elevation of the ALL (*arrow*). The bulbous segments of the separated spinal cord are identified showing minimal intrinsic edema (*dotted arrows*). The entire posterior ligamentous complex is disrupted as well (*asterisk*). **B:** Midcervical translocation. Sagittal CT MPR image in another patient shows complete separation of the C4 and C5 vertebral segments with complete obliteration of the spinal canal secondary to the degree of subluxation (*dotted line*). **C:** Sagittal T2-weighted MRI corresponding to (B) confirms the mechanical transection of the spinal cord by the corner of the dorsally displaced C5 fragment that obliterates the spinal canal (*arrow*). **D:** Midthoracic translocation in another patient who was thrown from a motorcycle. Sagittal T2-weighted MRI with fat suppression shows the acute angulation and malalignment of the T7 and T8 segments with disruption of the all of the ligamentous complexes. The severed ends of the spinal cord are widened and edematous (*arrows*).

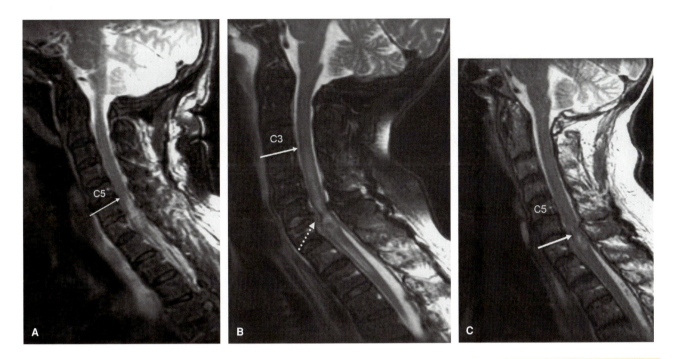

FIGURE 8-66. Transient ascension in neurologic level of injury (NLI) and therapeutic recovery correlated with MRI in a 68-year-old SCI patient. **A:** Sagittal T2-weighted MRI at the date of injury shows the upper boundary of spinal cord edema approximating the C5-6 interspace (C5 NLI). **B:** Spontaneous ascent in NLI to the C3 level, three days after admission. Repeat T2-weighted MRI shows that the edema now extends cephalad to approximately the C3-4 interspace and caudad to the T2-3 interspace. Note the disc herniation at the C6-7 level (*dotted arrow*). **C:** Marked reduction in lesion length after administration of high dose methylprednisolone. Sagittal T2-weighted image obtained ten days after steroid administration show reduction in spinal cord lesion which now is improved from the initial study. Patient's NLI also descended to C6 commensurate with the MRI findings.

hemorrhage, length of spinal cord edema, and spinal cord compression.

In a subsequent prognostic study, Flanders et al. (155) compared the MRI parameters of edema and hemorrhage to a standardized measurement of disability (the FIM). Four distinct motor scales from the FIM assessment were determined at the time of admission to rehabilitation and subsequently at discharge from rehabilitation. The individual motor scales included tasks related to self-care, sphincter control, mobility, and locomotion. Patients without spinal cord hemorrhage on MRI had significant improvement in self-care and mobility scores compared to patients with hemorrhage. The upper limit of the lesion (edema) correlated with admission and discharge self-care, admission mobility, and locomotion scores. Edema length correlated negatively with all FIM scores at admission and discharge. Moreover, at the time of admission to rehabilitation, all patients were completely dependant on equipment or caregivers to perform the FIM tasks. At the time of discharge, *only* patients with nonhemorrhagic MRI lesions improved to a modified dependence category.

Another clinical parameter that has tremendous bearing on neurologic function and potential for recovery is the neurologic level of injury (NLI). The NLI is deter-

mined by assessing the motor power and sensory function for myotomes and dermatomes that are innervated by adjacent spinal cord segments. By definition, the most caudal intact myotome or sensory dermatome is used to determine the NLI. Due to the linear organizational structure of the spinal cord, the NLI ascertained by clinical examination determines (by inference) the location of the lesion in the spinal cord. Since abnormal spinal cord tissue on MRI correlates with physiologic dysfunction, the anatomic location of the MRI relates to the NLI; the higher the signal changes on MRI extends up the spinal cord, the higher the NLI (Fig. 8-66).

Boghosian et al. (156) correlated the NLI with the anatomic location of the spinal cord lesions on the MRIs of 109 cervical spinal cord injured patients. The authors found a statistically significant correlation between the location of the upper margin of spinal cord edema and hemorrhage as well as the lesion epicenter. The upper boundary of hemorrhage showed a stronger correlation than either edema or lesion epicenter. The lesion length showed no statistical significance with NLI. Use of multiple regression analysis showed that the combination of lesion epicenter and edema length were the best predictors of NLI. Therefore, MRI measures may be used as an objective measure of the NLI when determination by clinical examination is either inaccurate or unavailable.

Recently, Boldin et al. (157) published a small prospective series of 29 SCI patients that compared an absolute measurement of the size of the injured segment on a postoperative MRI to the initial clinical examination and changes in long-term neurologic status. The authors also found that the presence of intramedullary hemorrhage had a higher association with a complete neurologic deficit and that patients with hemorrhages that measured greater than 4 mm in cranial-caudal length showed no clinical improvement at follow-up. Both the length of edema and hemorrhage were shown to be predictive variables for complete injuries. Patients with hemorrhages measuring <4 mm had incomplete injuries upon admission and showed clinical improvement at follow-up. Although their patient cohort was small and the authors were unable to control for time to clinical follow-up or time to imaging, their data suggest that there may be an absolute threshold for lesion size that predicts neurologic recovery.

In the only major study that minimizes the value of MRI in predicting neurologic recovery after SCI, Shepard and Bracken (158) compared the results of MRI studies in 191 cervical SCI patients from multiple institutions to motor and sensory evaluations obtained at admission and six weeks after injury. The authors reported no statistical difference in the presence of contusions or edema between complete and incomplete injuries. MRI studies that featured hemorrhage or contusion were more likely to be associated with lower initial motor, pain, and touch scores. Motor function recovery parameters were less in patients showing hemorrhage, contusion, and edema on MRI; however, the differences were not statistically significant. After controlling for the results of the initial clinical assessment, the authors found no added value of the MRI findings (cord hemorrhage, contusion, and edema) in predicting neurologic recovery. The validity of this ambitious study is questionable, especially in consideration of the number of other investigations that contradict these results. Although data from a large cohort of patients were collected for this study, there was no actual central review of *any* of the MRI examinations. The imaging protocol, scanner field strength, and overall image quality was not controlled for or assessed and the definitions of criteria of contusion, edema, and hemorrhage were never established.

Although there is an apparent relationship between spinal cord compression and neurologic injury, the methods for characterizing spinal cord compression, reduction in canal diameter following injury, and their relationship to neurologic deficit are inconsistent. Fehlings et al. (159) provided a critical, evidence-based analysis of existing radiologic literature that correlated the degree of posttraumatic spinal cord compression to neurologic deficit.

The studies that were evaluated contained both quantitative and qualitative assessments of spinal canal and spinal cord dimensions. Pre-existing midsagittal canal stenosis (developmental or congenital stenosis) was generally associated with more severe neurologic deficit following injury, notably when the midsagittal diameter of the spinal canal was 10 mm or less. There was a direct relationship between the severity of congenital stenosis (as defined by the Torg ratio) and the degree of neurologic function after injury in at least one study. The anteroposterior diameter of the spinal canal was significantly smaller in patients with complete injuries (10.5 mm) and in incomplete injuries (13.1 mm) compared to canal diameters in patients with no deficits (159). The sensitivity and specificity of canal diameter measurements to neurologic symptoms was high. In another study, Hayashi et al. (20) found that 30% of patients with severe spinal cord compression (defined as a two-thirds reduction in spinal cord diameter) had a complete motor deficit at the time of injury compared to 20% of patients with mild spinal cord compression (defined as less than one-third reduction in spinal cord diameter). More importantly, 90% of patients with mild spinal cord compression improved by one or more ASIA grades compared to 30% for patients with severe spinal cord compression.

Fehlings et al. (159) developed a standardized method for measuring midsagittal spinal canal compromise and spinal cord compression that is applicable to both CT and MRI. The authors found excellent agreement with CT and T1-weighted MRI images in determining canal compromise following injury. T2-weighted sagittal MRI provided the most reliable assessment of spinal cord compression. CT alone was a relatively poor predictor of spinal cord compression (98% specificity and 72% sensitivity). Overestimation of canal compromise occurred with MRI; however, agreement between CT and MRI in assessing canal narrowing in patients with pre-existent spondylosis was excellent. Spinal canal compromise on CT by 25% or more was 100% specific for spinal cord compression on MRI. The authors also identified a statistically significant difference in neurologic deficit for patients with and without spinal cord compression or spinal canal compromise.

EFFECTS OF METHYLPREDNISOLONE ON THE MAGNETIC RESONANCE IMAGING FINDINGS OF SPINAL CORD INJURY

Although there are several phase I clinical trials in progress for SCI, the only sanctioned medical therapy for SCI is the administration of high dose methylprednisolone (MPS) given within an 8-hour window after injury (161–163). Although the efficacy of MPS for SCI remains controversial, the drug is currently used

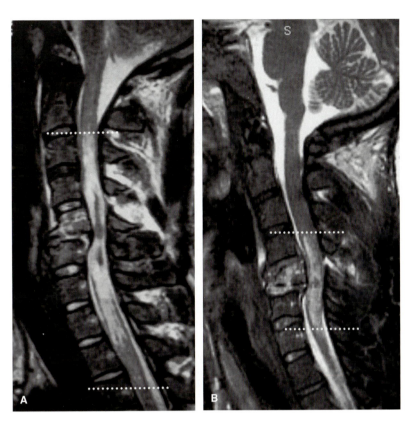

FIGURE 8-67. Difference in lesion morphology for two SCI patients with similar neurologic deficit (C5 ASIA A). **A:** T2-weighted sagittal MRI in a 20-year-old male not treated with MPS. **B:** T2-weighted sagittal MRI in a 29-year-old, MPS-treated SCI patient. Note that the overall lesion length and hemorrhage length is less in the MPS treated patient (*dotted lines*).

empirically at many trauma centers in the United States for this purpose. Moreover, while there is some experimental evidence that MPS can decrease the development intraparenchymal hemorrhage in a rodent model, there has been no direct evidence that a similar effect occurs in humans (164). Leypold et al. (165) recently compared the MRI findings of two cohorts of patients with ASIA type A injuries (motor and sensory complete); one group had received MPS within the therapeutic window prior to imaging and the other group did not receive steroids. The two groups were compared for the presence or absence of hemorrhage, the size of the hemorrhage, and the size of the surrounding edema. Multiple regression analysis was used to control for the effects of patient age, level of injury, and time period between injury and MRI as all three of these variables were found to have significant effects on edema length (Fig. 8-67). After correcting for these factors, it was determined that MPS administration did not have a significant effect on the mean length of spinal cord edema between treated and untreated subjects. However, there was a statistically significant difference in hemorrhage length between the treated and untreated groups and a larger proportion of treated patients had no evidence of hemorrhage in their lesions compared to the untreated group (not statistically significant). MPS could reduce the length of hemorrhage (on average) the equivalent of one half of a vertebral body height.

Several additional observations were derived from this data set: Age was noted to have a significant effect on presence/absence of intramedullary hemorrhage and on edema length. That is, the findings were more prevalent in younger patients. Alternatively, age had minimal effects on hemorrhage length. In addition, there was a significant relationship between the injury to imaging time interval and the length of the edema, such that a lesion would enlarge the equivalent of one third of a vertebral body height for every eight hours. This suggests that the MR lesion created in SCI is dynamic. This may be due in part to the evolution of the secondary phase of injury (166).

CONCLUSIONS

MRI has matured from a scientific curiosity to an essential part of the clinical armamentarium for assessment of the spinal injured patient. Although the traditional radiographic assessment and classification systems of spinal injury remain useful, MRI has eclipsed these other imaging methods because of its unique ability to demonstrate the soft tissue components of injury. In this regard, MRI is still the only imaging method that provides an objective assessment of the damaged spinal cord's internal architecture. As we look to the future, with implementation of novel medical and surgical therapies for spinal cord injury, MRI will continue to play an intimate role in the assessment of the SCI patient.

ACKNOWLEDGMENTS

We thank John F. Ditunno MD and Mary Patrick RN for their continuing support and critical input and the Regional Spinal Cord Injury Center of the Delaware Valley for clinical support.

REFERENCES

1. Allen BL, Ferguson RL, Lehmann TR, et al. A mechanistic classification of closed, indirect fractures and dislocations of the lower cervical spine. *Spine*. 1982;7(1):1–27.
2. McArdle CB, Crofford MJ, Mirfakhraee M, et al. Surface coil MRI of spinal trauma: preliminary experience. *Am J Neuroradiol*. 1986;7(5):885–893.
3. Weirich SD, Cotler HB, Narayana PA, et al. Histopathologic correlation of magnetic resonance imaging signal patterns in a spinal cord injury model. *Spine*. 1990;15(7): 630–638.
4. Wittenberg RH, Boetel U, Beyer HK. Magnetic resonance imaging and computed tomography of acute spinal cord trauma. *Clin Orthop*. 1990;260:176–185.
5. Chakeres DW, Flickinger F, Bresnahan JC, et al. MRI imaging of acute spinal cord trauma. *Am J Neuroradiol*. 1987;8(1):5–10.
6. Robertson PA, Ryan MD. Neurological deterioration after reduction of cervical subluxation; mechanical compression by disc tissue. *J Bone Joint Surg Br*. 1992;74B: 224–227.
7. Bondurant FJ, Cotler HB, Kulkarni MV, et al. Acute spinal cord injury. A study using physical examination and magnetic resonance imaging. *Spine*. 1990;15(3):161–168.
8. Flanders AE, Schaefer DM, Doan HT, et al. Acute cervical spine trauma: correlation of MRI imaging findings with degree of neurologic deficit. *Radiology*. 1990;177(1):25–33.
9. Kulkarni MV, McArdle CB, Kopanicky D, et al. Acute spinal cord injury: MRI imaging at 1.5T. *Radiology*. 1987;164(3):837–843.
10. Mirvis SE, Geisler FH, Jelinek JJ, et al. Acute cervical spine trauma: evaluation with 1.5-T MRI imaging. *Radiology*. 1988;166(3):807–816.
11. Tracy PT, Wright RM, Hanigan WC. Magnetic resonance imaging of spinal injury. *Spine*. 1989;14(3):292–301.
12. Beers GJ, Raque GH, Wagner GG, et al. MRI imaging in acute cervical spine trauma. *J Comput Assist Tomogr*. 1988;12(5):755–761.
13. Goldberg AL, Daffner RH, Schapiro RL. Imaging of acute spinal trauma: an evolving multi-modality approach. *Clin Imag*. 1990;14(1):11–16.
14. Flanders AE, Tartaglino LM, Friedman DP, et al. Magnetic resonance imaging in acute spinal injury. *Semin Roentgenol*. 1992;27(4):271–298.
15. Sett P, Crockard HA. The value of magnetic resonance imaging (MRI) in the follow-up management of spinal injury. *Paraplegia*. 1991;29(6):396–410.
16. Kerslake RW, Jaspan T, Worthington BS. Magnetic resonance imaging of spinal trauma. *Br J Radiol*. 1991;64: 386–402.
17. Goldberg AL, Rothfus WE, Deeb ZL, et al. The impact of magnetic resonance on the diagnostic evaluation of acute cervicothoracic spinal trauma. *Skeletal Radiol*. 1988;17(2): 89–95.
18. Kalfas I, Wilberger J, Goldberg A, et al. Magnetic resonance imaging in acute spinal cord trauma. *Neurosurgery*. 1988;23(3):295–299.
19. Larsson EM, Holtas S, Cronqvist S. Emergency magnetic resonance examination of patients with spinal cord symptoms. *Acta Radiol*. 1988;29(1):69–75.
20. Hayashi K, Yone K, Ito H, et al. MRI findings in patients with a cervical spinal cord injury who do not show radiographic evidence of a fracture or dislocation. *Paraplegia*. 1995;33(4):212–215.
21. Riviello JJ, Marks HG, Faerber EN, et al. Delayed cervical central cord syndrome after trivial trauma. *Pediatr Emerg Care*. 1990;6(2):113–117.
22. Pang D, Wilberger JE. Spinal cord injury without radiographic abnormalities in children. *J Neurosurg*. 1982;57:114–129.
23. Mendelsohn DB, Zollars L, Weatherall PT, et al. MRI of cord transection. *J Comput Assist Tomogr*. 1990;14(6): 909–911.
24. Goldberg AL, Rothfus WE, Deeb ZL, et al. Hyperextension injuries of the cervical spine. Magnetic resonance findings. *Skeletal Radiol*. 1989;18(4):283–288.
25. Gupta SK, Rajeev K, Khosla VK, et al. Spinal cord injury without radiographic abnormality in adults. *Spinal Cord*. October 1999;37(10):726–729.
26. Pope AM, Tarlov AR. *Disability in America: Toward a National Agenda for Prevention*. Washington, DC: National Academy Press; 1991.
27. Spinal cord injury: facts and figures at a glance. *J Spinal Cord Med*. 2000;23:51–53.
28. Mani RL. Potential hazard of metal-filled sandbags in MRI imaging. *Radiology*. 1992;182:286–287.
29. Brunberg JA, Papadopoulos SM. Technical note. Device to facilitate MRI imaging of patients in skeletal traction. *Am J Neuroradiol*. 1991;12(4):746–747.
30. Ballock RT, Hajed PC, Byrne TP, et al. The quality of magnetic resonance imaging, as affected by the composition of the halo orthosis. *J Bone Joint Surg Am*. 1989;71:431–434.
31. Shellock FG, Slimp G. Halo vest for cervical spine fixation during MRI imaging. *Am J Radiol*. 1990;154:631–632.
32. Shellock FG, Morisoli S, Kanal E. MRI procedures and biomedical implants, materials, and devices: 1993 update. *Radiology*. 1993;189:587–599.
33. Teitelbaum GP, Yee CA, Van Horn DD, et al. Metallic ballistic fragments: MRI imaging safety and artifacts. *Radiology*. 1990;175:855–859.
34. Smugar SS, Schweitzer ME, Hume E. MRI in patients with intraspinal bullets. *J Magn Reson Imaging*. January 1999;9(1):151–153.
35. Tartaglino LM, Flanders AE, Vinitski S, et al. Metallic artifacts on MRI images of the postoperative spine: reduction with fast spin-echo techniques. *Radiology*. 1994;190:565–569.
36. Flanders AE, Tartaglino LM, Friedman DP, et al. Application of fast spin-echo MRI imaging in acute cervical spine injury. *Radiology*. 1992;185(P):220.
37. Rockwell DT, Melhem ER, Bhatia RG. GRASE (gradient- and spin-echo) MR of the brain. *Am J Neuroradiol*. 1999;20(7):1381–1383.
38. Van Uijen CM, den Boef JH. Driven-equilibrium radiofrequency pulses in NMR imaging. *Mag Reson Med*. 1984; 1(4):502–507.
39. Griswold MA, Jakob PM, Chen Q, et al. Resolution enhancement in single-shot imaging using simultaneous acquisition of spatial harmonics (SMASH). *Magn Reson Med*. 1999;41:1236–1245.
40. Yousem DM, Atlas SW, Goldberg HI, et al. Degenerative narrowing of the cervical spine neural foramina: evaluation with high-resolution 3DFT gradient-echo MRI imaging. *Am J Neuroradiol*. 1991;12(2):229–236.
41. Perovitch M, Perl S, Wang H. Current advances in magnetic resonance imaging (MRI) in spinal cord trauma: review article. *Paraplegia*. 1992;30:305–316.
42. Schouman-Claeys E, Frija G, Cuenod CA, et al. MRI imaging of acute spinal cord injury: results of an experimental study in dogs. *Am J Neuroradiol*. 1990;11(5):959–965.

43. Terae S, Takahashi C, Abe S, et al. Gd-DTPA-enhanced MR imaging of injured spinal cord. *Clin Imaging.* 1997; 21(2):82–89.

44. Shimada K, Takahashi C, Satoru A, et al. Sequential MRI studies in patients with cervical cord injury but without bony injury. *Paraplegia.* 1995;33:573–578.

45. Nussbaum ES, Sebring LA, Wolf AL, et al. Myelographic and enhanced computed tomographic appearance of acute traumatic spinal cord avulsion. *Neurosurgery.* 1992;30:43–48.

46. Volle E, Assheuer J, Hedde JP, et al. Radicular avulsion resulting from spinal injury: assessment of diagnostic modalities. *Neuroradiology.* 1992;34:235–240.

47. Grossman MD, Reilly PM, Gillett T, et al. National survey of the incidence of cervical spine injury and approach to cervical spine clearance in U.S. trauma centers. *J Trauma.* 1999;47:684–690.

48. Wagner A, Albeck MJ, Madsen FF. Diagnostic imaging in fracture of lumbar vertebral ring apophyses. *Acta Radiol.* 1992;33:72–75.

49. Levitt MA, Flanders AE. Diagnostic capabilities of magnetic resonance imaging and computed tomography in acute cervical spinal column injury. *Am J Emerg Med.* 1991;9(2):131–135.

50. Tarr RW, Drolshagen LF, Kerner TC, et al. MRI imaging of recent spinal trauma. *J Comput Assist Tomogr.* 1987;11(3): 412–417.

51. Klein GR, Vaccaro AR, Albert TJ, et al. Efficacy of magnetic resonance imaging in the evaluation of posterior cervical spine fractures. *Spine.* April 15, 1999;24(8):771–774.

52. Baker LL, Goodman SB, Perkash I, et al. Benign versus pathologic compression fractures of vertebral bodies: assessment with conventional spin-echo, chemical shift, and STIR MRI imaging. *Radiology.* 1990;174:495–502.

53. Davis SJ, Teresi LM, Bradley WG, et al. Cervical spine hyperextension injuries: MRI findings. *Radiology.* 1991; 180(1):245–251.

54. Gardner E, Gray DJ. The back. In: Gardner E, Gray DJ, O'Rahilly Ronan, eds. *Anatomy.* 4th ed. Philadelphia: WB Saunders; 1975:508–540.

55. Saifuddin A, Green R, White J. Magnetic resonance imaging of the cervical ligaments in the absence of trauma. *Spine.* 2003;28:1686–1691.

56. Harris JH, Edeiken-Monroe B. *The Radiology of Acute Cervical Spine Trauma.* 2nd ed. Baltimore: Williams & Wilkins; 1987.

57. Edeiken-Monroe B, Wagner LK, Harris JH. Hyperextension dislocation of the cervical spine. *Am J Radiol.* 1986;146:803–808.

58. Regenbogen VS, Rogers LF, Atlas SW, et al. Cervical spinal cord injuries in patients with cervical spondylosis. *Am J Radiol.* 1986;146:277–284.

59. Pratt ES, Green DA, Spengler DM. Herniated intervertebral discs associated with unstable spinal injuries. *Spine.* 1990;15(7):662–666.

60. Dai L, Jia L. Central cord injury complicating acute cervical disc herniation in trauma. *Spine.* 2000;25:331–335.

61. Schaefer DM, Flanders A, Northrup BE, et al. Magnetic resonance imaging of acute cervical spine trauma: correlation with severity of neurologic injury. *Spine.* 1989;14:1090–1095.

62. Rizzolo SJ, Piazza MRI, Cotler JM, et al. Intervertebral disc injury complicating cervical spine trauma. *Spine.* 1991;16(6):187–189.

63. Harrington JF, Likavec MJ, Smith AS. Disc herniation in cervical fracture subluxation. *Neurosurgery.* 1991;29: 374–379.

64. Silberstein M, Tress BM, Hennessy O. Prediction of neurologic outcome in acute spinal cord injury: the role of CT and MRI. *Am J Neuroradiol.* 1992;13:1597–1608.

65. Rao SC, Fehlings MG. The optimal radiologic method for assessing spinal canal compromise and cord compression in patients with cervical spinal cord injury. Part I: An evidence-based analysis of the published literature. *Spine.* 1999;15:598–604.

66. El-Khoury GY, Whitten CG. Trauma to the upper thoracic spine: anatomy, biomechanics, and unique imaging features. *Am J Radio.* 1993;160:95–102.

67. Kulkarni MV, Bondurant FJ, Rose SL, et al. 1.5 tesla magnetic resonance imaging of acute spinal trauma. *Radiographics.* 1988;8(6):1059–1082.

68. Hackney DB, Asato LR, Joseph P, et al. Hemorrhage and edema in acute spinal cord compression: demonstration by MRI imaging. *Radiology.* 1986;161:387–390.

69. Rowed DW. Management of cervical spinal cord injury in ankylosing spondylitis: the intervertebral disc as a cause of cord compression. *J Neurosurg.* 1992;77:241–246.

70. Greiner FG, Orrison WW, King JN, et al. Vertebral artery injury association with cervical spine fractures. In: *Proceedings of the 29th Annual Meeting of the American Society of Neuroradiology.* Washington, DC; 1991:171.

71. Friedman DP, Flanders AE. Unusual dissection of the proximal vertebral artery: description of three cases. *AJNR.* 1992;13:283–286.

72. Biffl WL, Moore EE, Offner PJ, et al. Blunt carotid and vertebral arterial injuries. *World J Surg.* 2001;25:1036–1043.

73. Parbhoo AH, Govender S, Corr P. Vertebral artery injury in cervical spine trauma. *Injury Int J Care Injured.* 2001;32: 565–568.

74. Willis BK, Greiner F, Orrison WW, et al. The incidence of vertebral artery injury after midcervical spine fracture or subluxation. *Neurosurgery.* 1994;34:435–442.

75. Friedman DP, Flanders AE, Thomas C, et al. Vertebral artery injury after acute cervical spine trauma: rate of occurrence as detected by MR angiography and assessment of clinical consequences. *AJR.* 1995;164:443–447.

76. Biffl WL, Moore EE, Elliott JP, et al. The devastating potential of blunt vertebral arterial injuries. *Ann Surg.* 2000;23:672–681.

77. Giacobetti FB, Vaccaro AR, Bos-Giacobetti MA, et al. Vertebral artery occlusion associated with cervical spine trauma: a prospective analysis. *Spine.* 1997;22: 188–192.

78. Vaccaro AR, Klein GR, Flanders AE, et al. Long-term evaluation of vertebral artery injuries following cervical spine trauma using magnetic resonance angiography. *Spine.* 1998;23:789–794.

79. Torina PJ, Flanders AE, Carrino JA, et al. Incidence of vertebral artery thrombosis in cervical spine trauma: correlation with severity of spinal cord injury. *AJNR.* 2005;26: 2645–2651.

80. Miller PR, Fabian TC, Bee TK, et al. Blunt cerebrovascular injuries: diagnosis and treatment. *J Trauma.* 2001;51: 279–286.

81. Eachempati SR, Vaslef SN, Sebastian MW, et al. Blunt vascular injuries of the head and neck: is heparinization necessary? *J Trauma.* 1998;45:997–1004.

82. Greenberg MS. *Handbook of Neurosurgery.* 3rd ed. Lakeland, FL: Greenberg Graphics; 1994.

83. Matsura P, Waters RL, Adkins RH, et al. Comparison of computerized tomography parameters of the cervical spine in normal control subjects and spinal cord-injured patients. *J Bone Joint Surg.* 1989;71(2):183–188.

84. Tico N, Garcia-Ortun F, Ramirez L, et al. Traumatic spinal cord injury complicating ankylosing spondylitis. *Spinal Cord.* 1998;36(5):349–352.

85. Atlas SW, Regenbogen V, Rogers LF, et al. The radiographic characterization of burst fractures of the spine. *Am J Radio.* 1986;147:572–582.

86. Holdsworth F. Fractures, dislocations and fracture-dislocations of the spine. *J Bone Joint Surg Am.* 1970;52A: 1534–1551.

87. Denis F. The three column spine and its significance in the classification of acute thoracolumbar spinal injuries. *Spine.* 1983;8:817–831.

88. White AA III, Panjabi MM. *Clinical Biomechanics of the Spine.* Philadelphia: JB Lippincott; 1978.

89. McAfee PC, Yuan HA, Fredrickson BE, et al. The value of computed tomography in thoracolumbar fractures. *J Bone Joint Surg Am*. 1983;65:461–473.

90. Dorr L, Harvey J, Nickel V. Clinical review of the early stability of spine injuries. *Spine*. 1982;7(6):545–550.

91. Chiu WC, Haan JM, Cushing BM, et al. Ligamentous injuries of the cervical spine in unreliable blunt trauma patients: incidence, evaluation, and outcome. *J Trauma*. 2001;50:457–464.

92. White AA, Panjabi MM. Clinical biomechanics of the spine. Philadelphia: Lippincott; 1978.

93. Geck MJ, Yoo S, Wang JC. Assessment of cervical ligamentous injury in trauma patients using MRI. *J Spinal Disord*. 2001;14:371–377.

94. Insko EK, Gracias VH, Gupta R. Utility of flexion and extension radiographs of the cervical spine in the acute evaluation of blunt trauma. *J Trauma*. 2002;53:426–429.

95. Padayachee L, Cooper DJ, Irons S, et al. Cervical spine clearance in unconscious traumatic brain injury patients: dynamic flexion-extension fluoroscopy versus computed tomography with three-dimensional reconstruction. *J Trauma*. February 2006;60(2):341–345.

96. Cooper DJ, Ackland HM. Clearing the cervical spine in unconscious head injured patients—the evidence. *Crit Care Resusc*. September 2005;7(3):181–184.

97. Adams JM, Cockburn MI, Difazio LT, et al. Spinal clearance in the difficult trauma patient: a role for screening MRI of the spine. *Am Surg*. January 2006;72(1):101–105.

98. Haba H, Taneichi H, Kotani Y, et al. Diagnostic accuracy of magnetic resonance imaging for detecting posterior ligamentous complex injury associated with thoracic and lumbar fractures. *J Neurosurg*. 2003;99:20–26.

99. Lee H, Kim H, Kim D, et al. Reliability of magnetic resonance imaging in detecting posterior ligament complex injury in thoracolumbar spinal fractures. *Spine*. 2000;25: 2079–2084.

100. Vaccaro AR, Madigan L, Schweitzer ME, et al. Magnetic resonance imaging analysis of soft tissue disruption after flexion-distraction injuries of the subaxial cervical spine. *Spine*. 2001;26:1866–1872.

101. Carrino JA, Manton GL, Morrison WB, et al. Posterior longitudinal ligament status in cervical spine bilateral facet dislocations. *Skeletal Radiol*. 2006;35(7):510–514.

102. Stabler A, Eck J, Penning R, et al. Cervical spine: postmortem assessment of accident injuries—comparison of radiographic, MR imaging, anatomic, and pathologic findings. *Radiology*. 2001:221:340–346.

103. Frank JB, Lim CK, Flynn JM, et al. The efficacy of magnetic resonance imaging in pediatric cervical spine clearance. *Spine*. 2002;27:1176–1179.

104. Harrison JL, Ostlere SJ. Diagnosing purely ligamentous injuries of the cervical spine in the unconscious trauma patient. *Br J Radiol*. 2004;77:276–278.

105. Hogan GJ, Mirvis SE, Shanmuganathan K, et al. Exclusion of unstable cervical spine injury in obtunded patients with blunt trauma: is MR imaging needed when multidetector row CT findings are normal? *Radiology*. October 2005;237(1):106–113.

106. Sliker CW, Mirvis SE, Shanmuganathan K. Assessing cervical spine stability in obtunded blunt trauma patients: review of medical literature. *Radiology*. March 2005; 234(3):733–739.

107. Wilmink JT, Patijn J. MR imaging of alar ligament in whiplash-associated disorders: an observer study. *Neuroradiology*. October 2001;43(10):859–863.

108. Kaale BR, Krakenes J, Albrektsen G, et al. Whiplash-associated disorders impairment rating: neck disability index score according to severity of MRI findings of ligaments and membranes in the upper cervical spine. *J Neurotrauma*. April 2005;22(4):466–475.

109. Gatehouse PD, He T, Hughes SP, et al. MR imaging of degenerative disc disease in the lumbar spine with ultrashort TE pulse sequences. *MAGMA*. 2004;16(4): 160–166.

110. Meyer PR. Fractures of the thoracic spine: T1 to T10. In: Meyer PR, ed. *Surgery of Spine Trauma*. New York: Churchill Livingstone; 1989:525–571.

111. Rand RW, Crandall P. Central cord syndrome in hyperextension injuries of the cervical cord. *J Bone Joint Surg*. 1962;44:1415–1422.

112. Pang D. Spinal cord injury without radiographic abnormality in children, 2 decades later. *Neurosurgery*. 2004;55:1325–1343.

113. Shimada K, Tokioka T. Sequential MR studies of cervical cord injury: correlation with neurological damage and clinical outcome. *Spinal Cord*. 1999;37(6):410–415.

114. Ohta K, Fujimura Y, Nakamura M, et al. Experimental study on MRI evaluation of the course of cervical spinal cord injury. *Spinal Cord*. 1999;37:580–584.

115. Marciello M, Flanders AE, Herbison GJ, et al. Magnetic resonance imaging related to neurologic outcome in cervical spinal cord injury. *Arch Phys Med Rehabil*. 1993;74: 940–946.

116. Flanders AE, Spettell CM, Tartaglino LM, et al. Forecasting motor recovery after cervical spinal cord injury: value of MR imaging. *Radiology*. 1996;201:649–655.

117. Schaefer DM, Flanders AE, Osterholm JL, et al. Prognostic significance of magnetic resonance imaging in the acute phase of cervical spine injury. *J Neurosurg*. 1992;76(2): 218–223.

118. Silberstein M, Tress BM, Hennessy O. Delayed neurologic deterioration in the patient with spinal trauma: role of MRI imaging. *Am J Neuroradiol*. 1992;13:1373–1381.

119. Ramon S, Dominquez R, Ramirez L, et al. Clinical and magnetic resonance imaging correlation in acute spinal cord injury. *Spinal Cord*. 1997;35(10):664–673.

120. Pollard ME, Apple DF. Factors associated with improved neurologic outcomes in patients with incomplete tetraplegia. *Spine*. 2003;28:33–39.

121. Hackney DB, Finkelstein SD, Hand CM, et al. Postmortem magnetic resonance imaging of experimental spinal cord injury: magnetic resonance findings versus in vivo functional deficit. *Neurosurgery*. 1994;35(6):1104–1011.

122. Hackney DB, Ford JC, Markowitz RS, et al. Experimental spinal cord injury: imaging the acute lesion. *AJNR Am J Neuroradiol*. 1994;15(5):960–961.

123. Hackney DB, Ford JC, Markowitz RS, et al. Experimental spinal cord injury: MR correlation to intensity of injury. *J Comput Assist Tomogr*. 1994;18(3):357–362.

124. Croul SE, Flanders AE. Neuropathology of human spinal cord injury. *Adv Neurol*. 1997;72:317–323.

125. Ford JC, Hackney DB, Joseph PM. A method for in vivo high resolution MRI of rat spinal cord injury. *Magn Reson Med*. 1994;31:218–223.

126. LeMay DR, Fechner KP, Zelenock GB et al High resolution magnetic resonance imaging of the rat spinal cord. *Neurol Res*. 1996;18(5):471–474.

127. Falconer JC, Narayana PA, Bhattacharjee MB, et al. Quantitative MRI of spinal cord injury in a rat model. *Magn Reson Med*. 1994;32(4):484–491.

128. Duncan EG, Lemaire C, Armstrong RL, et al. High-resolution magnetic resonance imaging of experimental spinal cord injury in the rat. *Neurosurgery*. 1992;31: 510–519.

129. Bilgen M, Abbe R, Liu S. et al. Spatial and temporal evolution of hemorrhage in the hyperacute phase of experimental spinal cord injury: In vivo magnetic resonance imaging. *Magn Reson Med* 2000;43:594–600.

130. Metz GA, Curt A, van de Meent H, et al. Validation of the weight-drop contusion model in rats: a comparative study of human spinal cord injury. *J Neurotrauma*. 2000;17(1): 1–17.

131. Cotler HB, Kulkarni MV, Bondurant FJ. Magnetic resonance imaging of acute spinal cord trauma: preliminary report. *J Orthop Trauma*. 1988;2(1):1–4.

132. Sato T, Kokubun S, Rijal KP, et al. Prognosis of cervical spinal cord injury in correlation with magnetic resonance imaging. *Paraplegia*. 1994;32:81–85.

133. Blackwood W. Vascular disease of the central nervous system. In: Blackwood W, McMenemey WH, Meyer A, et al., eds. *Greenfield's Neuropathology*. Baltimore: Williams & Wilkins; 1963:71–115.

134. DiTunno J, ed. *Standards for Neurological and Functional Classification of Spinal Cord Injury*. 4th ed. Chicago: American Spinal Injury Association; 1992.

135. Tator CH, Rowed DW, Schwartz ML, eds. *Sunnybrook Cord Injury Scales for Assessing Neurological Injury and Neurological Recovery in Early Management of Acute Spinal Cord Injury*. New York: Raven Press; 1982.

136. Ditunno JF. Functional assessment measures in CNS trauma. *J Neurotrauma*. 1992;9:5301–5305.

137. Spiller, WG. Thrombosis of the cervical anterior median spinal artery: syphilitic acute anterior poliomyelitis. *J Nerv Ment Dis*. 1909;36:601–613.

138. Austin G, Rouhe S, Horn N. Vascular diseases of the spinal cord. In: Austin G, ed. *The Spinal Cord*. Springfield, IL: Charles C Thomas; 1972:455–469.

139. Hughes J, Brownell B. Cervical spondylosis complicated by anterior spinal artery thrombosis. *Neurology*. 1964; 14:1073.

140. Hughes J, Brownell B. Spinal cord ischemia due to arteriosclerosis. *Arch Neurol*. 1966;15:189–202.

141. Schneider RC, Cherry GL, Pantek HE. The syndrome of acute central cervical spinal cord injury. *J Neurosurg*. 1954;11:546–577.

142. Schneider, RC, Thompson JM, Bebin J. The syndrome of the acute central cervical spinal cord injury. *J Neurol Neurosurg Psychiatry*. 1958;21:216–227.

143. Taylor AR. The mechanism of injury to the spinal cord in the neck without damage to the vertebral column. *J Bone Joint Surg Br*. 1951;33:543–547.

144. Quencer RM, Bunge RP. The injured spinal cord: imaging, histopathologic clinical correlates, and basic science approaches to enhancing neural function after spinal cord injury. *Spine*. 1996;21:2064–2066.

145. Austin, G. *The Spinal Cord: Basic Aspects and Surgical Considerations*. Springfield, Il: Charles C Thomas; 1961.

146. St. John JR, Rand CW. Stab wounds of the spinal cord. *Bull Los Angeles Neurol Soc*. 1953;18:1–24.

147. Haymaker W. *Bing's Local Diagnosis in Neurological Diseases*. 15th ed. St. Louis: CV Mosby; 1969.

148. Hartwell JB. An analysis of 133 fractures of the spine treated at the Massachusetts General Hospital. *Boston Med Surg J*. 1917;177:31–41.

149. Frankel HL, Hancock DO, Hyslop G. The value of postural reduction in the initial management of closed injuries of the spine with paraplegia and tetraplegia. *Paraplegia*. 1969;7:179–192.

150. Hamilton BB, Fuhre MJ, eds. *Rehabilitation Outcomes: Analysis and Measurement*. Baltimore: Brooks; 1987: 137–147.

151. Hamilton BB, Laughlin JA, Fiedler RC, et al. Interrater reliability of the seven level functional independence measure (FIM). *Scand J Rehab Med*. 1994;26:115–119.

152. Yamashita Y, Takahashi M, Matsuno Y, et al. Chronic injuries of the spinal cord: assessment with MRI imaging. *Radiology*. 1990;175(3):849–854.

153. Yamashita Y, Takahashi M, Matsuno Y, et al. Acute spinal cord injury: magnetic resonance imaging correlated with myelopathy. *Br J Radiol*. 1991;64(759):201–209.

154. Selden NR, Quint DJ, Patel N, et al. Emergency magnetic resonance imaging of cervical spinal cord injuries: clinical correlation and prognosis. *Neurosurgery*. 1999;44:785–792.

155. Flanders AE, Spettell CM, Friedman DP, et al. The relationship between the functional abilities of patients with cervical spinal cord injury and the severity of damage revealed by MR imaging. *AJNR*. 1999;20:926–934.

156. Boghosian G, Leypold BG, Sharma DK, et al. Predicting the neurological level of injury with MRI following cervical spinal cord injury. *Radiology (240P?) p ?*

157. Boldin C, Raith J, Fankhauser F. Predicting neurologic recovery in cervical spinal cord injury with postoperative MR imaging. *Spine*. 2006;31(5):554–559.

158. Shepard MJ, Bracken MB. Magnetic resonance imaging and neurological recovery in acute spinal cord injury: observations from the National Acute Spinal Cord Injury Study 3. *Spinal Cord*. 1999;37:833–837.

159. Fehlings MG, Rao SC, Tator CH, et al. The optimal radiologic method for assessing spinal canal compromise and cord compression in patients with cervical spinal cord injury. Part II: Results of a multicenter study. *Spine*. 1999;24(6):605–613.

160. Kang, Figgie MP, Bohlman HH. Sagittal measurements of the cervical spine in subaxial fractures and dislocations. *J Bone Joint Surg*. 1994;76:1617–1628.

161. Bracken MB, Shepard MJ, Collins WF, et al. A randomized controlled trial of methylprednisolone or naloxone in the treatment of acute spinal cord injury: results of the Second National Acute Spinal Cord Injury Study. *N Engl J Med*. 1990;322:1405–1411.

162. Bracken MB, Shepard MJ, Collins WF, et al. Methylprednisolone or naloxone in the treatment of acute spinal cord injury: one year follow up results of the Second National Acute Spinal Cord Injury Study. *J Neurosurg*. 1992;76: 23–31.

163. Young W, Bracken MB. The Second National Acute Spinal Cord Injury Study. In: Jane J, Torner J, Anderson D, et al., eds. *NIH Central Nervous System Status Report*. New York: Mary Ann Liebert; 1991:5429–5451.

164. Taoka Y, Okajima K, Uchiba M, et al. Methylprednisolone reduces spinal cord injury in rats without affecting tumor necrosis factor-alpha production. *J Neurotrauma*. 2001; 18(5):533–543.

165. Leypold BG, Flanders AE, Schwartz ED, et al. The impact of methylprednisolone on lesion severity following spinal cord injury. In press, *Spine*.

166. Flanders AE, Leypold B, Sharma D, et al. Dynamic characteristics of acute spinal cord injury: is absolute lesion length affected by delay in MR imaging? *Radiology*. 2005;237(P):669.

Imaging of Pediatric Spinal Injury

Avrum N. Pollock and Stephen M. Henesch

In children, fractures and severe injuries to the spine are relatively rare and represent between 1% and 10% of injuries reported by various authors (1–5). Spinal fractures in children represent between 1% and 2% of all pediatric fractures (6). Compared with adults, spinal trauma is relatively rare in pediatric patients; however, the mortality rate is higher in children as a result of associated injuries (7,8). The anatomy and biomechanics of the growing spine, which include larger head size relative to body size, greater flexibility of the spine and supporting structures, incomplete ossification, as well as greater elasticity and compressibility of the bone, produce failure patterns different from those seen in adults. Anatomic differences between the pediatric and adult cervical spine are prominent until approximately 8 years of age and persist to a lesser degree until approximately 12 years of age (9–14). By the time a child is age 8 to 10 years of age, his or her spine has reached near adult size. Younger children present an additional challenge, as they are developmentally unable to communicate crucial symptoms. Furthermore, the physical examination can be limited by lack of cooperation in an anxious, crying child.

SPINAL DEVELOPMENT

Differing spinal levels demonstrate variability in their development, and awareness of these developmental and anatomic variants is essential in detecting true abnormalities in the pediatric spine. Avellino et al. (15) noted that among the most common factors for misdiagnosis of cervical spine injuries were unfamiliarity with the pediatric spine and failure to recognize normal variants. Spinal development in the upper cervical vertebrae is different from that of the lower cervical vertebrae (Fig. 9-1). The C1 vertebra develops from three ossification centers (body and two neural arches) (Fig. 9-1A). Anomalies occur when these centers either fail to develop or fail to fuse. The posterior arch normally fuses by the age of three. C2 develops from four ossification centers (body, odontoid, and two neural arches) (Fig. 9-1B) that are present at birth and also fuse by the age of three. The body and odontoid are joined by the dentocentral synchondrosis, and the body and neural arches are joined by two neurocentral synchondroses. The remainder of the lower cervical spine vertebrae develop with three primary centers of ossification (two neural arches and one vertebral centrum) that

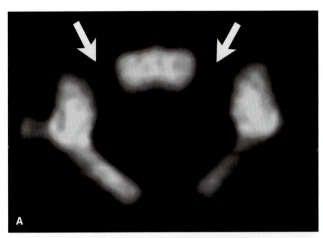

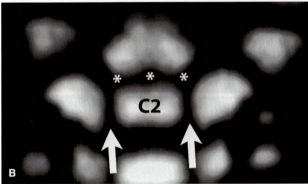

FIGURE 9-1. Normal age appropriate synchondroses. One-month-old female status postfall from height. Axial CT of the upper cervical spine at the level of C1 **(A)**, and coronal CT reconstructions at the level of C2 **(B)** demonstrate the early normal anatomic appearance of the vertebral bodies prior to fusion of the synchondroses. Note the paired neurocentral synchondroses (*arrows*) joining the body and neural arches in both C1 (A) and C2 (B), and the dentocentral synchondrosis (*asterisks*) joining the body and odontoid process of C2 (B).

are joined by two neurocentral synchondroses, which fuse by the time a child is 3 to 6 years of age. The vertebrae of the cervical and thoracic spine also have five secondary ossification centers (one spinous process, two transverse processes, and two ring apophyses). In addition to these five secondary centers, the lumbar spine has two additional centers corresponding to the mamillary processes.

IMAGING MODALITIES

Radiographs (Plain Films)

Radiographs of the cervical spine remain the initial imaging modality of choice for children of all ages following trauma. The *Guidelines for the Management of Acute Cervical Spine and Spinal Cord Injuries* published by the American Association of Neurological Surgeons/Congress of Neurologic Surgeons (16) suggest, however, that these

films may not be necessary in children following trauma who are alert, conversant, have no neurologic deficit, no midline or cervical tenderness, no painful distracting injury and are not intoxicated; these criteria are those that have been used by the National Emergency X-Ray Utilization Study (NEXUS) (17). This recommendation has been based in part in a study by Viccellio et al. (18) who applied the NEXUS criteria to the pediatric population and noted that application of these findings could reduce cervical spine imaging in children by up to 20%. In this study, however, there were few injured patients below the age of 9, and none were under the age of 2, which would suggest caution in applying these criteria to patients nine and younger.

In those patients who undergo radiography, an adequate lateral view is essential when evaluating this region as this view alone has 79% sensitivity for spinal injury (19). In the same study, a three-view radiographic series was shown to have a sensitivity of 94%. In the pediatric age group, prevertebral soft tissue swelling is a poor predictor of underlying abnormality and is often dependent on the degree of neck flexion and adequate inspiratory effort. An odontoid view should not even be attempted unless a child is old enough to follow commands, which in our experience occurs by approximately 5 years of age (20). Any suggestion of an abnormality on radiographs or any clinically suspicious area that is not properly visualized on radiographs warrants a focused computed tomography (CT) scan of the level in question, as well as one level above and below the level of suspected fracture (Fig. 9-2).

The role of flexion-extension radiography in the pediatric population has been controversial. Dwek and Chung (21) performed a retrospective review of 247 children who underwent flexion-extension radiography following standard static cervical spine imaging and found that if the standard views were normal, flexion-extension films did not find abnormalities and were therefore of "questionable use." Ralston et al. (22) also found that flexion-extension views were unlikely to be abnormal if standard radiographs showed no acute abnormality or isolated loss of lordosis (22). They also noted that flexion-extension views were of "limited usefulness" in confirming ligamentous injury in those patients with significant acute abnormalities on standard radiographs. However, they did note that flexion-extension radiographs could help rule out ligamentous injury in patients with suspicious findings on radiographs for occult ligamentous injury, including segmental kyphosis, prevertebral soft tissue swelling, and equivocal subluxation.

Computed Tomography

Complete CT scanning of the entire cervical spine, which may be the norm in adults, is not warranted in the child,

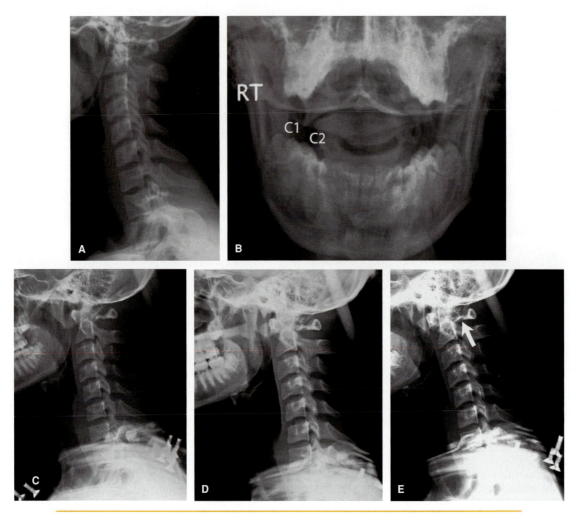

FIGURE 9-2. Right Jefferson (C1) fracture. Seventeen-year-old involved in a football injury 1 week earlier secondary to a head-on tackle. Lateral **(A)** and attempted open-mouth view **(B)** of the cervical spine were obtained 1 week after the initial injury. Lateral cervical spine views were also obtained approximately 3 weeks after the injury **(C)**, 5 weeks after injury **(D)**, and approximately 6 weeks after injury **(E)**. (*continued*)

given the additional radiation dose to the thyroid. The thyroid gland has an increased sensitivity to radiation in the growing child, and thus a similar radiation dose per gram of weight of tissue has a greater potential for developing fatal cancer later in life (23,24). Furthermore, the use of blanket trauma protocols increases the number of studies performed without a significant increase in injury identification, thus increasing cost without improving outcome (25).

The standard multidetector CT (MDCT) technique of imaging the cervical spine consists of thin (0.6 to 1.3 mm) axial helically acquired images, which can then be further broken down to thinner increments, thereby optimizing reconstructed images in the sagittal and coronal planes. Images are routinely reviewed on soft tissue and bone algorithms/windows.

Hernandez et al. (26) retrospectively evaluated 606 pediatric patients under the age of 5 who were evaluated

for cervical spine injury. Of these patients, 76% were cleared by plain films and clinical exam; of the remaining 24% (147 patients), only 2.7% (4 patients) demonstrated new traumatic findings, which in retrospect appeared to have been visible on plain films. Adelgais et al. (27) demonstrated that the use of screening CT for cervical spine injury in the pediatric population increased radiation dosage without decreasing either the time of the patient in the emergency department or reducing sedation usage. Therefore, considering the increased risk of cancer, CT should be used sparingly as a screening modality for cervical spine trauma in the pediatric population. Keenan et al. (28), however, identified subgroups that may benefit from screening CT without increasing radiation dose or cost. One such subgroup was patients with high risk for cervical spine trauma, including those unrestrained passengers in motor vehicle accidents with head trauma and Glasgow Coma Scale less than 8, for which

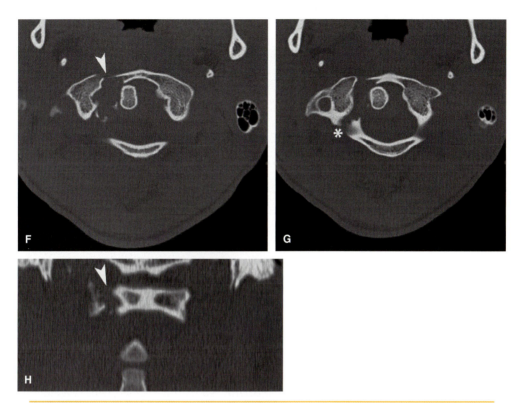

FIGURE 9-2. (*CONTINUED*) Also obtained were axial CT images of the cervical spine at the level of injury at 1-week postinjury **(F)** and ~6 weeks of postinjury **(G)**, with coronal reconstruction images of the cervical spine **(H)** obtained at 1-week postinjury. Although not completely visible on the lateral view of the early study (A), the open-mouth view (B) demonstrates splaying of the lateral masses of C1 with respect to C2, suggesting disruption of the ring of C1. Follow-up images up to 6 weeks postinjury (E) demonstrate lucency in the posterior arch of C1 (*arrow in E*). Axial images of the cervical spine (F,G) demonstrate disruption of the cortex of the anterior arch of C1 on the right (*arrowhead in F*) as well as the posterior arch C1 on the right (*asterisk in G*). The anterior arch injury is demonstrated on the reconstruction coronal images (*arrowhead in H*).

initial spine CT at time of cranial CT did not increase cost or radiation dose. It is worth noting that in pediatric patients with traumatic spinal injury, craniocerebral injury is the most common associated injury (29).

Magnetic Resonance Imaging

As children are more likely to have nonosseous cervical spine injuries than adults, magnetic resonance imaging (MRI), with its superior evaluation of soft tissue structures, would potentially be useful in the pediatric population. There have been relatively few articles, however, that address this issue. Keiper et al. (30) found that MRI could detect soft tissue abnormalities (including edema/ligamentous injury, spinal cord contusion, extra-axial hemorrhage, vertebral body subluxation/distraction occult fracture or disc protrusion) in 31% of patients who had normal radiographs or CTs and presented either with persisting or unexplained symptoms, signs of injury or instability not entirely explained by plain films, or with need for further evaluation of the extent of soft tissue injury not characterized by plain films.

Standard MRI technique, performed on a 1.5 Tesla system, consists of T1- and T2-weighted sagittal and axial imaging, as well as a sagittal short tau inversion recovery (STIR) and fat-saturated T2-weighted sequences.

A gradient echo susceptibility sequence can also be performed to assess for the possibility of blood products. If vertebral artery injury is suspected, additional axial fat-saturated T1-weighted images are required, with time-of-flight magnetic resonance angiography (TOF MRA) to assess the patency of the vertebral arteries.

Flynn et al. (31) found that MRI altered plain film diagnoses in 34% of patients who underwent the study in order to define the diagnosis or clear the cervical spine, because plain films and physical evaluation were inconclusive; they maintained that MRI was their imaging modality of choice in clearing the cervical spine for obtunded, intubated, or uncooperative children. A similar recommendation for obtunded and intubated pediatric patients is made by Frank et al. (32) who noted that MRI resulted in earlier clearing of the cervical spine with resultant cost savings of $7,000 per patient. Other indications for MRI are potential spinal cord birth injuries (33) and spinal cord injury without radiographic abnormality (SCIWORA).

Spinal Cord Injury without Radiographic Abnormality

SCIWORA is far more common in younger children than in older children, and is far more common in the cervical spine than it is in the thoracolumbar region (34). SCIWORA is found in 30% to 40% of children with spinal cord injury (35) and was originally described with regard to plain radiographs, but has grown to include CT scans, and in most cases has excluded MRI. A substantial number of children with neurologic deficits, however, show no evidence of abnormality on either MRI or somatosensory-evoked potential (SSEP). Several studies have shown that the main predictor of long-term outcome in SCIWORA patients is the neurologic status at admission, in that only patients presenting with mild to moderate initial deficits attain full recovery (36–38). Abnormalities visualized on MRI have more recently been shown to surpass clinical neurologic status with regard to prognosis, specifically with regard to cord concussion (39). In select cases, patients who have normal MRI examinations in the setting of complete sensorimotor paralysis have improved completely within 2 days (40). The agility of the pediatric spine creates the potential for serious spinal injuries in the setting of apparently normal initial radiographic evaluation. Therefore, it has been suggested that all patients with SCIWORA should obtain an MRI (35).

UPPER CERVICAL SPINE INJURIES (OCCIPITAL, C1, AND C2)

Distraction Injuries

Spines of neonates, infants, and young children are especially vulnerable to distraction injuries (Figs. 9-3–9-8) secondary to ligamentous injury/disruption in the upper cervical spine. Eleraky et al. (41) demonstrated that in children <9 years old, 78% of cervical spine injuries were in the upper cervical spine (occiput-C2) and 68% had either subluxation without fracture or SCIWORA. This contrasts with older children (ages 10 to 16) in which 70% sustained lower cervical spine fractures and 80% of the children in this group had fractures or a fracture with subluxation. Most distraction injuries in children occur before 5 years of age, with the vast majority occurring prior to 6 months of age (42,43); however, it has been reported that atlanto-occipital dislocation is more common in the 5- to 9-year-old age range (44). This predilection for upper cervical spine injuries in younger children

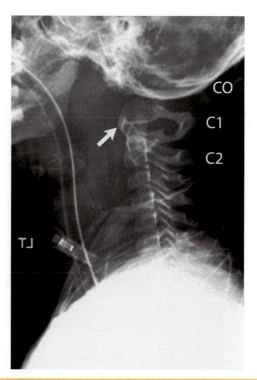

FIGURE 9-3. C0-1 distraction. Nine-year-old pedestrian hit by a car. Single lateral view of the cervical spine demonstrates increased distance between the occiput (C0) and C1, as well as between C1 and C2. Note the marked prevertebral soft tissue swelling. The arch of C1 (*arrow*) is rotated off of the odontoid process of C2.

may be due to a combination of factors. One may be the relatively larger head mass which results in a higher center of gravity. Additionally, spinal immaturity and ligamentous laxity, which may be beneficial for lower cervical spine, may not be able to withstand the sheer forces in the upper cervical spine (7). Spinal distraction injuries are rare in children, however, they are often fatal, due to associated high cervical spinal and brainstem injury leading to respiratory and cardiac arrest (45,46). In those patients who survive, they may be quadriplegic, as Leventhal (47) demonstrated that the spinal cord ruptures beyond a mere 1/4 inch of forced lengthening. Additionally, there may be associated cranial nerve and vascular stretch injuries (46), as well as diffuse axonal injury supratentorially (45). Certain congenital and acquired pathologies, including Down syndrome, Klippel-feil syndrome, Grisel syndrome, neoplasms, and myogenesis, may predispose to these injuries due to a combination of ligamentous laxity and bony abnormalities in the upper cervical spine (41).

As with adults, diagnosis of atlanto-occipital distraction (or disassociation) (AOD) may be made by plain film using Powers ratio (BC:OA), which is the distance between the basion and posterior arch of C1 (BC) divided by the distance between the opisthion and anterior arch of the atlas (OA).

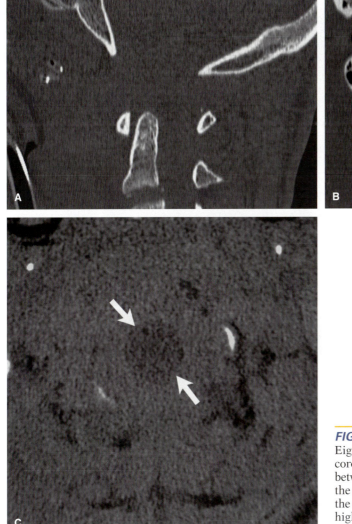

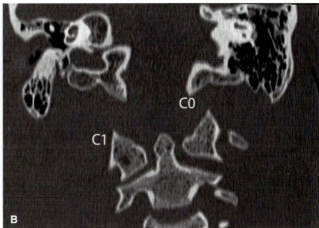

FIGURE 9-4. Vertical distraction of the atlanto-occipital joint. Eighteen-year-old hit by car. Sagittal CT reconstruction **(A)**, coronal CT reconstruction **(B)** demonstrate increased distance between the occiput (labeled C0) and C1. Axial CT at the level of the gap between the occiput and C1 shows low attenuation of the cervical spinal cord (*arrows*) with respect to the surrounding high attenuation, representing hemorrhage within the sub-arachnoid space around the upper cervical spinal cord.

A ratio >1.0 is considered diagnostic for AOD, with 0.77 being the mean for a normal population (46). The basion-dental interval (BDI) may also be used, with a measurement of >10 to 12.5 mm considered abnormal (46,48). Although other authors have found the BDI measurement to be unreliable in children (49), Bulas et al. (48), however, reported that in a series of 11 children with AOD, all had a BDI >14 mm and only six had a Powers ratio >1.0. Kenter et al. (46) suggest that both measurements be taken in patients with suspected AOD. CT with sagittal and coronal reformations may make the diagnosis easier as bony landmarks may be better visualized (Figs. 9-3, 9-4). Additionally, subarachnoid hemorrhage (SAH), which is seen in over 50% of patients with AOD, can also be visualized (Figs. 9-4, 9-8). This finding of infratentorial subarachnoid is important when reviewing cranial CTs following trauma, as <2% of traumatic brain injury results in infratentorial

SAH; thus the presence of this findings should prompt further evaluation for spinal injury (50). MRI may also be utilized to directly evaluate ligamentous injury as well as spinal cord parenchymal and vascular injury (Figs. 9-5, 9-7). Sun et al. (51) used MRI evaluation of ligamentous injury to define a new measure for detecting tectorial membrane injury from plain films. They found that in patients with tectorial membrane injury, the ratio of C1-2:C2-3 inter-spinous distances was >2.5 (Fig. 9-5).

Occipital-atlanto-axial Instability

The atlanto-occipital joint allows extension and flexion, which in turn causes an anterior translation of C1 on C2. Movement >5 mm and 3 mm, in a child less than and >8 years old respectively, indicates atlanto-axial instability, which is suggestive of ligamentous laxity and possible

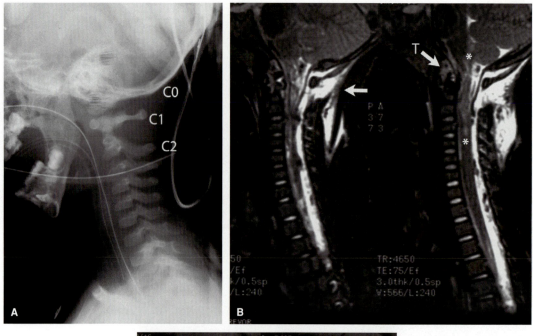

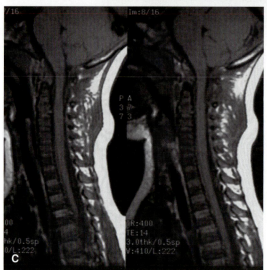

FIGURE 9-5. Atlanto-occipital disassociation with ligamentous injury and spinal cord edema. Three-year-old unrestrained motor vehicle accident passenger, ejected from car. Lateral cervical spine view **(A)**, sagittal T2-weighted MRI **(B)**, and sagittal T1-weighted image **(C)** of the cervical spine demonstrate an increase in the atlanto-occipital distance (C0-1) and the C1-2 distance, with soft tissue swelling posteriorly (*unlabeled arrow in B*). Increased T2 signal is seen within the upper cervical spinal cord extending from the cervical-medullary junction to the C3 level (*asterisks in B*), in keeping with spinal cord injury, likely secondary to distraction and disruption of the cervical spinal cord. An additional sign of instability is that of injury to the tectorial membrane (*arrow labeled T in B*), which is the superior extension of the posterior longitudinal ligament and comes in close approximation to the dens of C2 and the clivus.

transverse ligament disruption. In equivocal cases, flexion and extension views have shown to be of some benefit, as opposed to their acquisition in clearly normal cases, where they have not shown to be beneficial (52). As noted above, many processes can cause ligamentous laxity, and thus atlanto-axial instability can also be seen in the nontrauma setting, most commonly with Trisomy 21 (Fig. 9-9), but

also in spondyloepiphyseal dysplasia and mucopolysaccharidoses.

Pseudosubluxation

Pseudosubluxation, or normal physiologic displacement of C2 on C3, and to a lesser extent C3 on C4, can mimic

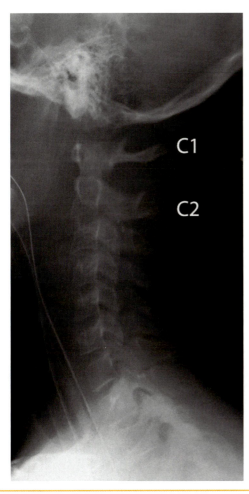

FIGURE 9-6. C1-2 distraction injury. Thirteen-year-old hit by car. Lateral view of the cervical spine demonstrates increased in distance between the posterior elements of C1 and C2, consistent with a C1-2 distraction type injury.

the appearance of a true cervical spine injury (Fig. 9-10). However, studies have shown that ~40% of children under the age of 8 demonstrate pseudosubluxation at the C2-3 level (53). The spinolaminar line is a line drawn from the anterior aspect of the spinous process of C1 to the anterior aspect of the spinous process of C3. When the anterior edges of the respective spinous processes line up to within 1.5 mm of each other on both flexion and extension views, this confirms the pseudosubluxation, and consequently rules out suspected true injury (54). This is not the case with a true cervical spine injury associated with displacement/subluxation (Fig. 9-11). A measurement of >2 mm is definitely abnormal, indicating a true injury, while a measurement of 1.6 to 1.9 mm is considered indeterminate (54).

Rotatory Subluxation

A previously normal child with persistent refusal to turn the head to one side or the other, or with fixed rotation

after even a presumed trivial trauma, raises suspicion for atlanto-axial rotatory fixation/subluxation or fixed rotation of C1 on C2. Dynamic CT scan is the imaging modality of choice, in which the neck is first imaged in its rotated position of comfort (i.e., neutral) and is subsequently imaged with the neck actively rotated by the patient, maximally toward both shoulders respectively, in order to evaluate the motion of the anterior arch of C1, with respect to the odontoid process of C2. An unchanged C1 and C2 relationship indicates rotatory subluxation, toward the side on which the patient is unable to rotate the midline fissure of C1 beyond the median raphe of the odontoid process of C2 (i.e., is unable to subtend an angle beyond the midline of the odontoid process of C2 [Figs. 9-12, 9-13]). Additional anterior or posterior displacement is indicative of a highly unstable injury.

Jefferson Fracture

Fractures of C1 are uncommon in children. Jefferson fractures (Fig. 9-2) are most often the result of an axial load from above, or due to the head hitting the ground (i.e., secondary to a diving injury). CT is the most sensitive diagnostic modality for imaging ring fractures of C1. Unlike adults with a double break, children may have a single bony fracture with a hinge on the synchondrosis (55).

Odontoid Fractures

Odontoid fractures are less often detected as an acute finding in children than in adults. The varied appearance of the odontoid process of C2 often leads to confusion, secondary to the appearance of the synchondroses, which can be further magnified in the presence of certain syndromes (i.e., Morquio, spondyloepiphyseal dysplasia, Klippel-Feil, and so forth) (Figs. 9-14–9-17). However, the incidence of nonunion may be as high as 62% if not promptly diagnosed and treated (56). Anterior tilt of the odontoid is worrisome for serious injury in the setting of acute spinal trauma. The clinical picture in cases of odontoid injury is very important, as it is extremely rare to have an injury to this region without significant pain (57). MRI may be slightly more sensitive in the setting of acute injury with respect to bone marrow edema indicative of fracture. However, CT is otherwise the standard cross-sectional modality for acute injuries and is used for classification as well as in the identification of more chronic injuries to this region. Imaging of this region can often be obtained nonacutely following immobilization.

Anderson and D'Alonzo (58) classified odontoid fractures into three types. Type I odontoid fractures are the least worrisome of the three, most often heal on their own without treatment, and are theorized to represent

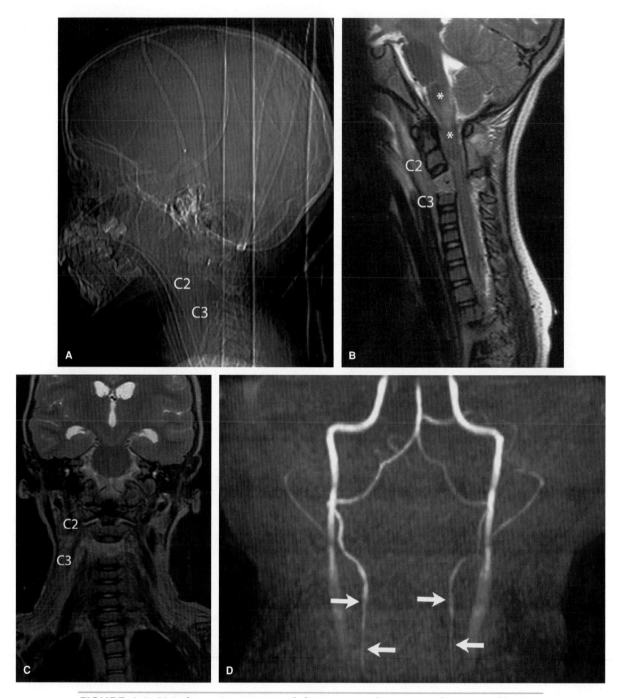

FIGURE 9-7. C2-3 distraction injury with ligamentous disruption. Three-year-old status post–motor vehicle accident, with spinal shock. Sagittal scout image from CT **(A)** demonstrates distraction of C2 upon C3. Sagittal **(B)** and coronal **(C)** T2-weighted MRI confirm the distraction injury and shows prevertebral soft tissue swelling, posterior interspinous ligamentous signal abnormality, and signal abnormality within the cervical-medullary junction region (*asterisks in B*). Anterior view of maximum intensity projection from neck three-dimensional time-of-flight MRA **(D)** demonstrates attenuated appearance of the vertebral arteries bilaterally, in keeping with stretching of these vessels (*arrows*) due to the distraction injury.

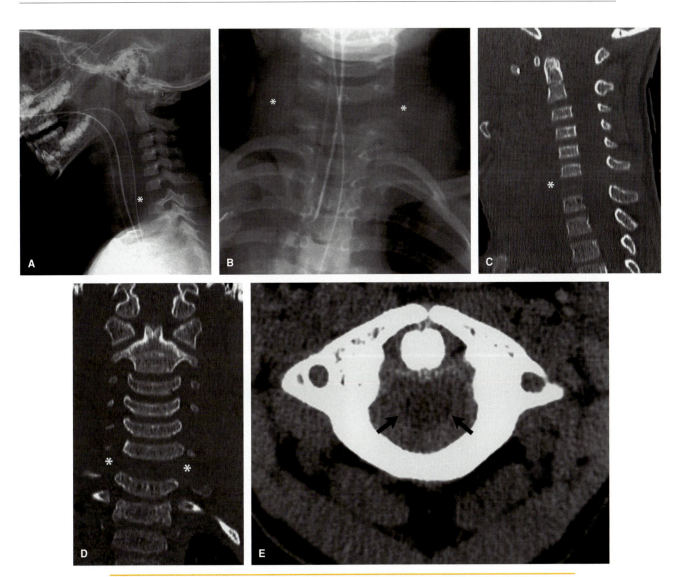

FIGURE 9-8. C6-7 distraction injury. Six-year-old pedestrian hit by car. Lateral **(A)** and frontal **(B)** views of the cervical spine demonstrate a nasogastric and endotracheal tube that obscures the prevertebral soft tissues, despite obvious soft tissue swelling identified on the CT sagittal reconstructed image **(C)**. A gap (*asterisks in A and B*) is seen between the expected location of the C6 and C7 vertebral bodies, in keeping with a distraction type injury. This finding is reconfirmed on the sagittal and coronal (*asterisks in C and D*) CT reconstructions. Axial CT **(E)** demonstrates the relative low attenuation of the spinal cord (*black arrows*) surrounded by relative high attenuation within the subarachnoid space, in keeping with cord edema and extra axial hemorrhage respectively.

an avulsion fracture related to the alar ligament (Fig. 9-18). The os odontoideum, which is often the result of old trauma, vascular insufficiency to the tip of the odontoid, or a congenital anomaly, as well as the entity of odontoid hypoplasia, may at times additionally complicate the scenario (Fig. 9-19). Type II fractures represent transverse fractures that extend into the odontoid base and often result in nonunion. Sagittal and coronal reconstructed CT images are essential in making this diagnosis, as these fractures are often missed in the axial plane (Figs.

9-20, 9-21). Type III odontoid fractures extend into the body of C2 and are a common injury in children under the age of 7 (Fig. 9-22). They are most often physeal type fractures traversing the dentocentral synchondrosis (59) (Fig. 9-23). Acute fracture through the dentocentral synchondrosis at the junction of the vertebral body and dens is a phenomenon unique to young children (Fig. 9-24). Until it has fully fused at approximately 7 years old, the synchondrosis is an inherent area of weakness through the bone (60,61). An acute distracting neck injury, such

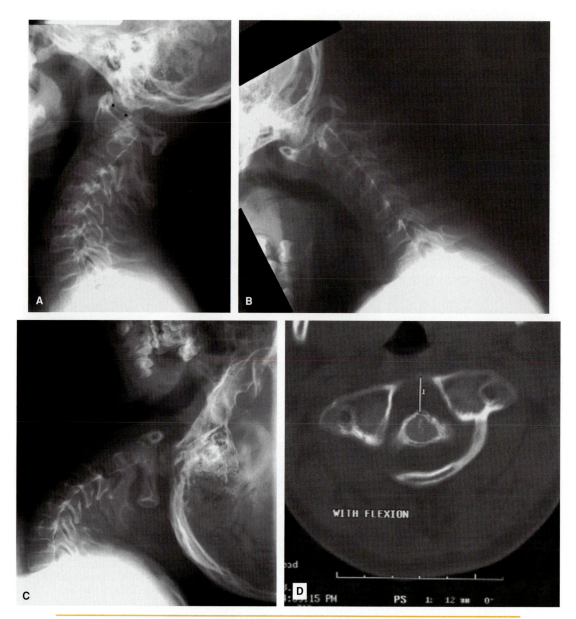

FIGURE 9-9. Atlanto-axial instability. Nine-year-old with Trisomy 21. Neutral **(A)**, flexion **(B)**, and extension **(C)** lateral views of the cervical spine were obtained, which demonstrate marked increase in anteroposterior (AP) distance (*asterisks*) between the odontoid and the posterior arch of C1. This is reconfirmed on the axial CT **(D)** performed at the time of flexion, with a distance between the anterior arch of C1 and the odontoid (*indicated by white line*) of ~12 mm. This greatly exceeds the upper limits of acceptable measurement of 5 mm in a child.

as in a restrained child in a car seat during a high-speed collision, can disrupt this synchondrosis. This fracture is unstable and can cause spinal cord injury. Reduction and treatment with immobilization result in high fusion rates (61).

Hangman fractures (Figs. 9-25, 9-26) are rare in children and usually do not present with neurologic deficit because the disruption actually expands the spinal canal at C2 (62). Halo or collar immobilization is often adequate for treatment.

LOWER CERVICAL SPINE INJURIES (SUBAXIAL)

Subaxial Spinal Injury

In the pediatric population, subaxial cervical spine fractures occur more commonly in older children. Typical fractures in this region are often due to vertebral body compression fractures, or facet fractures, and dislocations secondary to hyperflexion mechanisms (55) (Figs. 9-27–9-30). Injuries to this region in younger children are

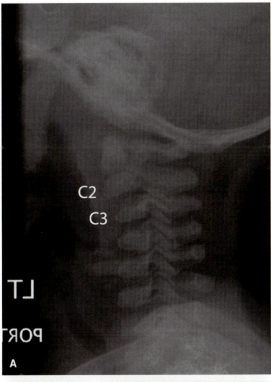

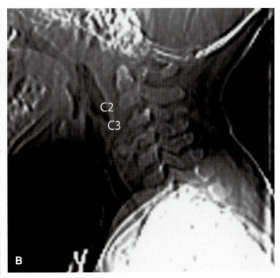

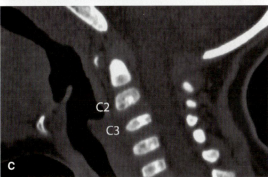

FIGURE 9-10. C2 upon C3 pseudosubluxation. Six-year-old involved in a motor vehicle accident with mental status changes. Lateral cervical spine view **(A)** demonstrates apparent subluxation of C2 upon C3. This is seen to neutralize on the scout view from the cervical spine CT **(B)** and is reconfirmed on the sagittal reconstruction images **(C)**, which demonstrate normal alignment of C2 with respect to C3.

often not radiographically evident and are due to ligamentous injuries. MRI is often adept in elucidating ligamentous injury from flexion or extension injuries (Figs. 9-31–9-33). Although more common in the upper cervical spine, distraction injuries may also occur at lower levels in the cervical spine (Figs. 9-7, 9-8). Difficult to diagnose synchondrotic fractures, occasionally the result of severe extension injuries, may present with displacement in the period beyond the acute setting. Isolated wedge compression fractures in younger children are also occasionally seen (Fig. 9-34). In older children, the types of injuries in this region parallel those of adults (Fig. 9-35).

Thoracolumbar Spinal Injury

Thoracic spine fractures in children most often represent solitary compression fractures caused by falls from a height (Figs. 9-36, 9-37). However, Murray et al. (63)

reported that only 2% of pediatric patients who fell from a height >15 feet sustained spinal injury. The remainder is caused by sporting (i.e., trampoline) and swimming injuries. Less than 10 degrees of wedging requires bed rest and resumption of activities as tolerated, while over 10 degrees of wedging (and up to 50 degrees) associated with a Risser stage of <3, requires immobilization in hyperextension for 2 months, followed by bracing for over a year (64). Surgical stabilization is recommended when compression is >50%, for lateral compression >15 degrees, or in adolescents near skeletal maturity (65). Lateral radiographs are often key in diagnosing compression fractures.

Classification systems for thoracolumbar spine fractures in children have not been proposed, and neither the three-column theory of Denis (66) nor the comprehensive

(text continues on page 268)

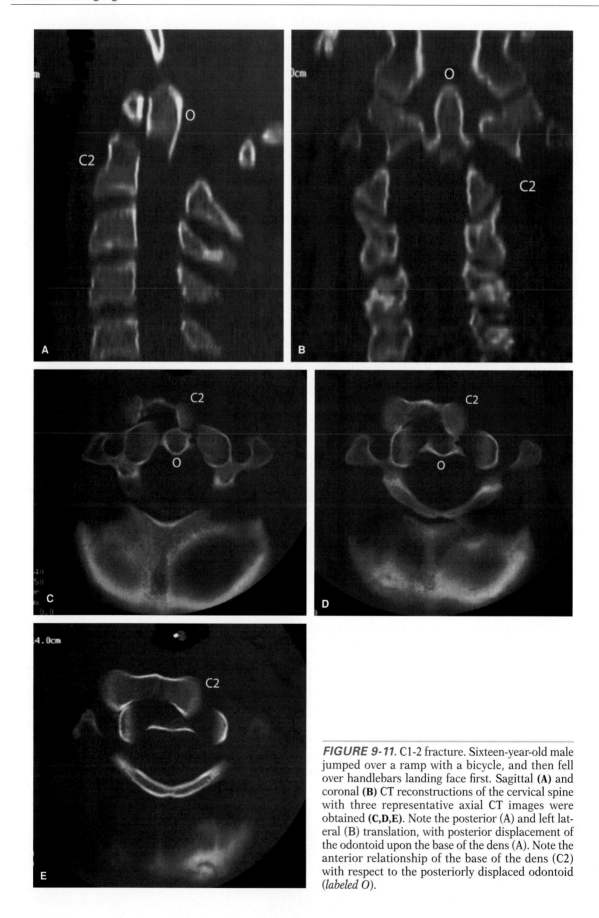

FIGURE 9-11. C1-2 fracture. Sixteen-year-old male jumped over a ramp with a bicycle, and then fell over handlebars landing face first. Sagittal **(A)** and coronal **(B)** CT reconstructions of the cervical spine with three representative axial CT images were obtained **(C,D,E)**. Note the posterior (A) and left lateral (B) translation, with posterior displacement of the odontoid upon the base of the dens (A). Note the anterior relationship of the base of the dens (C2) with respect to the posteriorly displaced odontoid (*labeled O*).

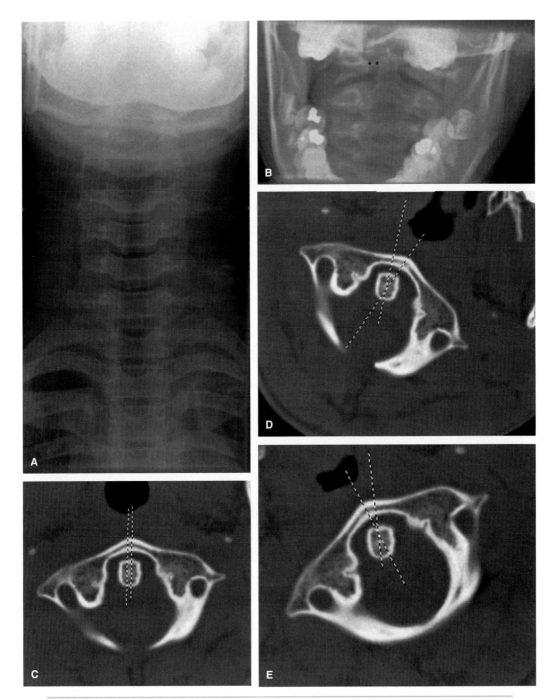

FIGURE 9-12. Normal rotatory subluxation study with no evidence of subluxation. Thirteen-year-old who tried to crack his own neck, now with pain on the right and with head turned to the left. Frontal (A) and open-mouth views (B) demonstrate some head tilt to the left (A), and normal relationship of lateral masses of C1 to C2, with some apparent widening of the distance between the lateral mass of C1 and the odontoid on the right (*asterisks in B*). In order to assess the ability of C1 to normally rotate upon C2, a line is drawn both through the midline raphe of C1 and the midline sagittal point of the odontoid process of C2 (dens). The angles subtended by the anterior arch of C1 upon the odontoid process of C2, in the neutral, rightward rotational, and leftward rotational positions are assessed. Normally, the anterior arch of C1 should be able to subtend an angle beyond the sagittal midpoint of the dens (i.e., beyond 0 degrees), with both rightward and leftward head turning. With rotatory subluxation this is usually easily accomplished to the symptomatic side of suspected fixation, but is not possible toward the opposite side, due to fixation and limitation of rotation beyond the midline. In this patient with absence of rotatory subluxation, note is made of a neutral relationship of the anterior arch of C1 with respect to the odontoid on the neutral view (C). The patient is able to subtend an angle beyond the midline both with rotation to the left (D) and with rotation to the right (E). The findings in (A) and (B) are therefore representative of changes related to muscle spasm/splinting, secondary to torticollis.

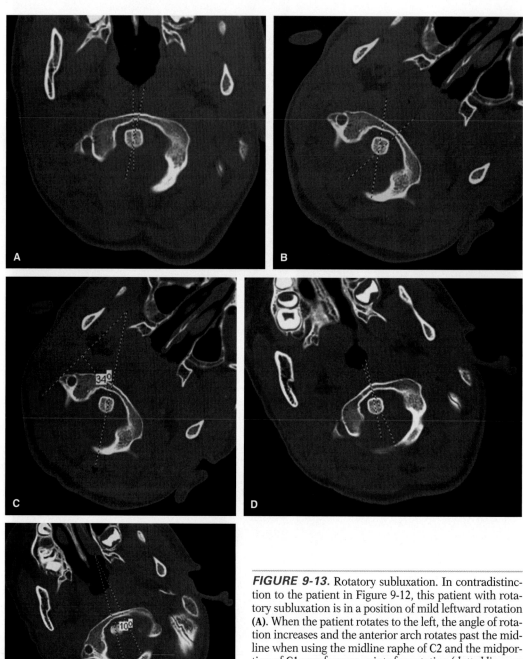

FIGURE 9-13. Rotatory subluxation. In contradistinction to the patient in Figure 9-12, this patient with rotatory subluxation is in a position of mild leftward rotation **(A)**. When the patient rotates to the left, the angle of rotation increases and the anterior arch rotates past the midline when using the midline raphe of C2 and the midportion of C1 as reference points for rotation (*dotted lines on images B and C*). When rotating to the right, however, the angle of rotation is decreased and the patient is unable to mobilize the anterior arch of C1 beyond the midline to the right (*dotted lines on images D and E*).

classification of Magerl et al. (34) has been validated for the pediatric population. The more severe burst, flexion distraction, Chance, lateral compression, and rotational injury high energy spinal fractures are most often the result of motor vehicle accidents, including lap-belt injuries (Figs. 9-38–9-42). The Chance-type fracture, a flexion-distraction injury, is a horizontal fracture extending from the anterior to the posterior elements, either involving osseous or discoligamentous structures. Although

associated intra-abdominal injury remains a concern in the setting of Chance fractures, this association reported in a multicenter review was demonstrated in only 33% of cases, most often identified by CT (67) (Fig. 9-43). Spondylolysis and spondylolisthesis are most often seen after sporting injuries, likely from hyperextension, and are more common in older children (Fig. 9-44). Evaluation of

(text continues on page 299)

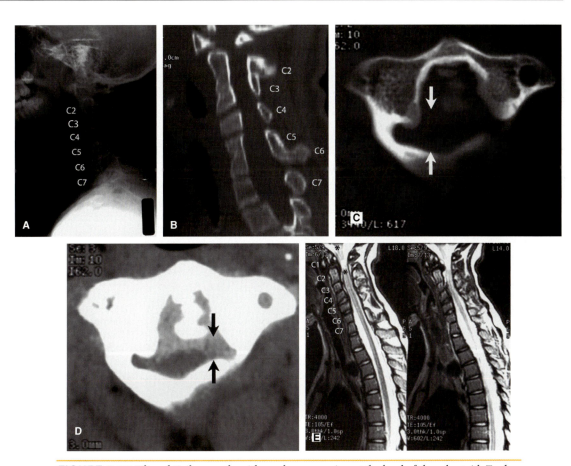

FIGURE 9-14. Klippel-Feil anomaly with cord compression at the level of the odontoid. Twelve-year-old with minor trauma, noted to be quadriplegic on examination. Lateral view of the cervical spine **(A)** demonstrates abnormal fusion of the vertebral bodies and posterior elements at multiple levels. This is confirmed on the sagittal CT reconstruction **(B)** with fusion at C2-3 and C5-6. Axial bone window **(C)** and soft tissue window **(D)** from the same CT examination demonstrate marked anteroposterior (AP) narrowing of the spinal canal (*arrows*). Note the compression of the spinal cord on the soft tissue window (D). Sagittal T2-weighted images of the cervical spine from MRI **(E)** demonstrate the narrowing of the spinal canal (*asterisks*) at the level of the above noted abnormality. There is abnormal signal intensity within the spinal cord, again suggestive of spinal cord injury or myelomalacia. Note the fusion abnormalities of the vertebral bodies.

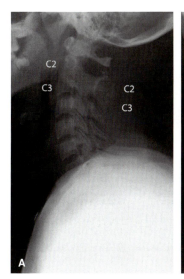

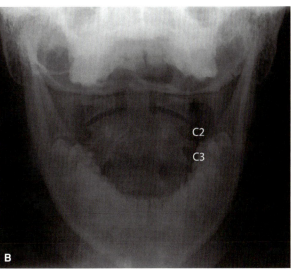

FIGURE 9-15. C2-3 posterior fusion anomaly. Pedestrian versus automobile. Frontal **(A)** and open-mouth view **(B)** demonstrate abnormal bony fusion of the C2 and C3 vertebral bodies with absence of an intervertebral disc and nonseparation of the posterior elements of C2 and C3. Note the apparent overgrowth of the bone posteriorly, which is secondary to fusion of two adjacent vertebral segments.

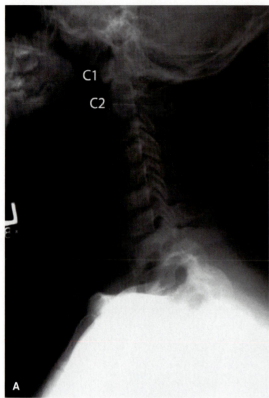

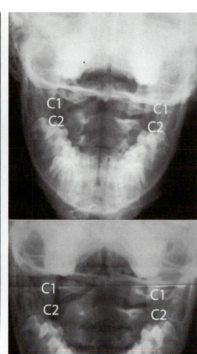

FIGURE 9-16. Anomalous C2 variant. Ten-year-old with minor neck trauma. Lateral **(A)** and two open-mouth views **(B)** demonstrate an anomalous C2 vertebral body. Note the hypoplasia of the left half of the C2 vertebral body, with caudal displacement of the left lateral mass of C1 with respect to its counterpart on the right.

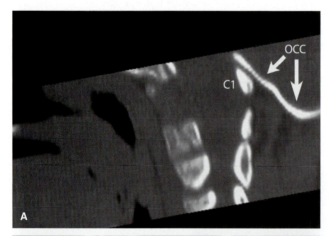

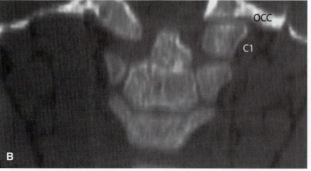

FIGURE 9-17. Occipitalization of the C1 vertebral body with the appearance of upward invagination of the cervical spine. Three-year-old status postfall. Sagittal **(A)** and coronal **(B)** CT reconstructions demonstrate abnormal C1 posterior element fusion to the base of the occiput (OCC) (A), and abnormal fusion of the lateral mass of C1 to the left half of the occiput (OCC) (B). This leads to lack of mobility at this level and upward displacement of the odontoid toward the level of the foramen magnum.

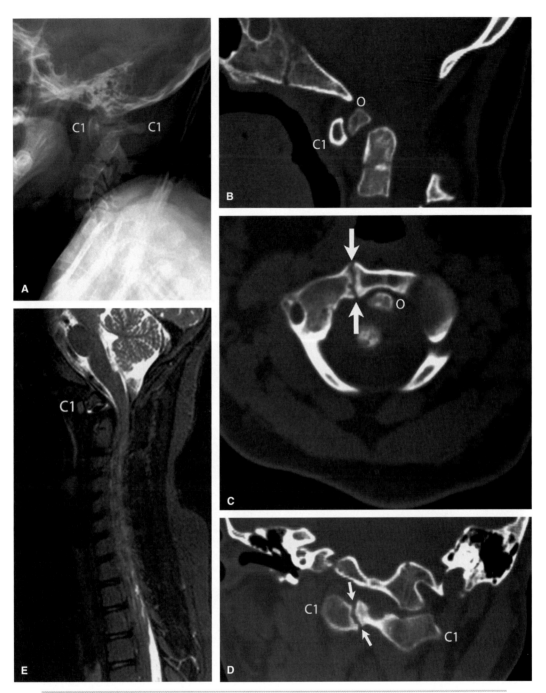

FIGURE 9-18. Dysmorphic C1-2 junction, secondary to congenital abnormality (os odontoideum) versus old trauma (type I odontoid fracture). Seven-and-a-half-year-old Trisomy 21 patient status postfall. Lateral view of the cervical spine **(A)** demonstrates abnormal lordosis of the cervical spine. The anterior arch of C1 is displaced anteriorly and the posterior arch of C1 is high riding. Sagittal reconstruction image obtained from the axial CT **(B)** reconfirms anterior placement of the anterior arch of C1. The tip of the odontoid (*labeled O*) is ventrally displaced and moves in conjunction with the anterior arch of C1. Axial CT **(C)** confirms the above-noted findings. Additionally, there is an abnormal bony partial nonunion of the anterior arch of C1 visualized (*arrows in C*), which is reconfirmed on the coronal reconstruction image **(D)** from the same CT (*arrows in D*). Sagittal T2-weighted image through the cervical spine **(E)** demonstrates no significant soft tissue abnormality or signal abnormality within the marrow at C1-2, suggesting there is no acute injury present.

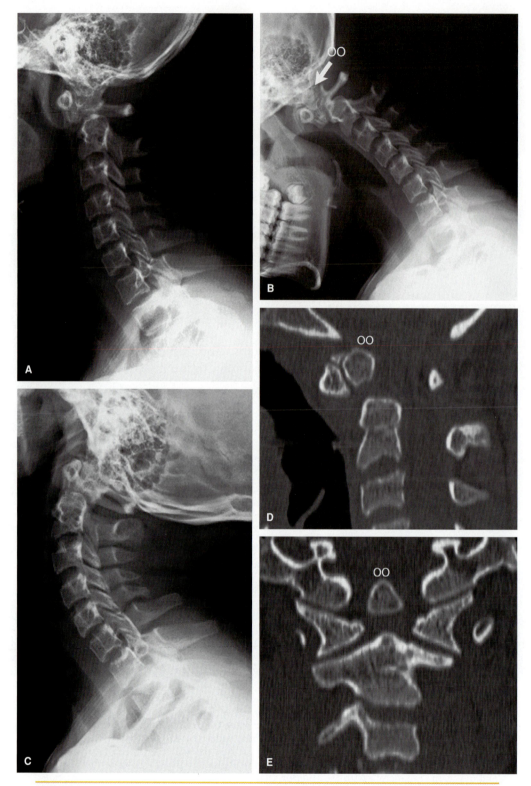

FIGURE 9-19. Os odontoideum with C1 on C2 subluxation. Fourteen-and-a-half-year-old male with lower extremity spasticity and C1-2 instability. Neutral (**A**), flexion (**B**), and extension (**C**) views of the cervical spine demonstrate an abnormal tip of the odontoid in keeping with an os odontoideum (*labeled OO*). The odontoid appears to move as a unit with the anterior arch of C1. Sagittal (**D**) and coronal (**E**) CT reconstructions confirm the findings of the plain film, with a gap between the base of the odontoid and the os odontoideum, which is closely related to the anterior arch of C1. (*continued*)

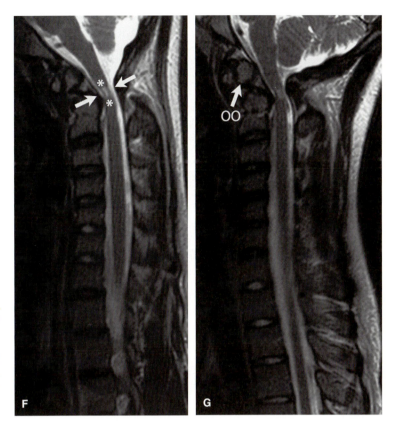

FIGURE 9-19. (*CONTINUED*) Sagittal flexion (**F**) and extension (**G**) T2-weighted MRIs of the spine demonstrate narrowing of the spinal canal (*arrows in F*) in the anteroposterior (AP) dimension. Note the abnormal signal intensity within the upper spinal cord at the cervical-medullary junction, in keeping with myelomalacia (*asterisks in F*), most likely secondary to abnormal mobility at the cranial cervical junction.

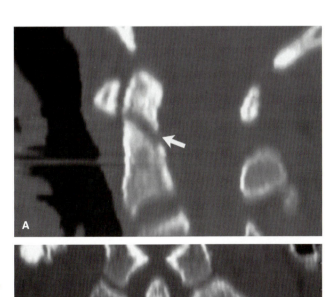

FIGURE 9-20. Type II odontoid fracture. Sixteen-year-old with neck trauma. Sagittal (**A**) and coronal (**B**) CT reconstruction images of the cervical spine demonstrate an obliquely oriented fracture line (*arrows*) through the midodontoid just above the level of the dentocentral synchondrosis, with no displacement, in keeping with a type II odontoid fracture.

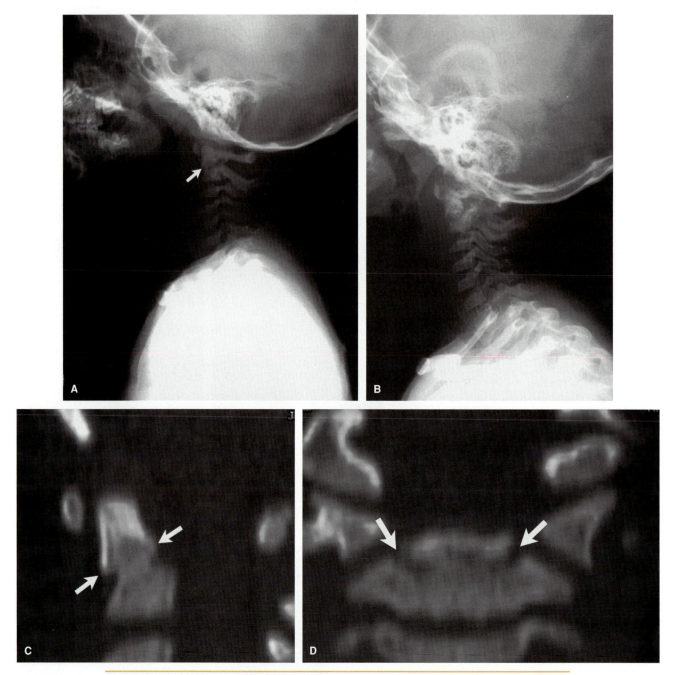

FIGURE 9-21. Type II odontoid fracture. Three-year-old jumped out of bed, now with neck pain. Lateral cervical spine views **(A,B)**, sagittal CT reconstruction **(C)**, and coronal CT reconstruction **(D)**, demonstrate a fracture (*arrows*) through the odontoid just above the level of the synchondrosis, with forward flexion of the odontoid process upon the base of C2.

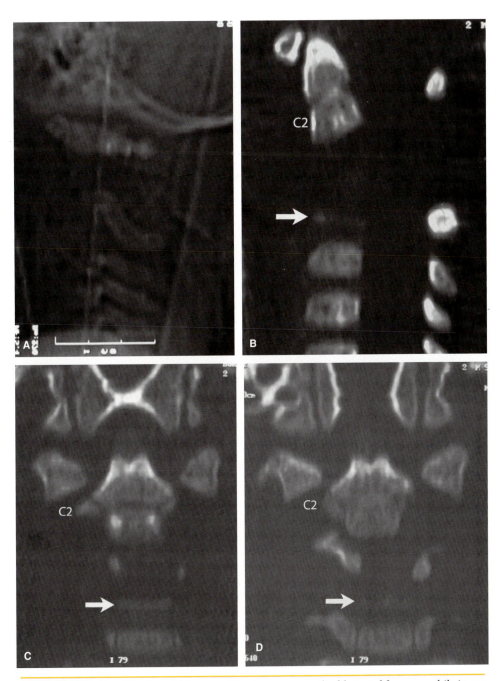

FIGURE 9-22. Type III odontoid fracture. Twenty-seven-month-old ejected from car while in car seat, with resultant quadriplegia and downbeat nystagmus. Lateral scout view from CT **(A)**, sagittal CT reconstruction **(B)**, and sequential coronal CT reconstruction images **(C,D,E,F)**, as well as sagittal STIR from MRI **(G)**, demonstrate a fracture through the lower most aspect of C2 (*arrows in B,C,D*) with marked distraction and kyphotic deformity, prevertebral and posterior soft tissue swelling, and marked signal abnormality within the cervical cord (*asterisks in G*), in keeping with cervical cord disruption. Disruption of the posterior longitudinal ligament, as indicated by the increased T2 signal along the posterior soft tissues (*arrows in G*), is indicative of an unstable injury. (*continued*)

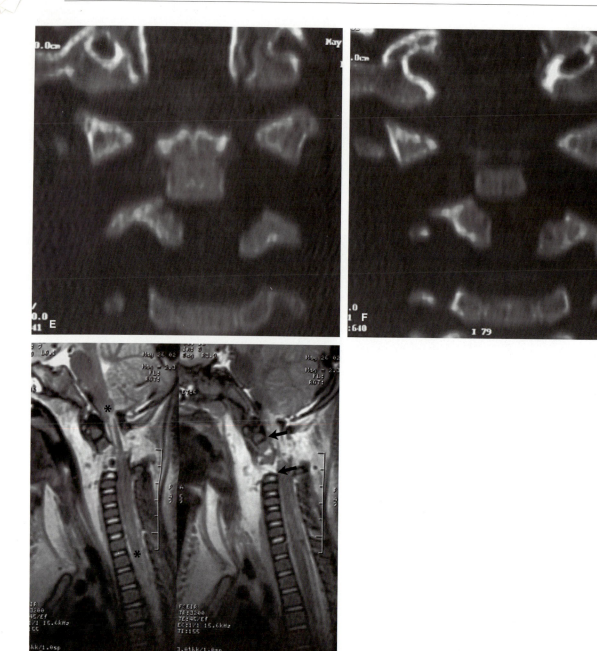

FIGURE 9-22. *(CONTINUED).*

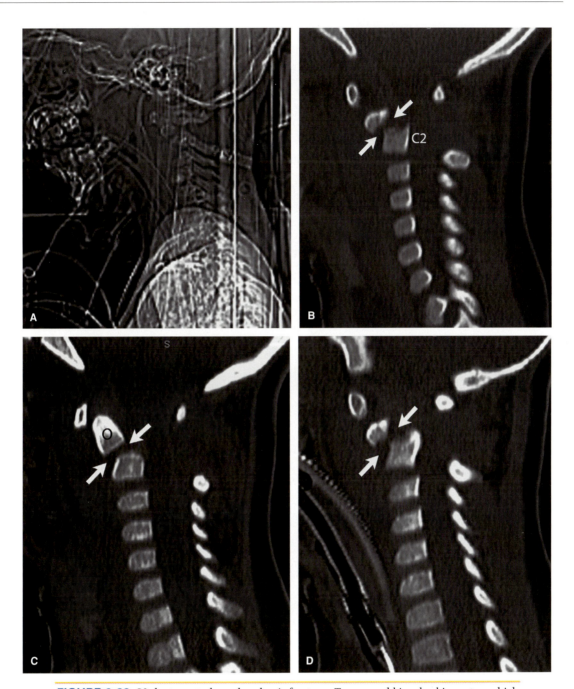

FIGURE 9-23. C2 dentocentral synchondrosis fracture. Two-year-old involved in motor vehicle accident, with resultant C-spine injury and flaccid paralysis. Lateral scout view from the cervical spine CT **(A)**, sagittal reconstruction images from right **(B)**, to midline **(C)**, to left **(D)**, and axial CT **(E)** demonstrate a fracture (*arrows*) through the odontoid (*labeled O in C*) with ventral displacement of the odontoid upon the base of C2 at the level of the dentocentral synchondrosis. Also seen is an increase in distance between the posterior arches of C1 and C2. The findings are reconfirmed on sagittal T2-weighted images on the cervical spine **(F)**. Note the ventral tilt of the odontoid, the signal abnormality within the cervical cord (*asterisks*), and the prevertebral and posterior soft tissue swelling (*labeled STS*), suggestive of ligamentous disruption. (*continued*)

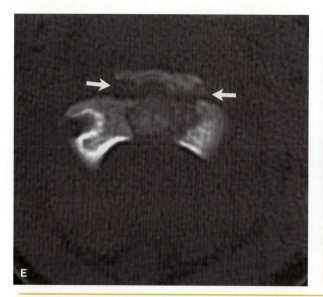

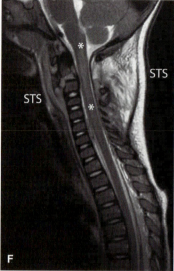

FIGURE 9-23. (CONTINUED).

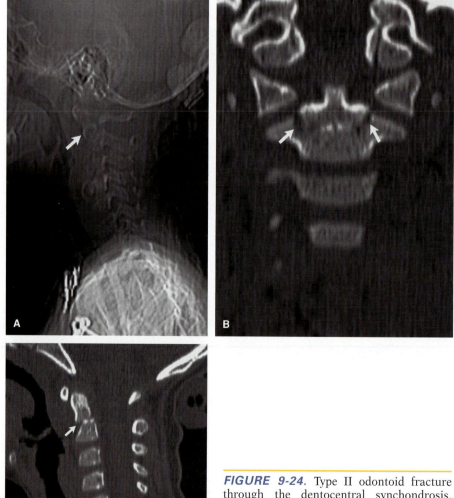

FIGURE 9-24. Type II odontoid fracture through the dentocentral synchrondrosis. Three-year-old fell off of bed. Lateral scout view from cervical spine CT **(A)**, coronal CT reconstruction **(B)**, and sagittal CT reconstruction **(C)** demonstrate a fracture through the base of the odontoid at the level of the dentocentral synchondrosis (*arrows*) in keeping with a type II odontoid fracture.

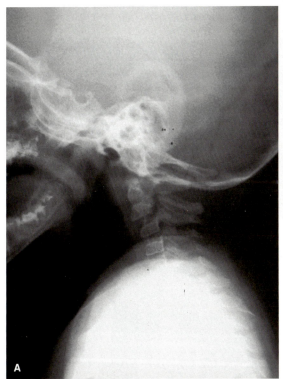

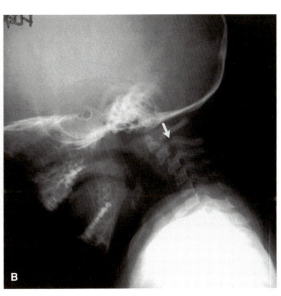

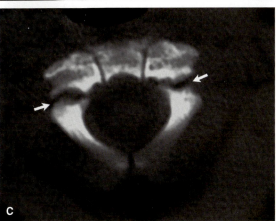

FIGURE 9-25. Bilateral C2 pedicle fracture (hangman fracture). Eleven-month-old status postfall. Lateral neutral view of the cervical spine **(A)** and flexion view **(B)**, as well as axial CT image **(C)** through the level of injury, demonstrate bilateral C2 pedicle fractures (*arrows in B and C*).

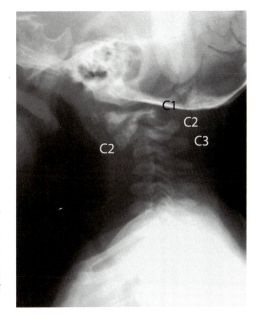

FIGURE 9-26. C2 Hangman fracture. Ten-month-old with questionable neck trauma. Single lateral view of the cervical spine demonstrates marked kyphotic deformity of the upper cervical spine at the level of C2. Note the disruption in the posterior elements of C2 with resultant anterior displacement of C2 upon C3. There is anterior translation of the C2 vertebral body upon C3. Note the marked anterior displacement of posterior arch of C1 with respect to the posterior arch of C2, with anterior displacement of the posterior spinal-laminar line.

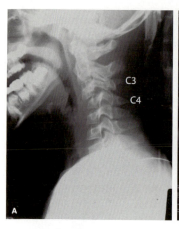
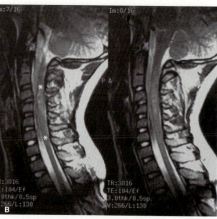

FIGURE 9-27. C3-4 jumped facet with associated with cord contusion. Eight-year-old flipped over on all-terrain-vehicle (ATV); now quadriplegic postaccident. Lateral cervical spine view **(A)** demonstrates marked anterior displacement of C3 upon C4. Note the anterior overriding of the facet of C3 upon C4. Sagittal T2-images (postreduction) through the spine at the level of injury **(B)** demonstrate abnormal increased signal within the spinal cord (*asterisks*) and loss of the normal cervical lordosis.

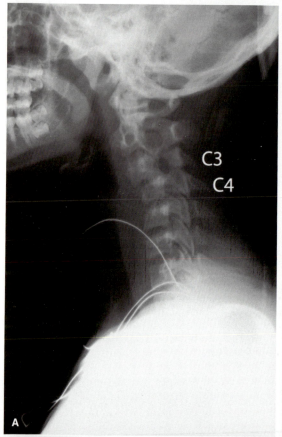

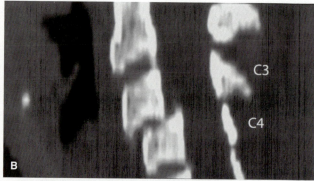

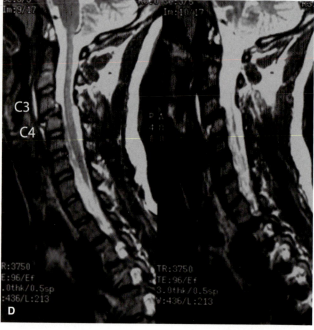

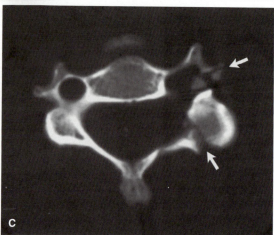

FIGURE 9-28. C3-4 posterior element fracture with unilateral jumped facet. Thirteen-year-old in a motor vehicle accident and thrown from driver's seat. Lateral cervical spine view **(A)**, sagittal CT reconstruction **(B)**, axial CT from level of injury **(C)**, and sagittal T2-weighted images from MRI **(D)** demonstrate a fracture through the posterior elements on the left (*arrows in C*), with resultant anterior displacement of C3 upon C4 (A,B,D), and narrowing of the spinal canal to the left of midline (D). Unilateral jumped facet is inferred by visualization of the entire neural foramen of C3 and the apparent rotation below this level as visualized on the lateral view (A).

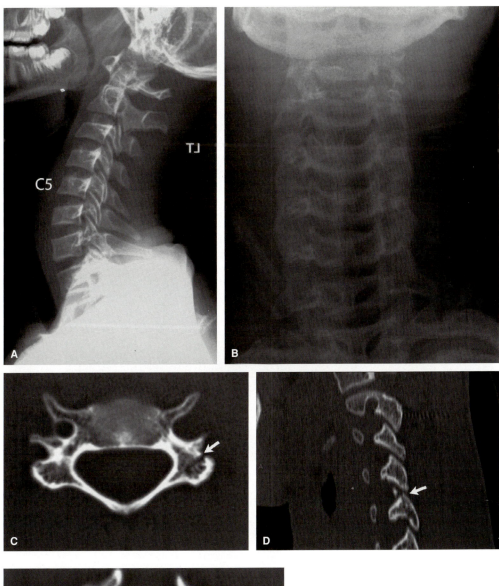

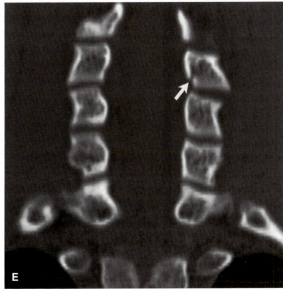

FIGURE 9-29. Left C5 facet fracture with perched facet. Thirteen-year-old status post–motor vehicle accident with focal point tenderness at the midcervical region. Lateral (**A**), anteroposterior (**B**), axial CT (**C**), and sagittal CT reconstruction (**D**), as well as coronal CT reconstruction (**E**), demonstrate a fracture through the left facet and lamina of C5 (*arrow in C*), with a small bony fragment seen on the sagittal reconstruction (*arrow in D*). Facet fracture is confirmed on the coronal image (*arrow in E*).

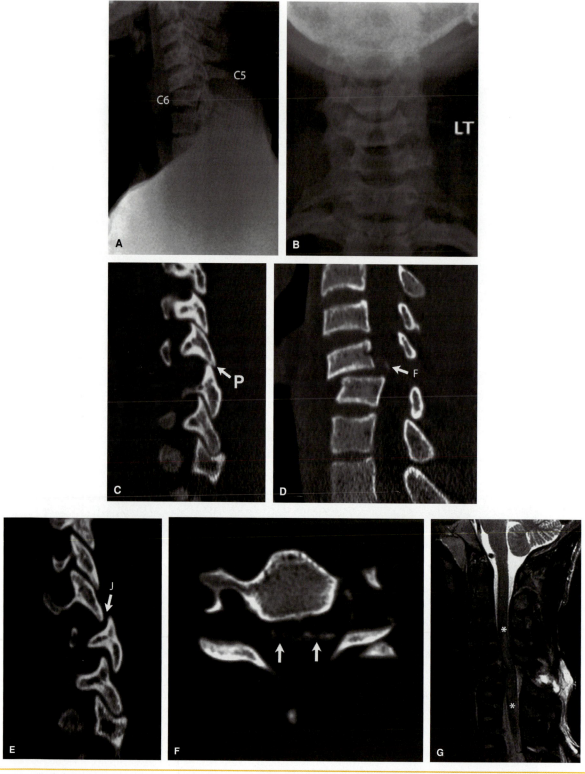

FIGURE 9-30. Left jumped facet, right perched facet, at the C5-6 level. Seventeen-year-old status postwrestling injury now with incomplete quadriplegia. Lateral **(A)** and anteroposterior **(B)** views demonstrate malalignment of the cervical spine at the level of C5-6. Sagittal CT reconstructions from left to right **(C,D,E)** demonstrate perching *(labeled P)* of the right C5-6 facet (C), a jumped *(labeled J)* left facet of the same level (E), and a small posterior bony fragment *(labeled F)* noted on sagittal reconstruction images (D). This fracture is reconfirmed on the axial CT **(F)** bone windows *(arrows in F)*. Sagittal T2-weighted image of the cervical spine **(G)** demonstrates marked compromise of the spinal canal at this level, with posterior soft tissue swelling and abnormal increased signal intensity. Abnormal increased signal abnormality is seen within the spinal cord *(asterisks in G)*, indicative of spinal cord injury.

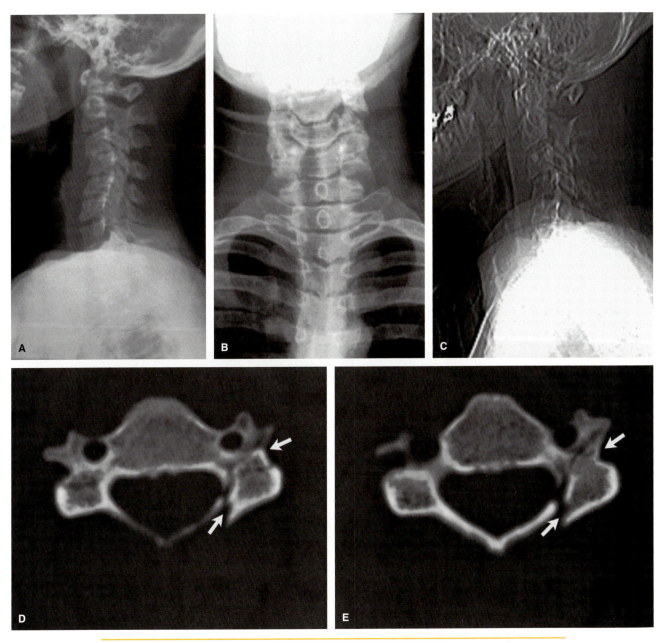

FIGURE 9-31. Comminuted left C4 fracture involving the pedicle, lamina, and transverse process. Fell out of wheelchair. Lateral **(A)** and anteroposterior **(B)** views of the cervical spine demonstrate kyphotic deformity at the C3-4 level, which is confirmed on the sagittal localizing view of the cervical spine **(C)**. Representative axial bone images through C4 **(D,E,F)** demonstrate the fracture (*arrows*) through the posterior elements of C4 on the left. (*continued*)

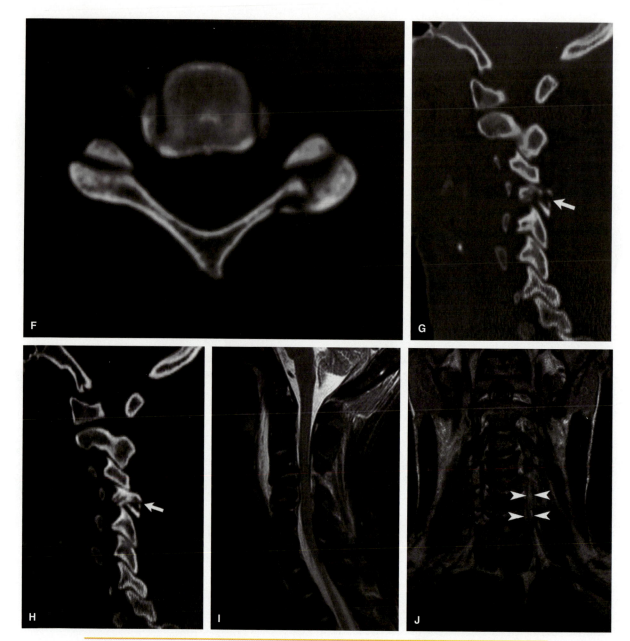

FIGURE 9-31. (*CONTINUED*) This is confirmed on the sagittal CT reconstruction bone images
(G,H). Sagittal short tau inversion recovery (STIR) **(I)**, and coronal T2 **(J)** MRI demonstrate prevertebral soft tissue swelling and kyphotic deformity, as well as narrowing of the spinal canal in
the anteroposterior dimension, best visualized on the sagittal STIR image (I). Of note, there is
absence of flow void within the left vertebral artery as visualized on the coronal T2-weighted
image (*arrowheads in J*), in keeping with a vertebral artery dissection.

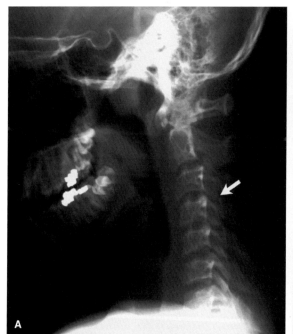

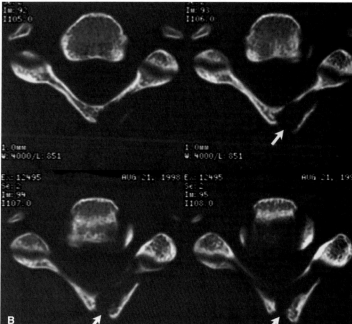

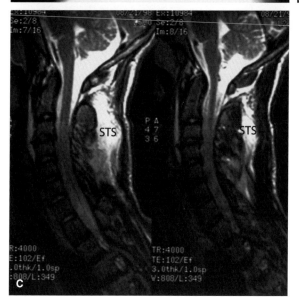

FIGURE 9-32. C4 laminar fracture. Fourteen-year-old fell over handlebars. Lateral cervical spine **(A)**, axial CT images through the areas of interest **(B)**, and sagittal T2-weighed images through the area of interest **(C)** demonstrate a left-sided C4 laminar fracture (*arrows in B*), with prevertebral swelling and marked posterior soft tissue swelling (STS) (C). Note the subtle cortical disruption as visualized on the lateral view of the cervical spine (*arrow in A*).

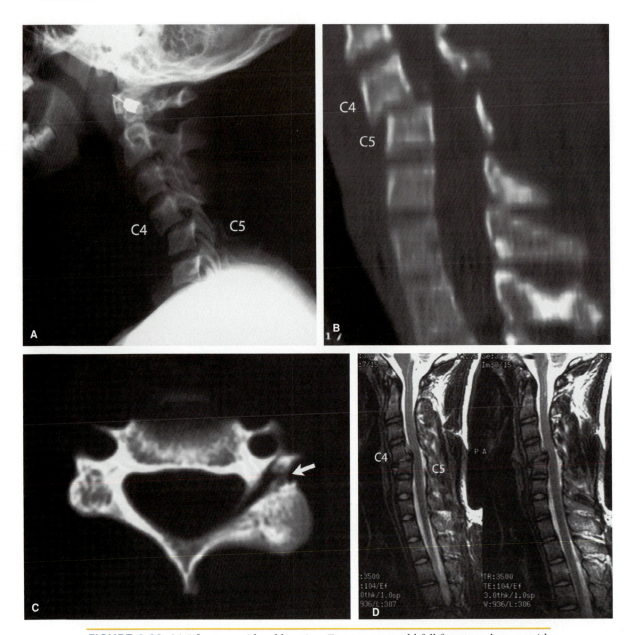

FIGURE 9-33. C4-5 fracture with subluxation. Fourteen-year-old fell from porch, now with bilateral arm weakness. Lateral view of the cervical spine **(A)** demonstrates marked anterolisthesis of C4 upon C5. This is reconfirmed on sagittal CT reconstruction **(B)**. Note the fracture line *(arrow)* through the posterior elements of C4 as visualized on axial CT **(C)**. Sagittal T2-weighted images through the cervical spine **(D)**, demonstrate kyphotic deformity at the level of injury with associated compromise of the spinal canal in the anteroposterior dimension.

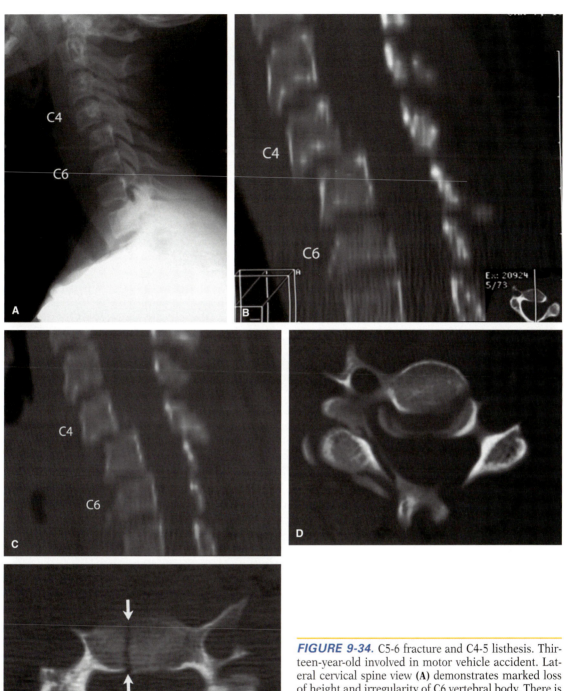

FIGURE 9-34. C5-6 fracture and C4-5 listhesis. Thirteen-year-old involved in motor vehicle accident. Lateral cervical spine view **(A)** demonstrates marked loss of height and irregularity of C6 vertebral body. There is loss of the normal cervical lordosis. Sagittal CT reconstruction demonstrate C4 on C5 anterolisthesis **(B,C)** as well as loss of height of the C6 vertebral body. Axial CT **(D)** demonstrates the anterolisthesis of C4 upon C5, and a fracture of the C6 vertebral body is confirmed on axial CT (*arrows in E*) with extension into the posterior elements on the right.

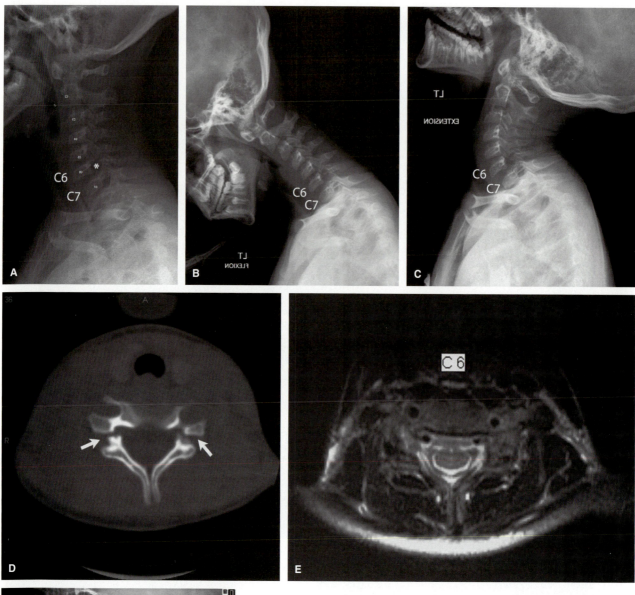

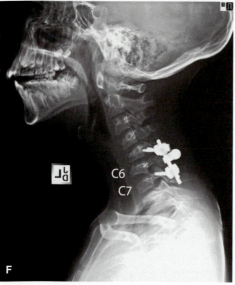

FIGURE 9-35. Old bilateral C6 pars fractures with spondylosis (not to be mistaken for an acute injury). Thirteen-year-old male ran into stop sign, now with headache and neck pain. Neutral lateral (**A**), flexion lateral (**B**), and extension lateral (**C**) images of cervical spine demonstrate anterolisthesis of C6 on C7. A fracture line is seen on the lateral view (*asterisk in A*). This is confirmed on the axial CT bone window (**D**) as bilateral lucent lines (pseudofacet sign) (*arrows*) through the bilateral posterior elements; this finding is similar to that seen with pars defects in the lumbar spine. No acute marrow signal abnormality is noted on the axial T2-weighted MRI of the spine, indicating that there is no acute fracture (**E**). Lateral view of the cervical spine (**F**) demonstrates postoperative fixation of the injury with loss of the normal cervical lordosis, but with relative reduction of the previously noted anterolisthesis of C6 upon C7.

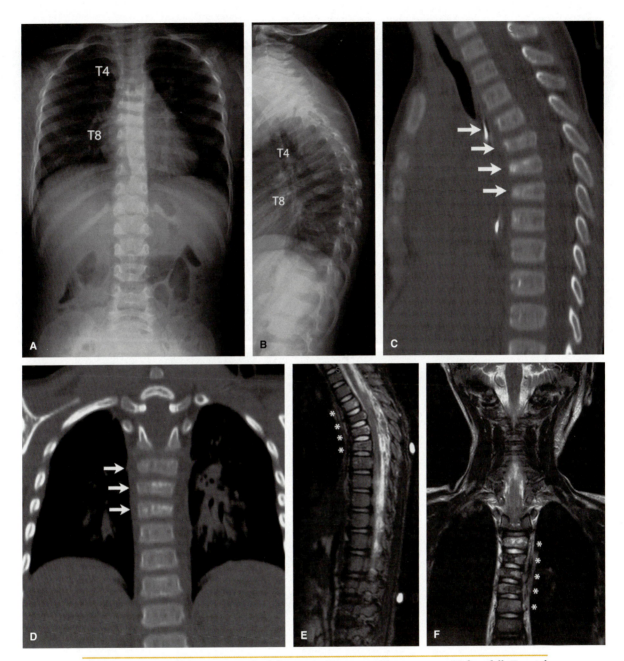

FIGURE 9-36. Midthoracic vertebral fractures. Two-year-old status post–12-foot fall. Frontal (**A**) and lateral (**B**) views of the thoracic spine demonstrate loss of height in the midthoracic vertebral bodies from T4 through to T8. This is reconfirmed on the sagittal CT reconstruction (**C**) and the coronal CT reconstruction (*arrows*) (**D**). Marrow edema and loss of height of the vertebral bodies is noted on sagittal T2 (**E**) and coronal T2 (**F**) weighted MRI (*asterisks mark levels of abnormal vertebral bodies*).

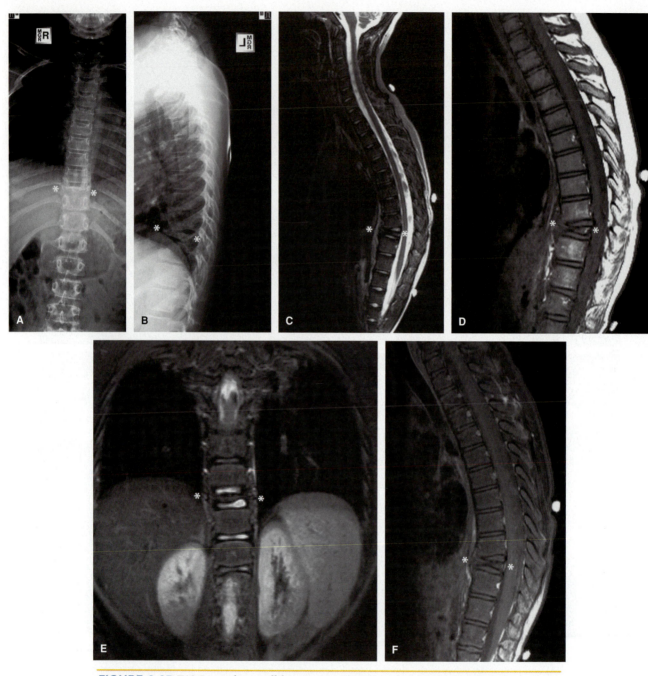

FIGURE 9-37. T10 Langerhans cell histiocytosis (LCH) with associated pathologic fracture. Eight-and-a-half-year-old with T10 compression fracture secondary to LCH. Frontal **(A)** and lateral **(B)** views of the thoracic spine demonstrate loss of the height of the T10 vertebral body (*asterisks*). This is confirmed on a sagittal T2-weighted MRI **(C)** and further demonstrated on sagittal T1 **(D)** and coronal short tau inversion recovery (STIR) **(E)** MRI of the thoracic spine. Postcontrast T1-weighted MRI **(F)** demonstrates no significant abnormal contrast enhancement. This is typical of a vertebra plana (flattened vertebra) seen with LCH, and is essentially a pathologic fracture through an area of abnormal bone, not to be mistaken for a posttraumatic fracture of the thoracic spine.

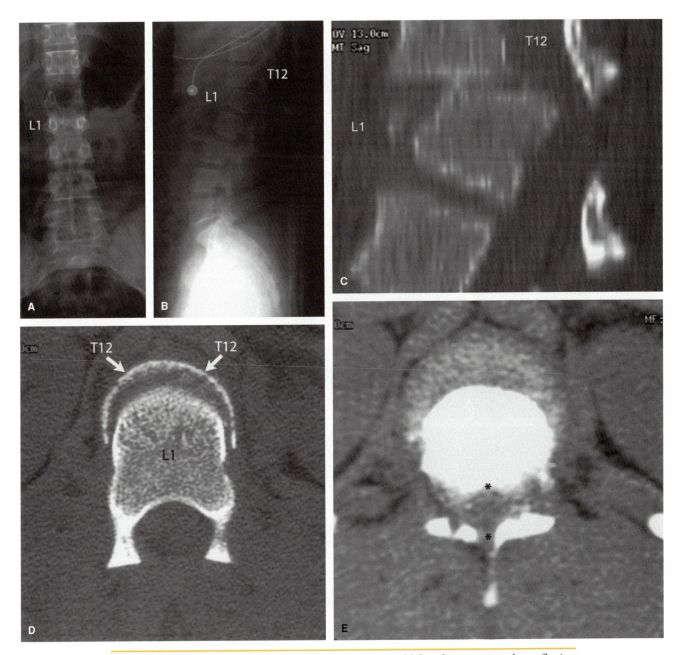

FIGURE 9-38. Fracture-dislocation of L1. Eleven-year-old female status post hyperflexion injury sustained on a trampoline after being fallen upon by another child. Frontal **(A)** and lateral **(B)** views of the lumbar spine demonstrate anterolisthesis of T12 upon L1 and splaying of the spinous processes of T12 with respect to L1, secondary to a hyperflexion injury with resultant fracture-dislocation. This is confirmed on the sagittal reconstruction CT image **(C)**. Axial CT image **(D)** demonstrates the outline of the cortex of the T12 vertebral body above with respect to the more posterior located L1 vertebral body below. Axial soft tissue window from CT of the lumbar spine **(E)** demonstrates narrowing of the lumbar spinal canal (*asterisks*) at the level of the fracture-dislocation.

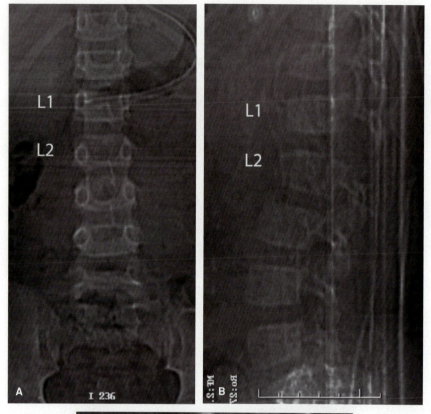

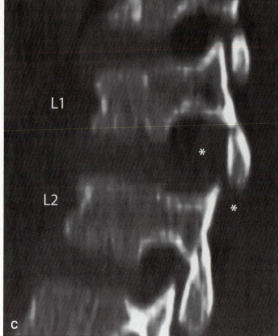

FIGURE 9-39. L1 upon L2 perched facets. Eight-year-old restrained rear seat passenger. Frontal **(A)** and lateral **(B)** CT scout views of the lumbar spine demonstrate abnormal relationship of the L1 upon the L2 vertebral body with increase in distraction of the L1 vertebral body from the L2 vertebral body. Sagittal reconstruction CT image **(C)** demonstrates an increase in distance between the L1 and L2 vertebral bodies, with perching of the facet (*asterisks*) of L1 above upon L2 below. The patient also sustained a duodenal injury, not demonstrated in this figure.

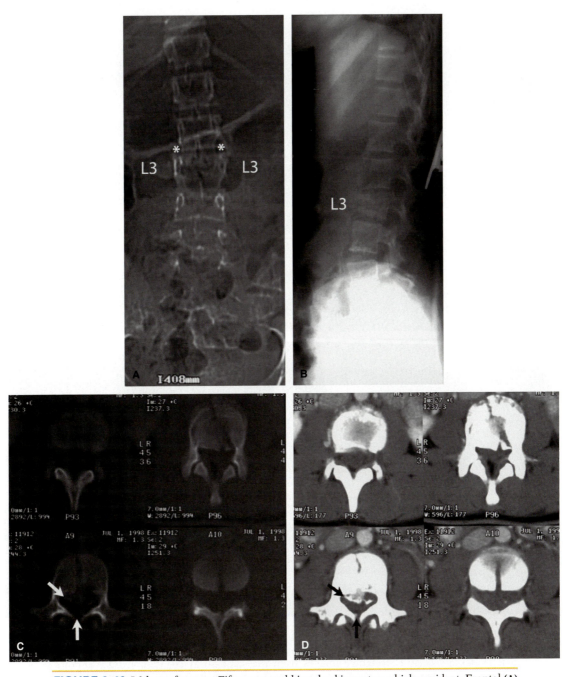

FIGURE 9-40. L3 burst fracture. Fifteen-year-old involved in motor vehicle accident. Frontal **(A)** and lateral **(B)** views of the lumbar spine demonstrate abnormal configuration to the L3 verte-bral body with increase in the interpediculate distance of L3 (*asterisks in A*) and loss of height of the L3 vertebral body as visualized on the lateral view of the lumbar spine **(B)**. Axial bone win-dow from CT **(C)** and soft tissue window from the same CT **(D)** demonstrate the narrowing of the spinal canal (*arrows*) at the level of the burst fracture. (*continued*)

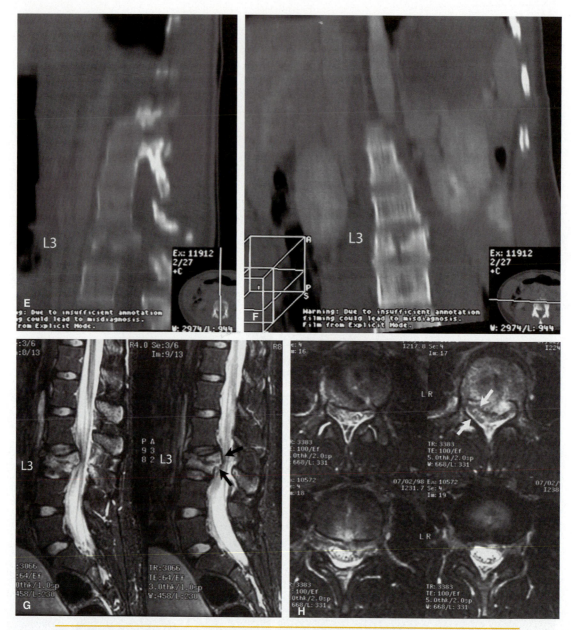

FIGURE 9-40. (*CONTINUED*) Sagittal reconstruction (**E**) and coronal CT reconstruction (**F**) redemonstrate the fracture as seen on the plain films. Sagittal T2-weighted image of the lumbar spine (**G**) and axial T2-weighted images from the same study (**H**) demonstrate abnormal increased signal intensity and configuration of the L3 vertebral body with a retropulsed fragment (*arrows in G*) seen narrowing the spinal canal in the anteroposterior dimension (*arrows in H*).

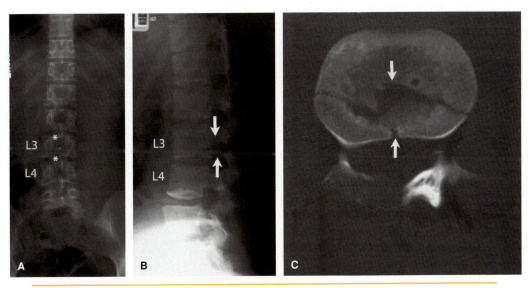

FIGURE 9-41. L3 Chance fracture. Sixteen-year-old involved in motor vehicle accident. Frontal **(A)** and lateral **(B)** views of the lumbar spine demonstrate an increase in the distance between the spinous processes of L3 and L4 on the frontal view *(asterisks in A)* and a posterior fracture/split through the lower L3 vertebral body into the posterior elements *(arrows in B)*. This is confirmed on the axial CT **(C)**.

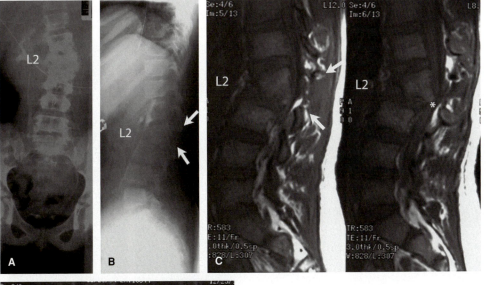

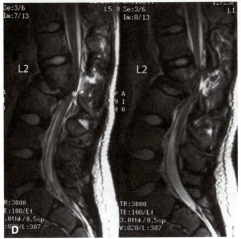

FIGURE 9-42. L2 Chance fracture. Ten-year-old rear seat passenger restrained by lap belt. Frontal **(A)** and lateral **(B)** views of the lumbar spine demonstrate malalignment of the lumbar spine at the L2 level with a convex leftward scoliosis (A) and kyphotic deformity (B) at the L2 level. Note the posterior opening of the spinal elements at L2 *(arrows in B)*. The findings are reconfirmed on sagittal T1-weighted **(C)** and sagittal T2-weighted **(D)** MRI. Note the kyphotic deformity, the retropulsed bony fragment *(asterisks)*, and the compromise of the spinal canal at this level.

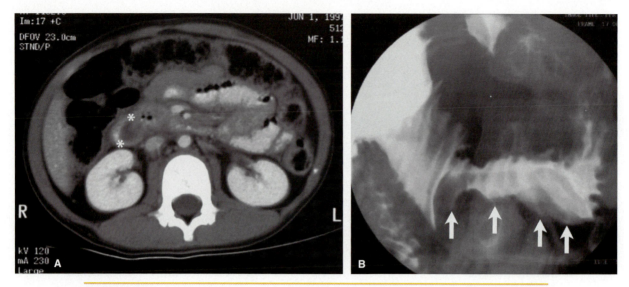

FIGURE 9-43. Duodenal hematoma. Rear seat passenger who sustained a lap belt injury. Axial contrast enhanced CT **(A)** and prone image from single contrast upper GI examination **(B)**, in a different patient than in Figures 9-41 and 9-42, but with a similar mechanism, demonstrate a hematoma within the duodenal wall (low attenuation region on CT) (*asterisks in A*), with contour abnormality along the inferior portion of the duodenum (*arrows*) on the upper GI examination **(B)**. This is a not an uncommon type of injury with lap-belt-type injuries in which children also sustain Chance-type fractures.

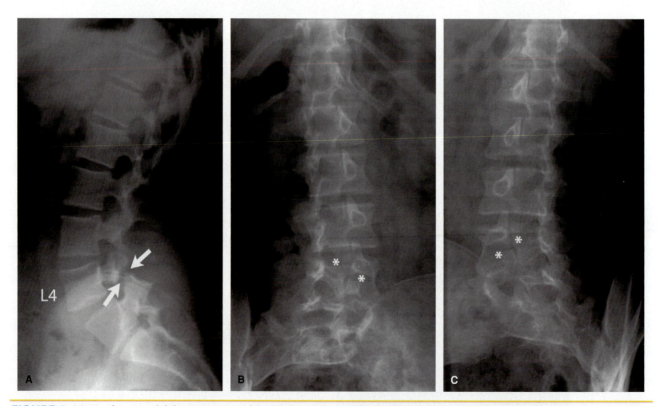

FIGURE 9-44. Lumbar spondylolysis. Imaging of the lumbar spine in four separate patients with low back pain, two with L4 spondylolysis **(A,B,C,D,E)** and two with L5 spondylolysis **(F,G,H,I,J,K)** demonstrates the multimodality approach to imaging when assessing for spondylolysis/spondylolisthesis. Conventional lumbar radiographs, including lateral and bilateral obliques (A,B,C) nicely demonstrate the bony break (*arrows in A*) within the region of the bilateral L4 pars interarticularis, with the infraction seen in the region of the so-called Scotty dog (*asterisks in B and C*). (*continued*)

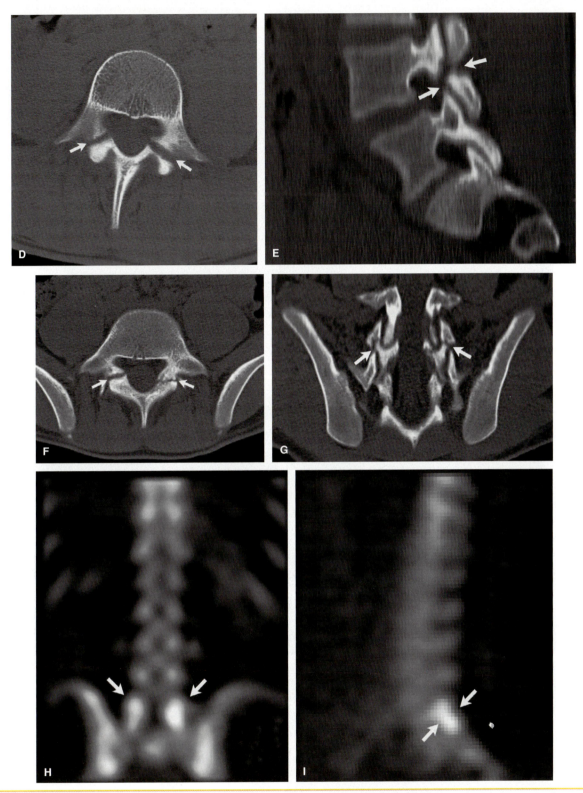

FIGURE 9-44. (*CONTINUED*) Axial (D) and sagittal (E) CT reconstruction through the level of the right pars interarticularis in a second patient with L4 spondylolysis demonstrate the fractures (*arrows in D and E*) within the region of the bilateral pars interarticularis, the so-called pseudofacet sign as seen on the axial image, which is confirmed on the sagittal reconstruction image. CT (F,G) and nuclear medicine single photon emission computed tomography (SPECT) bone scan (H,I) in a patient with L5 spondylolysis again demonstrate the pseudofacet sign (*arrows*) in the region of the L5 bilateral pars interarticularis (F), confirmed on coronal reconstruction image (G). Focal areas of radiotracer uptake (*arrows*) in the region of the L5 pars interarticularis are nicely demonstrated on the coronal (H) and sagittal (I) tomographic views from bone SPECT examination. Although not the modality of choice when imaging for spondylolysis, MRI can adequately demonstrate the area of involvement by its increased T2 signal secondary to bone marrow edema at the site of infraction, as indicated by arrows in a sagittal T2-weighted image with fat saturation (J), and axial T2-weighted image at the level of the L5 pars interarticularis (K). (*continued*)

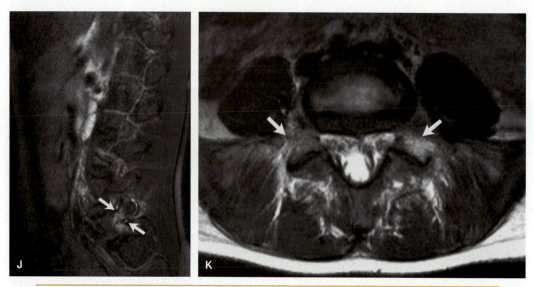

FIGURE 9-44. (CONTINUED).

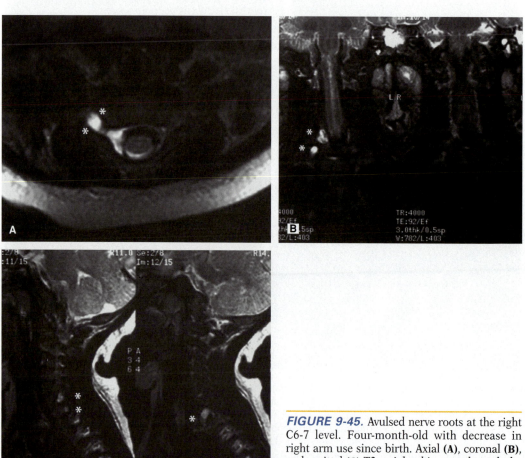

FIGURE 9-45. Avulsed nerve roots at the right C6-7 level. Four-month-old with decrease in right arm use since birth. Axial **(A)**, coronal **(B)**, and sagittal **(C)** T2-weighted images through the cervical spine demonstrate abnormal outpouching of cerebrospinal fluid (*asterisks*) at the level of the neural foramina, in keeping with avulsed nerve roots and resultant pseudomeningocele.

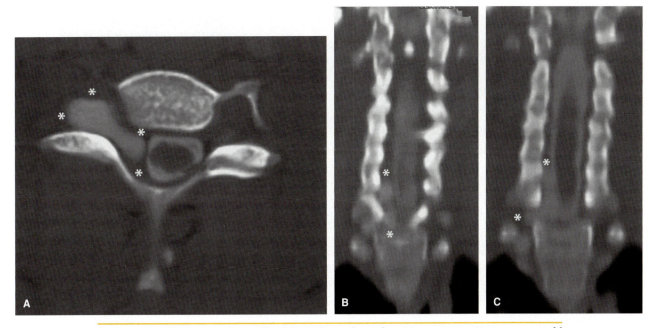

FIGURE 9-46. Pseudomeningocele of the right C6 through to T1 nerve roots. Fourteen-year-old status post–all-terrain-vehicle accident (ATV) now with right arm and neck pain. Axial images from CT myelogram **(A)** and coronal CT reconstruction from the same study **(B,C)** demonstrate abnormal filling of the nerve root sleeve (*asterisks*) in the lower cervical region in keeping with an avulsed nerve root, with contrast filling the post traumatic pseudomeningocele.

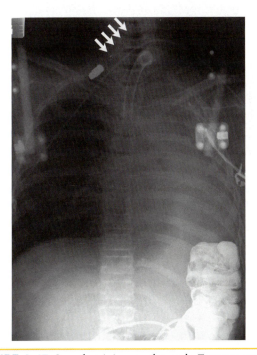

FIGURE 9-47. Gun shot injury to the neck. Fourteen-year-old playing with gun, accidentally discharged, with resultant C-spine injury, cervical spinal cord disruption, and quadriplegia. Single frontal view of the chest demonstrates a bullet within the right apical region. Note the trajectory of the bullet with fragments of lead (*arrows*) seen coursing from the top left to the bottom right of the patient's cervical spine.

high energy injuries requires initial CT imaging if abnormalities are seen on plain film, and requires MRI if neurologic deficit is present and no radiographic abnormality is apparent on plain radiographs (31).

OTHER INJURY TYPES

Nerve Root Avulsions

Nerve root avulsions are another dimension of spinal injury, which often presents with persisting pain or focal nerve root deficit following injury. Brachial plexus birth injury occurs in ~0.5 to 2 in 1,000 live births (68), with most injuries in the upper plexus (C5-6) as well as C7. Although the prognosis is good for the majority of patients, recovery is slow and patients with poorer prognosis who may benefit from surgical intervention, need to be identified. Imaging is an important part of a battery of tests designed to predict outcome. On imaging, the presence of a pseudomeningocele may indicate that nerve root avulsion has occurred, which would alert the surgeon to the possibility that the corresponding nerve root may not be available for reconstruction (69). The presence of a large diverticulum or pseudomeningocele seen on CT myelography or MRI was almost universally diagnostic for identifying a nerve root avulsion; however, smaller diverticulum were only 60% accurate in predicting a nerve root avulsion

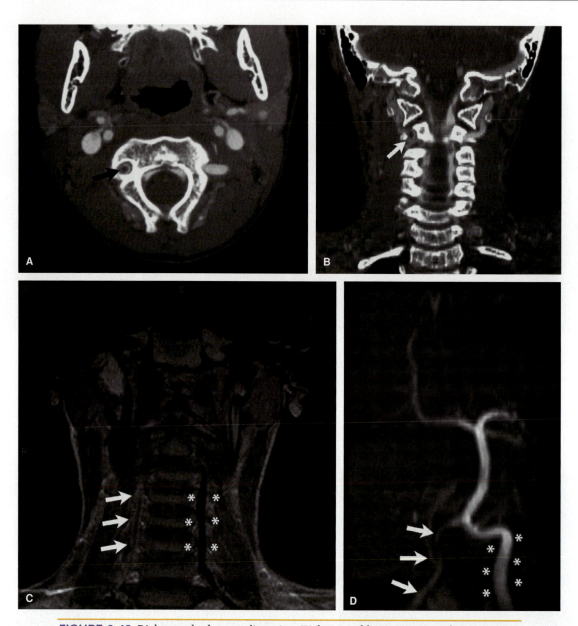

FIGURE 9-48. Right vertebral artery dissection. Eight-year-old status post–neck trauma, now with sudden onset of ataxia and resultant right cerebellar stroke. Axial CT angiogram **(A)**, and coronal CT reconstruction from CT angiogram **(B)** demonstrate a filling defect within the expected location of the right vertebral artery within the foramen transversarium (*arrows*). This is confirmed on coronal fat-saturation T1-weighted MRI **(C)** where there is a visualized left vertebral artery flow void (*asterisks*), with a markedly diminished visualized right vertebral artery flow void (*arrows*). Three-dimensional time-of-flight MRA of the posterior circulation **(D)** demonstrates thinning of the right vertebral artery throughout (*arrows*). This is confirmed on gadolinium enhanced MRA of the neck **(E)** where there is poor visualization of the right vertebral artery (*arrows*). Direct catheter angiogram **(F)** of the same patient further outlines the absence of proper filling of the right vertebral artery (*arrows*) as compared to its counterpart on the left (*asterisks*).

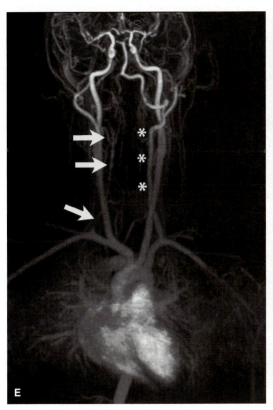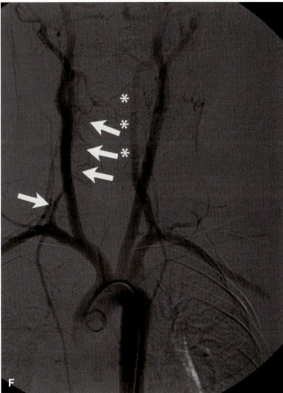

FIGURE 9-48. (CONTINUED).

(70). Although CT myelography may better visualize the nerve roots than MRI, the less-invasive nature of MRI makes it the study of choice (Fig. 9-45). In addition to birth trauma, pseudomeningoceles can also occur in the setting of pediatric spinal trauma (Fig. 9-46) (71). In the lumbar spine these most often accompany pelvic or lumbar fractures and are associated with high velocity accidents, but may also occur without associated fractures (72).

Penetrating Trauma

Violent injuries, including direct trauma from firearms (Fig. 9-47), are the etiology for 23% of spinal cord injuries up to age 15 (73).

Vascular Injury

Although vertebral artery dissections in the pediatric population are rare, one of the more common etiologies is trauma, which can result in intracranial pathology (Fig. 9-48) such as vertebrobasilar stroke (74,75). In a study of adult and pediatric patients with seat belt injury signs, 3% were noted to have associated carotid artery injuries. However, there were no arterial injuries in the pediatric population, and the authors suggest further study in determining whether algorithms that propose angiograms or CTA in the presence

of seat belt signs and abnormal physical exam are appropriate in the pediatric population (76).

REFERENCES

1. Anderson JM, Schutt AH. Spinal injury in children: A review of 156 cases seen from 1950 through 1978. *Mayo Clin Proc.* 1980;55:499–504.
2. Hamilton MG, Myles ST. Pediatric spinal injury: review of 174 hospital admissions. *J Neurosurg.* 1992;77:700–704.
3. Osenbach RK, Menezes AH. Pediatric spinal cord and vertebral column injury. *Neurosurgery.* 1992;30:385–390.
4. Rekate HL, Theodore N, Sonntag VK, et al. Pediatric spine and spinal cord trauma. State of the art for the third millennium. *Childs Nerv Syst.* 1999;15:743–750.
5. Dickman CA, Zabramski JM, Hadley MN, et al. Pediatric spinal cord injury without radiographic abnormalities: report of 26 cases and review of the literature. *J Spinal Disord.* 1991;4:296–305.
6. Anderson PA, Montesano PX. Morphology and treatment of occipital condyle fractures. *Spine.* 1988;13(7):731–736.
7. Nitecki S, Moir CR. Predictive factors of the outcome of traumatic cervical spine fracture in children. *J Pediatric Surg.* 1994;29:1409–1411.
8. Dowd MD, Keenan HT, Bartton SL. Epidemiology and prevention of childhood injuries. *Crit Care Med.* 2002;20:385–392.
9. Swischuk L. Anterior displacement of C2 in children: physiologic or pathologic? *Radiology.* 1977;122:759–763.
10. Swischuk L. The cervical spine in childhood. *Curr Probl Diagn Radiol.* 1984;13:1–26.

11. Cattell HS, Filtzer DL. Pseudosubluxation and other normal variations of the cervical spine in children. *J Bone Joint Surg.* 1965;47A:1295–1309.

12. Harris JH, Jr. Mirvis SE, eds. The normal cervical spine. In: *The Radiology of Acute Cervical Spine Trauma.* 3rd ed. Baltimore: Williams & Wilkins; 1996:1–76.

13. Fesmire FM, Luten RC. The pediatric cervical spine: developmental anatomy and clinical aspects. *J Emerg Med.* 1989;7:133–142.

14. Kriss VM, Kriss TC. Imaging of the cervical spine in infants. *Pediatr Emerg Care.* 1996;13:44–49.

15. Avellino AM, Mann FA, Grady MS, et al. The misdiagnosis of acute cervical spine injuries and fractures in infants and children: the 12-year experience of a level I pediatric and adult trauma center. *Child Nerv Syst.* 2005;21:122–127.

16. Hadley MN, Walters BC, Grabb PA, et al. Guidelines for the management of acute cervical spine and spinal cord injuries. *Clin Neurosurg.* 2002;49:407–498.

17. Hadley MN, Walters BC, Grabb PA, et al. Management of pediatric cervical spine and spinal cord injuries. *Neurosurgery.* 2002;50:S85–S99.

18. Viccellio P, Simon H, Pressman BD, et al. A prospective multicenter study of cervical spine injury in children. *Pediatrics.* 2001;108:E20.

19. Baker C, Kadish H, Schunk JE. Evaluation of pediatric cervical spine injuries. *Am J Emerg Med.* 1999;17:230–234.

20. Buhs C, Cullen M, Klein M, et al. The pediatric trauma c-spine: is the odontoid view necessary? *J Pediatr Surg.* 2000; 35:947–997.

21. Dwek JR, Chung CB. Radiography of cervical spine injury in children: are flexion-extension radiographs useful for acute trauma? *AJR Am J Roentgenol.* June 2000;174(6):1617–1679.

22. Ralston ME, Chung K, Barnes PD, et al. Role of flexion-extension radiographs in blunt pediatric cervical spine injury. *Acad Emerg Med.* 2001;8:237–245.

23. Frush DP, Donnelly LF, Rosen NS. Computed tomography and radiation risks: what pediatric health care providers should know. *Pediatrics.* 2003;112(4):951–957.

24. Brenner DJ. Estimating cancer risks from pediatric CT: going from the qualitative to the quantitative. *Pediatr Radiol.* 2002;32:228–231.

25. Fraenkel L, Lavalley M, Felson D. The use of radiographs to evaluate shoulder pain in the ED. *Am J Emerg Med.* 1998;16: 560–563.

26. Hernandez JA, Chupik C, Swischuk LE. Cervical spine trauma in children under 5 years: productivity of CT. *Emerg Radiol.* 2004;10(4):176–178.

27. Adelgais KM, Grossman DC, Langer SG, et al. Use of helical computed tomography for imaging the pediatric cervical spine. *Acad Emerg Med.* 2004;11:228–236.

28. Keenan HT, Hollingshead MC, Chung CJ, et al. Using CT of the cervical spine for early evaluation of pediatric patients with head trauma. *AJR Am J Roentgenol.* 2001;177(6):1405–1409.

29. Cirak B, Ziegfeld S, Knight VM, et al. Spinal injuries in children. *J Pediatr Surg.* April 2004;39(4):607–612.

30. Keiper MD, Zimmerman RA, Bilaniuk LT. MRI in the assessment of the supportive soft tissues of the cervical spine in acute trauma in children. *Neuroradiology.* 1998;40: 359–363.

31. Flynn JM, Closkey RF, Mahboubi S, et al. Role of magnetic resonance in the assessment of pediatric cervical spine injuries. *J Pediatr Orthop.* 2002;22(5):573–577.

32. Frank JB, Lim CK, Flynn JM, et al. The efficacy of magnetic resonance imaging in pediatric cervical spine clearance. *Spine.* 2002;27:1176–1179.

33. Caird MS, Reddy S, Ganley TJ, et al. Cervical spine fracture-dislocation birth injury: prevention, recognition, and implications for the orthopaedic surgeon. *J Pediatr Orthop.* 2005;25(4):484–486.

34. Magerl F, Aebi M, Gertzbein SD, et al. A comprehensive classification of thoracic and lumbar injuries. *Eur Spine J.* 1994;3(4):184–201.

35. Pang D. Spinal cord injury without radiographic abnormality in children. 2 decades later. *Neurosurgery.* 2004;55(6):1325–1342; discussion 1342–1343.

36. Hadley MN, Zabramski JM, Browner CM, et al. Pediatric spinal trauma: review of 122 cases of spinal cord and vertebral column injuries. *Contemp Neurosurg.* 1988;10:1–6.

37. Osenbach RK, Menezes AH. Spinal cord injury without radiographic abnormality in children. *Pediatric Neurosci.* 1989;15:168–175.

38. Pang D, Pollack IF. Spinal cord injury without radiographic abnormality in children: the SCIWORA syndrome. *J Trauma.* 1989;29:654–664.

39. Quencer RM. The injured spinal cord: Evaluation with magnetic resonance and intraoperative sonography. *Radiol Clin North Am.* 1988;26:1025–1045.

40. Grabb PA, Pand D. Magnetic resonance imaging in the evaluation of a spinal cord injury without radiographic abnormality in children. *Neurosurgery.* 1994;35:406–414.

41. Eleraky MA, Theodore N, Adams M, et al. Pediatric cervical spine injuries: report of 102 cases and review of the literature. *J Neurosurg.* 2000;92(1 Suppl):12–17.

42. Burke DC. Traumatic spinal paralysis in children. *Paraplegia.* 1974;11:268–276.

43. Glasuer FE, Cares HL. Biomechanical features of traumatic paraplegia in infancy. *J Trauma.* 1973;13:166–170.

44. Partrick DA, Bensard DD, Moore EE, et al. Cervical spine trauma in the injured child: a tragic injury with potential for salvageable functional outcome. *J Pediatr Surg.* 2000;31: 1571–1575.

45. Meyer PG, Meyer F, Orliaguet G, et al. Combined high cervical spine and brain stem injuries: a complex and devastating injury in children. *J Pediatr Surg.* 2005;40:1637–1642.

46. Kenter K, Worley G, Griffin T, et al. Pediatric traumatic atlanto-occipital dislocation: five cases and a review. *J Pediatr Orthop.* 2001;21:585–589.

47. Leventhal HR. Birth injuries of the spinal cord. *J Pediatr.* 1960;56:447–453.

48. Bulas DI, Fitz CR, Johnson DL. Traumatic atlanto-occipital dislocation in children. *Radiology.* 1993;188(1):155–158.

49. Deliganis AV, Baxter AB, Hanson JA, et al. Radiologic spectrum of craniocervical distraction injuries. *Radiographics.* 2000;20:S237–S250.

50. Przybylski GJ, Clyde BL, Fitz CR. Craniocervical junction subarachnoid hemorrhage associated with atlanto-occipital dislocation. *Spine.* 1996;21:1761–1769.

51. Sun PP, Poffenbarger GJ, Durham S, et al. Spectrum of occipitoatlantoaxial injury in young children. *J Neurosurg.* (Spine I) 2000;93:28–39.

52. Dwek JR, Chung CB. Radiography of cervical spine injury in children: are flexion-extension radiographs useful for acute trauma? *Am J Roentgenol.* 2000;174(6):1617–1619.

53. Cattell HS, Filtzer DL. Pseudosubluxation and other normal variations of the cervical spine in children. *J Bone Joint Surg Am.* 1965;47:1295–1309.

54. Swischuk LE. *Emergency Imaging of the Acutely Ill or Injured Child. The Spine and the Spinal Cord.* 4th ed. Philadelphia: Lippincott Williams & Wilkins; 2000:532–587.

55. Vialle LR, Vialle E. Pediatric spine injuries. *Injury.* 2005;36(suppl 2):B104–112.

56. Levine AM, Edwards CC. Fractures of the atlas. *J Bone Joint Surg.* 1991;73A:680–691.

57. Reynolds R. Pediatric spinal injury. *Curr Opin Pediatr.* 2000;12(1):67–71.

58. Anderson LD, D'Alonzo RT. Fractures of the odontoid process of the axis. *J Bone Joint Surg.* 1974;56A:1663–1674.

59. Blockey NJ, Purser DW. Fractures of the odontoid process of the axis. *J Bone Joint Surg.* 1956;38B:794–817.

60. Griggiths S. Fracture of the odontoid process in children. *J Pediatr Surg.* 1972;7:680–683.

61. Sanderson SP, Houten JK. Fracture through the C2 synchondrosis in a young child. *Pediatr Neurosurg.* 2002;36: 277–278.

62. Kleinman PK, Shelton YA. Hangman's fracture in an abused infant: imaging features. *Pediatr Radiol.* 1997;27: 776–777.

63. Murray JA, Chen D, Velmahos GC, et al. Pediatric falls: is height a predictor of injury and outcome? *Am Surg.* 2000;66: 863–865.

64. Pouliquen JC, Kassis B, Glorion C, et al. Vertebral growth after thoracic or lumbar fracture of the spine in children. *J Pediatr Orthop*. 1997;17(1):115–120.

65. Crawford AH. Operative treatment of spine fractures in children. *Orthop Clin North Am*. 1990;21(2):325–339.

66. Denis F. The three column spine and its significance in the classification of acute thoracolumbar spinal injuries. *Spine*. 1983;8(8):817–831.

67. Tyroch AH, McGuire EL, McLean SF, et al. The association between Chance fractures and intra-abdominal injuries revisited: a multicenter review. *Am Surg*. 2005;71(5): 434–438.

68. Yilmaz K, Caliskan M, Oge E, et al. Clinical assessment, MRI, and EMG in congenital brachial plexus palsy. *Pediatr Neurol*. 1999;21:705–710.

69. Piatt JH Jr. Birth injuries of the brachial plexus. *Pediatr Clin North Am*. 2004;51:421–440.

70. Waters PM. Update on management of pediatric brachial plexus palsy. *J Pediatr Orthop*. 2005;25:116–126.

71. Miller SF, Glasier CM, Griebel ML, et al. Brachial plexopathy in infants after traumatic delivery: evaluation with MR imaging. *Radiology*. 1993;189(2):481–484.

72. Hans FJ, Reinges MH, Krings T. Lumbar nerve root avulsion following trauma: balanced fast field-echo MRI. *Neuroradiology*. 2004;46(2):144–147.

73. *Annual Report for the Model Spinal Cord Injury Care Systems*. National Spinal Cord Injury Center. Birmingham: University of Alabama Press; 2005.

74. Kim SH, Kosnik E, Madden C, et al. Cerebellar infarction from a traumatic vertebral artery dissection in a child. *Pediatr Neurosurg*. 1997;27:71–77.

75. Ganesan V, Chong WK, Cox TC, et al. Posterior circulation stroke in childhood: risk factors and recurrence. *Neurology*. 2002;59:1552–1556.

76. Rozycki GS, Tremblay L, Feliciano DV, et al. A prospective study for the detection of vascular injury in adult and pediatric patients with cervicothoracic seat belt signs. *J Trauma*. 2002;52:618–624.

Postoperative Spinal Imaging

Ashwini D. Sharan, Hana Choe, and Laura Snyder

The goal of this chapter is to present a surgeon's approach to management of the postsurgical spinal trauma patient and inherent complications. The abnormal postoperative findings that require further investigation are reviewed, such as spinal deformity, nonunion, graft-failure, pseudoarthrosis, and instability. Also, unexpected neurologic deficits or unresolved pain mandate an evaluation in an acute, subacute, or chronic setting. In many instances, imaging studies are helpful in confirming the existence of postoperative complications such as hematomas, infection, pseudomeningocele, or arachnoiditis. Other chronic sequelae such as syringomyelia, myelomalacia, and spinal cord tethering are discussed in Chapter 11.

IMMEDIATE POSTOPERATIVE EVALUATION

Before the patient leaves the operating room, graft position and operative levels must be confirmed radiographically. Radiographs in both anteroposterior (AP) and lateral views are excellent for grossly assessing spinal alignment, hardware placement, and positioning of interbody and graft material (Figs. 10-1–10-3). Radiographs also provide a good, reliable, and reproducible means to follow normal sagittal balance, kyphosis, and translation. An abnormality in any one of these measures may

warrant further intervention. Malpositioned hardware may be surgically modified before concluding the procedure, or may lead to supplemental imaging in the immediate postoperative period (Fig. 10-4). Immediate postoperative radiographs serve as a reference point in the event of hardware failure or delayed posttraumatic deformity.

All postoperative spine patients must be neurologically assessed while in the surgical recovery area to determine that there has been no deterioration in preoperative neurologic status (i.e., new motor weakness or sensory disturbance). In addition, spine surgery patients are commonly assessed in the operative suite for inadvertent neurologic damage by monitoring motor and sensory evoked potentials. These physiologic parameters are followed closely during surgery and may influence surgical technique to avoid further neurologic injury.

ASSESSMENT OF FUSION/ GRAFT STABILITY

Whenever possible, during interval follow-up, the fused segment of the spine should be evaluated with radiographs obtained with the patient upright and compared with those performed immediately after surgery. Weight bearing is an important part of the postoperative assessment as it can provide early indication of progressive deformity and

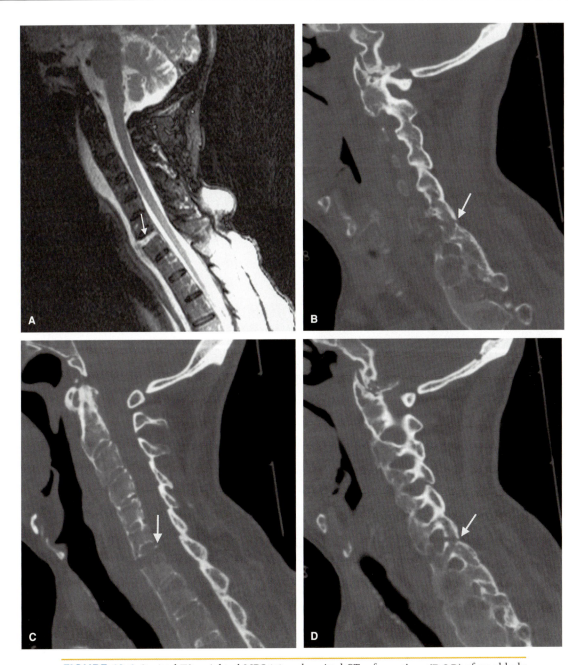

FIGURE 10-1. Sagittal T2 weighted MRI **(A)** and sagittal CT reformations **(B,C,D)** of an elderly gentleman with ankylosing spondylitis who sustained a C6-7 cervical extension injury resulting in a fracture that extended through the superior endplate of the C7 vertebral body (*white arrow in B, C, D*). There is T2 signal through the disc and vertebral body (*white arrow in A*). The patient had a two-staged posterior instrumented fixation with lateral mass screws and anterior interbody graft placement with a radiolucent bioabsorbable plate. (*continued*)

instability at the fusion site. The Cobb angle (Fig. 10-5) is usually used as a measure of the curvature of the spine at the fracture site. The angle between intersecting lines drawn perpendicular to the top of the top vertebrae above the fracture site and the bottom of the bottom vertebrae is the Cobb angle. A minor change in the angle may suggest progression of kyphosis and the need for surgical intervention and fur-

ther stabilization. Moreover, extreme kyphosis, inadequate correction of kyphotic deformity, or subluxation has been cited to cause strut graft failure. Graft fracture, malposition, and dislodgment are obvious evidence of failure of the surgical construct. Furthermore, the vertebral body onto which the graft is seated can fracture, especially in the setting of pre-existent osteoporosis. If this occurs when the fracture is

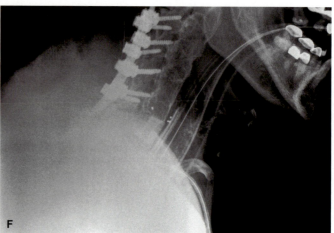

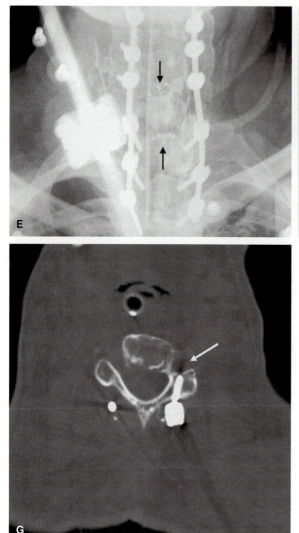

FIGURE 10-1. *(CONTINUED)* Note on the anteroposterior (AP) **(E)** and lateral **(F)** radiographs, only the radiopague screws are apparent, which reveal the orientation of the invisible, radioluscent plate (*black arrows in E*). Also, the trajectory of the third left lateral mass screw is inadequately visualized in the AP radiographs (E). An axial CT **(G)** shows the screw to be acceptably short of the vertebral foramen (*arrow*).

minimally displaced and the graft position is still satisfactory, immobilization with a halo vest and close observation may be all that is required. If no further displacement occurs and there is no kyphosis, the fracture is likely to heal spontaneously. However, many times, strut graft failure results in the implantation of a longer graft and extending the fusion one more level. If questions remain regarding the quality of the bone or stability of the construct, supplemental posterior stabilization is recommended.

UTILITY OF DYNAMIC IMAGING IN THE POSTOPERATIVE PERIOD

Dynamic images are functional radiographs obtained in at least two extremes of normal physiologic motion (e.g., flexion and extension) to provide critical information regarding presence stability. Dynamic images are of limited usefulness in the immediate postoperative period for several reasons: (a) surgical manipulation of the

spine is associated with pain and muscle spasm, which limit the normal range of movement and act as a brace to stabilize the spine; and (b) patients are commonly immobilized with external orthotic devices such as a halo vest, hard cervical collar, or thoracolumbo-sacral orthotic (TLSO) brace. Thus, dynamic imaging may only be useful many months later. Sequential flexion-extension x-ray films are useful for the assessment of strut graft failure.

COMPUTED TOMOGRAPHY IN THE POSTOPERATIVE SPINE

Computed tomography (CT) scans are informative postoperatively particularly after deployment of instrumentation to precisely define hardware positions in relation to the pedicles or lateral masses. In general, spinal hardware malposition does not correlate with neurologic complications; however, identification of an osseous breech warrants

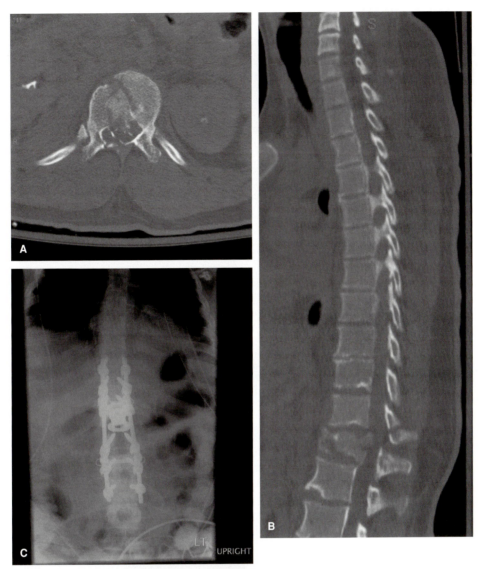

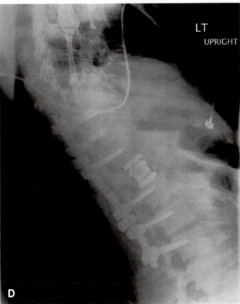

FIGURE 10-2. Axial CT image **(A)** and sagittal CT reformation **(B)** of an 18-year-old man after a motor vehicle accident sustaining a T12 comminuted burst fracture. The ensuing images show a standard pedicle screw construct with an expandable cage device on anteroposterior (AP) **(C)** and lateral **(D)** radiographs. Of particular note to the surgeon is to look for the screws to transverse through the pedicles and not cross the midline of the vertebral body on the AP image. Additionally, with the presence of such an extensive amount of hardware, it is exceedingly difficult on x-ray imaging to detect the presence of arthrodesis or bone bridging across the facet joint or the vertebral body; the absence of movement does not necessarily translate into the presence of the former.

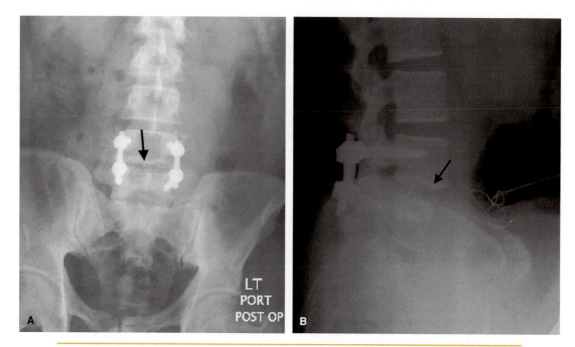

FIGURE 10-3. Anteroposterior (**A**) and lateral (**B**) radiographs of a patient with an L4-5 laminectomy and fusion with instrumentation at the L4 and L5 pedicles bilaterally with an interbody radiolucent graft packed with bone between the L4 and L5 vertebral body. Note the four radiopague dots marking the boundaries of the radiolucent graft (*black arrows in A and B*).

investigation and sometimes intervention. A medial breech of the pedicle from inaccurate pedicle screw placement can potentially compromise the spinal canal and contents (spinal cord or cauda equina), and an inferior cortex pedicle breach places the nerve root at risk for injury. A lateral breech of a cervical lateral mass screw might encroach upon the vertebral artery, while a lateral breech of a thoracic pedicle screw may compromise the aorta. A screw that is inadvertently placed through an adjacent disc space may result in injury to that disc. These findings may be visible on radiographs, but a CT scan with reconstruction of the images gives better anatomical delineation of the hardware as well the relationship of the hardware to the normal anatomy. Moreover, the higher in-plane resolution afforded with modern multidetector CT equipment actually minimizes the image degradation commonly associated with imaging of metallic hardware. If a clinically significant malposition is identified, then the patient may need to return to the operating room to have the hardware repositioned.

MAGNETIC RESONANCE IMAGING IN POSTOPERATIVE SPINE TRAUMA

Magnetic resonance imaging (MRI) is used in the examination of both the early and late postoperative spine when the patient has recurrent or persistent symptoms or new deficits. When decompression of the spinal cord is the

goal of surgical intervention, a postoperative MRI is a necessary assessment tool to evaluate the adequacy of decompression, the integrity of spinal cord and canal anatomy, as well as to gain insight into the patient's functional prognosis. High bandwidth MRI techniques tend to decrease metallic artifact after arthrodesis and improve image quality. Even with these image improvements, there is often sufficient artifact from the instrumentation to obscure soft tissue details in the neural foramina (Fig. 10-6).

POSTOPERATIVE COMPLICATIONS IN SPINAL TRAUMA

Patients with spinal trauma are subject to the additional comorbidities associated with multisystem trauma. Thus, while the average length of stay for all causes of hospital admissions is 4.9 days, the average length of initial hospitalization following spinal cord injury (SCI) in acute care units is 19 days. This extended hospitalization for the typical SCI patient is attributed to the severity of the initial injuries and the inherent comorbidities associated with loss of normal physiologic functions.

Acute Complications

The most devastating complication of spinal trauma is the development of a new neurologic deficit. When the

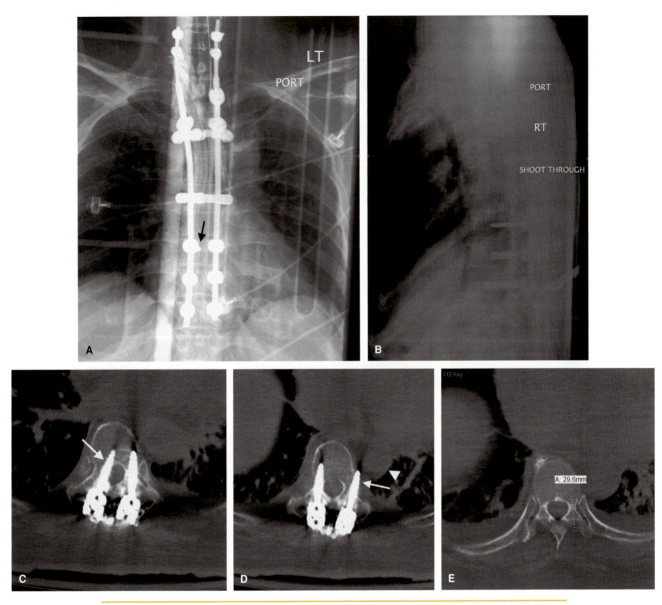

FIGURE 10-4. Malpositioned hardware. Postoperative anteroposterior (AP) **(A)** and lateral **(B)** radiographs from a female undergoing an anterior corpectomy and cervicothoracic fusion. The lateral radiograph shows good positioning of the pedicle screws. However, in the AP radiograph, the third pedicle screw from the bottom on the right appears to divert towards the midline (*black arrow in A*). Axial CT image **(C)** reveals the screw to be in the canal (*white arrow in C*). No adverse event was experienced by the patient, but the screw was later operatively removed by the surgeon. Additionally, the plain x-rays do not reveal any other obvious problems with the hardware. Axial CT scan also reveal a lateral trajectory of the second from the bottom left pedicle screw (*white arrow in D*). The concern is its proximity to the aorta (*white arrowhead in D*). Planning on a preoperative CT scan **(E)** can allow measurement of the distance from the aorta in a very lateral positioned aorta.

neurologic deficit occurs immediately following the surgical intervention or shortly thereafter, the etiology is likely due to iatrogenic spinal cord injury, ischemia, or bleeding. The deficit may result from direct injury to the spinal cord or nerve roots or may occur secondary to a vascular injury, such as injury to the vertebral artery. Sudden onset of spinal cord compression from a hematoma or retained disc or bony fragment can also produce late neurologic complications. Direct surgical causes of neurologic injury include malalignment of the vertebral column, malposition of the hardware, anesthetic-related fluctuations in the blood pressure, or a postoperative hematoma/fluid collection (Fig. 10-7).

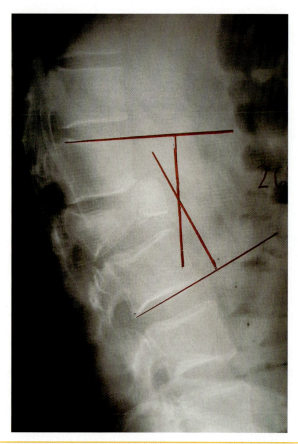

FIGURE 10-5. Cobb angle. This patient has a L2 burst fracture. The patient remained neurologically intact and was managed successfully with a brace. Lateral radiograph demonstrates how the Cobb angle is measured. Parallel lines are traced from the adjacent vertebral endplates above and below the fractured segment. Perpendicular lines from these represent the Cobb angle. Progressive changes in the Cobb angle may reflect progressive kyphosis, implying the loss of spinal stability. It should be noted that this measurement can have a 3- to 5-degree interobserver variability.

Hypotension and Ascending Spinal Cord Injury

Harrop et al. (1) found that 12 of 186 or 6% of patients with American Spinal Injury Association Impairment Scale (ASIA) A complete spinal cord injuries worsened in the first 30 days after injury. Progression of the injury characteristically occurred along a temporal continuum and was classified into three discrete time intervals: *early*, *delayed*, and *late deterioration*. *Early* deterioration (<24 hours) is typically related to traction and immobilization. National spinal cord injury data suggest that the use of standardized resuscitative protocols have improved the incidence of early deterioration in victims of spinal cord injuries. In contrast to early deterioration, *delayed* deterioration occurs between 24 hours and 7 days from time of injury, often as a result of sustained hypotension in patients with fracture dislocations.

SCI patients are predisposed to hypotension due to loss of normal vasomotor tone in the peripheral arterioles and subsequent pooling of blood in the peripheral vasculature. Therefore, the first line of treatment for vasomotor hypotension is volume resuscitation. Given that there is evidence for secondary ischemic injury in SCI patients, maintaining appropriate blood pressure to perfuse the injured spinal cord is paramount. Less well known is the optimal pressure to sustain perfusion to the spinal cord, and there is no clear way to measure spinal cord perfusion (2). Vale et al. (3) treated a series of patients with acute SCI with fluid and vasopressors to achieve a mean arterial pressure (MAP) of 85 mm Hg for a minimum of 7 days and reported favorable neurologic outcomes. However, the chosen MAP was arbitrary and the study uncontrolled; thus, the optimal value remains unknown.

Acute SCI, in particular cervical SCI, patients are especially prone to hemodynamic instability (2). This occurs when sympathetic fibers exiting the spinal cord in the thoracic region are interrupted. Parasympathetic outflow becomes unopposed, which results in cardiac arrhythmias and hypotension. The most common arrhythmia seen is bradyarrhythmia, which further exacerbates hypoperfusion and loss of sympathetic tone. Arrhythmias appear to be most common within the first 14 days after injury and are more common in neurologically complete injuries (4).

Ascending spinal cord injury is the rare instance in which a patient spontaneously ascends in their neurologic level of injury. In the acute period, this can occur within the first few days after the initial injury. Though many etiological factors have been implicated in ascending spinal cord injury, the cause frequently remains elusive. One factor that is consistently implicated has been the maintenance of blood perfusion in the first 48 to 72 hours after injury and particularly during surgery. Intraoperative events that cause new deficits are rare and may be monitored during surgery with electrophysiological motor and sensory feedback. Further, strict adherence to minimum blood pressure or MAP parameters with aggressive fluid or cardiac vasopressor administration can often prevent untoward events. Anecdotal reports have described adverse changes in intraoperative electrophysiological monitoring that returns to baseline levels with aggressive fluid resuscitation and maintenance of MAPs to at least greater than or equal to 85 mm Hg.

Postoperative Hematoma

It is extremely difficult to obtain absolute hemostasis in the postsurgical bed. Tissue changes from the initial traumatic injury and surgical dissection will cause venous blood to drain from epidural veins, decorticated bony edges, and manipulated muscles. Hemorrhages of this type

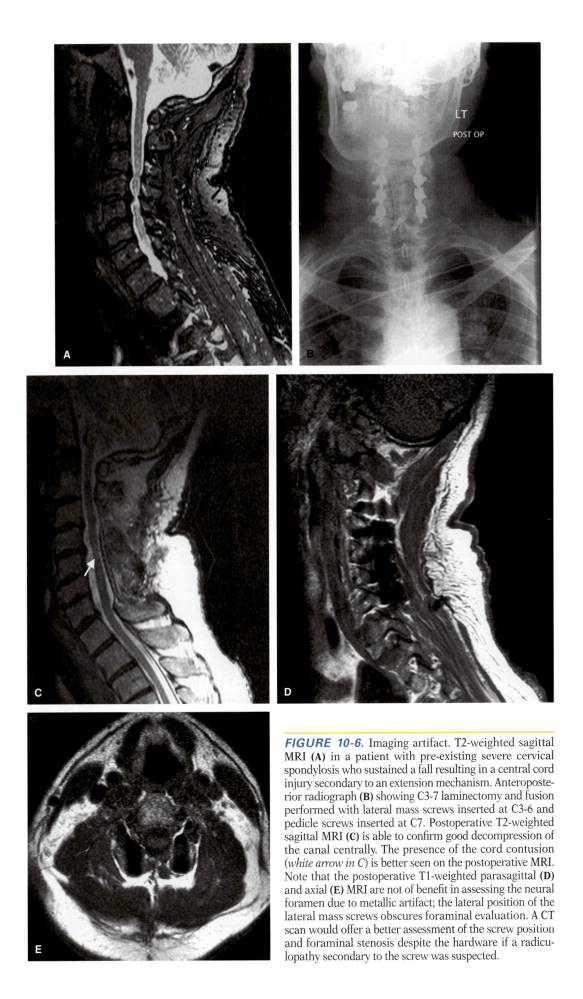

FIGURE 10-6. Imaging artifact. T2-weighted sagittal MRI **(A)** in a patient with pre-existing severe cervical spondylosis who sustained a fall resulting in a central cord injury secondary to an extension mechanism. Anteroposterior radiograph **(B)** showing C3-7 laminectomy and fusion performed with lateral mass screws inserted at C3-6 and pedicle screws inserted at C7. Postoperative T2-weighted sagittal MRI **(C)** is able to confirm good decompression of the canal centrally. The presence of the cord contusion (*white arrow in C*) is better seen on the postoperative MRI. Note that the postoperative T1-weighted parasagittal **(D)** and axial **(E)** MRI are not of benefit in assessing the neural foramen due to metallic artifact; the lateral position of the lateral mass screws obscures foraminal evaluation. A CT scan would offer a better assessment of the screw position and foraminal stenosis despite the hardware if a radiculopathy secondary to the screw was suspected.

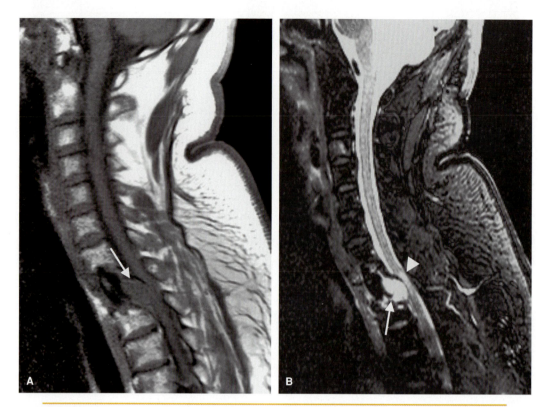

FIGURE 10-7. Post-operative fluid collection. This patient had an anterior cervical corpectomy and graft placed. After the graft was positioned and prior to extubation, the patient experienced changes in electrophysiological monitoring of evoked potential. She awoke unable to move her legs. An emergent MRI was obtained. Sagittal T1-weighted **(A)** and T2-weighted **(B)** images show that there is fluid dorsal to the graft causing compression of the spinal cord (*white arrows in A and B*). Additionally, there are T2-weighted signal changes apparent in the spinal cord, suggestive of spinal cord injury (*white arrowhead in B*). (*continued*)

typically do not progress to symptomatic hematomas as a small bleeding vein will likely tamponade from the pressure of the surrounding soft tissue structures. Nevertheless, there will always appear to be some blood in the postoperative surgical bed, and delayed epidural hematomas can develop. Risk factors identified in the development of epidural hematomas include prior surgery with resultant scarring, multilevel laminectomies, ankylosing spondylitis, and preoperative coagulopathy (5,6).

A new neurologic deficit, whether immediate or delayed, mandates follow-up imaging on an emergent or urgent basis, in accordance with the acuity of the deterioration. The outcome of spinal epidural hematomas is purportedly influenced by two factors: the accuracy of the diagnosis and the time interval between the onset of symptoms and surgical decompression (7). The more rapid the decompression, the better the therapeutic outcome. Imaging confirmation of an epidural hematoma is best verified with MRI. In instances where MRI is not available or is contraindicated, myelography with postmyelography CT is the best second imaging approach. In certain instances of high clinical suspicion

and when the change in neurologic status is substantial, surgical exploration without imaging may be favored over delays imposed by emergent imaging. In one study, emergent surgical decompression of a spinal epidural hematoma within 12 hours of progression to complete paraplegia provided full resolution of the symptoms, while symptom duration of 72 hours or greater did not improve after surgical intervention (8). Although most epidural hematomas will occur within 24 hours of the surgery, in one report, hematoma developed >3 days after the index procedure (9). The most common presenting symptom was severe, sharp pain radiating down to the extremities with neurologic deterioration. In all cases, MRI was used to document the presence of an epidural hematoma. Surgical evacuation with improvement in symptoms occurred in 4 out of 6 patients (9).

It should be noted that we have seen CSF leaks underlying an epidural hematoma which the patient was clinically completely asymptomatic (Fig. 10-8). Thus, the radiographic relevance of a postoperative hematoma must be made in light of the clinical scenario.

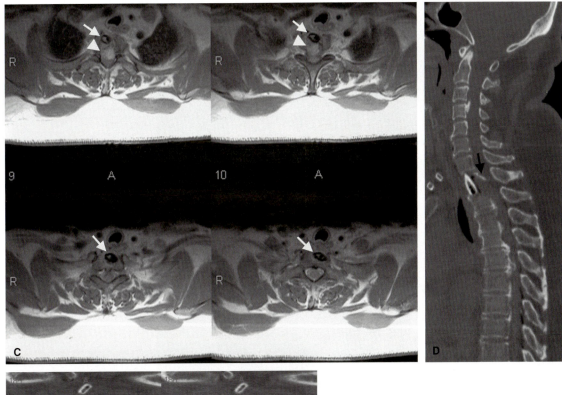

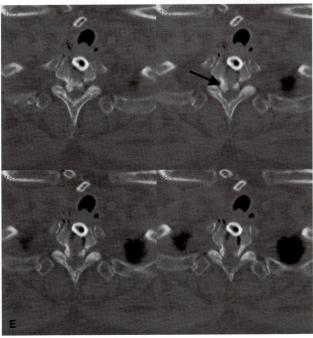

FIGURE 10-7. *(CONTINUED)* T2-weighted axial images **(C)** show appropriate anterior position of the graft *(white arrows)* and the corpectomy defect *(white arrowheads)*. Prior to returning to the operating room, the surgeon elected to also obtain a CT scan of the cervical spine. Intraoperatively, a cerebral spinal fluid leak was noted, and it was not clear how that may have resulted in neurologic deterioration. Sagittal reformats **(D)** and axial CT images **(E)** shows prominent osteophytes *(black arrows in D and E)* remaining behind the superior aspect of the corpectomy defect. The patient returned to the operating room for further decompression.

Subacute Complications

Infection

The diagnosis and management of a postoperative infection is complex. A constellation of clinical findings supplemented by radiographic evidence can suggest the diagnosis, but frequently a patient will need a tissue biopsy to identify the pathogen. The incidence of infection in the postoperative spinal trauma patient has been documented to be as high as 9.4% (10). The immobilized postsurgical patient is susceptible to urinary tract infections secondary to Foley catheters and urinary stasis, prolonged ventilator dependence, pneumonia, and atelectasis with prolonged bed rest, deep venous thrombosis, and wound infections. A patient's nutritional status is a key factor in the risk of development of an infection. The clinical parameters most

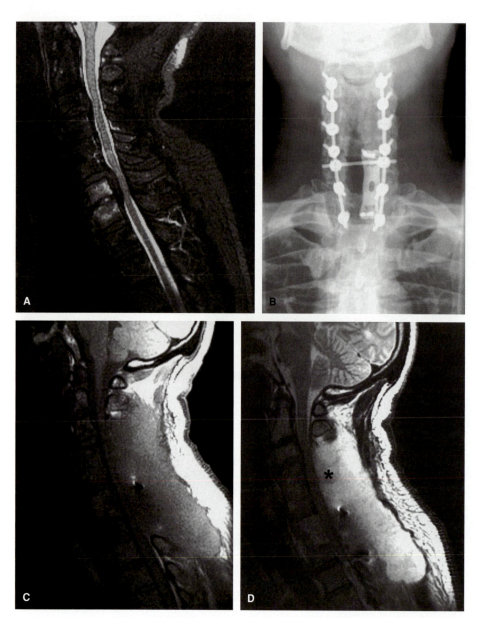

FIGURE 10-8. Epidural hematoma. T2-weighted sagittal image **(A)** in a patient with cervical spondylosis and stenosis who underwent a C7 anterior discectomy with posterior C3-T1 laminectomy and fusion as seen on postoperative anteroposterior radiograph **(B)**. The patient had improved strength immediate postoperatively and was discharged uneventfully on postoperative day 2. Patient had a routine postoperative MRI to assess the decompression on the spinal cord. The MRI reveals what appears to be a large compressive epidural hematoma (*asterisk in D*), as seen on T1-weighted sagittal **(C)** and T2-weighted **(D)** images.

commonly used to assess the nutritional status of surgical patients are the serum albumin level and the total lymphocyte count (TLC). Serum albumin is an index of visceral protein mass, and decreased levels are associated statistically with poor wound healing, postoperative infectious, complications, mortality, and immune suppression (11). The total lymphocyte count is a marker of immune competence and is decreased in malnourished patients. Malnutrition depresses immunity by impairing chemotaxis and phagocytosis. Serum albumin <3.5 g/dL and TLC <1,500 to 2,000 cells/mm3 are considered by most authors to represent clinical malnutrition. Moreover, SCI patients tend to be in a highly catabolic state after spinal cord injury, which exacerbates the malnutrition and sets the stage for poor wound healing and postoperative wound infections.

About 75% of spinal cord injury patients (primarily young, otherwise healthy men), become malnourished in the postoperative period as studied with serum albumin and TLC parameters. Further, postoperative complications occurred only in patients who were malnourished ($p = 0.001$) and not in those nutritionally replete. There was also a statistically significant relationship between nutritional status and the need for prolonged (>24 hours) intubation ($p = 0.016$) whereby all patients with prolonged intubation were malnourished.

Interestingly, Galandiuk et al. (12) showed that the use of high-dose methylprednisolone (MPS) as part of the treatment for SCI was not related significantly to the incidence of postoperative complications and did not increase the number of complications experienced by patients during their hospitalizations. However, pneumonia

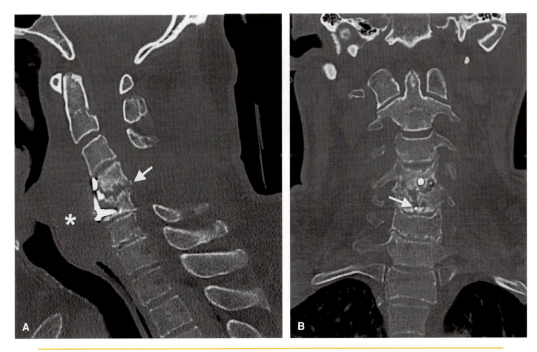

FIGURE 10-9. Postoperative infection. Sagittal **(A)** and coronal **(B)** CT reformations in a patient status postfusion and laminectomies at C4-5. Prevertebral swelling is seen on the sagittal image consistent with prevertebral abscess (*asterisk in A*), and erosions associated with discitis are visualized at C4-5 (*white arrow in A*). Also seen are lucencies around the screws, likely due to loosening associated with infection (*white arrow in B*).

was both more frequent and severe in MPS-treated patients. Though MPS treated patients did have an initially higher earlier boost, in some host defense parameters, they rapidly declined and the subsequent response was both blunted and delayed. In addition, the length of hospital stay was longer in MPS-treated patients than in patients not treated with steroids (44.4 days versus 27.7 days, respectively; $p = 0.065$) and 79% of patients treated with MPS had pneumonia compared with an incidence of 50% for patients that did not receive the treatment ($p = 0.614$).

The presence of fevers is not diagnostic of a wound infection, and in fact, patients with spinal cord injuries have been documented to have fevers of unknown origin (13,14). A patient with discitis or osteomyelitis typically presents with fever and back pain "out of proportion" to the surgery within 12 weeks of surgery. The incision may be tender and blood cultures may be positive for bacteria. Elevated erythrocyte sedimentation rate (ESR) and C-reactive protein (CRP) are sensitive for discitis and infection, though variance in the ESR and CRP in the initial postoperative period has been described (15).

Although CT may be helpful in evaluating infection involving spinal hardware (Fig. 10-9), postcontrast MRI is the study of choice in detecting discitis and the attendant complications, including epidural and paraspinal abscess (16,17). In general, intervertebral disc space enhancement, annular enhancement, and vertebral body enhance-

ment suggest spondylodiscitis (Fig. 10-10). Other changes related to discitis seen on MRI include loss of disc height, intradiscal high signal intensity on T2W images, endplate erosion, and vertebral marrow edema (16). An epidural abscess is seen as a central nonenhanced region surrounded by enhancing inflammatory tissue. An infected paravertebral fluid collection may appear similarly (18). The normal postoperative disc and postoperative surgical bed may also exhibit gadolinium enhancement. This emphasizes the point that clinicians must rely on a complete evaluation of the patient, including laboratory values such as elevated sedimentation rate, CRP, total lymphocyte count, and white blood cell count to make an accurate diagnosis.

Of surgical concern is the presence of deep tracking infections, abscess formation, discitis, and osteomyelitis. The former can be difficult to ascertain on imaging. The integrity of a competent fascial layer distinguishes a deep versus a superficial infection. The distinction is important because a superficial infection or cellulitis can be adequately treated with antibiotics. Unfortunately, surgical exploration of the wound is the only definitive assessment of the competency of the fascial layer. Therefore, many surgeons will treat a deep postoperative infection through irrigation and debridement (I&D) and externalized drains. Removal of the implanted instrumentation (i.e., hardware) is generally not an option (and typically not necessary). The process of incision and drainage alone

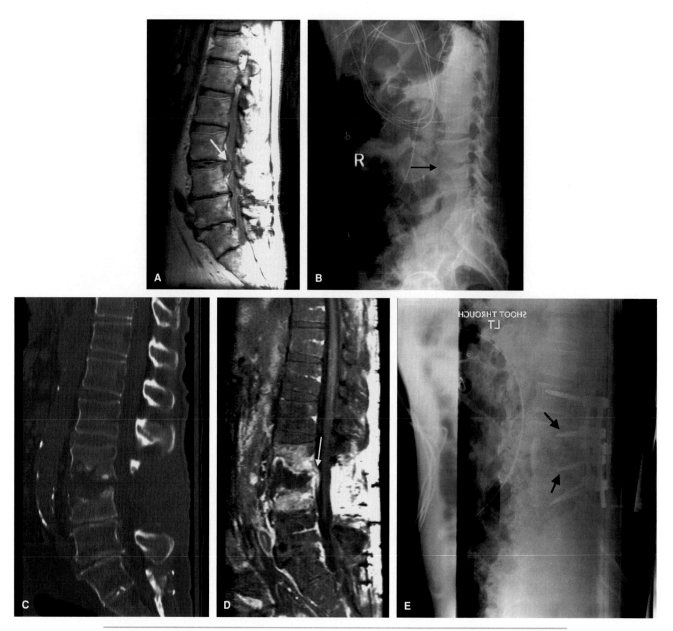

FIGURE 10-10. Postoperative infection. **A:** This patient had a left-sided extruded L3-4 herniated disc as seen on the sagittal T1-weighted images (*white arrow*). He had a persistently draining wound for 3 weeks, which was oversewn multiple times. He presented again with increasing back pain and elevated C-reactive protein and sedimentation rates without a fever or white blood cell count. **B:** A lateral radiograph suggests destruction of the inferior L3 and superior L4 endplate (*black arrow*), which is further confirmed on the sagittal CT reformation **(C)**. A gadolinium enhanced T1-weighted sagittal MRI **(D)** reveals destructive osteomyelitis and discitis with enhancement around the destroyed L3-4 disc space as well as within the adjacent vertebral bodies. Note extension to the epidural space (*white arrow in D*). The patient had an anterior lumbar debridement, interposition of an autologous iliac crest bone graft spanning L3 and L4, and stabilization with posterior pedicle screws from L2-4. Note on lateral radiograph **(E)** that short pedicle screws (*black arrows*) were used at L3 and L4 (compare to L2 and L5) because of the severe bony destruction.

may break up the purulent collection sufficiently to reduce the bacterial load. Since the process of fusion (i.e., arthrodesis), requires implantation of small fragments of cancellous bone along the bony prominences, these unincorporated bone fragments serve as a nidus for ongoing

infection and must be debrided and removed. An untreated infection may proceed to form an epidural abscess that has the potential to compress the neural elements and produce an ascending thrombophlebitis of the epidural venous plexus resulting in ischemia to the spinal cord. Therefore, I&D of the wound in conjunction with antibiotics is the most effective strategy for treating deep postoperative infections.

Chronic Complications of the Postoperative Spine

Other types of complications can arise in the postoperative period between 1 week and 1 year after surgery. The most frequent type of delayed complication often affects the integrity of hardware or graft material and therefore will present as an alteration in spinal alignment from the immediate postoperative period. A full imaging assessment is often necessary when graft failure is suggested, with a determination of whether proper fusion has been achieved or pseudoarthrosis exists. CT is often useful in this assessment and will help to determine whether revision surgery is required. A delayed presentation of neurologic progression will usually require assessment with MRI.

Delayed Deformity

A delayed posttraumatic deformity is one of the most challenging complications to correct after spinal trauma surgery (19). A posttraumatic kyphotic deformity may occur anywhere in the spine, most often due to inadequate initial treatment or inadequate immobilization techniques. Delayed instability may result in progressive deformity, pain, or increased neurologic deficit. When inadequate immobilization is suspected, progressive deformity occurs due to occult instability and continued exposure to physiologic stresses (20). Risk factors that are associated with increased risk for posttraumatic deformity include prior laminectomy and a short segment fusion. In one study, improved spinal alignment was achieved when at least five levels or more were incorporated into the fusion and when a posterior laminectomy was not performed (20).

The mechanism of injury and the stability of the three spinal columns theorized in the thoracolumbar spine are factors that influence the surgical treatment and together, affect the development of posttraumatic deformity. Injuries affecting primarily the anterior and middle bony column will rarely develop late progressive deformity with the use of appropriate immobilization. However, even with the use of proper immobilization, when the injury includes disruption of the posterior column structures, the kyphotic deformity may gradually progress over time (19). Therefore, burst flexion-compression injuries or flexion-distraction injuries, which affect the posterior column, are particularly prone to posttraumatic deformity. This is more common at the thoracolumbar junction where the absence of a complete rib cage offers limited secondary support and may even occur at the cervical-thoracic junction.

Radiographic criteria of delayed deformity include progressive spinal kyphosis. Specifically in the thoracic spine, abnormal kyphotic angulation is defined by ≥30 degrees angulation or 50% loss of vertebral body height. Surgical intervention is recommended if the kyphotic deformity is progressive over time or there is new onset or progression of neurologic deficits. Once progressive kyphosis is identified, the treatment of posttraumatic deformity follows the same basic biomechanical principles of re-establishing the integrity of the compromised spinal column so that spinal stability can be restored.

Nonunion

One etiology of late posttraumatic spinal deformity is the lack of development of a mechanically competent fusion between the adjacent segments, referred to as nonunion. Nonunion often presents clinically as increasing pain localized to the surgical site with radiographic evidence of instrumentation fatigue and bone nonhealing. In long-segment fibular grafts, the process of fusion often takes 1 to 2 years and occurs by "creeping substitution," beginning at the endplates and extending toward the midportion of the strut graft. Creeping substitution is a term used to describe the osteoclast mediated revascularization process that occurs to transform avascular grafted material into strong cortical bone. Initially, bone resorption precedes new bone formation; therefore, bone strut grafts are relatively weak and are susceptible to delayed fracture with normal loading of the cervical spine when external bracing is discontinued early. Current practice recommends supplemental support with additional posterior fusion and instrumentation.

The diagnosis and treatment of nonunion should be pursued aggressively. Nonunion in the presence of an anterior cervical fixation device carries the additional risk of screw fracture or migration with associated esophageal penetration, mediastinitis, and death. Moreover, a deep infection can mimic or be the cause of a symptomatic nonunion.

An initial radiograph is usually the first imaging study obtained to evaluate for arthrodesis. Radiographic criteria used to assess strut graft fusion include the presence of bone trabeculae crossing the disc spaces, absence of radiolucent lines at the graft-host junction, and <2 mm of motion between adjacent spinous processes on flexion-extension views.

The reported rate of nonunion of spine fusions performed with allograft bone (donor bone) is 41% to 62% compared to 5% (single level fusion) and 17% to 27% (multilevel fusion) with autograft bone (bone acquired from the graft recipient) (21,22).

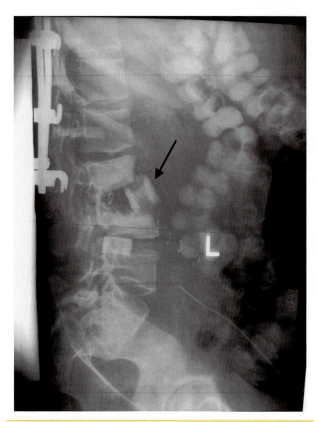

FIGURE 10-11. Graft dislodgement. Lateral radiograph shows dislodgement of an L2-3 humeral allograft (*black arrow*) after the patient underwent an anterior L3 corpectomy. There clearly is a lack of apposition of the superior graft with the L2 endplate.

Implant Failure

Strut grafts are long segments of bone used in fusion procedures. Because of their size they are susceptible to migration, angulation, fracture, nonunion, and instrument failure (Figs. 10-11,10-12). Instrument failure may be due to excessive force at the implant bone junction, technical errors, poor implant selection, weak and osteoporotic bone, or from poor patient compliance with postoperative bracing. Bone graft–related complications in the early postoperative period include graft dislodgment, fracture, or collapse. High complication rates of up to 60% have been reported when struts grafts are incorporated in multilevel cervical corpectomy and reconstruction (23). For example, failure rates of 9% are reported in patients with a two-level anterior corpectomy, fusion, and plating procedure, while the same procedure performed at three cervical levels has a 50% failure rate (24,25).

Implant dislodgment is the most commonly reported complication, resulting in posttraumatic deformity after posterior instrumentation. Moreover, graft dislodgment is reported in 5% to 50% of multilevel corpectomy patients when stand-alone grafts have been used without plating. Thirty percent to 50% of the complications in these multi-

level cases are due to graft- and instrumentation-related causes and carry a significant reoperation rate (23,26). Patients with anterior graft dislodgment may present with difficulty swallowing or breathing. Anterior grafts are weaker in compression and may collapse, resulting in a kyphotic deformity that requires strut graft revision. Alternatively, posterior graft displacement may cause new-onset neurologic deficits.

Patients with early- or late-onset graft fracture usually present with neck pain. Patients with significant fracture displacement require a revision of the strut graft and instrumentation or additional posterior fusion and fixation. Interestingly, graft fracture is reported to occur more frequently when the graft is harvested with an osteotome instead of a saw. All forms of strut graft failure must be addressed surgically.

Pseudoarthrosis

One of the main goals of spinal surgery is to achieve fusion. A successful bony fusion implies that contiguous bone has bridged across a particular motion segment in the spine, either in the intervertebral disc space, across the transverse processes in the thoracolumbar spine or the lateral masses in the cervical spine, or through the facets. A pseudoarthrosis is defined as the "absence of bridging bone between adjacent vertebra," or the lack of bridging bone to a graft or motion across a fused joint (27).

Bohlman et al. (28) concluded that motion and the presence of chondro-osseous spurs at the level of a pseudoarthrosis may contribute to residual nerve root compression that can cause postoperative neck or arm pain. Phillips et al. (unpublished data, North American Spine Society meeting, 1996) reported that one-third of patients with symptomatic pseudoarthrosis initially had symptom-free intervals following surgery despite radiographic evidence of pseudoarthrosis. They developed symptoms after a subsequent traumatic event, suggesting that a fibrous union may have been disrupted.

Radiographs are the initial imaging study of choice to diagnosis a postoperative pseudarthrosis in the spine. Although the combination of dynamic flexion-extension or lateral bending films may confirm the existence of a fusion, radiographs can be insufficient in a symptomatic patient. Dynamic films are useful for detection of gross instability; however, they can be relatively insensitive to the presence of a subtle pseudoarthrosis. The measurement of the change in distance between the spinous processes is more reproducible and accurate than the Cobb method (angle measurement to assess scoliosis) for making the diagnosis of pseudoarthrosis. Moreover, the radio-opaque hardware frequently obscures the view to adequately confirm the presence of bridging bone. Conventional tomography, CT, and scintigraphy scanning may be necessary in questionable cases.

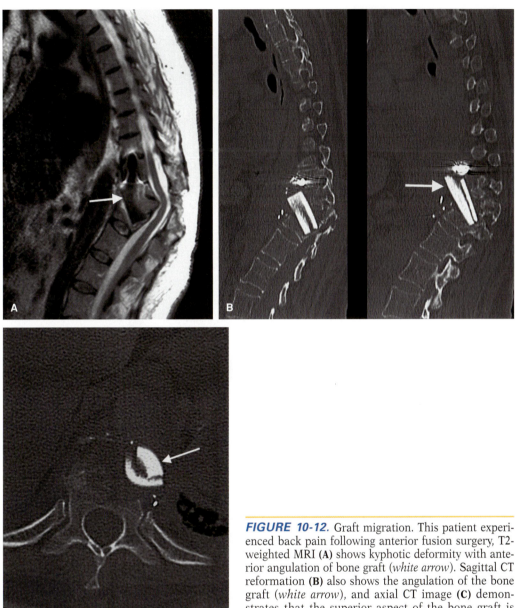

FIGURE 10-12. Graft migration. This patient experienced back pain following anterior fusion surgery, T2-weighted MRI (**A**) shows kyphotic deformity with anterior angulation of bone graft (*white arrow*). Sagittal CT reformation (**B**) also shows the angulation of the bone graft (*white arrow*), and axial CT image (**C**) demonstrates that the superior aspect of the bone graft is located in the left-sided paravertebral soft tissues (*white arrow*).

Conventional tomography increases the accuracy of diagnosis of pseudoarthrosis to 96% over plain radiography. However, CT, which affords the highest spatial resolution as well as multiplanar and three-dimensional reformations, is probably the most useful imaging modality for identifying the presence of contiguous bone and confirming arthrodesis; this modality has proven useful in the diagnosis of pseudoarthrosis. MRI has also been advocated as a method to identify motion segments at a fusion site (29).

Technetium bone scan and single-photon emission computed tomography (SPECT) have also been used to detect pseudoarthrosis. SPECT scanning involves the use of a tomographic camera to remove three-dimensional superimposition from images derived from an injectable radiotracer, thereby improving image contrast and offering more complete spatial information than conventional bone scans. A site of pseudoarthrosis may reveal increased uptake of the injected radiotracer (30). However, the false positive rate is high before 1 year and the sensitivity and specificity of SPECT has been reported to be low at 0.50 and 0.58, respectively (30–32).

Imaging findings suggestive of implant failure include loosening or breakage of screws, radioluscency ("halo") around screws (Fig. 10-13), broken fixation plates, and changes in the spinal alignment. These imaging findings suggest that there is continued motion of the spinal elements despite the presence of rigid instrumentation (i.e.,

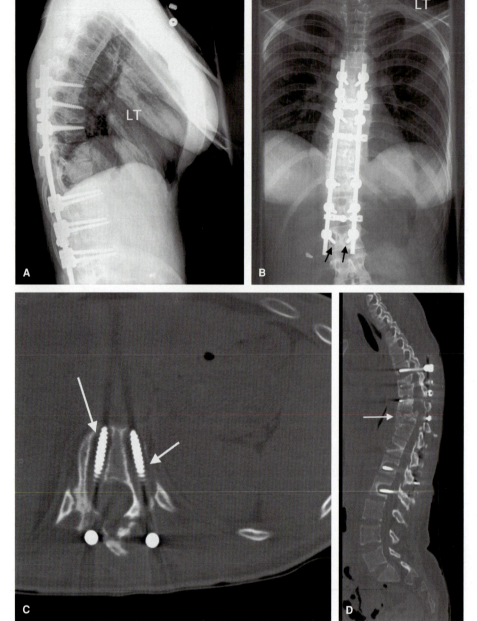

FIGURE 10-13. Pseudoarthrosis. This 20-year-old female was in a rollover motor vehicle accident and presented 2 years after having undergone a posterior T7-L2 pedicle screw fixation for a T10 fracture dislocation. She presented with a skin boil and no other symptoms. Lateral radiograph **(A)** shows relatively good positioning of the hardware. The pedicle screws are too long. In general the goal of a pedicle screw is to lay approximately two thirds within the vertebral body. The anteroposterior radiograph **(B)** clearly shows halos around every pedicle screw (*black arrows at L2*), suggesting continued motion and remodeling around the screw. **C:** The lucencies around the screws are more apparent on axial CT image (*white arrows*), and the lack of bony growth across the fractured T10 segment on sagittal CT **(D)** reformation (*white arrow*) confirms the pseudoarthrosis.

a motion segment). The abnormal motion indicates that the majority of the load has been transferred to the implant, which then leads to fatigue failure. However, the identification of pseudoarthrosis does not automatically necessitate surgical intervention. Many patients with such findings remain largely asymptomatic or complain of mild axial back or neck symptoms. It is unclear if rigid fusion is always necessary for a good surgical result. Current thinking suggests that even when a patient demonstrates imaging manifestations of pseudarthrosis, the

patient may still progress to arthrodesis over time. A solid surgical fusion can easily take years to achieve.

Cerebrospinal Fluid Leak and Pseudomeningocele

Although it is an infrequent occurrence, cerebrospinal fluid (CSF) leakage as a result of laceration to the dural membrane inadvertently created at surgery can pose potentially serious clinical problems including pseudomeningocele

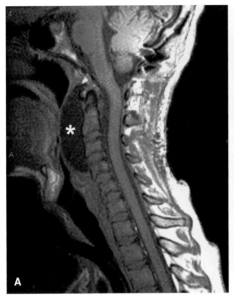
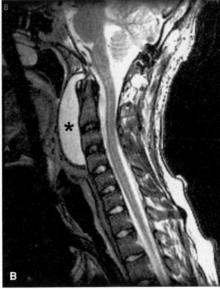

FIGURE 10-14. Anterior pseudomeningocele. A young man suffered an atlanto-occipital dislocation and underwent an occiput-C2 fusion. He presented 2 months later with increasing difficulty swallowing. T1-weighted **(A)** and T2-weighted **(B)** sagittal images from a follow-up MRI of his neck revealed an extremely large anterior pseudomeningocele (*asterisks in A and B*). The patient was treated with a lumbar drain successfully.

formation, CSF fistula formation, meningitis, and arachnoiditis with subsequent chronic pain. Spontaneous post-traumatic dural tears have been reported to occur in 7.7% of all spine fractures, are more common in the lumbar area, and are frequently associated with neurologic deficits (33).

The incidence of dural tears often is not reported because of the lack of morbidity associated with most cases, but such tears are generally reported to occur in 0% to 13.7% of spinal surgeries. The reported prevalence of iatrogenic dural tears is 1% to 17% in series ranging from five to 450 patients (34).

The patient with a dural tear is likely to experience postural headache with a combination of nausea, vomiting, pain or tightness in the neck or back, dizziness, diplopia, photophobia, tinnitus, and blurred vision. A persistent CSF leak also places the patient at risk for developing meningitis or arachnoiditis. In most cases, the dural tear can be detected intraoperatively by the presence of clear fluid emanating from the thecal sac. Obvious tears should be repaired at the time of the operation before closure (35). A watertight closure may be attempted using nonabsorbable sutures in either a running or interrupted technique with the application of fibrin glue on the tear to promote the seal. However, a small dural tear may remain undetected or may not be properly repaired at the time of surgery. Persistent leakage of CSF through the dural tear results in a loss of CSF volume, decreasing the brain's supporting cushion, which is aggravated by upright positioning and relived in the recumbent position. Conservative management of dural tears advises that patients remain flat in bed for 4 to 7 days to reduce symptoms and facilitate healing. However, some authors advocate reoperation to repair and seal the dural tear. Patients may ambulate immediately after surgery but should be cautioned to lay flat if they develop symptoms. In some instances, leaking CSF from the dural tear may drain through the surgical tract and form a cutaneous CSF fistula, which becomes a conduit for infection. When simple suturing or fibrin glue fails to seal the leak, other surgical methods may then be employed such as use of either a muscle or a fat graft to plug the hole. Fibrin or collagen-based substitutes help create a water-tight seal around the tear. In recurrent leaks, a watertight fascial closure can be prepared to create a controlled pseudomeningocele, which typically tends to heal over time.

A focal CSF collection in the paraspinal soft tissues from a dural tear is known as a pseudomeningocele (PSM) (Figs. 10-14, 10-15, 10-16). These encapsulated cerebrospinal fluid collections develop extra-durally as a result of dural tears and may develop soon after surgery or trauma. One report describes a pseudomeningocele, which developed 10 years after surgery and still remained asymptomatic (36). Pseudomeningoceles form fluctuant masses at the incision site and can be a cause of chronic back pain, persistent headache, and less commonly, nerve root entrapment (37–40). The incidence of symptomatic PSM after laminectomy was 2% in 400 patients (37). In a report where postoperative leaks of cerebrospinal fluid developed, the majority had persistent cerebrospinal-fluid fistulas, while only one developed a late symptomatic pseudomeningocele. In our experience, most pseudomeningoceles do not require surgical treatment as long as the fascia and dermis heal. In general, when a symptomatic pseudomeningocele is identified early, repair is usually successful. The long-term clinical outcomes of an untreated, asymptomatic pseudomeningocele are not known.

Postoperative fluid collections are common after surgery and usually represent seromas or asymptomatic

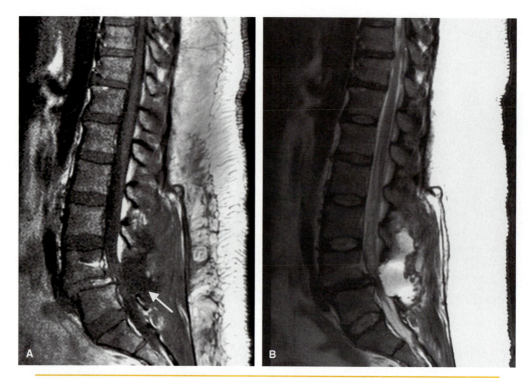

FIGURE 10-15. Cerebral spinal fluid leak. This man had a L4-5 laminectomy and pedicle screw fusion for lumbar stenosis and spondylolisthesis. He had postoperative postural headaches and T1-weighted **(A)** and T2-weighted **(B)** sagittal MRI reveals a fluid collection (*white arrow in A*), which is consistent with a cerebral spinal fluid leak. Note that the fascia appears to be in continuity. He was successfully managed with bed rest and lumbar drain.

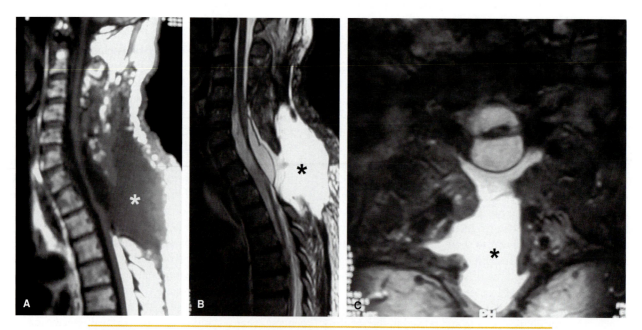

FIGURE 10-16. Postoperative pseudomeningocele. After laminectomy and expansile duraplasty, T1-weighted sagittal **(A)**, T2-weighted sagittal **(B)**, and T2-weighted axial **(C)** MRI show a fluid collection is seen in the dorsal soft tissues (*asterisks in A, B, and C*). It can be difficult to distinguish a pseudomeningocele from a seroma. Note the lack of mass effect on the thecal sac/cord. Patients with a spinal leak will typically have positional headaches indicative of low intracranial pressure. (Images courtesy of Dr. Steven Falcone, University of Miami.)

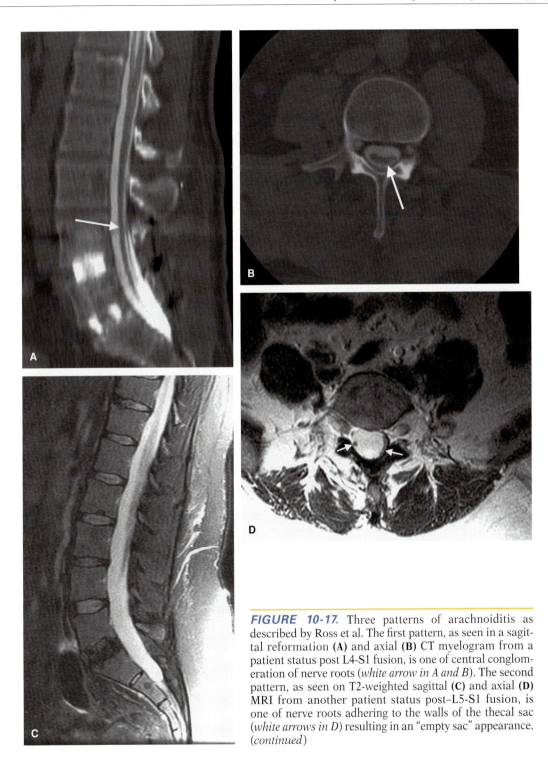

FIGURE 10-17. Three patterns of arachnoiditis as described by Ross et al. The first pattern, as seen in a sagittal reformation **(A)** and axial **(B)** CT myelogram from a patient status post L4-S1 fusion, is one of central conglomeration of nerve roots (*white arrow in A and B*). The second pattern, as seen on T2-weighted sagittal **(C)** and axial **(D)** MRI from another patient status post–L5-S1 fusion, is one of nerve roots adhering to the walls of the thecal sac (*white arrows in D*) resulting in an "empty sac" appearance. (*continued*)

postoperative hematoma. However, since CSF fistulas or pseudomeningoceles may require further management or may be associated with arachnoiditis, nerve root entrapment, or tethered cord, it is important to be able to identify these problematic lesions accurately. MRI is the principal imaging tool for this application because of its superior soft tissue resolution compared with CT. MRI can usually help localize the site of leakage and

the extent of the PSM (41). Distinguishing between pseudomeningocele and a seroma in the early postoperative period can be difficult as both types of collections can contain a mixture of serum and fluid. However, seromas generally resolve spontaneously in the early postoperative period, while pseudomeningoceles will persist and demonstrate a signal that is isointense to CSF on all MRI sequences. The presence of postural headaches is

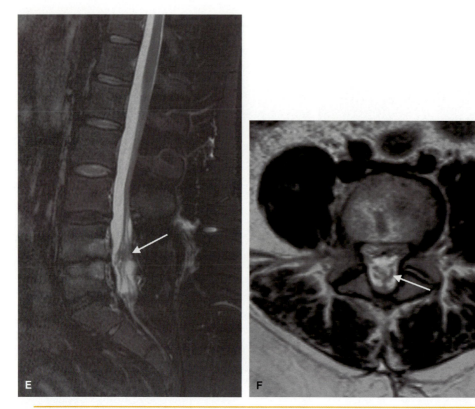

FIGURE 10-17. (*CONTINUED*) The third pattern, as seen on T2-weighted sagittal (**E**) and axial (**F**) MRI from another patient status post–L4-5 laminectomies, is one of soft tissue obliterating the majority of the subarachnoid space (*white arrow in E and F*). (Ross JS, et al. MR imaging of lumbar arachnoiditis. *AJR Am J Roentgenol.* 1987;149(5):1025–1032.)

usually associated with PSM. In equivocal cases, it may be necessary to confirm a dural leak using CT myelography (42). CT scanning can localize a CSF fistula tract or PSM. Several reports describe the utility of postmyelogram CT to diagnose CSF fistula or pseudomeningoceles in the cervical spine (43–45) lumbar spine (39), and sacral spine, which developed after traumatic transverse sacral fracture (46).

Arachnoiditis

Spinal arachnoiditis is described as a nonspecific, inflammatory process affecting the nonvascular arachnoid membrane of the spinal cord or cauda equina (47). This condition is thought to arise as a result of irritation to the membrane and causes the arachnoid layer to become thickened and adherent to the dura and pia mater (48). Initially, spinal arachnoiditis was thought to be caused by infections, particularly in the early 20th century, due to the spread of syphilis, tuberculosis, and pyogenic bacteria (49,50). Further, postmyelography arachnoiditis was commonly associated with the intrathecal injection of oil-based or ionic water–soluble contrast medium (51); the incidence has declined with the use of nonionic water–soluble contrast for myelograms. Though chronic

infection may still be a causative factor, late noninfectious causes have become more common. Additionally, the rapid growth and utilization of spinal surgery parallel a surge in postsurgical arachnoiditis.

Postoperatively, arachnoiditis can be the source of recurrent pain or progressive neurologic deficits. The clinical presentation includes burning and constant leg and low back pain worsened by activity (47,52). Sphincter disturbance, most commonly urinary frequency, urgency, and, occasionally, incontinence were reported in 20% of patients (53). Burton (54) reports little motor weakness with arachnoiditis but emphasizes paravertebral muscle spasms and limited range of motion in the trunk.

MRI is an important tool when the postoperative patient has chronic or recurrent symptoms and is often the first imaging study obtained. When MRI was developed, many studies were conducted to assess the reliability and accuracy of MRI in detecting disease entities. MRI findings correlated well with those seen on myelography or postmyelography CT scans (55). Earlier studies found CT myelography to be superior to MRI in detecting arachnoiditis (51), but more recent studies indicate that MRI may be as good or better than CT myelography at detecting and accurately diagnosing arachnoiditis (56,57).

Three distinct patterns of arachnoiditis induced changes were described by Ross et al. (57) (Fig. 10-17). The first pattern showed central conglomerations of nerve roots in the thecal sac. In the second pattern, the nerve roots were clumped and attached peripherally to the meninges; there were no subarachnoid roots, giving the appearance of the empty tube similar to that seen on myelography. The third pattern showed an increased soft tissue signal within the thecal sac, obliterating the major part of the subarachnoid space centrally. Using these findings, MRI was able to accurately diagnose moderate to severe arachnoiditis.

Arachnoiditis is an important entity to recognize both clinically and radiographically. It can be the cause of chronic debilitating pain and suffering. Though it may result from iatrogenic intervention by use of contrast for myelograms or after extradural surgery, there is little surgical treatment to ameliorate the effects of nerve root clumping. Thus, recognition of the radiographic evidence of arachnoiditis would guide proper treatment of these patients and circumvent unnecessary surgical intervention.

CONCLUSION

There are many facets of postoperative spinal imaging. More studies will be needed to establish the clinical significance of the postoperative imaging. Awareness of the complications from spinal surgery and the familiarity with the nuances of the surgical procedure, however, will assist in interpreting relevant imaging findings. It is essential to understand that symptomatology may not correlate directly with a single imaging study, and often multiple modalities may still provide significant relevant information in the management of the postoperative spinal patient.

REFERENCES

1. Harrop JS, Sharan AD, Vaccaro AR, et al. The cause of neurologic deterioration after acute cervical spinal cord injury. *Spine*. February 2001;26(4):340–346.
2. Ball P. Critical care of spinal cord injury. *Spine*. 2001;26 (24S):S27–S30.
3. Vale FL, Burns J, Jackson AB, et al. Combined medical and surgical treatment after acute spinal cord injury: results of a prospective pilot study to assess the merits of aggressive medical resuscitation and blood pressure measurement. *J Neurosurg*. 1997;87:239–246.
4. Lehmann KG, Lane JG, Peipmeier JM, et al. Cardiovascular abnormalities accompanying acute spinal cord injury in humans: incidence time course and severity. *J Am Coll Cardiol*. 1987;10:46–52.
5. Kou J, Fischgrund J, Biddinger A, et al. Risk factors for spinal epidural hematoma after spinal surgery. *Spine*. 2002;27(15):1670–1673.
6. Teo HE, Peh WC, Tan SB. Percutaneous drainage of a postoperative intraspinal hematoma using a Tuohy needle. *Skeletal Radiol*. 2003;32(10):603–607.
7. Lawton MT, Porter RW, Heiserman JE, et al. Surgical management of spinal epidural hematoma: relationship between surgical timing and neurological outcome. *J Neurosurg*. 1995;83(1):1–7.
8. Alexiadou-Rudolf C, Ernestus RI, Nanassis K, et al. Acute nontraumatic spinal epidural hematomas. An important differential diagnosis in spinal emergencies. *Spine*. 1998;23(16): 1810–1813.
9. Uribe J, Moza K, Jimenez O, et al. Delayed postoperative spinal epidural hematomas. *Spine J*. 2003;3(2):125–129.
10. Blam OG, Vaccaro AR, Vanichkachorn JS, et al. Risk factors for surgical site infection in the patient with spinal injury. *Spine*. 2003;28(13):1475–1480.
11. Donigi R, Gnes F, Bonera A, et al. Nutrition and infection. *J Parenter Enteral Nutr*. 1979;3:62.
12. Galandiuk S, Rague G, Appel S, et al. The two edged sword of large dose steroids for spinal cord trauma. *Ann Surg*. 1993;218: 419–425.
13. Colachis SR, Otis S. Occurrence of fever associated with thermoregulatory dysfunction after acute traumatic spinal cord injury. *Am J Phys Med Rehabil*. 1995;74(2):114–119.
14. Beraldo PS, Neves EG, Alves CM, et al. Pyrexia in hospitalised spinal cord injury patients. *Paraplegia*. 1993;31(3):186–191.
15. Schulitz KP, Assheuer J. Discitis after procedures on the intervertebral disc. *Spine*. 1994;19(10):1172–1177.
16. Babar S, Saifuddin A. MRI of the post-discectomy lumbar spine. *Clin Radiol*. 2002;57(11):969–981.
17. Rothman SL. The diagnosis of infections of the spine by modern imaging techniques. *Orthop Clin North Am*. 1996; 27(1):15–31.
18. Ross JS. Magnetic resonance imaging of the postoperative spine. *Semin Musculoskelet Radiol*. 2000;4(3):281–291.
19. Vaccaro A, Silber J. Post-traumatic spinal deformity. *Spine*. 2001;26:S111–S118.
20. Keene J, Lash E, Kling TJ. Undetected post-traumatic instability of "stable" thoracolumbar fractures. *J Orthop Trauma*. 1988;2:202–211.
21. Fernyhough J, White J, LaRocca H. Fusion rates in multilevel cervical spondylosis comparing allograft fibula and autograft fibula in 126 patients. *Spine*. 1991;16(S10): 561–564.
22. Zdeblick T, Ducker T. The use of freeze-dried allograft bone for anterior cervical fusions. *Spine*. 1991;16:726–729.
23. Foley KT, DiAngelo DJ, Rampersaud YR, et al. The in vitro effects of instrumentation on multi-level cervical strut-graft mechanics. *Spine*. 1999;24(22):2366–2376.
24. Vaccaro AR, Falatyn SP, Scuderi GJ, et al. Early failure of long segment anterior cervical plate fixation. *J Spinal Disord*. 1998;11(5):410–415.
25. Sasso RC, Ruggiero RA Jr., Reilly TM, et al. Early reconstruction failures after multi-level cervical corpectomy. *Spine*. 2003;28(2):140–142.
26. DiAngelo D, Foley K, Vossel K. Anterior cervical plating reverses load transfer through multi-level strut-grafts. *Spine*. 2000;25:783–795.
27. Phillips CD, Kaptain GJ, Razack N. Depiction of a postoperative pseudomeningocele with digital subtraction myelography. *AJNR Am J Neuroradiol*. 2002;23(2):337–338.
28. Bohlman HH, Emery SE, Goddfellow DB, et al. Robinson anterior cervical discectomy and arthrodesis for cervical radiculopathy: long-term follow-up of one hundred and twenty-two patients. *J Bone Joint Surg Am*. 1993;75(9): 1298–1307.
29. Zinreich SJ, Long DM, Davis R, et al. Three-dimensional CT imaging in post-surgical "failed back" syndrome. *J Comput Assist Tomogr*. 1990;14(4):574–580.
30. Slizofski WJ, Colier BD, Flatley TJ, et al. Painful pseudarthrosis following lumbar spinal fusion: detection by combined SPECT and planar bone scintigraphy. *Skeletal Radiol*. 1987; 16(2):136–141.
31. McMaster MJ, James JI. Pseudoarthrosis after spinal fusion for scoliosis. *J Bone Joint Surg Br*. 1976;58(3): 305–312.

32. Albert TJ, Pinto M, Smith MD, et al. Accuracy of SPECT scanning in diagnosing pseudoarthrosis: a prospective study. *J Spinal Disord*. 1998;11(3):197–199.

33. Keenen T, Antony J, Benson D. Dural tears associated with lumbar burst fractures. *Orthop Trauma*. 1990;4(3): 243–245.

34. Wang JC, Bohlman HH, Riew KD. Dural tears secondary to operations on the lumbar spine. Management and results after a two-year-minimum follow-up of eighty-eight patients. *J Bone Joint Surg Am*. 1998;80(12):1728–1732.

35. Eismont FJ, Wiesel SW, Rothman RH. Treatment of dural tears associated with spinal surgery. *J Bone Joint Surg Am*. 1981;63(7):1132–1136.

36. Paolini S, Ciappetta P, Piattella MC. Intraspinous post-laminectomy pseudomeningocele. *Eur Spine J*. 2003;12(3): 325–327.

37. Teplick JG, Peyster RG, Teplick SK, et al. CT Identification of postlaminectomy pseudomeningocele. *AJR Am J Roentgenol*. 1983;140(6): 1203–1206.

38. Schumacher HW, Wassmann H, Podlinski C. Pseudo-meningocele of the lumbar spine. *Surg Neurol*. 1988;29(1): 77–78.

39. Hadani M, Findler G, Knoler N, et al. Entrapped lumbar nerve root in pseudomeningocele after laminectomy: report of three cases. *Neurosurgery*. 1986;19(3):405–407.

40. Lee KS, Hardy IM II. Postlaminectomy lumbar pseudo-meningocele: report of four cases. *Neurosurgery*. 1992;30(1): 111–114.

41. Murayama S, Numaguchi Y, Whitecloud TS, et al. Magnetic resonance imaging of post-surgical pseudomeningocele. *Comput Med Imaging Graph*. 1989;13(4):335–339.

42. Gundry CR, Fritts HM. Magnetic resonance imaging of the musculoskeletal system: the spine. *Clin Orthop Relat Res*. 1998;346:262–278.

43. Hanakita J, Kinuta Y, Suzuki T. Spinal cord compression due to postoperative cervical pseudomeningocele. *Neurosurgery*. 1985;17(2):317–319.

44. Maiuri F, et al. Postoperative cervical pseudomeningocele. *Neurochirurgia (Stuttg)*. 1988;31(1):29–31.

45. Horowitz SW, Azar-Kia B, Fine M. Postoperative cervical pseudomeningocele. *AJNR Am J Neuroradiol*. 1990;11(4): 784.

46. Hadley MN, Carter LP. Sacral fracture with pseudo-meningocele and cerebrospinal fluid fistula: case report and review of the literature. *Neurosurgery*. 1985;16(6):843–846.

47. Heary RF, Northrup BE, Barolat G. Arachnoiditis. In: Benzel EC, ed. *Spine Surgery, Techniques, Complication Avoidance and Management*. Vol. 2, 2nd ed. Philadelphia: Elsevier Churchill Livingstone; 2005:2205.

48. Ransford AO, Harries BJ. Localised arachnoiditis complicating lumbar disc lesions. *J Bone Joint Surg Br*. 1972;54(4):656–665.

49. Burton CV, ed. Adhesive arachnoiditis. In: Youmans JR, ed. *Neurological Surgery*. 3rd ed. Philadelphia: WB Saunders, 1990:2856–2863.

50. Grahame R, et al. Toward a rational therapeutic strategy for arachnoiditis. A possible role for d-penicillamine. *Spine*. 1991;16(2):172–175.

51. Karnaze MG, et al. Comparison of MR and CT myelography in imaging the cervical and thoracic spine. *AJR Am J Roentgenol*. 1988;150(2):397–403.

52. Benner B, Ehni G. Spinal arachnoiditis. The postoperative variety in particular. *Spine*. 1978;3(1):40–44.

53. Guyer DW, Wiltse LL, Eskay ML, et al. The long-range prognosis of arachnoiditis. *Spine*. 1989;14(12):1332–1341.

54. Burton CV. Lumbosacral arachnoiditis. *Spine*. 1978;3(1): 24–30.

55. Delamarter RB, Ross JS, Masaryk TJ, et al. Diagnosis of lumbar arachnoiditis by magnetic resonance imaging. *Spine*. 1990;15(4):304–310.

56. Fitt GJ, Stevens JM. Postoperative arachnoiditis diagnosed by high resolution fast spin-echo MRI of the lumbar spine. *Neuroradiology*. 1995;37(2):139–145.

57. Ross JS, Masaryk TJ, Modic MT, et al. MR imaging of lumbar arachnoiditis. *AJR Am J Roentgenol*. 1987;149(5): 1025–1032.

Imaging of the Previously Injured Spinal Cord

Steven Falcone

Up to 95% of acute spinal cord injury (SCI) patients will survive their initial hospitalization (1). This is primarily attributable to improved treatment of spine injury and associated injuries in the field, advances in spinal surgery, and improved recognition and treatment of associated medical conditions. Once past the acute stage, survival will greatly depend on the degree and success of rehabilitation therapy and psychological counseling. Major advances in the management of some of the long-term health medical complications of SCI patients such as bacterial infection related to urinary sepsis, pressure sores, pulmonary infections, and pulmonary emboli have been the primary contributor to improved survival and better quality-of-life for these patients.

Substantial improvement in the survival of the SCI patient has occurred over the recent years. Ten-year survival is inversely related to the severity and level of neurological injury. Patient survival at 10 years is 98% if neurologically normal, 91.8% if an incomplete paraplegic, 90.9% if a complete paraplegic, 86.2% if an incomplete quadriplegic, and 78.2% for a complete quadriplegic (2).

This improved survival leads to a heightened awareness of the neurological issues that are prevalent in this patient population. It has been found that 5% to 10% of

patients with a spinal cord injury may suffer worsening motor or sensory function, increasing pain, or dysautonomia (3). Other studies have shown that posttraumatic myelopathy can occur in 0.3% to 3.2% of chronically injured spinal cord patients, and that these changes may ensue as early as 2 months after injury to as late as 36 years after injury (4,5). If a paraplegic or quadriplegic patient presents with an ascending neurologic level, with loss of motor or sensory function, or with increasing pain, it is important to determine if there is a treatable cause and then make an attempt to preserve or regain function. Progressive myelopathy may be seen with a cord cyst, myelomalacia, and cord tethering (4). However, other less commonly described causes include arachnoiditis, cord compression secondary to spinal instability or bone fragments narrowing the canal, cord tethering, loculated subarachnoid cysts with resultant cord compression, cord atrophy, and microcystic spinal cord degeneration/gliosis (4). Imaging plays a key and crucial role in the evaluation of these patients.

There are essentially five imaging modalities/procedures that may prove useful in the evaluation of the previously injured spinal cord patient who presents with neurological deterioration. These include plain film radiography, computed tomography (CT), myelography with plain film and CT, magnetic resonance imagery (MRI), and intraoperative sonography/ultrasound.

INDICATIONS FOR IMAGING AND IMAGING TECHNIQUES

In SCI patients, either complete or incomplete, the continued preservation of existing sensory or motor neurological function is important to the existing quality-of-life and the prevention of medical complications. For example, the patient may be able to move the thumb and index fingers of one of their hands that might allow for the operation of a motorized wheelchair. Any loss of this motor skill might result in a loss of independence and function. In addition, the loss of sensation of one area of the body that was previously preserved could result in an increased incidence of injury or pressure sores in this part of the body.

Imaging is indicated in those patients who suffer new loss of neurological function, new spasticity or loss of tone, ascending neurological deficit, and pain. The choice of imaging modality depends on many factors, but the combination of plain radiography and MRI can provide the needed information in most instances. In those instances where MRI is contraindicated or when metal artifact precludes sufficient MRI evaluation, CT with or without myelography may be necessary.

Plain radiography of the cervical spine is still an invaluable tool for evaluating the previously injured spinal cord patient. Many spinally injured patients have undergone previous surgery and plain radiographs are useful to check the position of any metallic hardware or bone grafts, to evaluate for signs of metallic hardware loosening, to assess healing of bone grafts, to check the position of graft material, and to look for signs of infection. In both the operated and unoperated spine, plain radiographs are useful to evaluate alignment and to assess for the presence of bony fragments within the canal. Recently, however, the emergence of multidetector CT with multiplanar reconstruction has relegated plain radiography to a slightly less important position in the workup of these patients. Multidetector CT with multiplanar reconstruction is at least as good if not better in the evaluation of the parameters discussed above. Plain radiography, however, is still used and may be best suited for the evaluation of spinal stability.

Delayed instability may be encountered in up to 20% of patients with hyperflexion sprain injury (6). A clinical definition of spinal stability is "the ability of the spine under physiologic loads to limit patterns of displacement so as not to damage or irritate the spinal cord or nerve roots and in addition prevent incapacitating deformity or pain due to structural damage" (7,8). Spinal instability would therefore be the inability of the spine to limit patterns of displacement. Regarding radiographic evaluation, instability may be present when one of the following are encountered: (a) obvious dislocations and fracture dislocations, (b) 3.5 mm of horizontal displacement on lateral radiograph, (c) >11-degrees kyphosis, (d) widened intervertebral disc space, or (e) splaying of spinous processes (8). Cervical spine flexion and extension radiographs in the previously injured spinal cord patient can provide information as to whether instability is present (Fig. 11-1).

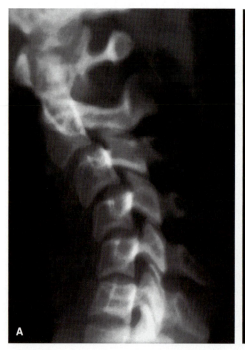
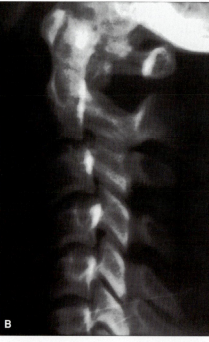

FIGURE 11-1. Hyperflexion sprain. **A:** Lateral plain radiograph in flexion reveals splaying of the spinous processes, abnormal angulation at C3-4, as well as anterolisthesis of C3 as compared to C4. **B:** Lateral plain radiograph in extension shows splaying of the spinous processes of C3-4 and C4-5 as compared to adjacent levels. As compared to flexion radiograph, there is persistent, but less anterolisthesis and angulation at C3-4, suggesting motion at this level that may be associated with ligamentous injury and instability. There is a fixed anterolisthesis at C2-3.

Multidetector helical CT with rapid data acquisition and multiplanar reformations can provide exquisite bone detail and information regarding bony anatomic relationships in the previously injured spinal cord patient including: (a) bony canal or neural foraminal narrowing, (b) spinal alignment, (c) location of bone graft and hardware, (d) determination of adequate fusion, and (e) endplate erosion in the setting of discitis. In addition to standard sagittal and coronal reformations, oblique sagittal reformation may improve confidence in the assessment of neural foraminal stenosis (9).

CT of the postoperative patient who has metallic spinal fixation can be difficult given the associated streak artifacts that can limit evaluation of the implant as well as obscure or distort adjacent anatomy. The streak artifacts occur because the density of the metal is beyond the normal range that can be handled by the computer, resulting in incomplete attenuation profiles (10). X-ray beam hardening, partial volume, and aliasing further compound streak artifacts (10). Reduction of metallic artifact can be accomplished by many methods including increasing the kVp, decreasing the slice thickness, and utilizing various postprocessing algorithms (10). Multidetector CT with the capability of performing submillimeter slices can help to limit this artifact and provides better images than were obtained with single slice methods (10).

MRI has nearly replaced myelography in the evaluation of patients with spinal disease because it is noninvasive, does not use ionizing radiation, is less expensive, is less time consuming, and provides greater contrast resolution. Myelography still plays a role in select patients, particularly when high spatial resolution is necessary. A study by Bartynski and Lin (11) indicates that a myelographic study is useful and better than MRI in predicting lateral recess stenosis in the setting of degenerative disease. Myelography may also be useful in the evaluation of spinal leaks. By convention, its use in this setting is primarily limited to those patients who cannot undergo MRI.

A complete quality myelographic examination should include the combination of fluoroscopic observation, the acquisition of plain radiographic images, and postmyelography CT. Multidetector CT with the application of isotropic voxels allows for exquisite multiplanar reformations that can enhance evaluation. In the previously injured spinal cord patient, it may be useful to perform postmyelographic CT immediately after the myelogram and 4 hours after the myelogram (12). This delayed CT can be helpful to detect spinal cord cysts with contrast diffusing into the cyst on delayed evaluation (12).

MRI has proven extremely useful in the evaluation of patients who develop delayed or progressive neurologic deficits months to years after acute spinal injury (3,13). MRI is particularly well suited for detection of the pathology encountered in these patients due to its superb contrast resolution and multiplanar capabilities. These pathologies include spinal cord cysts, spinal cord tethering/myelomalacia, and spinal cord compression related to bony deformities or disc herniations.

Special conditions or patient needs may be present when attempting to perform an MRI in the previously injured spinal cord patient. The presence of uncontrollable muscle spasms, ferromagnetic hardware, and respiratory difficulties can negatively affect image quality. It is important that the imager work closely with the patient and the referring physician to provide sufficient medical therapy before imaging so that satisfactory images are obtained. The application of fast scanning techniques and those techniques that reduce susceptibility in the presence of metallic hardware may also be necessary.

T1-weighted and T2-weighted sequences in both the axial and sagittal planes are needed in the complete evaluation of these patients. The use of T2-weighted fast spin echo sequences may decrease magnetic susceptibility artifact in these patients who have often undergone previous surgery with titanium plates or wires in place. Moreover, increasing the receiver bandwidth on fast spin echo sequences can markedly improve the visualization of tissues adjacent to hardware (14). As compared to the acute setting, a T2* sequence is not as useful in the previously injured patient because the detection of blood is not of prime consideration. Additionally, because these patients commonly have metallic hardware, the T2* sequence can be problematic because of susceptibility effects (Fig. 11-2). The addition of a conventional proton density spin echo sagittal sequence can be also beneficial in distinguishing between a confluent spinal cord cyst and myelomalacia. An additional sequence that we routinely employ in the previously injured spinal cord patient is a cerebral spinal fluid (CSF) flow study. Phase contrast CSF cine-flow studies are useful in the confirmation and diagnosis of posttraumatic and postoperative spinal cord tethering with or without subarachnoid cyst formation. CSF flow studies can also be useful in the determination of spinal cord cyst pulsatility (15).

Advanced MRI strategies that are currently in routine use in the brain, such as diffusion weighted imaging, perfusion studies, spectroscopy, and magnetization transfer, are not routinely used in the clinical setting for spinal cord lesions. As MRI hardware improves, these techniques may be used for the evaluation of spinal cord pathology. These advanced techniques may prove to be helpful in the clinical setting as diffusion-weighted imaging with apparent diffusion coefficient (ADC) maps have been shown to detect cystic lesions within spinal cord gray matter following experimental spinal cord injury before they were seen on conventional T1- and T2-weighted images (16).

Intraoperative spinal sonography is a modality that is not widely used in the community; however, it can provide invaluable information to the surgeon while operating

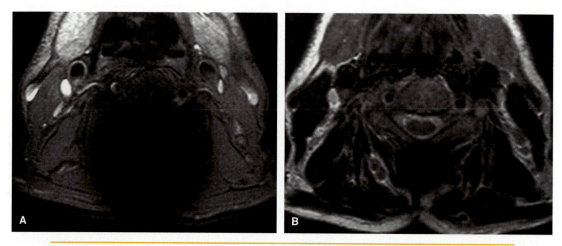

FIGURE 11-2. Metal artifact. **A:** T2-weighted gradient echo axial image of the spine is nondiagnostic due to the susceptibility artifact caused by the metal fusion hardware associated with the posterior arch. **B:** T2-weighted fast spin echo axial image at the same level results in a significant reduction in the metallic artifact with resulting diagnostic image of the spinal canal.

on the previously injured spinal cord patient (17). Although the clinical presentation in conjunction with preoperative imaging determines who will ultimately be operated on, intraoperative sonography can play an important role in improving surgical outcome (17). Since the introduction of ultrasound into the operating room in 1982 (18), high-resolution spinal sonography has provided the spinal surgeon with a view never before possible. Intraoperative spinal sonography provides a 360-degree circumferential view of the operative field, allowing the surgeon to precisely depict and view the canal contents directly opposite the exposure. The surgeon, for example, can view the ventral canal from a posterior approach. Intraoperative sonography provides real-time evaluation that can help limit or minimize damage to neural tissue and can help determine if an adequate result has been achieved. Intraoperative sonography might be critical in distinguishing between a confluent cyst and microcystic myelomalacia and is extremely useful in the evaluation of the patient who is undergoing cyst decompression and cord untethering to determine if adequate cyst decompression and untethering has been achieved. Additionally, intraoperative sonography is useful in the determination of adequate canal decompression of stenotic regions.

A portable sonographic machine equipped with preset parameters, high-resolution (7 to 10 MHz) sector, curved array, or linear transducers on a long cord, are satisfactory for image acquisition (17). The transducer and attached cord are placed in a sterile sheath along with sterile gel that serves as an acoustic couplet between the transducer and sterile sheath. Many patients undergo spinal surgery in the prone position and therefore are examined from a posterior approach (17). This must be kept in mind when correlating the sonographic images with the preoperative imaging. Once the surgeon retracts the paraspinal muscles and performs the laminectomy, sterile water can be poured into the operative field to serve as an acoustic path. The tip of the draped transducer is then placed in the water bath, and scanning of the spinal canal and its contents in the transverse and longitudinal planes commences.

Prior to further surgical manipulation, the initial images are reviewed for the pertinent findings and are correlated with the preoperative images. Based on the initial findings, the surgical plan may or may not be altered (17). The progress of surgery is monitored with sonography, and changes are made to the operative approach when necessary. Upon completion of the surgery, final sonographic images are taken to document the results of surgery (17).

There are some limitations to sonography, some of which are unique to intraoperative sonography. A major limitation of intraoperative spinal sonography is the sonographic window. The extent of the laminectomy or amount of bone removed ultimately determines the field of view. Intraoperative sonography cannot be used with microsurgical techniques because a window of at least 1.5 cm by 1 cm is necessary for adequate visualization of the canal and its contents. Bone is not the only substance that may interfere with the transmission of sound waves and obscure the anatomy of interest. Calcification of the dura mater, bullet fragments, and Gelfoam can all obscure anatomic detail. Small amounts of Gelfoam can be confused with pathologic processes, and, therefore, it is desirable to remove all Gelfoam from the operative field prior to scanning.

CLINICAL PRESENTATION AND PATHOPHYSIOLOGY OF POSTTRAUMATIC MYELOPATHY

In spinally injured patients, delayed or late deterioration of neurological function has been referred to as posttraumatic myelopathy or progressive myelopathy (19). This clinical syndrome has been described using various terms that refer to the clinical syndrome or the pathologic etiology, including chronic injury of the central cervical spinal cord (20), posttraumatic syringomyelia (21,22), ascending cystic degeneration of the cord (23,24), posttraumatic progressive myelopathy (13), posttraumatic cystic myelopathy (25), progressive posttraumatic cystic myelopathy (26), and progressive posttraumatic myelomalacic myelopathy (PPMM) (4). The presenting symptoms of these entities may be indistinguishable. The most common pathologic etiologies underlying posttraumatic myelopathy may be divided into the categories of spinal cord cysts and myelomalacia.

Spinal Cord Cysts

Posttraumatic spinal cord cysts affect as many as 3.2% of spinal cord injured patients and up to 8% of patients with complete quadriplegia (27). The incidence is on the rise for a variety of reasons that include increasing survival of SCI patients and improved visualization of the spinal cord with MRI (27). The time of symptom onset after injury ranges from 2 months to 30 years (28), with the most common initial complaint being pain (29). Other presenting symptoms include sensory loss, motor weakness, increased or decreased spasticity, autonomic dysreflexia, hyperhidrosis (above level of injury), sphincter loss or sexual dysfunction, Horner syndrome, respiratory insufficiency, and death (28). The classic sensory dysfunction is a distal loss of pain and temperature sensation with preservation of proprioceptive sensation and light touch (30).

The terminology of cystic cavities in the cord can be confusing. Hydromyelia refers to those cavities that are ependymal lined, syringomyelia to glial lined cavities, and syringohydromyelia to either a combined or indeterminate cyst. Imaging often cannot distinguish between these cysts, and hence the general term spinal cord cyst (or syrinx) may be used for all cysts other than those lesions that are clearly related to a dilated central canal. The most frequently reported pathologic feature of syringomyelia is cavitation of the gray matter adjacent to or directly involving the central canal with an associated inner layer of gliotic tissue (31,32).

In a monograph published in 1973, Barnett (33) proposed a classification scheme for syringomyelia based on a variety of clinical and experimental observations and studies. This scheme has five divisions: (a) communicating syringomyelia (syringohydromyelia) subdivided into those associated with developmental anomalies at the foramen magnum and posterior fossa contents and those associated with acquired skull base abnormalities, (b) syringomyelia as a late sequel to trauma (posttraumatic cystic myelopathy), (c) syringomyelia associated with spinal cord tumors, (d) syringomyelia as a sequel to arachnoiditis confined to the spinal canal, and (e) idiopathic syringomyelia.

The pathogenesis for the development and growth of posttraumatic cysts remains controversial. It is likely that there are many contributing factors to the development and progression of posttraumatic spinal cord cysts. Cavitation of the spinal cord after trauma is a common pathologic change, as demonstrated by magnetic resonance studies and pathologic series (34–37). Posttraumatic spinal cord cyst formation can also be divided into two steps: initial cavity formation followed by cyst extension. Causal factors preceding initial cavity formation may include liquefaction of intraparenchymal hematoma, ischemia due to tethering, arterial or venous obstruction, release of intracellular lysosomal enzymes and excitatory amino acids, and mechanical damage from cord compression. Tethering of the spinal cord also figures prominently in initial cavitation (38).

Blockage of CSF flow has been proposed by Williams (39) as an explanation for spinal cord cyst formation and extension. One of the problems with this theory is that it requires a pressure differential between the ventricular system and spinal subdural space during valsalva maneuver, and subsequently Williams et al. (40) stressed that the majority of cases of traumatic syringomyelia had no evidence of a posterior fossa abnormality that may cause the blockage of CSF flow. It is likely that scar formation within the subarachnoid space plays a vital role in cyst formation and expansion. The tethered cord (which is commonly dorsal in location because of patient recumbency following injury) disrupts CSF flow in the subarachnoid space. The normal motion of the cord and CSF during the cardiac cycle is disrupted. The lack of cord motion results in stress forces that are transmitted to the cord and may initiate cavitation (41) (Fig. 11-3).

Several theories have been proposed to explain rostral or caudal cyst extension. Turbulent CSF flow around a tethered cord may expand a cyst via similar forces that contributed to initial formation. A ball valve connection between the subarachnoid space and the cyst may allow entrance but not egress of CSF into the cyst, resulting in expansion (38). Disturbed CSF flow has been the basis of the "slosh" and "suck" theories, in which valsalva-like activity causes increased epidural venous flow, resulting in increased pressure around the cord that cannot be dissipated because of interruptions in the normal CSF flow patterns (5,38). This circulatory disruption can result in pressure dissociation between the upper and lower

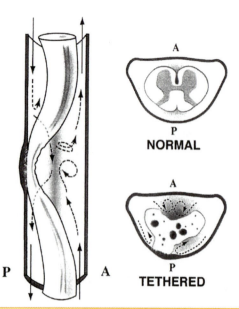

FIGURE 11-3. Diagram of spinal cord tethering. Longitudinal drawing of spinal canal shows tethering of spinal cord posteriorly with thickening of dura, resulting in turbulent CSF flow. Axial drawings of spinal canal compare normal cord with tethered cord. Turbulent CSF flow contributes to progressive damage at level of spinal cord tethering, and early cystic changes are seen within cord parenchyma. A, anterior; P, posterior. (Reproduced from Schwartz ED, Falcone S, Quencer RM, et al. Posttraumatic syringomyelia: pathogenesis, imaging, and treatment. *AJR.* 1999;173:487–492, with permission.)

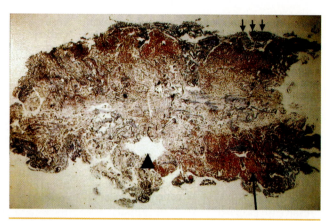

FIGURE 11-4. Histopathologic transverse section through a posttraumatic myelomalacic spinal cord at the C4 level. This trichrome stain demonstrates an area of abnormal red staining which represents and astrocytosis (*long arrow*). In the center of the cord there is a loose matrix of blood vessels and astrocytes. Dorsally is a microcyst (*arrowhead*). The pia-arachnoid is abnormally thickened by blue staining connective tissue (*short arrows*). (Reproduced from Falcone S, Quencer RM, Green BA, et al. Progressive posttraumatic myelomalacic myelopathy (PPMM): imaging and clinical features. *AJNR.* 1994;15(4): 747–754, with permission.)

compartments of the subarachnoid space. Distensile pressure pulse waves transmitted within the epidural veins during valsalva maneuvers associated with coughing and sneezing can, in concert with the pressure dissociation, expand the cyst within the spinal cord (40). CSF may initially enter from the Virchow-Robin spaces, or the dorsal root entry zone, and then enter the cyst by transmural fluid migration (42,43).

Myelomalacia

PPMM is a less well-studied clinical entity first described in 1994 (4). Patients present with signs and symptoms of a progressive posttraumatic myelopathy without an associated confluent spinal cord cyst. Myelomalacia or "soft cord" is characterized by microcysts, reactive astrocytosis, and thickening of the pia-arachnoid at histology (4) (Fig. 11-4). Intraoperative observations may reveal associated cord tethering by fibrous adhesions and thickening of the overlying dura. Recognition of posttraumatic myelomalacia prior to an operation may be important because untethering of the spinal cord may lead to clinical improvement (4). PPMM may represent a continuum of interrelated disease processes that precede formation of a confluent cyst.

IMAGING APPEARANCE OF LATE SEQUELAE OF SPINAL CORD INJURY

The lack of clinical distinction between cystic and noncystic posttraumatic myelopathy necessitates that imaging play a key role in the evaluation of these patients (4,13,44–46). MRI is the preferred imaging modality in the evaluation of these patients (3). Less common causes of posttraumatic myelopathy, such as cord compression from malalignment, herniated disc, osteophytes (Fig. 11-5), and arachnoid cysts, are also readily detectable by MRI. Progressive neurologic deterioration can also result from accelerated neuronal death or apoptosis that may be seen as spinal cord atrophy with MRI.

Quencer et al. (3) demonstrated the benefit of MRI compared to immediate and delayed CT myelography in differentiating spinal cord cysts from myelomalacia. It was found that MRI more accurately demonstrated the intramedullary abnormalities in the injured spinal cord than did delayed CT myelography because the former could separate myelomalacia from a posttraumatic spinal cord cyst, a differentiation that was frequently difficult with CT. In addition to the usual drawbacks of the invasive nature of myelography, both false positive and false negative cases of spinal cord cysts were found with CT myelography.

Spinal Cord Cysts

Spinal cord cysts typically follow CSF signal intensity on all imaging sequences (3) (Fig. 11-6). CSF pulsation

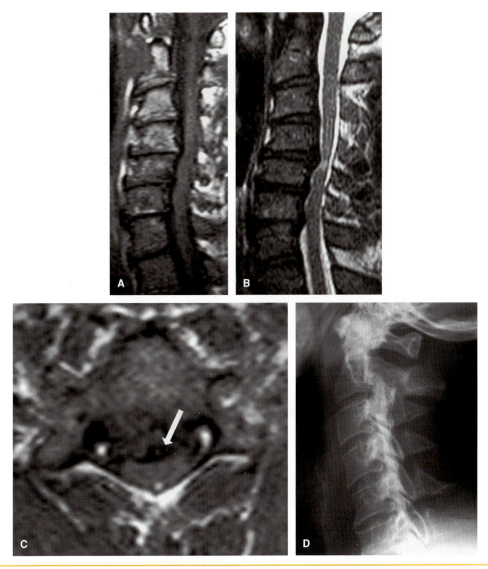

FIGURE 11-5. Ossification of the posterior longitudinal ligament (OPLL). T1-weighted sagittal **(A)** and T2-weighted sagittal **(B)** images reveal compression of the ventral aspect of the cord with T2 weighted images revealing abnormal increased signal intensity in the spinal cord parenchyma at C4-5 suggestive of injury. On the sagittal images, low signal intensity band is suspicious for a continuous ossification in the ventral subarachnoid space, which is better depicted on the T1-weighted axial image **(C)** (*arrow*). Lateral plain radiography **(D)** also depicts the ossified posterior longitudinal ligament.

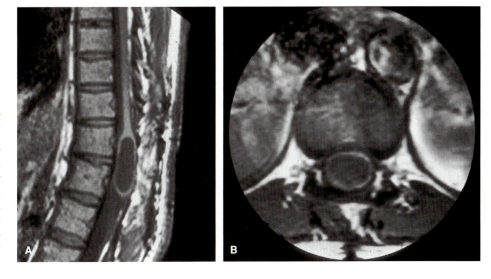

FIGURE 11-6. Simple posttraumatic spinal cord cyst. This patient, who was previously injured many years prior, was developing an increased inability to walk. T1-weighted sagittal **(A)** and axial **(B)** images reveal an expansile spinal cord cyst of the conus. There is also evidence of a prior laminectomy in the posterior soft tissues.

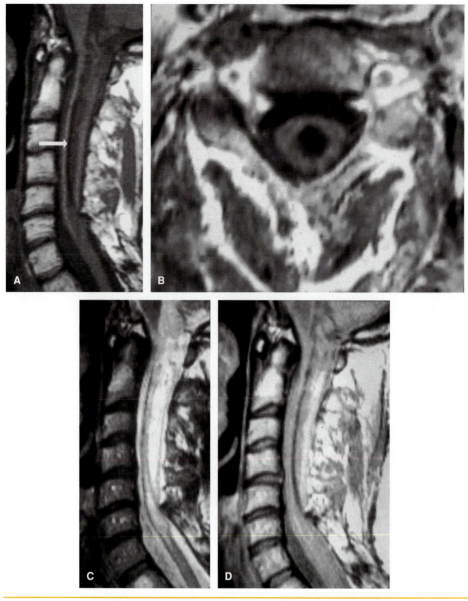

FIGURE 11-7. Simple cervical cord posttraumatic cyst with myelomalacia. The cervical cord is noted to be expanded, with central low signal intensity on T1 weighted sagittal **(A)** and axial **(B)** images, and high signal intensity on T2 weighted sagittal image **(C)**. A catheter is noted to be lying in the ventral aspect of the cyst, best seen as linear low signal intensity in the T1 weighted sagittal image (*A, arrow*). The proton density image **(D)** reveals that the posterior aspect of the signal abnormality is brighter than CSF and is most compatible with myelomalacia; the more ventral aspect has signal intensity of CSF and is compatible with a simple cyst. This cannot be clearly discerned by analysis of the T1-weighted and T2-weighted images.

induced signal loss or flow-related enhancement may be seen in large pulsatile cysts varying the MRI signal intensity (47). Rarely, alteration of cyst signal intensity can also result from an elevated protein content compared to CSF. Most cord cysts contain a well-defined border that easily demarcates them from the surrounding cord parenchyma on T1-weighted images. These margins, however, may not always be well defined, particularly those portions of the posttraumatic spinal cord cyst that are located at the injury site (3), as the intervening parenchyma may be significantly distorted as a result of previous hemorrhage, gliosis, and scarring (Fig. 11-7). Posttraumatic spinal cord

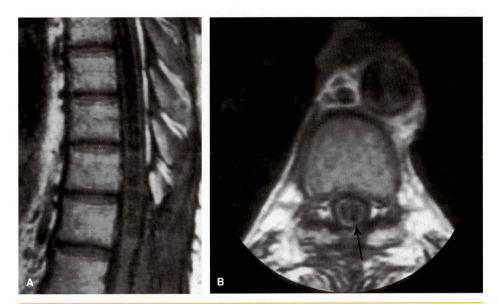

FIGURE 11-8. Septated posttraumatic cyst. T1-weighted sagittal **(A)** and axial **(B)** in a patient who is status postlamincetomy and shunting of a spinal cord cyst several years previously, now presents with progressive myelopathy. There are multiple glial bands within this septated cyst as seen on the sagittal image. Axial image reveals a "double-barreled" cyst with a catheter on the left (*arrow*). The thoracic spinal cord is expanded by this cyst.

cysts may be simple or complex with varying numbers of septations (Fig. 11-8). Identification of these septations may be important to the surgeon prior to shunting (Fig. 11-9). Posttraumatic spinal cord cysts may occur above, below, or at the site of initial injury. Cine images may demonstrate pulsatility within spinal cord cysts (48), and cysts that demonstrate pulsatility preoperatively may be more likely to expand over time (15) (Fig. 11-10). The postoperative cine evaluation may lend some help in determining the efficacy of surgery as demonstrated by Brugieres et al. (49) in a group of Chiari I patients in which high postoperative diastolic CSF flow velocities indicated a poor surgical outcome.

Myelomalacia

In the appropriate clinical setting, any noncystic, nonenhancing signal abnormality within the spinal cord, at the initial level of injury, likely represents an area of myelomalacia. Typically, T1-weighted images reveal signal intensity that is hypointense to normal spinal cord, however, greater in intensity than the CSF. T2-weighted images reveal corresponding hyperintensity within the spinal cord (Fig. 11-11). Differentiation from a cyst can be made with proton density images in which myelomalacia will not parallel CSF in signal intensity and instead will reveal isointense to hyperintense signal changes relative to normal spinal cord (4) (Fig. 11-12). In contradistinction to a spinal cord cyst, the margins of a myelomalacic cord are usually irregular and ill defined. At the site of myelomalacia, the spinal cord may be normal in size, atrophic, or expanded (Fig. 11-13). This expansion is thought to be associated with significant intradural scarring and a spinal cord that is adhered to the dura at multiple sites.

Spinal Cord Tethering

Cord tethering is usually a coexistent feature of myelomalacia. Using MRI, this tethering typically manifests as an asymmetric loss of the subarachnoid space, although it can be circumferential. Loss of the subarachnoid space is most commonly encountered dorsally, presumably due to the constant recumbency of these patients (4). Ventral tethering, however, is not uncommon (Fig. 11-14). Cord expansion likely results from a "pulling apart" of the spinal cord by fibrous adhesions. These adhesions can sometimes be directly visualized on MRI (4), and qualitative evaluation of phase contrast cine MRI may be useful in the confirmation and detection of cord tethering with loss of normal CSF flow patterns. After an untethering procedure, flow studies might be useful in the postoperative assessment of these patients to demonstrate reestablishment of CSF flow (Figs. 11-15, 11-16). In addition to fibrous adhesions, the spinal cord may appear tethered due to an anterior spinal cord herniation, which may be due to a tear of the dura from bony fragments following trauma (Fig. 11-17).

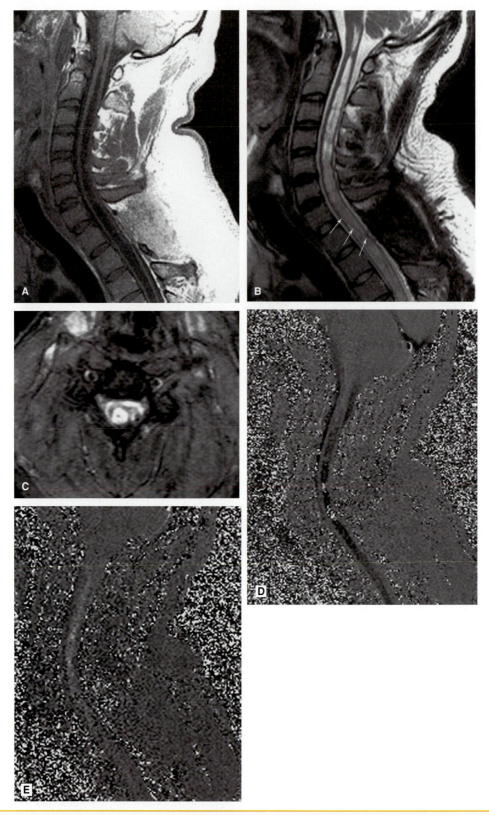

FIGURE 11-9. Re-expansion of posttraumatic cyst after cyst shunting. T1-weighted sagittal **(A)** and T2-weighted sagittal **(B)** reveal evidence of previous laminectomy at T1-2 for placement of a catheter for cyst decompression. The catheter is difficult to see on the sagittal images but is seen in **(B)** as a thin dark curvilinear region (*arrows*). The cyst extends to the brainstem where it is not expanded. Axial gradient echo image better depicts that there are two catheters in place and that the catheter on the right is not functioning as this cyst is complex without collapse of the right-sided component. Phase contrast cine evaluation in the sagittal plane **(D,E)** shows pulsation of the cyst (low signal intensity in D and high signal intensity in E) as well as attenuation of flow through the midcervical region likely related to cord expansion and effacement of the CSF space surrounding the spinal cord.

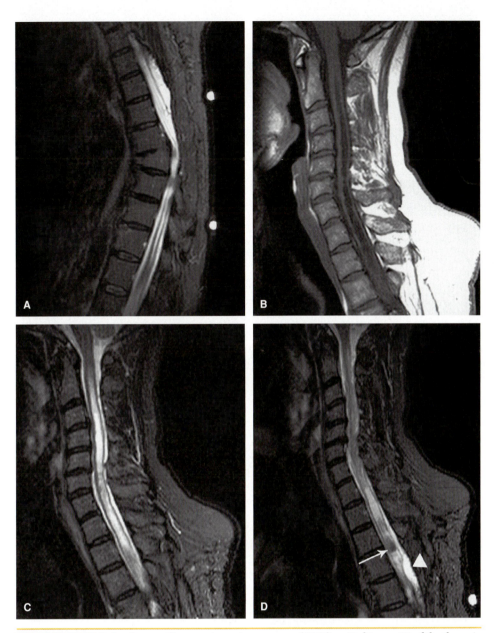

FIGURE 11-10. Pulsatile cyst. Short tau inversion recovery (STIR) sagittal image **(A)** of the thoracic spine demonstrates old midthoracic fracture with residual kyphosis and central canal narrowing related to bony retropulsion. A spinal cord cyst ascends and descends from the level of injury. T1-weighted sagittal **(B)** and STIR sagittal **(C)** of the cervical spine above the level of injury reveals the cephalad extent of the cyst to C2. STIR sagittal image slightly off midline **(D)** in the cervical region, but midline in the upper thoracic region reveals evidence of cyst pulsatility with low signal intensity (*arrow*). Also note the dorsal subarachnoid cyst (*arrowhead*). (*continued*)

Wallerian Degeneration

Following separation, or transection, from the cell body, the separated axon and myelin sheath degenerates (50). This process is referred to as Wallerian degeneration. It is important to distinguish the MRI changes of Wallerian degeneration from other chronic changes in the spinal cord.

Terae et al. (51) described six patients in which high signal intensity was observed on T2-weighted and proton density images in the dorsal columns cephalad to the primary injury site. No corresponding abnormality was identified on T1-weighted images. These signal alterations were seen 10 weeks to 12 months postinjury. In an examination of

(*text continues on page 340*)

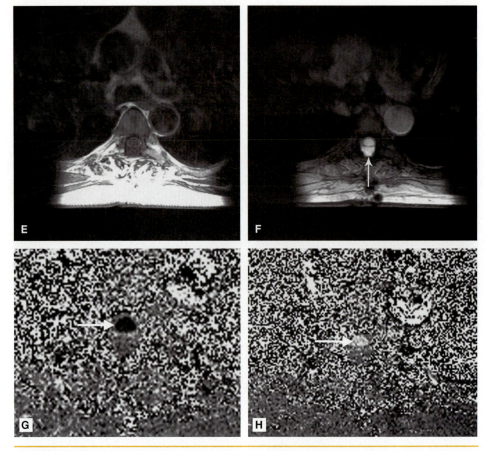

FIGURE 11-10. *(CONTINUED)* Axial T1-weighted **(E)** and gradient echo **(F)** in the upper thoracic spine best reveal evidence of prior laminectomy, a simple cord cyst, and expansile duraplasty *(arrow)*. Axial phase contrast cine images **(G,H)** through the cyst in the upper thoracic region and show pulsatility and flow within the cyst *(arrows indicating low signal intensity in G and high signal intensity in H)* with minimal flow in the subarachnoid space.

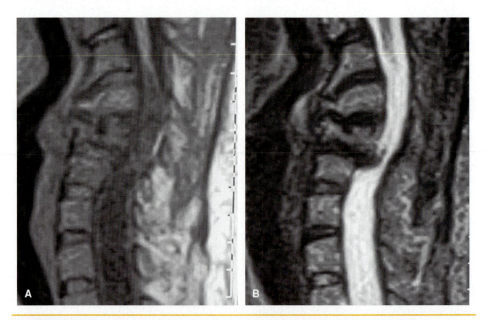

FIGURE 11-11. Kyphosis with cord compression, myelomalacia, and intramedullary cyst. T1-weighted sagittal **(A)** and T2-weighted sagittal **(B)** in this quadriplegic patient with deteriorating neurologic function shows a kyphotic deformity at the old fracture site with bony canal narrowing, microcystic myelomalacia at the injury site (mixed signal intensity in T1 weighted image and increased signal intensity in T2-weighted image), and an expansile cyst (CSF signal intensity on both T1-weighted and T2-weighted images) extending inferior to the original site of injury.

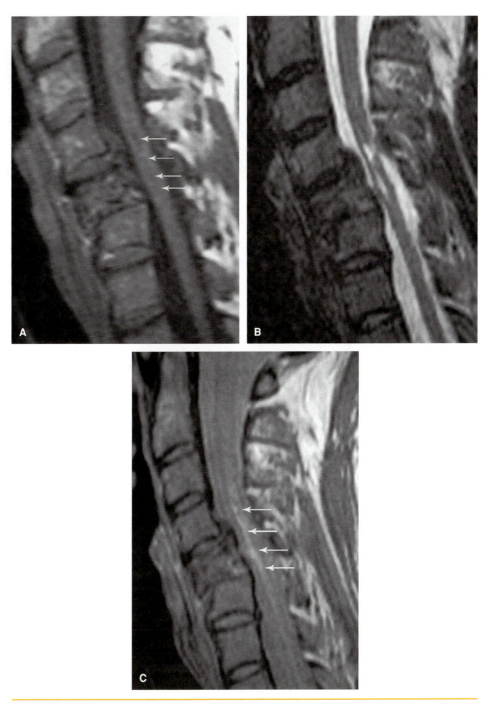

FIGURE 11-12. Myelomalacia. T1-weighted sagittal image **(A)** in this patient who suffered a spinal cord injury at C5 barely reveals a signal abnormality in the cord that is CSF equivalent (*arrows*). There is mild anterolisthesis of C4 relative to C5 with an old posttraumatic deformity of the C5 vertebral body and the spinal cord is atrophic from C4 to C6. T2-weighted sagittal image **(B)** shows corresponding high signal intensity. The proton density image **(C)**, however, reveals that the signal abnormality seen in A is hyperintense to CSF (*arrows*), most indicative of myelomalacia.

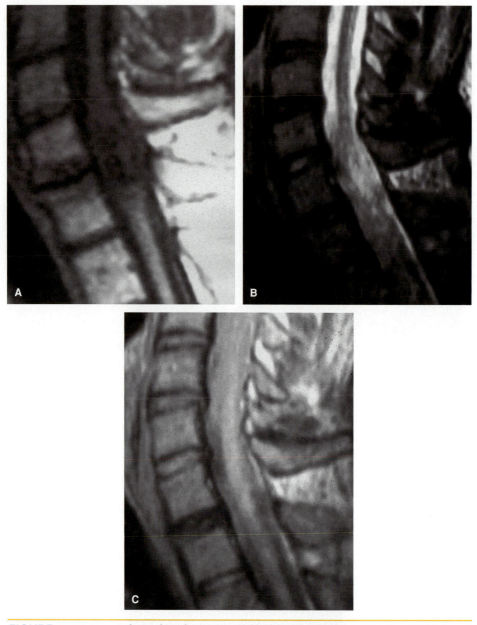

FIGURE 11-13. Expansile myelomalacia. T1-weighted sagittal **(A)**, T2-weighted sagittal **(B)**, and proton density sagittal **(C)** images reveal cord expansion of the midcervical spinal cord, likely the result of tethering bands in this patient who had previously undergone traumatic cord injury. The proton density image **(C)** deciphers the true nature of the cord expansion and signal. The majority of the expanded spinal cord is hyperintense to CSF on the PD image, as it is on the T1-weighted image (A), findings that are more compatible with myelomalacia rather than a confluent cyst. In addition, the margins of the cord lesion are not well defined, a finding more compatible with myelomalacia rather than a cyst.

postmortem spinal cords from patients who suffered a traumatic spinal cord injury, Becerra et al. (52) demonstrated that MRI could identify Wallerian degeneration by 7 weeks postinjury and could be visualized as increased signal intensity on both T1-weighted and T2-weighted images. Wallerian degeneration was seen below the primary injury site within the corticospinal tracts and above the injury site in the dorsal columns; these locations are expected as axons in the corticospinal tract and are descending, whereas axons in the posterior columns are ascending (Figs. 11-18, 11-19, 11-20).

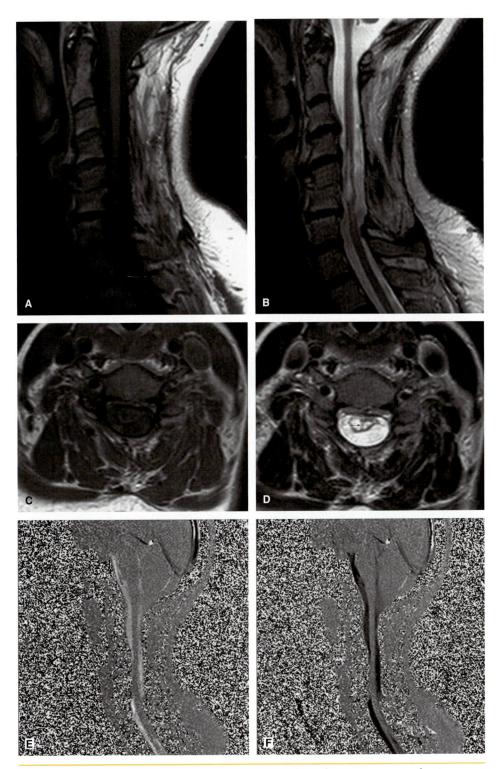

FIGURE 11-14. Anterior cord tethering. There is evidence for prior extensive laminectomy defect and anterior cervical fusion at C5-6. T1-weighted sagittal **(A)** and T2-weighted sagittal **(B)** show anterior cord tethering centered at C5-6 with an associated cord cyst. **(C,D)** axial T1-weighted and T2-weighted images reveals that the cyst is complex with a vertical band down the center (*arrow*). The cord is also seen to be ventrally tethered. Phase contrast cine sagittal **(E,F)** shows lack of flow in the ventral canal confirming the presence of ventral cord tethering. There is also attenuation of flow at the cervical thoracic junction where a change in curvature occurs.

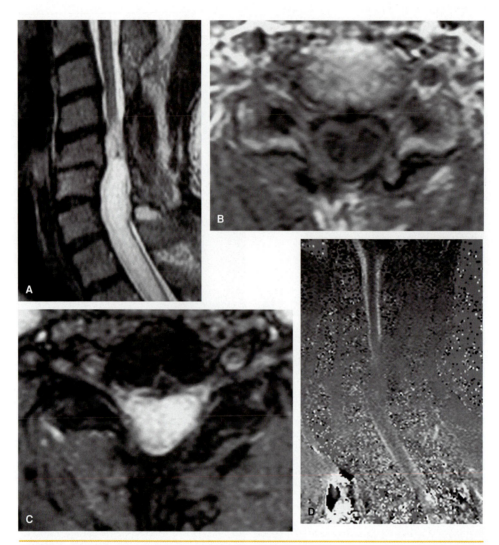

FIGURE 11-15. Pre- and postuntethering. T2-weighted sagittal **(A)**, T1-weighted axial **(B)**, T-2 weighted gradient echo axial **(C)** images reveal an expansile double barreled cervical thoracic spinal cord cyst. Single sagittal image from phase contrast CSF flow study **(D)** prior to untethering demonstrates attenuation of flow ventral and dorsal to the cord, as compared to the normal high signal bands seen ventral and dorsal to the spinal cord above and below the tethering. Note evidence of previous laminectomy in the posterior soft tissues. At surgery, dorsal tethering of the cord was encountered. The laminectomy was extended, the cord was untethered, and a widened dorsal subarachnoid space was created with placement of freeze dried dural allograft (expansile duraplasty). (*continued*)

Intraoperative Sonography

Intraoperative sonography is an invaluable tool in the surgical management of patients suffering from progressive posttraumatic myelopathy (17). Uses of this modality include assessing and confirming the levels of cord tethering, determining the success of cord untethering (Fig. 11-21), distinguishing between confluent cord cysts and myelomalacia, determining if a cord cyst has collapsed after cord untethering, and monitoring the placement of the shunt catheter and subsequent spinal cord cyst decompression (Fig. 11-22). If intraoperative sonography does not demonstrate the desired surgical result, modifications to the surgical approach can be made, such as lysing an additional scar, repositioning a shunt catheter, or placing an additional shunt catheter (17).

Posttraumatic spinal cord cysts have the typical anechoic appearance of cysts on intraoperative sonography. Myelomalacia, however, appears as a region of abnormal spinal cord echotexture with loss of the central echo (4). This abnormal echotexture may be hyperechoic or hypoechoic compared to the normal adjacent cord and it is not uncommon to see microcysts (4) (Fig. 11-23). The spinal

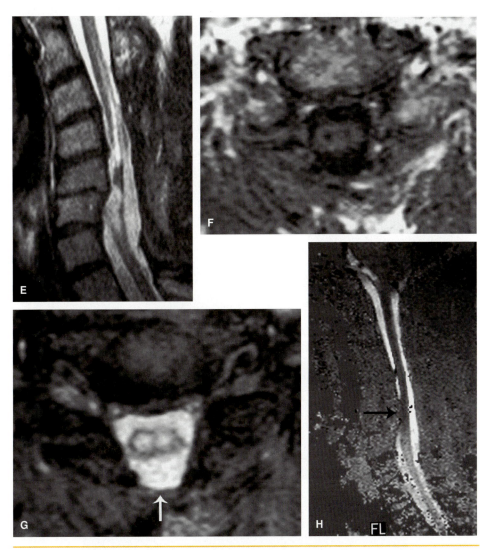

FIGURE 11-15. *(CONTINUED)* Postuntethering T2-weighted sagittal **(E)**, T1-weighted axial **(F)**, gradient echo axial **(G)** images shown at the same slice position and reveal that the cyst has collapsed and the spinal cord is no longer expanded. Note the dural graft with re-creation of the dorsal subarachnoid space (*arrow, G*). Sagittal image from CSF flow study **(H)** shows reconstitution of flow (high signal band now seen dorsal to the spinal cord at level of injury) with residual ventral tethering and loss of CSF flow at the kyphosis (*arrow*).

cord may also be expanded as the result of a "pulling apart" by intradural tethering bands, and it is important to sonographically distinguish a cyst from myelomalacia because surgical management may be different. In patients with a progressive posttraumatic myelomalacic myelopathy, lysis of surrounding spinal cord adhesions with untethering of the cord may result in clinical improvement. If cord untethering does not result in cyst decompression in a patient with progressive posttraumatic cystic myelopathy, then a cyst to peritoneal, or cyst to pleural, shunt may be placed.

In the posttraumatic setting, subarachnoid cysts are the result of arachnoid adhesions and intrathecal scarring with a ball valve phenomenon; CSF enters, but the egress is impeded (Fig. 11-24). Using intraoperative sonography, the presence of a subarachnoid cyst is confirmed by the presence of an anechoic extramedullary cyst that compresses the spinal cord. Septations may be present within these cysts.

SURGICAL TREATMENT OPTIONS

"There is little consensus among clinicians regarding the surgical management of posttraumatic syringomyelia, and many neurosurgeons contend that there is no effective surgical treatment"(5). This statement exemplifies the

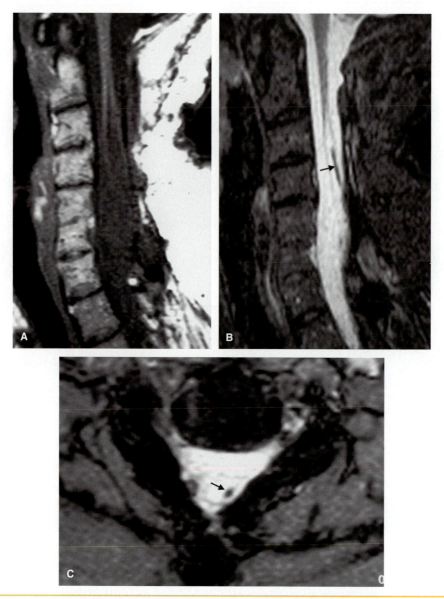

FIGURE 11-16. Retethering and cyst formation. T1-weighted sagittal **(A)** and T2 weighted sagittal **(B)** images reveals extensive cord expansion by a CSF signal intensity equivalent lesion in a patient status postprevious laminectomy and untethering of the spinal cord. There is minimal CSF dorsal or ventral to the cord form the mid- to lower cervical levels. A portion of an intramedullary shunt catheter is visualized on the sagittal T2 weighted image (*B, arrow*) and a T2-weighted axial image (*C, arrow*). (*continued*)

controversy regarding the treatment of posttraumatic syringomyelia. In 1994 Aschoff et al. (53) reported that although more than 3,000 operations had been reported for the treatment of syringomyelia, there continued to be no optimal treatment because of the variability in the types of cysts, multiple procedures on individual cases, and the lack of long-term follow-up. A recent study by Carroll and Brackenridge (54) in 2005 also noted that the "benefits of surgical management of [posttraumatic syringomyelia] are unclear." More studies documenting

the long-term results must be performed as it appears that long-term results of surgical therapy are less favorable than those after a limited postoperative observation period. What most agree on, however, is that asymptomatic cysts should not be operated upon.

The surgical management of syringomyelia dates back to 1892 when Abbe and Coley (55) reported the successful aspiration of a cyst after performing a laminectomy and opening the dura. Although the patient did not significantly improve, the importance of this report is that it

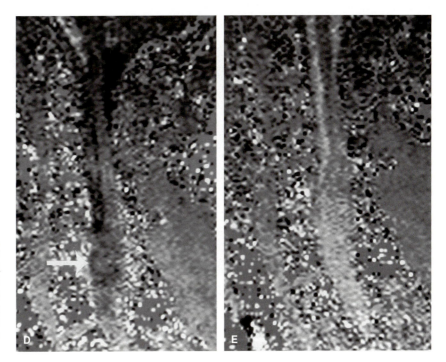

FIGURE 11-16. *(CONTINUED)* Cine CSF flow evaluation **(D,E)** confirms both ventral and dorsal tethering with lack of normal laminar CSF flow anterior and posterior to the cord, although there is some swirling CSF flow seen ventrally (*D, arrow*). There is near complete loss of flow dorsal to the cord below C3.

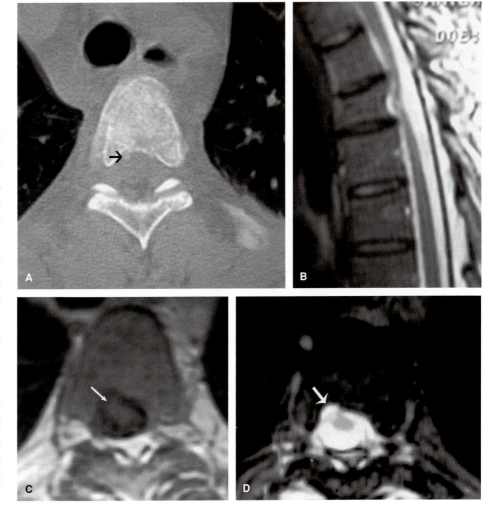

FIGURE 11-17. Anterior cord herniation. This patient presented 7 years after sustaining a traumatic injury at T4 with a progressive myelopathy. **A:** Axial CT at T4 reveals the chronic fracture deformity at T4 with a small spicule of bone (*arrow*) in the right ventral epidural space. Presumably, this contributed to a tear in the dura. **B:** T2-weighted sagittal image better depicts the compression fracture but also reveals anterior deviation of the spinal cord at the level of injury. The differential diagnosis at this point would be a dorsal posttraumatic arachnoid cyst compressing the cord versus a posttraumatic anterior cord herniation. Axial T1-weighted **(C)** and T-2 weighted gradient echo axial **(D)** images clinch the diagnosis by demonstrating that the cord is herniated through a defect in the right ventral dura (*arrows*). Note the small associated epidural CSF collection.

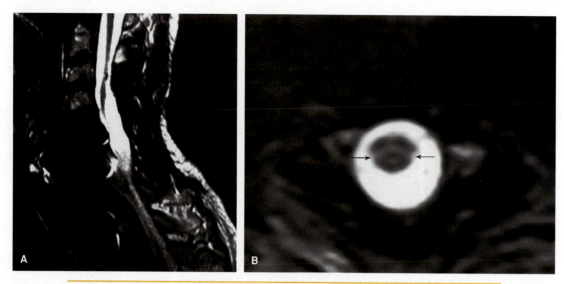

FIGURE 11-18. Wallerian degeneration in the lateral corticospinal tracts below the level of cord injury. T2-weighted fast spin echo sagittal **(A)** through the cervical spine shows evidence of previous laminectomies and anterior fusion with metal artifact. Also noted is ventral cord tethering and diffuse cervical cord atrophy most pronounced in the region of initial cord trauma. T2-weighted axial image of the thoracic cord **(B)** demonstrates increased signal intensity in the corticospinal tracts, indicative of Wallerian degeneration (*arrows*). (Reproduced from Latchaw RE, Falcone S, Saraf-Lavi E. Imaging of spinal trauma. In: Latchaw RE, Kurcharczyk J, Moseley ME, eds. *Imaging of the Nervous System: Diagnostic and Therapeutic Applications*. New York: Elsevier Mosby; 2005:1581–1625, with permission.)

revealed that syringomyelia could be approached surgically without morbidity (30). Good results following surgical intervention for a posttraumatic cyst were first obtained by Freeman (56) in 1959. He advocated surgical drainage as the treatment of choice. Since then, there have been various reports of many approaches to the treatment of posttraumatic cysts, including shunting to the subarachnoid or pleural space (57–61), reconstruction of the subarachnoid space with a surgical meningocele (62), and untethering with lysis of adhesions and recreation of the subarachnoid space with dural allograft with, or without, shunting of the cyst (63).

An operation in the presence of a posttraumatic spinal cord cyst may be considered in the presence of one or more signs and symptoms of a progressive posttraumatic cystic myelopathy with spinal cord cysts greater than a centimeter (5). The surgical management requires preoperative assessment of imaging features including: (a) the extent of the cyst, (b) the location of the cyst within the spinal cord parenchyma, (c) the identification of septations within the cyst, (d) the location of cord tethering, (e) the identification of an associated subarachnoid cyst, (f) the presence of cord compression, and (g) the presence of a fissure (Fig. 11-25). Untethering of the spinal cord and nerve roots is the first goal of treatment, along with reduc-

tion of any bony or soft tissue protrusions that may be compressing the neural elements. Once this is accomplished, cyst decompression may be seen with intraoperative ultrasound. If the cyst continues to remain expanded, shunting of the cyst may be performed (63).

In those patients who have the syndrome of a progressive posttraumatic myelopathy and imaging features of a myelomalacic and tethered cord, untethering of the cord may result in stability, improvement, or arrest of symptoms (4).

CONCLUSION

Due to increased survival and improved imaging techniques, we are encountering more patients who develop late sequelae of spinal cord injury. Posttraumatic cystic and noncystic myelopathy present with the same clinical picture, and MRI is the most helpful imaging study in distinguishing between these types of myelopathy and in the detection of other abnormalities that are frequently encountered in this patient population. Both preoperative and intraoperative imaging play an important role in surgical management; however, surgical management remains controversial, and further study is required to determine which patients might benefit from surgery.

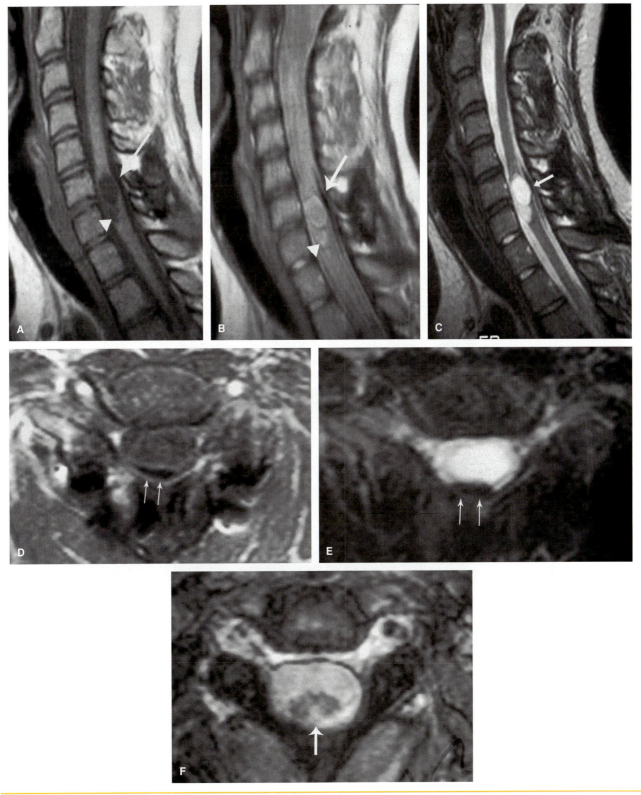

FIGURE 11-19. Posttraumatic cord cyst with rim of myelomalaica, posterior tethering, and Wallerian degeneration above the injury. T1-weighted sagittal image **(A)** reveals an expansile spinal cord cyst at C6-7. A less well-defined region of low signal intensity is seen along the ventral and inferior aspect of the main cyst. Also seen is a subtle focal region of low signal on the dorsal aspect of the cord (*arrow*). Proton density sagittal image **(B)** shows a hyperintense rim surrounding the cyst, including the inferior aspect of the lesion (*arrowhead*) most consistent with myelomalacia/gliosis surrounding the cyst. The dorsal low signal is much more evident (*arrow*). T2-weighted sagittal image **(C)** does not allow separation of the cyst and gliotic/myelomalacic border. Again seen is dorsal band of low signal intensity (*arrow*). T1-weighed axial **(D)** and T2-weighted fast spin echo axial **(E)** images best demonstrate the dorsal and lateral tethering with the dorsal band of low signal intensity likely representing thickening of the dorsal dura that is calcified or contains old blood (*arrows in D and E*). Note evidence of previous posterior fusion with metallic artifact, T2-weighted image above the level of injury **(F)** shows associated Wallerian degeneration in the dorsal column (*arrow*).

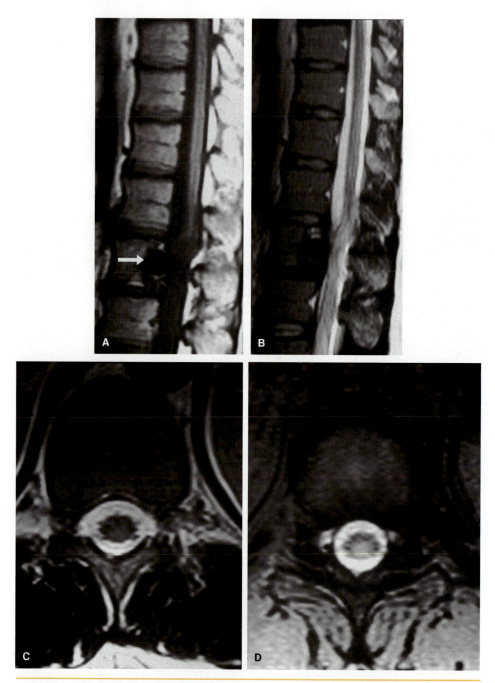

FIGURE 11-20. Wallerian degeneration above penetrating injury. T1-weighted sagittal **(A)** and T2-weighted sagittal **(B)** images show susceptibility artifact from a retained bullet fragment within the vertebral body of L1 (*arrow in A*). The conus is atrophic without obvious signal abnormality; however, the cauda equina nerve roots are clumped indicative of adhesive arachnoiditis. T2-weighted axial **(C)** and T2-weighted gradient echo axial **(D)** at T10-11 reveal increased signal in the dorsal columns consistent with Wallerian degeneration.

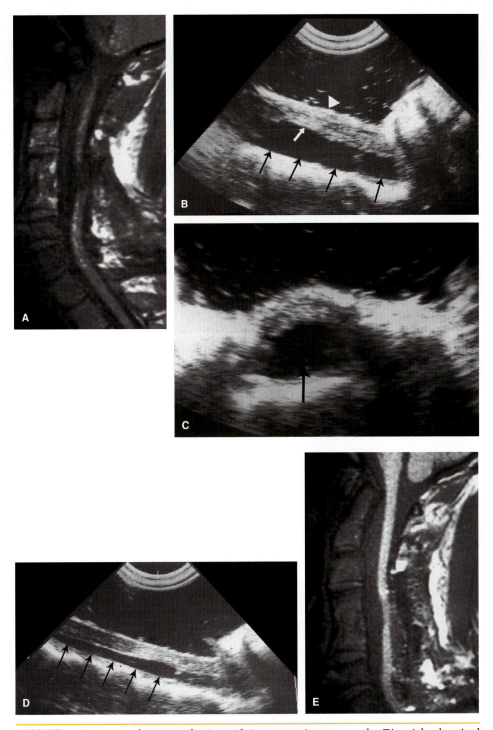

FIGURE 11-21. Pre- and postuntethering with intraoperative sonography. T1-weighted sagittal image **(A)** in this patient with previous anterior cervical discectomy and fusion (ACDF) and laminectomy demonstrates dorsal tethering of an atrophic spinal cord with abnormal hypointense signal indicative of myelomalacia. Preuntethering intraoperative ultrasound in the sagittal **(B)** and axial **(C)** planes shows the spinal cord tethered posteriorly against a thickened dura (*white arrowhead, B*) with abnormal increased echogenicity seen with spinal cord parenchyma (*white arrow, B*). The ventral subarachnoid space is asymmetrically widened (*black arrows, B and C*). Postuntethering intraoperative sagittal ultrasound **(D)** and sagittal T1-weighted MRI **(E)** reveals a more normal position of the subarachnoid space within the canal with a reduction in size of the ventral subarachnoid space (*black arrows, D*). (Reproduced in part from Falcone S, Quencer RM, Green BA, et al. Progressive posttraumatic myelomalacic myelopathy (PPMM): imaging and clinical features. *AJNR.* 1994;15(4):747–754, with permission.)

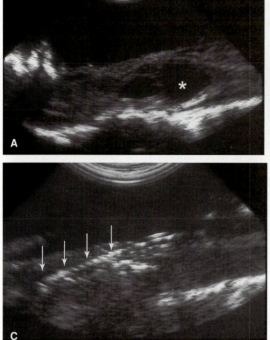

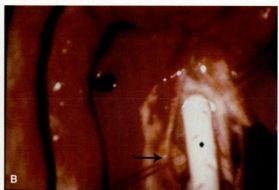

FIGURE 11-22. Shunt. Intraoperative sonography **(A)** demonstrates an anechoic posttraumatic spinal cord cyst (*white asterisk, A*) seen following posterior approach and laminectomy. Intraoperative photograph *(B)* showing the location of a small midline dorsal myelotomy through which a catheter is inserted (*black asterisk, B*). The dura is reflected laterally (*arrows*). Postcatheter insertion intraoperative sonography **(C)** reveals that the cyst has collapsed and the catheter is identified as a hyperechoic structure (*white arrows, C*).

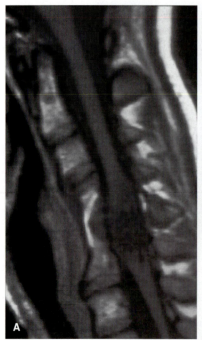

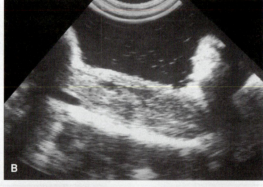

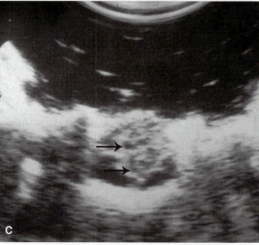

FIGURE 11-23. Expansile microcystic myelomalacia. T1-weighted sagittal image **(A)** reveals an expanded spinal cord with low signal intensity, although slightly hyperintense than CSF. The margins of the lesion are ill defined and irregular, typical of myelomalacia. Note that the cord abnormality is centered and directly opposite the anterior cervical discectomy and fusion (ACDF) at the site of previous traumatic spinal cord injury. Intraoperative sonography in the sagittal **(B)** and axial **(C)** planes following laminectomy from dorsal approach reveals thickening of the dura, expansion of the cord, dorsal tethering, and heterogenous hyperechoic signal with small anechoic microcysts (*arrows*). (Reproduced in part from Falcone S, Quencer RM, Green BA, et al. Progressive posttraumatic myelomalacic myelopathy (PPMM): imaging and clinical features. *AJNR*. 1994;15(4):747–754, with permission.)

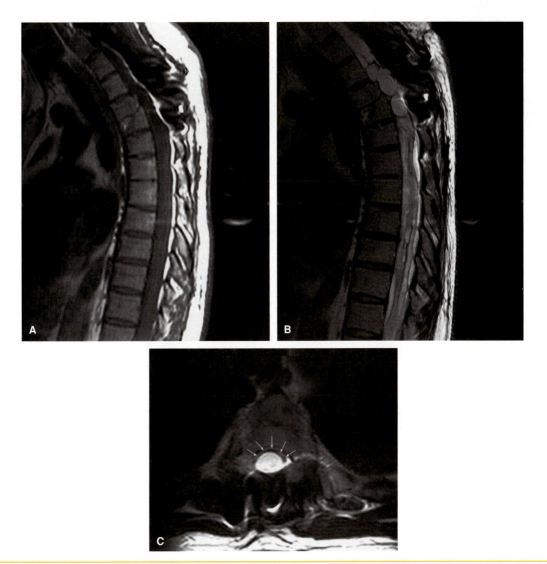

FIGURE 11-24. Posttraumatic subarachnoid cysts. This patient suffered a traumatic injury to the upper thoracic cord many years previously and underwent an instrumented fusion posteriorly; the patient presents with progressive neurologic deficit. T1-weighted sagittal image **(A)** shows the old fracture deformity, metal artifact posteriorly, and diffusely abnormal increased CSF equivalent signal within the upper thoracic spinal canal without visualization of a normal appearing spinal cord. T2-weighted fast spin echo sagittal **(B)** image demonstrates diffuse arachnoiditis with regions of old hemorrhage (foci of dark signal), increased intramedullary spinal cord signal intensity, and scattered subarachnoid cyst formation, most prominent in the upper thoracic region. Axial T2 weighted image **(C)** in the upper thoracic region suggests that the anterior displacement of the thinned and compressed spinal cord (*arrows*) is due to mass effect from a posteriorly located subarachnoid cyst, as opposed to anterior tethering.

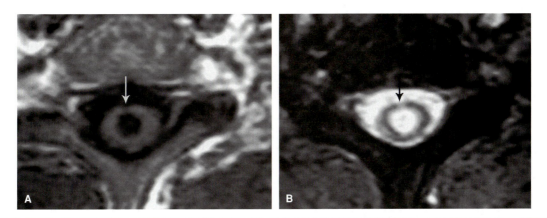

FIGURE 11-25. Posttraumatic spinal cord cyst with fissure. T1-weighted axial **(A)** and T2-weighted gradient echo axial **(B)** images in the lower cervical spinal reveal a simple, mildly expansile, spinal cord cyst that appears to communicate with the ventral subarachnoid space via a fissure (*arrows in A and B*).

REFERENCES

1. DeVivo MJ, Kartus PL, Stover SL, et al. Benefits of early admission to an organized spinal cord injury care system. *Paraplegia*. 1990;28:545–555.

2. Stover SL, Fine PR, eds. *Spinal Cord Injury: The Facts and Figures*. Birmingham: National Spinal Cord Injury Statistical Center, University of Alabama; 1986:58.

3. Quencer RM, Sheldon JJ, Post JMD, et al. Magnetic resonance imaging of the chronically injured cervical spinal cord. *AJNR* 1986;7:457–464.

4. Falcone S, Quencer RM, Green BA, et al. Progressive posttraumatic myelomalacic myelopathy (PPMM): imaging and clinical features. *AJNR*. 1994;15(4):747–754.

5. Green BA, Lee TT, Madsen PW, et al. Management of post-traumatic cystic myelopathy. *Top Spinal Cord Inj Rehabil*. 1997;2:36–46.

6. Harris JH, Mirvis SE, eds. *Hyperflexion Injuries*, 3rd ed. Baltimore: Williams & Wilkins; 1995:245–289.

7. White AA, Panjabi MM. *Clinical Biomechanics of the Spine*. Philadelphia: JB Lippincott; 1978.

8. White AA, Johnson RM, Panjabi MM, et al. Biomechanical analysis of clinical stability in the cervical spine. *Clin Orthop*. 1975;109:85–96.

9. Roberts CC, Troy MN, Krupinski EA, et al. Oblique reformation in cervical spine computed tomography: a new look at an old friend. *Spine*. January 15, 2003;28(2):167–170.

10. Barrett JF, Keat N. Artifacts in CT: recognition and avoidance. *RadioGraphics*. 2004;24:1679–1691.

11. Bartynski WS, Lin L. Lumbar root compression in the lateral recess: MR imaging, conventional myelography, and CT myelography comparison with surgical confirmation. *Am J Neuroradiol*. March 2003;24:348–360.

12. Quencer RM, Green BA, Eismont FJ. Posttraumatic spinal cysts: clinical features and characterization with metrizamide computed tomography. *N Radiol*. 1983;146:415–423.

13. Gebarski SS, Maynard FW, Garbrielsen TO, et al. Posttraumatic progressive myelopathy: clinical and radiologic correlation employing MR imaging, delayed CT metrizamide myelography, and intraoperative sonography. *Radiology*. 1985;157:379–385.

14. Tartaglino LM, Flanders AE, Vinitski S, et al. Metallic artifacts on MR images of the postoperative spine: reduction with fast spin-echo techniques. *Radiology*. 1994;190(2):565–569.

15. Post MJD, Quencer RM, Hinks RS, et al. Spinal CSF flow dynamics: qualitative and quantitative evaluation by cine MRI. Presented at the Annual Meeting of the American Society of Neuroradiology, March 24, 1989; Orlando, Fla.

16. Schwartz ED, Yezierski RP, Pattany PM, et al. Diffusion-weighted MR imaging in a rat model of syringomyelia after excitotoxic spinal cord injury. *Am J Neuroradiol*. 1999;20:1422–1428.

17. Montalvo BM, Quencer RM, Green BA, et al. Intraoperative sonography in spinal trauma. *Radiology*. 1984;153:125–134.

18. Dohrmann GJ, Rubin JM. Intraoperative ultrasound imaging of the spinal cord: syringomyelia, cysts and tumors: preliminary report. *Surg Neurol*. 1982;18:395–399.

19. Barnett HJM, Botterell EH, Jousse AT, et al. Progressive myelopathy as a sequel to traumatic paraplegia. *Brain*. 1965;89:159–178.

20. Schneider RC, Knighton R. Chronic neurological sequelae of acute trauma to the spine and spinal cord: Part III: the syndrome of chronic injury to the cervical spinal cord in the region of the central canal. *J Bone Joint Surg*. 1954;41A: 905–919.

21. Lyons BM, Brown DJ, Calvert JM, et al. The diagnosis and management of post traumatic syringomyelia. *Paraplegia*. 1987;25:340–350.

22. Oakley JC, Ojemann GA, Alvord EC. Posttraumatic syringomyelia: case report. *J Neurosurg*. 1981;55:276–281.

23. Watson N. Ascending cystic degeneration of the cord after spinal cord injury. *Paraplegia*. 1981;19:89–95.

24. Nurick S, Russell JA, Deck MDF. Cystic degeneration of the spinal cord following spinal cord injury. *Brain*. 1970;93:211–222.

25. Griffiths ER, McCormick CC. Posttraumatic syringomyelia (cystic myelopathy). *Paraplegia*. 1981;19:81–88.

26. Seibert CE, Creisbach JN, Swanson WB, et al. Progressive posttraumatic cystic myelopathy: neuroradiologic evaluation. *AJR*. 1981;136(1):161–165.

27. Green BA, Quencer RM, Post MJD, et al. A review of 100 patients surgically treated for progressive post-traumatic cystic myelopathy. *J Neurosurg*. 1990;72:353A.

28. Biyani A, El Masry WS. Post-traumatic syringomyelia: a review of the literature. *Paraplegia*. 1994;32:723–731.

29. Rossier AB, Foo D, Shillito J, et al. Progressive late post traumatic syringomyelia. *Paraplegia*. 1981;19:96–97.

30. Madsen PW, Falcone S, Bowen BC, et al. Post-traumatic syringomyelia. In: Levine A, Eismont F, Garfin S, et al., eds. *Spine Trauma*. Philadelphia: Saunders; 1998:608–629.

31. Walshe FMR. Developmental anomalies: syringomyelia and syringobulbia (status dysraphicus). In: *Diseases of the Nervous System*. 11th ed. Baltimore: Williams and Wilkins; 1970.

32. Williams B. Current concepts of syringomyelia. *Br J Hosp Med*. 1970;4:331–342.

33. Barnett HJM. The epilogue. In: Barnett HJM, Foster JB, Hudgson P, eds. I. London, Eng: WB Saunders; 1973.

34. Backe HA, Betz RR, Mesgarzadeh M, et al. Post-traumatic spinal cord cysts evaluated by magnetic resonance imaging. *Paraplegia*. 1991;29:607–612.

35. Bunge RP, Puckett WR, Becerra JL, et al. Observations on the pathology of human spinal cord injury. In: Seil FJ, ed. *Advances in Neurology*. Vol 59. New York: Raven Press, Ltd; 1996:75–89.

36. Squier MV, Lehr RP. Post-traumatic syringomyelia. *J Neurol Neurosurg Psychiatry*. 1994;57:1095–1098.

37. Wozniewicz B, Filipowicz K, Swiderska SK, et al. Pathophysiological mechanism of traumatic cavitation of the spinal cord. *Paraplegia*. 1983;21:312–317.

38. Schwartz ED, Falcone S, Quencer RM, et al. Posttraumatic syringomyelia: pathogenesis, imaging, and treatment. *AJR*. 1999;173:487–492.

39. Williams B. The distending force in the production of "communicating syringomyelia." *Lancet*. 1969;2:189–193.

40. Williams B, Terry AF, Jones F, et al. Syringomyelia as a sequel to traumatic paraplegia. *Paraplegia*. 1981;19:67–80.

41. Klekamp J, Batzdorf U, Samii M, et al. Treatment of syringomyelia associated with arachnoid scarring caused by arachnoiditis of trauma. *J Neurosurg*. 1997;86:233–240.

42. Ball MJ, Dayan AD. Pathogenesis of syringomyelia. *Lancet*. 1972;2:799–801.

43. Williams B. Pathogenesis of post-traumatic syringomyelia (editorial). *Br J Neurosurg*. 1992;6:517–520.

44. MacDonald RL, Findlay JM, Tator CH. Microcystic spinal cord degeneration causing posttraumatic myelopathy. Report of two cases. *J Neurosurg*. 1988;68:466–471.

45. Fox JL, Wener L, Drennan DL, et al. Central spinal cord injury: magnetic resonance imaging confirmation and operative considerations. *Neurosurgery*. 1988;22:340–347.

46. Stevens JM, Olney JS, Kendall BE. Posttraumatic cystic and non-cystic myelopathy. *Neuroradiology*. 1985;24:48–56.

47. Enzmann DR, O'Donohue J, Ubin JB, et al. CSF pulsations within non-neoplastic spinal cord cysts. *AJNR*. 1987;8:517–525.

48. Quencer RM, Post JMD, Hinks RS. Cine MR in the evaluation of normal and abnormal CSF flow: intracranial and intraspinal studies. *Neuroradiology*. 1990;32(5):371–391.

49. Brugieres P, Idy-Peretti I, Clement I, et al. CSF flow measurement in syringomyelia. *AJNR*. 2000;21:1785–1792.

50. Waller AV. Experiments on the section of the glosso pharyngeal and hypoglossal nerves of a frog, and observations of the alterations produced thereby in the structure of their primitive fiber. *Philos Trans R Soc Lond Biol*. 1850;140:423–429.

51. Terae S, Taneichi H, Abumi K. MRI of Wallerian degeneration of the injured spinal cord. *J Comput Assist Tomogr.* 1993;17:700–703.

52. Becerra JL, Puckett WR, Hiester ED, et al. MR-pathologic comparisons of Wallerian degeneration in spinal cord injury. *AJNR.* 1995;16:125–133.

53. Aschoff A, Donauer E, Huwel N, et al. Evaluation of syrinx surgery: a critical comment on requirements for reliable follow-up studies. *Acta Neurochir (Wien).* 1993;123:224–225.

54. Carroll AM, Brackenridge P. Post-traumatic syringomyelia: a review of the cases presenting in a regional spinal injuries unit in the north east of England over a 5-year period. *Spine.* May 15, 2005;30:1206–1210.

55. Abbe R, Coley W. Syringo-myelia: operation-exploration of cord-withdrawal of fluid-exhibition of patient. *J Nerv Ment Dis.* 1892;19:512–520.

56. Freeman LW. Ascending spinal paralysis: case presentation. *J Neurosurg.* 1959;16:120–122.

57. Edgar R, Quail P. Progressive posttraumatic cystic and non cystic myelopathy. *Br J Neurosurg.* 1994;8:7–22.

58. Hida K, Iwasaki Y, Imamura H, et al. Posttraumatic syringomyelia: its characteristic magnetic resonance imaging findings and surgical management. *Neurosurgery.* 1994;35:886–891.

59. Rossier AB, Foo D, Shillito J, et al. Posttraumatic cervical syringomyelia: incidence, clinical presentation electrophysiological studies, syrinx protein and results of conservative and operative treatment. *Brain.* 1985;108:439–461.

60. Rossier AB, Werner A, Wildi E, et al. Contribution to the study of late cervical syringomyelic syndromes after dorsal or lumbar traumatic paraplegia. *J Neurol Neurosurg Psychiatry.* 1968;31:99–105.

61. Shanon N, Symon L, Logue V, et al. Clinical features, investigation and treatment of posttraumatic syringomyelia. *J Neurosurg Psychiatry.* 1981;44:35–42.

62. Sgouros S, Williams B. A critical appraisal of drainage in syringomyelia. *J Neurosurg.* 1995;82:1–10.

63. Lee TT, Alameda GJ, Camilo E, et al. Related articles: surgical treatment of post-traumatic myelopathy associated with syringomyelia. *Spine.* December 15, 2001;26(suppl 24): S119–127.

Experimental

Experimental Therapies for Spinal Cord Injury

Marion Murray

INTRODUCTION: THE PROBLEMS OF SPINAL CORD INJURY

Many factors conspire to prevent repair and recovery after spinal injury. The intact adult spinal cord contains inhibitory molecules that cause collapse of growth cones, which are the elongating tips that begin to emerge from damaged axons, thus preventing regenerative sprouting. The injury itself creates a hostile environment; the entrance of inflammatory cells and release of toxic compounds from injured cells lead to a secondary expansion of the injury. The glial scar, a barrier to regeneration, then develops. The adult central nervous system (CNS) neuron is itself poorly equipped to regenerate. These neurons, unlike peripherally projecting neurons, do not readily express genes needed for axonal elongation and, in addition, they are more vulnerable to axotomy and thus may demyelinate, atrophy, or die when injured. These pathological changes may diminish functional contributions by intact collaterals of damaged neurons even to circuits not directly affected by the injury (Fig. 12-1).

These daunting obstacles are yielding to a series of novel research directions. Many of the barriers to regeneration, whether intrinsic or extrinsic to the neuron, and whether normally present or associated with the injury, can now be at least partially breached. Although treatments directed to individual components have led to only incremental improvements in regeneration and recovery of function, there is hope that appropriate combinations of treatments targeted at mechanistically different impediments will ultimately result in a substantially greater extent of recovery and repair. We are looking not for a magic bullet but perhaps for a magic fusillade.

EXPERIMENTAL INJURY PARADIGMS

The search for the most appropriate animal model for developing and validating spinal cord injury (SCI) treatments has focused on those that more closely mimic injuries seen in the clinic, such as contusion or compression injuries. These are incomplete injuries that often leave the dura intact and spare, to a variable extent, white matter while destroying much of the gray matter at the injury site. Other models include surgical lesions that interrupt specific white matter tracts, or funiculi, and thus permit a more focused mechanistic investigation of the effects of injury and treatment on identified pathways. The type of injury model that is most appropriate is, of course, dependent on the questions being asked, but is

INJURED SPINAL CORD

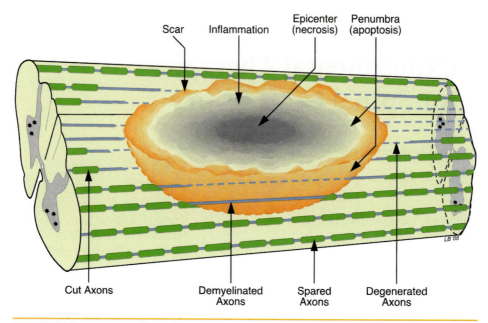

FIGURE 12-1. Diagram of spinal cord following a contusion injury. A contusion injury induces hemorrhage and may or may not damage the dura. The epicenter is characterized by necrotic cell death and the lesion expands (secondary injury) into a penumbra region, with additional cell death due to apoptosis. The secondary injury is associated with entry of inflammatory cells and toxicity from dying spinal cord cells. Ultimately, the area of injury is surrounded by a dense glial scar. The injury destroys some axons, and damages others, leading to demyelination. Cut axons often retract (dieback). Some axons are usually spared by a contusion injury.

likely to progress from the more analytical approach to the more clinically relevant (1).

The emphasis over the past decade has been on demonstrating efficacy of single treatments as measured with one or more outcome measures. One of the encouraging features of the research being carried out currently is the development and validation of a range of outcome measures that may include axonal growth, neuroprotection, and behavioral measures targeting different functions. Anatomical repair has been assessed by evidence of axonal growth, using tracing methods to estimate increased density or distance of growth; both regeneration and sprouting have shown stimulation through various treatments. Neuroprotection has been evaluated by lesion size to estimate effects on secondary damage, or by cell counts of surviving axotomized neurons to estimate rescue from retrograde degeneration; some treatments have resulted in decreased lesion size and others have shown rescue of neurons distant from but axotomized by the lesion. Functional improvement has usually been evaluated using one or more behavioral measures. Most commonly, tests of overground locomotion have been used, and a variety of treatments have shown improvement in motor function. More recently, in response to the needs

articulated by SCI patients, treatments that may ameliorate autonomic disorders (e.g., bladder, bowel, sexual dysfunction, or neuropathic pain) are being emphasized.

There has been no shortage of positive findings from experimental studies. The emphasis in the next decade will be on determining efficacy of individual treatments from different laboratories and in developing combinatorial treatments that target different mechanisms.

NEW TREATMENTS FROM THE LABORATORY

Rescuing Injured Neurons

Necrosis

Necrosis is the form of cell death resulting from external insults, including physical injury, glutamate toxicity, and ischemia, and is the primary cause of cell death following CNS trauma. In CNS injury, the cells in the core of the injury site undergo necrosis (Fig. 12-1), are resistant to treatments, and are probably unsalvageable. The cysts that develop once necrotic tissue is phagocytosed constitute additional barriers to repair.

Apoptosis

Apoptosis is the form of cell death that is amenable to treatment. Neurons in the penumbra, adjacent to the epicenter of the injury (Fig. 12-1), may escape necrosis but remain susceptible to apoptosis. These neurons can be rescued by antiapoptotic treatments, such as inhibitors to caspases, which are enzymes (cysteine proteases) expressed following injury that can kill cells by cleaving critical repair and homeostatic proteins as well as cytoskeletal proteins (2). The effect of diminishing apoptosis would be a decrease in the secondary expansion of the lesion and thus an improvement in the prospects for recovery. In the adult CNS, apoptosis is mediated through pathways both extrinsic and intrinsic to the neuron (3) (Fig. 12-2). Treatments to be administered acutely that will detoxify the environment, and thus diminish apoptotic cell death, are currently under active investigation.

The extrinsic apoptotic process is initiated by binding of ligands (e.g., tumor necrosis factor, TNFa) to death receptors located on the neuronal membrane that mediate apoptosis. Intrinsic apoptosis results from mitochondrial damage triggered by ischemia, stress, excitotoxicity, elevated intracellular calcium (Ca^{++}), and other insults. Both intrinsic and extrinsic apoptotic pathways activate caspase cascades leading to degradation of structural proteins, DNA, and ultimately death. These are parallel and interacting death mechanisms, and their relative importance may differ according to neuronal types (Fig. 12-2). Neurons contain a default apoptotic pathway, normally inhibited by extrinsically supplied trophic factors that bind to trophic factor receptors and block apoptosis; there is also an intracellular pathway that blocks the apoptotic pathway. Apoptosis can be suppressed by using decoy proteins that block death receptors or inhibition of pro-apoptotic proteins by apoptotic brakes (e.g., activated protein C [APC], proteins from the B-cell leukemia/lymphoma-2 [Bcl2], or heat shock protein [HSP] families, as well as enzymes such as heme oxygenase) (3). Apoptosis can also be suppressed by providing therapeutic levels of trophic factors that activate survival pathways (4) or caspase inhibitors that act further downstream. Animal research has therefore identified several promising approaches that result in greater survival of vulnerable injured neurons at the site of injury. Nevertheless, there has not yet been successful translation of these therapies to the clinic. The variety of targets and pathways suggests redundancy and increases the likelihood that combined approaches may be needed.

Other strategies to diminish secondary injury include suppressing inflammation. In the acute post-injury phase, there is strong up regulation of genes involved in inflammation (5,6). Although inflammatory responses to SCI clearly contribute to secondary damage, nonselective suppression of inflammation has not proven useful, perhaps because beneficial effects of the inflammatory response are also eliminated. Methylprednisolone, for example, is an anti-inflammatory, antioxidant steroid approved for use in human SCI patients but whose benefits have been questioned (7–9). Given the complex cascade of bioactive molecules that are released upon injury, it is not surprising that components of the inflammatory process may promote repair; therefore, the inhibition of inflammatory events might have deleterious consequences. Studies of optic nerve injury have shown that apoptosis is reduced and regeneration is enhanced by several interventions that are mediated by a macrophage-derived factor whose release is stimulated by injury (10). Kipnis et al. (11) have proposed that boosting reactive T cells, normally considered to be deleterious, can confer protective autoimmunity and improve function after spinal cord injury and, indeed, clinical trials are under way to test that hypothesis. A study that attempted to replicate those laboratory findings, however, instead showed that T cells activated by SCI are pathological effector cells that impair spontaneous functional recovery and exacerbate tissue injury

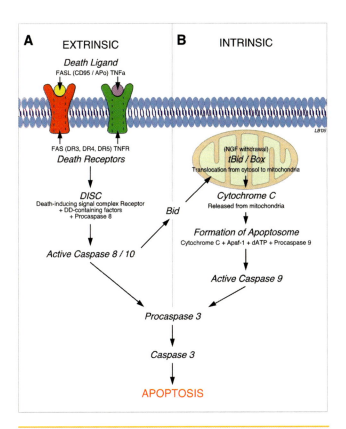

FIGURE 12-2. Extrinsic and intrinsic pathways leading to apoptosis. **A:** Extrinsic pathways involve binding of a death ligand to death receptors, with subsequent activation of caspases leading to apoptosis. **B:** The intrinsic pathway is engaged by the activated caspases, leading to apoptosis. The pathways may thus converge within the cell. Identification of the components of the pathways, some of which are indicated here, provides targets for pharmacological intervention.

(12). Further, macrophage infiltration and phagocyte-mediated degeneration of myelin following SCI result in exposure of axons to inhibitory molecules that contribute to dieback of injured axons (13). The discovery that cellular and molecular events thought to be inhibitory to repair may also have positive effects is a recurrent theme as research progresses. Thus, more targeted approaches may be needed to focus on specific deleterious effects while preserving beneficial effects of treatments.

There are several examples of more targeted approaches. Following injury, integrin molecules on the cell surface of leukocytes bind to endothelial cell adhesion molecules, resulting in infiltration of neutrophils and entry of hematogenous monocyte macrophages at the injury site; this inflammatory response can result in significant secondary tissue damage. Blockade of an integrin receptor, cd11d/cd18, with monoclonal antibodies following SCI diminishes this inflammatory response, and, if this treatment is applied within the first 48 hours after the injury, there is reduced secondary damage, stimulated axonal growth, and improved outcome with decreased autonomic dysreflexia, decreased neuropathic pain, and improved hindlimb function (14). Another target is the blockade of glutamate receptors. Levels of excitatory amino acids such as glutamate rise rapidly to toxic levels after SCI, leading to neuronal death, glial death, and delayed expansion of the injury. The potent and highly specific antagonist 2,3-dihydroxy-6-nitro-7-sulfamoyl-benzo(f)quinoxaline (NBQX) is a subset of glutamate receptors, the alpha-amino-3-hydroxy-5-methyl-4-isoxazole propionate (AMPA) receptors (15), and, when administered soon after SCI, results in reduced functional impairment on a range of outcome measures and stimulated axonal growth (16,17), presumably through a protective effect that results in greater sparing of spinal tissue.

Death at a Distance

Axotomized CNS neurons whose cell bodies are located at a distance from the injury may undergo retrograde degenerative changes. These may include moderate or severe atrophy as well as death of the axotomized neuron. There is controversy about whether some neurons actually die or simply atrophy below the level of resolution; nevertheless, it is likely that axotomized neurons that are severely atrophic will not contribute to useful function even if some of their collateral projections to other targets survive. The retrograde degenerative changes appear to be apoptotic in nature and thus amenable to treatment. Disappearance of Clarke or red nucleus neurons following axotomy with spinal hemisection has been prevented by transplanting fetal spinal cord tissue, by cell grafts that produce neurotrophic factors (NTFs), and by direct injection into the injured spinal cord of the antiapoptotic molecule Bcl-2 or NTFs such as brain-derived neurotrophic

factor (BDNF) or neurotrophin-3 (NT-3). These treatments rescue most of the neurons that would otherwise disappear as well as prevent much of the atrophy (18). Delivery of large amounts of BDNF directly into the red nucleus can rescue axotomized neurons even after chronic injuries (19). There are thus a number of plausible approaches to decreasing apoptosis, preserving damaged neurons, and decreasing secondary injury; other intracellular pathways that contribute to neuronal death are being examined and many have shown promising results. Comparative tests will be needed to determine which are the more effective. What is not known is whether these rescued neurons remain functional. This will probably require electrophysiological analyses, which have not yet been done. An important corollary of this is the observation that despite the very promising preclinical work, clinical trials with antiapoptotic molecular approaches have not proven successful.

Countering the Hostile Environment

The pioneering work from the Schwab laboratory focused attention on the inhibitory nature of CNS myelin and its role in blocking axonal outgrowth (20–22). The inhibitory molecules associated with CNS myelin are those encountered initially by a regenerative sprout and are primarily responsible for the abortive nature of regenerative sprouting. Huang et al. (23) blocked myelin-associated inhibitors by injecting a vaccine against myelin to stimulate the animal's own immune system to produce antibodies to these inhibitors. These mice showed dramatic regeneration of corticospinal axons after a hemisection with recovery of hindlimb function. Over the past few years, the mechanisms by which myelin inhibition acts to prevent regenerative growth have begun to be understood. Three inhibitors associated with myelin (NogoA, myelin-associated protein [MAG], and oligodendrocyte myelin glycoprotein [OMgp]) have been identified. These are structurally different molecules but surprisingly all bind to the same receptor, NgR, which is located on the neuronal membrane and results in inhibition of axonal regeneration. The NgR itself requires transmembrane coreceptors, one of which is the p75 receptor (24). Activation of the p75 receptor leads to downstream activation of the GTPase RhoA, and its target Rho dependent kinase (ROCK) (Fig. 12-3). This Rho-ROCK intracellular pathway acts on the intracellular cytoskeletal proteins actin and myosin, resulting in collapse of the growth cone. The importance of this line of research is in the identification of additional targets for pharmacological intervention. NogoA can be blocked by antibodies (e.g., NEP 1-40), and this leads to regenerative growth and recovery of function (25).

The injured CNS is even more inhibitory to axonal growth than the intact CNS. A contrary perspective on the

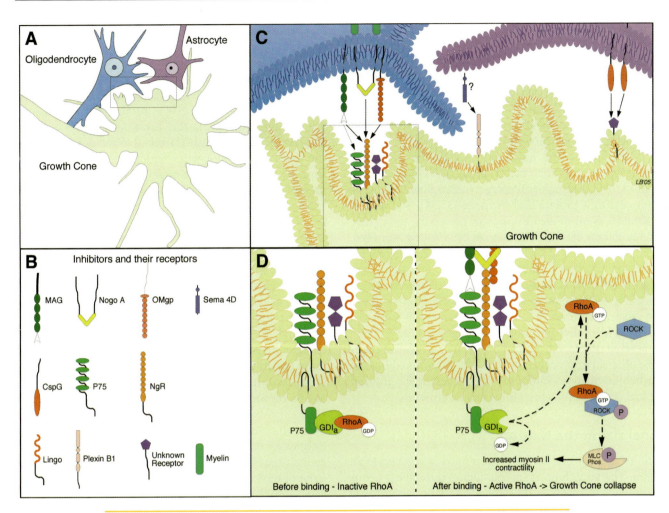

FIGURE 12-3. Inhibitory molecules associated with oligodendroglia and astrocytes produce growth cone collapse. **A:** Following injury, the growth cone must extend into an inhibitory environment provided by oligodendrocytes and astrocytes. **B:** Several inhibitors associated with oligodendrocytes and astrocytes have been identified and **C:** receptors for these molecules have been localized to the growth cone membrane. It is still unclear, however, whether the Semaphorin (Sema 4D) on the astrocyte membrane (*indicated by question mark*) links to the Plexin B1 receptor at the growth cone. **D:** Binding to the receptors actives the RhoA pathway, which leads to growth cone collapse and failure of regenerative sprouting. Blockade of receptors for the glial cell inhibitors, or of the RhoA pathway, is associated with increased regeneration and recovery of function.

role of myelin in prevention of axonal growth is offered by Raisman (26). He distinguishes between the observed collapse of the growth cone in culture and the possibility that myelin-based inhibition in vivo may be a mechanism that guides, and thus facilitates, axonal growth through the highly structured environment of the developing CNS. He suggests that reactive astrocytes are the greater villain among the environmental inhibitors. Astrocytes become activated in response to inflammatory cytokines, begin to secrete inhibitory proteoglycans, for example, chondroitin sulphate proteoglycan (CSPG), and establish a dense glial scar (27). These proteoglycans are inhibitory to axon outgrowth in the uninjured adult CNS and a major inhibitory contributor to the glial scar. The scar,

which develops within a week or two following injury, thus provides both biochemical and mechanical barriers to injured axons. In the past few years, we have increased our understanding of these inhibitory events, and therapies that diminish their inhibitory activity are being developed (28). CSPG is normally present in the CNS, however, it is produced in greater quantities by reactive astrocytes. CSPG acts through unknown receptors on the neuron to activate the protein kinase C (PKC) pathway; blockade of PKC activity by intrathecal administration of a specific inhibitor, Go6976, will promote regeneration (29). CSPG thus evokes inhibition of axonal growth using a signaling pathway that is different from that employed by myelin inhibitors. It does not produce generalized growth cone collapse, as does RhoA, but instead retraction of those short processes on the growth cone that contact the CSPG (30,31). CSPG can be degraded by chondroitinase ABC (ChABC), an enzyme that partially digests the molecule and thus renders it less inhibitory. Delivery of ChABC into an injured spinal cord has been shown to elicit regeneration of corticospinal axons and to support functional recovery (32).

The glial scar also has beneficial functions. Reactive astrocytes contribute to repair of the blood-brain barrier, reduce the inflammatory response, limit cellular degeneration, and thus protect healthy tissue (33,34). The search, therefore, is on to identify ways of preserving the beneficial functions of reactive astrocytes by targeting more specific contributions to their role in blocking axonal growth.

Given the many contributors to the nonpermissive environment of the adult CNS, it is not surprising that blocking only one set of inhibitors has but modest effects on repair or recovery of function. As the range of inhibitors is being identified and ways of countering some of them are being developed, we can expect combinatorial pharmacological approaches to be useful in diminishing the influence of these inhibitory molecules in the injured spinal cord and thus permitting axonal growth.

Energizing the Neuron

Adult CNS neurons are poorly equipped to regenerate an axon. The growth program that guides developing axons is difficult to access in the adult. Modifying the intrinsic growth potential of the neuron is an important component of a strategy to improve repair. Certain proteins expressed by genes associated with axon regeneration, such as growth-associated protein-43 (GAP-43), tubulin, and membrane proteins, are up regulated by successfully regenerating peripheral nervous system (PNS) neurons. These genes show little response to axotomy in CNS neurons. In the PNS, Schwann cells provide trophic factors that nurture the regenerating PNS neuron and re-establish the genetic program for axonal growth. An inadequate supply of trophic factors in the adult CNS may be a major cause of the difference in regenerative capability between PNS and CNS neurons. The neurotrophins bind to their receptors in the CNS through Trk receptors and an essential coreceptor, p75. Interestingly, p75 also activates the RhoA (35) and the Nogo receptors (36), pathways that cause growth cone collapse. This shared requirement for the coreceptor suggests a competition for access to the coreceptor by neurotrophins that may induce regeneration and inhibitory factors that prevent it; this competition may further limit CNS regeneration. Increasing the supply of neurotrophins to the CNS can improve axonal outgrowth. Indeed provision of trophic factors to the injured spinal cord, either exogenously or through transplantation of cells engineered to secrete trophic factors, is adequate to elicit modest growth of CNS axons, accompanied in some cases by recovery of function (37–41). There remain questions of duration and amounts of neurotrophins needed. Treatments that include exogenous administration of large quantities of neurotrophins appear to be more successful in eliciting regenerative growth, but controlling the duration of NTF secretion may also be important. It is likely that repair processes in the injured CNS may occur within a limited window of time. Thus it may be necessary to develop methods of turning off the expression of the neurotrophins. These methods are being developed for cells genetically modified to produce neurotrophins using regulatory elements to control the expression of the transgene.

Successful axonal regeneration mediated by trophic factors binding to the appropriate receptors on the injured neuron is known to elicit an up regulation of a specific set of regeneration associated genes, including transcription factors, GAP-43, and cytoskeletal proteins. Although it is intuitively obvious that coordinated changes in expression of a great many genes at different times postinjury would be required for efficient regrowth of an axon, the likelihood is that the entire pattern need not be reproduced (42). Still the pattern and nature of gene expression is only poorly understood at present. This will certainly change with the advent of microarray technology that will eventually allow the discovery of the genetic requirements (5,43–45) and, with the development of molecular methods to regulate the expression of genes introduced into the damaged CNS.

A conditioning lesion, in which a sensory axon is injured and then later a second injury is made proximal to the first, is a well-established method to increase regenerative growth by dorsal root axons. Interestingly, this can be mimicked by increasing the intracellular concentration of the cyclic Adenosine MonoPhosphate (cAMP) (46,47). The cAMP is a second messenger that couples extracellular signaling to changes in gene expression that contribute to neuronal plasticity and acts to promote neurite growth. Normally levels of intracellular cAMP expression in neurons are high during development and then diminish once developmental growth has ceased (48). The cAMP pathway, in fact, is one of the targets of neurotrophins. Increasing cAMP levels in neuronal cell bodies after axotomy in the adult has been shown to elicit a partial regenerative response by increasing expression of components of the axonal cytoskeleton (e.g., alpha-I and beta-III tubulin isotypes) (49). Increasing cAMP in the cell body or providing trophic factors that engage the cAMP pathway can counter the inhibition mediated by the inhospitable CNS environment, and thus shift the metabolic balance of an injured neuron toward axonal growth (47,50). More practically, systemic injection of rolipram (AG Scientific), an inhibitor of the enzyme that degrades cAMP, has been a successful strategy for promoting regeneration and recovery of function. When rolipram is administered after SCI, together with a transplant of fetal spinal cord (51), Schwann cells or olfactory ensheathing cells (52), or NT-3 (53), regeneration and, in some cases, recovery of function is demonstrated.

We know that axotomized CNS neurons normally elaborate only feeble growth cones that soon collapse. Although the growth cone is specialized for elongation, the collapse occurs when the inadequate growth cone meets the hostile CNS environment. The collapse of the growth cone is driven by activation of the Rho-ROCK pathway, which regulates actin filament polymerization, assembly, and disassembly and the interaction of actin with myosin (54). The collapse can be prevented by blocking the Rho-ROCK pathway. The potential for developing pharmacological treatments is being eagerly explored. RhoA, a small GTPase molecule, can be blocked by a permeable C3 transferase, and ROCK can be blocked by another small molecule, Y27632. Inhibition of this pathway by either means has been associated with axonal growth and with recovery of function (50,55,56). The functional improvements occur early, which suggests that these treatments may also provide some degree of neuroprotection (Fig. 12-3).

The good news is that CNS neurons can be encouraged to regenerate their axons within the injured CNS by stimulation of existing growth programs or by blocking pathways that promote collapse within the neuron. Long-distance regeneration has so far been a more elusive goal and one that is likely to require additional interventions. David and Aguayo (57), in their early work, noted that while lesioned CNS axons would grow almost indefinitely in a peripheral nerve graft, they ceased growth once they re-entered the CNS. An unresolved question is whether guidance cues are present or indeed necessary for directed growth, and another is whether reinnervation of normal targets is required for restoration of some function. Liu et al. (38) showed regeneration of some rubrospinal axons several segments distal to a transplant of fibroblasts modified to secrete BDNF. The regenerating axons elongated in the lateral funiculus in the location of the degenerated rubrospinal tract. This implied either that guidance cues are present or that regenerating axons preferentially elongate along degenerated, demyelinated pathways. Menei et al. (58) were successful in creating a trail of exogenously delivered BDNF distal to a Schwann cell graft that elicited longer regeneration (59). Similarly, Lu et al. (53) showed that NT-3 injections rostral to a lesion could elicit regeneration of sensory axons following treatment with both cAMP injections and stromal cell transplants.

Chronic Spinal Cord Injury

Treatments that will improve repair and recovery after chronic injury are particularly important in view of the large number (250,000 in the United States) of chronically injured patients. The challenges are even greater than for acute injuries (60). Neurons may have died or atrophied severely, and injured, but surviving, axons may have retracted or become demyelinated. Thus, the normally inadequate neuron becomes even less able to mount a growth response. A dense scar has formed at the injury site that surrounds a cystic cavity creating a more impenetrable barrier. Experiments studying transplantation strategies that are effective when initiated within 2 weeks showed little or no regeneration or recovery of function when instituted 6 (61) or 8 (62) weeks postoperatively. There are indications, however, that some repair processes can be instituted under certain circumstances weeks or months postinjury. Thus, the chronically injured neuron may have greater needs but still possess the capacity to respond to growth factors and to elongate. Chronically injured and greatly atrophied red nucleus neurons can respond to large doses of trophic factors applied directly to the cell bodies by regenerating axons into a peripheral nerve graft (19), although the provision of equally large doses of trophic factors (63) or the transplantation of fibroblasts modified to produce BDNF (61) into the injury site in the spinal cord is considerably less effective. Nevertheless, recent work has suggested a more optimistic scenario. Providing neurotrophins and a peripheral nerve graft, which provides a permissive environment for regeneration, can also lead to axonal growth even after chronic injury (64).

The presence of a dense scar may impede the injured CNS from receiving benefits of treatment in chronic injuries. Debridement and removal of the scar will, however, reinjure the spinal cord. Exogenous provision of BDNF or glial derived growth factor (GDNF) into an injury site 4 weeks postinjury was shown to stimulate regeneration of rubrospinal axons into a peripheral nerve graft, and the GDNF treatment led to up regulation of two regeneration-associated genes, beta-II tubulin and GAP-43; these findings indicate that chronically axotomized neurons remained sensitive to trophic factors and can mount a regenerative response (65). Interestingly, when the scar is removed and the rubrospinal axons reinjured, a more rapid and heightened expression of regeneration associated genes was seen in red nucleus neurons (66). Thus the second injury caused by the debridement may have acted as a conditioning injury and reinvigorated the chronically injured neuron.

Engineering a New Spinal Cord

Following spinal cord injury, normal compensatory responses create a new spinal cord with different ways of processing input and generating output (67). Severe spinal cord injury leads to dorsal root sprouting into the dorsal horn caudal to the lesion (68,69), modification of spinal reflexes (70), up regulation of receptors (67,71–73), changes in motor neuron dendritic architecture (74), and alterations at the neuromuscular junction. It is possible that some of these responses can be harnessed and used to promote recovery of function. Spinal cord repair achieved by interventions such as cellular transplantation may also entail formation of additional novel pathways by further stimulating sprouting or regeneration. Improving the extent of functional recovery through these interventions is likely to entail learning to use the new circuitry, perhaps through repetitive training paradigms.

Sprouting

Axonal sprouting can result in the development of new intraspinal circuits in adult rats following spinal injury. There are different types of sprouting (Fig. 12-4). Collateral sprouting occurs when one pathway converging on a shared target is injured and the uninjured pathway forms new terminals to occupy freed synaptic space; compensatory sprouting refers to formation of additional collaterals proximal to the site of injury; regenerative sprouting is the abortive attempt of an injured axon to form successful growth cones at the site of injury. Elegant studies have shown compensatory sprouting of lesioned corticospinal axons that contacted propriospinal neurons, forming a novel pathway (75). Over a period of 3 months, contacts with propriospinal neurons that bridged the lesion were maintained and others were lost. Long propriospinal neurons arborized on lumbar motor neurons, creating yet another novel pathway. In another study animals with a corticospinal lesion were treated with an antibody that neutralizes a myelin inhibitor (76). Tracing experiments showed that collateral sprouting from rubrospinal tract axons innervated corticospinal targets, concomitant with restoration of precision movements of the forelimb and digits. In another set of experiments, recovery of function following injury to the dorsal corticospinal tract was attributable to collateral sprouting of axons in the ventral corticospinal tract (77). The mechanisms by which axonal growth from undamaged neurons can be enhanced or modulated are not understood but it is likely that some of the same interventions that stimulate regenerative sprouting may also stimulate collateral or compensatory sprouting (78). Sprouting in fact may account for much of the recovery of function that occurs following injury (79,80). Some of the recovery may, of course, be maladaptive, for example, dorsal root sprouting is likely to contribute to neuropathic pain and to autonomic dysreflexia that develops after SCI (68,79).

Transplantation Strategies

The modern era of CNS regeneration studies was pioneered by experiments from David and Aguayo (57) that

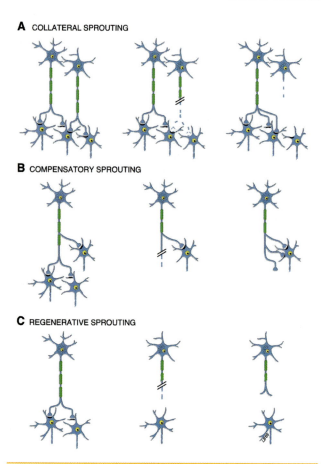

FIGURE 12-4. Types of sprouting. Formation of new axonal processes and synaptic terminals can occur following injury to the adult CNS. **A:** Collateral sprouting indicates development of new collaterals by undamaged CNS neurons that will innervate target cells that receive a convergent projection from a damaged pathway. **B:** Compensatory sprouting indicates formation of additional collaterals above the level of axonal damage that acts to increase the density of innervation to targets rostral to the site of injury. **C:** Regenerative sprouting, normally abortive, represents the attempt of an injured neuron to reform an injured axon.

showed that the permissive environment of a peripheral nerve was adequate to induce long-distance regeneration by CNS axons into a peripheral nerve graft. The limitation was that when the peripheral nerve was inserted into the CNS, the axons that had regenerated into the graft could penetrate only a small extent into the spinal cord parenchyma, and recovery was correspondingly limited.

These experiments with peripheral nerve grafts stimulated further studies in which cells or neural tissue were transplanted directly into the lesion sites. This approach has been among the most successful in treatment of spinal cord injury. If cells transplanted into a lesion site survive, they provide a potential for forming a bridge across which host axons can grow. This requires that the bridge be permissive for growth, and a variety of cell types

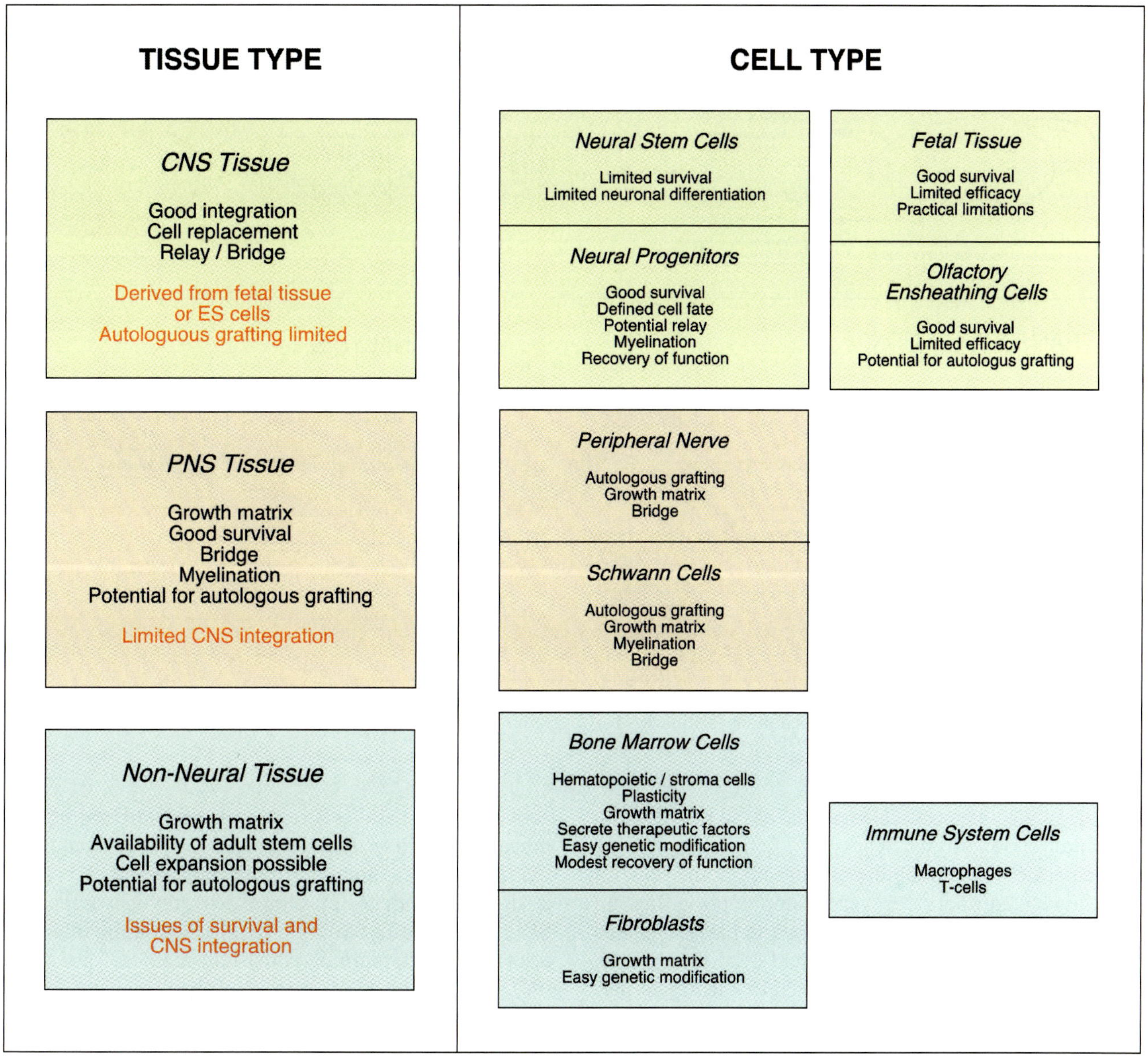

TISSUE TYPE

CNS Tissue

Good integration
Cell replacement
Relay / Bridge

Derived from fetal tissue
or ES cells
Autologuous grafting limited

PNS Tissue

Growth matrix
Good survival
Bridge
Myelination
Potential for autologous grafting

Limited CNS integration

Non-Neural Tissue

Growth matrix
Availability of adult stem cells
Cell expansion possible
Potential for autologous grafting

Issues of survival and
CNS integration

CELL TYPE

Neural Stem Cells

Limited survival
Limited neuronal differentiation

Neural Progenitors

Good survival
Defined cell fate
Potential relay
Myelination
Recovery of function

Fetal Tissue

Good survival
Limited efficacy
Practical limitations

Olfactory Ensheathing Cells

Good survival
Limited efficacy
Potential for autologus grafting

Peripheral Nerve

Autologous grafting
Growth matrix
Bridge

Schwann Cells

Autologous grafting
Growth matrix
Myelination
Bridge

Bone Marrow Cells

Hematopoietic / stroma cells
Plasticity
Growth matrix
Secrete therapeutic factors
Easy genetic modification
Modest recovery of function

Fibroblasts

Growth matrix
Easy genetic modification

Immune System Cells

Macrophages
T-cells

FIGURE 12-5. Candidates for cellular transplants. A number of cells and tissues from CNS, PNS, and nonneural sources have been evaluated as candidates for therapeutic transplants. None so far meet all of the requirements for success, but most have shown some efficacy in animal trials.

have been shown to be permissive. If the cells are neural in origin, they may be able to replace neurons or glial cells lost by the injury. Despite their potential, however, fetal spinal cord tissue and stem cells raise political and ethical issues. Additionally, there are issues of availability in the case of fetal spinal cord tissue. Nevertheless, the potential value of stem cells and lineage-restricted precursors ensures that they will continue to be the source of intense interest. There are downsides, however, as transplantation is an invasive strategy. If scar removal is necessary, surviving host tissue may also be destroyed. If transplants are not autologous, immunosuppression will

be necessary. Nevertheless, transplantation, often combined with other treatments, has provided the most promising results so far and thus the choice of cell to transplant has been the object of considerable attention (Fig. 12-5). Despite the number and diversity of cell types used, the procedures by which the cells are obtained and prepared and the types of analysis are similar (Fig. 12-6).

Training the Spinal Cord

The injured spinal cord can be trained using operant conditioning methods to increase or decrease the magnitude

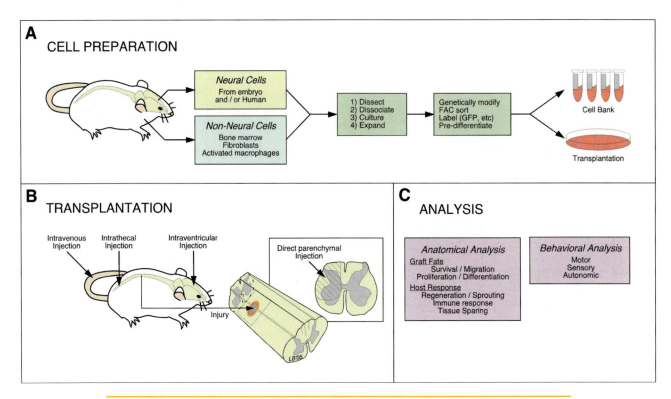

FIGURE 12-6. Procedure for therapeutic transplants. Schemata of **(A)** the procedures in animal studies for isolating cellular candidates for transplants, **(B)** the transplant procedures, and **(C)** outcome analysis.

of the H-reflex, the electrical analogue of the monosynaptic spinal tendon stretch reflex (81). Activity dependent plasticity offers the possibility of entraining other central pathways to support recovery. Simply providing an enriched environment has been shown to have beneficial effects for rats with brain and spinal cord injury (82). These environments can be structured to encourage particular movements (e.g., by forelimb foraging or locomotion on a running wheel). The equivalent of an enriched environment for patients, of course, would be structured physical therapy of the appropriate type and duration, although the most useful treatment may be limited by cost considerations that drive some current health care practices. The optimal treatment, extent, duration, task-specific nature, intensity, and the possibility that some treatments will be deleterious remain to be thoroughly evaluated (83–86). The clinical use of task-specific partial weight–supported locomotion is being evaluated in several centers. The value of physical training in promoting recovery of function, particularly in the case of incomplete injuries, has been repeatedly demonstrated both in animal studies and clinically (87,88). The beneficial effects of exercise are due to the increased expression of trophic factors in spinal cord and muscle (89) and also to activity-dependent changes evoked by specific patterns of movements within spinal circuits. Locomotor training activates reflex locomotor circuits and provides increased

activity to the pathways responsible for alternating limb movements. These treatments also restore normal BDNF mRNA levels in spinal cord and muscle and reverse the atrophy of dendrites on motor neurons that occur after SCI (74). Repetitive robotic treadmill training offers the possibility of developing consistent methods of training (90). Adaptive plasticity appears to be dependent on sensory feedback, and specific types of training may be required to guide certain kinds of recovery. Rats and cats with spinal injuries respond differently to step training and stand training (67), and rats with contusion injuries develop hypersensitivity to somatic stimulation (allodynia), which can be eliminated by some kinds of training (treadmill) but not others (stand training) (91).

The biological basis of activity-dependent modifications has been extensively studied (67). The success of these approaches appears to be based on several mechanisms. First, intrinsic spinal circuits have the capacity to drive complex tasks, including locomotion, even after spinal injury has removed descending controls. One such intrinsic circuit is the central pattern generator (CPG), which is a group of interneurons in the lumbosacral spinal cord that generates alternating hindlimb movement. Activity of the CPG is normally modulated both by supraspinal pathways that are lost and by afferent pathways that may be enhanced following spinal injury. Exogenous delivery of neurotransmitters associated with these modulating pathways, such as serotonin or serotonin agonists, has been associated with improved locomotor function (92–94). Second, plastic changes occur in response to the injury, which include sprouting of spared pathways, changes in dendritic architecture, and up regulation of receptors on target cells partially denervated by the injury. Serotonergic (71,72,95), noradrenergic (96,97), and gamma-aminobutyrate (GABA) (67) receptors are among those that have been shown to up regulate in lumbar spinal cord following injury, and administration of agonists or antagonists can improve function by acting on sensitized neurons deprived of their descending projections (71,79,95,98–100). Third, plastic changes occur at the cellular level in response to specific patterns of activity (101) (Fig. 12-7).

Bypassing the Injury

It remains unrealistic at this time to imagine that a severely damaged spinal cord can be repaired with restoration of normal pathways and full recovery of function. Ways of bypassing the injury to target spinal cord caudal to the injury and thus to promote function are being developed. A biological bypass has been described in which a thoracic nerve is disconnected and the cut end inserted into the spinal cord caudal to transection lesion. The thoracic motor axons regenerated through the nerve into the ventral horn, intermediate zone, and dorsal horn at the lumbar level and formed novel synapses in the lumbosacral motor circuits (102). The distances in which these motor axons grew in the lumbosacral cord, while small, appeared to be sufficient to mediate function, as stimulation of the nerve evoked contraction of back and leg muscles. Since the motor neurons are rostral to the lesion, they remain under descending control, thus allowing for the possibility of providing voluntary control over lumbosacral circuits newly innervated by these axons. Other strategies take a more neuroprosthetic approach using assistive devices that restore function lost as a result of neurological damage (103,104). The burgeoning field of

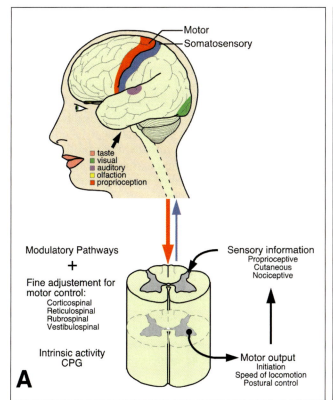 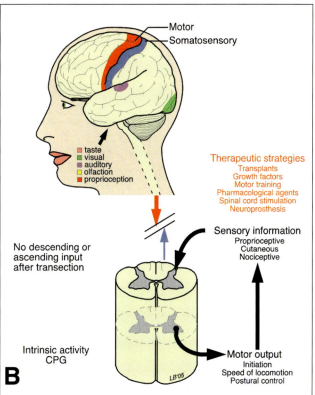

FIGURE 12-7. Spinal transection creates a new spinal cord. Spinal transection results in considerable modification of the circuitry caudal to the lesion. Some of these changes may contribute to the deficits, while others may provide opportunities for therapeutic interventions. **A:** The intact spinal cord receives control and modulation from supraspinal systems and sensory input from primary afferents, which determines the activity of spinal circuits, including the central pattern generator. **B:** After SCI, descending pathways are lost, their denervated receptors up regulate, and afferent pathways are enhanced, leading to hyperexcitable reflexes. Strategies targeting independent mechanisms are the bases of potential treatments.

neuroengineering is developing CNS-machine interfaces that will permit bypassing the injury site (105,106) with direct intraspinal stimulation of selective motor pools (107) or interneuronal circuits (108). Electrical stimulation of spinal circuits using chronically implanted microwires has yielded functional movements in intact cats, and perhaps could be used in animals with spinal injuries (109). These devices, along with combination therapies to improve repair, have the potential to greatly increase the useful function that can be restored after injury (Fig. 12-8).

Combination Therapies

Individual treatments targeted at the many impediments to spinal cord repair have provided proof of principle for

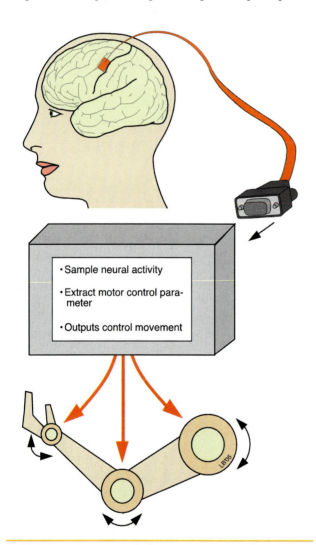

FIGURE 12-8. Bypassing the transection. An alternative to interventions promoting repair is provided through utilization of brain-machine interfaces, in which motor commands issuing from cortical regions can be recognized by electrode arrays, processed using a computer, and the output used to control movement by robotic devices.

these strategies. Individually, however, only modest improvements in function are usually seen in animal models. Long-distance regeneration is rarely reported, and the improvements in function, which are usually greater after smaller lesions, may be due primarily to other processes (behavioral compensation, sprouting, or neuroprotection) rather than regeneration. Developing methods to stimulate long-distance regeneration is an important goal and may be associated with the next step in qualitative improvements in functional recovery. The greater requirements for successful treatment in chronic injuries also need to be understood.

Rational combination therapies, directed at several mechanistically distinct targets, are being investigated. Individual treatments that have shown promise include: (a) pharmacological treatments that diminish apoptosis; (b) enhancing the growth potential of neurons, either pharmacologically (modulating cAMP levels), or by provision of trophic factors (exogenous administration or transplantation of cells genetically modified to secrete neurotrophic factors); (c) cellular transplantation to fill the lesion site and provide a pathway for growing axons (fibroblasts, stromal cells, Schwann cells, olfactory ensheathing cells, fetal spinal cord, neural stem cells or precursors); (d) pharmacological blockade of environmental inhibitors (myelin proteins, CSPG); (e) enhancing activity-dependent plasticity by structured motor training; (f) delivery of agonists or antagonists to target neurons partially denervated and sensitized by removal of descending input; and (g) neuroprostheses. Combining these approaches is complex and can be technically difficult, but these procedures are beginning to identify appropriate paradigms for a coordinated therapeutic approach to spinal injury. Indeed these combinatorial approaches have in several cases demonstrated greater functional improvement than single interventions.

SUMMARY

Are Animal Models Useful?

It is interesting that many of the animal studies reviewed here report not only some degree of repair (regeneration, sprouting, or neuroprotection) but also improvement in function. It needs to be emphasized that the repair processes may so far be modest and that the recovery of function in animal models is also often modest and may not translate into useful function in a human with severe spinal injury. Nevertheless, these improvements can point to promising strategies that can be developed to become parts of successful treatment plans.

Recovery of Function

It is significant that many researchers now include a range of functional evaluations as outcome measures, although there are at present few standards that will allow comparisons across laboratories. Recovery of function, in fact, has been described for the majority of studies reviewed here. We know that the effects of interventions that promote axonal growth may extend beyond the local circuitry because recent studies have shown recovery of hindlimb function associated with injury and treatment at the cervical (94,110) or thoracic (39) level. The mechanisms that account for the recovery need to be explored. More importantly, means of evaluating recovery reported under different conditions are lacking. Finally, most of the experimental paradigms use rodents, and issues of scale are not addressed. Examination of therapies in animals with spinal cords comparable in size to humans (e.g., cats or primates) will be required to provide convincing evidence of the value of these interventions. Pharmacological therapy has been useful in animal studies, but similar strategies proved to be less effective in humans (67). Administration of noradrenergic agonists induces locomotion in spinal cats (99,111) but may have a depressing effect on electromyography (EMG) activity in SCI patients engaged in treadmill locomotion (112). Of course, delivery of transmitter agents may have different effects on different systems. Noradrenergic antagonists are effective in improving bladder function, and when combined with transplanted cells are even more effective (79). It remains to be determined whether these antagonists would have untoward effects on other functions that would limit their usefulness.

Repair

The effects of neuroprotection treatments for stroke models in a variety of mammalian models have shown more efficacy in small mammalian models than in humans (113). Similarly, development of clinical trials for CNS injury based on neurotrophins has been largely unsuccessful (114), perhaps in part because of secondary side effects that may not be observed in animals. In addition, a local and regulated supply of neurotrophins will undoubtedly be required, and indeed such procedures are being developed. Finally, more detailed knowledge of signal transduction pathways activated by neurotrophins is likely to provide better targets for interventions.

Combination Therapy

The challenges of combination therapy include identifying the most appropriate mix of interventions. This will require evaluation of individual contributions to neuroprotection, axonal growth, and perhaps, most important, recovery of a range of functions (53,100,115,116). Receiving FDA approval for combinatorial treatments is likely to provide additional challenges.

Major advances have been made and trials are under way, yet the magic fusillade remains to be discovered.

REFERENCES

1. Kwon BK, Oxland TR, Tetzlaff W. Animal models used in spinal cord regeneration research. *Spine*. 2002;27(14): 1504–1510.
2. Moskowitz MA, Lo EH. Neurogenesis and apoptotic cell death. *Stroke*. 2003;34(2):324–326.
3. Benn SC, Woolf CJ. Adult neuron survival strategies—slamming on the brakes. *Nat Rev Neurosci*. 2004;5(9): 686–700.
4. Himes B, Tessler A. Neuroprotection from cell death following axotomy. In: Ingolia N, Murray, M, eds. *Axonal Regeneration in the Central Nervous System*. New York: Marcel Dekker; 2001:477–504.
5. Bareyre FM, Schwab ME. Inflammation, degeneration and regeneration in the injured spinal cord: insights from DNA microarrays. *Trends Neurosci*. 2003;26(10):555–563.
6. Nakamura M, Houghtling RA, MacArthur L, et al. Differences in cytokine gene expression profile between acute and secondary injury in adult rat spinal cord. *Exp Neurol*. 2003;184(1):313–325.
7. Bartholdi D, Schwab ME. Methylprednisolone inhibits early inflammatory processes but not ischemic cell death after experimental spinal cord lesion in the rat. *Brain Res*. 1995;672(1–2):177–186.
8. Haghighi SS, Agrawal SK, Surdell D Jr, et al. Effects of methylprednisolone and MK-801 on functional recovery after experimental chronic spinal cord injury. *Spinal Cord*. 2000;38(12):733–740.
9. Bracken MB, Holford TR. Neurological and functional status 1 year after acute spinal cord injury: estimates of functional recovery in National Acute Spinal Cord Injury Study II from results modeled in National Acute Spinal Cord Injury Study III. *J Neurosurg*. April 2002;96(suppl 3):259–266.
10. Yin Y, Cui Q, Li Y, et al. Macrophage-derived factors stimulate optic nerve regeneration. *J Neurosci*. 2003;23(6): 2284–2293.
11. Kipnis J, Mizrahi T, Hauben E, et al. Neuroprotective autoimmunity: naturally occurring CD4+CD25+ regulatory T cells suppress the ability to withstand injury to the central nervous system. *Proc Natl Acad Sci USA*. 2002;99(24): 15620–15625.
12. Jones TB, Ankeny DP, Guan Z, et al. Passive or active immunization with myelin basic protein impairs neurological function and exacerbates neuropathology after spinal cord injury in rats. *J Neurosci*. 2004;24(15):3752–3761.
13. McPhail LT, Stirling DP, Tetzlaff W, et al. The contribution of activated phagocytes and myelin degeneration to axonal retraction/dieback following spinal cord injury. *Eur J Neurosci*. 2004;20(8):1984–1994.
14. Gris D, Marsh DR, Oatway MA, et al. Transient blockade of the CD11d/CD18 integrin reduces secondary damage after spinal cord injury, improving sensory, autonomic, and motor function. *J Neurosci*. 2004;24(16):4043–4051.
15. Park E, Velumian AA, Fehlings MG. The role of excitotoxicity in secondary mechanisms of spinal cord injury: a review with an emphasis on the implications for white matter degeneration. *J Neurotrauma*. 2004;21(6):754–774.
16. Wrathall JR, Teng YD, Choiniere D. Amelioration of functional deficits from spinal cord trauma with systemically administered NBQX, an antagonist of non-N-methyl-D-aspartate receptors. *Exp Neurol*. 1996;137(1):119–126.
17. Wrathall JR, Teng YD, Marriott R. Delayed antagonism of AMPA/kainate receptors reduces long-term functional deficits resulting from spinal cord trauma. *Exp Neurol*. 1997;145(2 pt 1):565–573.
18. Himes BT, Liu Y, Solowska JM, et al. Transplants of cells genetically modified to express neurotrophin-3 rescue

axotomized Clarke's nucleus neurons after spinal cord hemisection in adult rats. *J Neurosci Res*. 2001;65(6): 549–564.

19. Kwon BK, Liu J, Messerer C, et al. Survival and regeneration of rubrospinal neurons 1 year after spinal cord injury. *Proc Natl Acad Sci USA*. 2002;99(5):3246–3251.

20. Hunt D, Coffin RS, Anderson PN. The Nogo receptor, its ligands and axonal regeneration in the spinal cord: a review. *J Neurocytol*. 2002;31(2):93–120.

21. Filbin MT. Myelin-associated inhibitors of axonal regeneration in the adult mammalian CNS. *Nat Rev Neurosci*. 2003;4(9):703–713.

22. Schwab ME. Nogo and axon regeneration. *Curr Opin Neurobiol*. 2004;14(1):118–124.

23. Huang DW, McKerracher L, Braun PE, et al. A therapeutic vaccine approach to stimulate axon regeneration in the adult mammalian spinal cord. *Neuron*. 1999;24(3):639–647.

24. Kaplan DR, Miller FD. Axon growth inhibition: signals from the p75 neurotrophin receptor. *Nat Neurosci*. 2003;6(5): 435–436.

25. GrandPre T, Li S, Strittmatter SM. Nogo-66 receptor antagonist peptide promotes axonal regeneration. *Nature*. 2002;417(6888):547–551.

26. Raisman G. Myelin inhibitors: does NO mean GO? *Nat Rev Neurosci*. 2004;5(2):157–161.

27. Kinouchi R, Takeda M, Yang L, et al. Robust neural integration from retinal transplants in mice deficient in GFAP and vimentin. *Nat Neurosci*. 2003;6(8):863–868.

28. Tom VJ, Steinmetz MP, Miller JH, et al. Studies on the development and behavior of the dystrophic growth cone, the hallmark of regeneration failure, in an in vitro model of the glial scar and after spinal cord injury. *J Neurosci*. 2004;24(29):6531–6539.

29. Sivasankaran R, Pei J, Wang KC, et al. PKC mediates inhibitory effects of myelin and chondroitin sulfate proteoglycans on axonal regeneration. *Nat Neurosci*. 2004;7(3): 261–268.

30. Snow DM, Lemmon V, Carrino DA, et al. Sulfated proteoglycans in astroglial barriers inhibit neurite outgrowth in vitro. *Exp Neurol*. 1990;109(1):111–130.

31. Hynds DL, Snow DM. Neurite outgrowth inhibition by chondroitin sulfate proteoglycan: stalling/stopping exceeds turning in human neuroblastoma growth cones. *Exp Neurol*. 1999;160(1):244–255.

32. Bradbury EJ, Moon LD, Popat RJ, et al. Chondroitinase ABC promotes functional recovery after spinal cord injury. *Nature*. 2002;416(6881):636–640.

33. Bush TG, Puvanachandra N, Horner CH, et al. Leukocyte infiltration, neuronal degeneration, and neurite outgrowth after ablation of scar-forming, reactive astrocytes in adult transgenic mice. *Neuron*. 1999;23(2):297–308.

34. Faulkner JR, Herrmann JE, Woo MJ, et al. Reactive astrocytes protect tissue and preserve function after spinal cord injury. *J Neurosci*. 2004;24(9):2143–2155.

35. Yamashita T, Tohyama M. The p75 receptor acts as a displacement factor that releases Rho from Rho-GDI. *Nat Neurosci*. 2003;6(5):461–467.

36. Wang KC, Kim JA, Sivasankaran R, et al. P75 interacts with the Nogo receptor as a co-receptor for Nogo, MAG and OMgp. *Nature*. 2002;420(6911):74–78.

37. Grill R, Murai K, Blesch A, et al. Cellular delivery of neurotrophin-3 promotes corticospinal axonal growth and partial functional recovery after spinal cord injury. *J Neurosci*. 1997;17(14):5560–5572.

38. Liu Y, Kim D, Himes BT, et al. Transplants of fibroblasts genetically modified to express BDNF promote regeneration of adult rat rubrospinal axons and recovery of forelimb function. *J Neurosci*. 1999;19(11):4370–4387.

39. Coumans JV, Lin TT, Dai HN, et al. Axonal regeneration and functional recovery after complete spinal cord transection in rats by delayed treatment with transplants and neurotrophins. *J Neurosci*. 2001;21(23):9334–9344.

40. Ramer MS, Bishop T, Dockery P, et al. Neurotrophin-3-mediated regeneration and recovery of proprioception following dorsal rhizotomy. *Mol Cell Neurosci*. 2002;19(2): 239–249.

41. Zhou L, Baumgartner BJ, Hill-Felberg SJ, et al. Neurotrophin-3 expressed in situ induces axonal plasticity in the adult injured spinal cord. *J Neurosci*. 2003;23(4): 1424–1431.

42. Bomze HM, Bulsara KR, Iskandar BJ, et al. Spinal axon regeneration evoked by replacing two growth cone proteins in adult neurons. *Nat Neurosci*. 2001;4(1):38–43.

43. Aimone JB, Leasure JL, Perreau VM, et al. Spatial and temporal gene expression profiling of the contused rat spinal cord. *Exp Neurol*. 2004;189(2):204–221.

44. Velardo MJ, Burger C, Williams PR, et al. Patterns of gene expression reveal a temporally orchestrated wound healing response in the injured spinal cord. *J Neurosci*. 2004; 24(39):8562–8576.

45. Zhang KH, Xiao HS, Lu PH, et al. Differential gene expression after complete spinal cord transection in adult rats: an analysis focused on a subchronic post-injury stage. *Neuroscience*. 2004;128(2):375–388.

46. Neumann S, Woolf CJ. Regeneration of dorsal column fibers into and beyond the lesion site following adult spinal cord injury. *Neuron*. 1999;23(1):83–91.

47. Neumann S, Bradke F, Tessier-Lavigne M, et al. Regeneration of sensory axons within the injured spinal cord induced by intraganglionic cAMP elevation. *Neuron*. 2002; 34(6):885–893.

48. Cai D, Qiu J, Cao Z, et al. Neuronal cyclic AMP controls the developmental loss in ability of axons to regenerate. *J Neurosci*. 2001;21(13):4731–4739.

49. Han PJ, Shukla S, Subramanian PS, et al. Cyclic AMP elevates tubulin expression without increasing intrinsic axon growth capacity. *Exp Neurol*. 2004;189(2):293-302.

50. Cai D, Deng K, Mellado W, et al. Arginase I and polyamines act downstream from cyclic AMP in overcoming inhibition of axonal growth MAG and myelin in vitro. *Neuron*. 2002;35(4):711–719.

51. Nikulina E, Tidwell JL, Dai HN, et al. The phosphodiesterase inhibitor rolipram delivered after a spinal cord lesion promotes axonal regeneration and functional recovery. *Proc Natl Acad Sci USA*. 2004;101(23):8786–8790.

52. Bunge MB, Pearse DD. Transplantation strategies to promote repair of the injured spinal cord. *J Rehabil Res Dev*. 2003;40(4 suppl 1):55–62.

53. Lu P, Yang H, Jones LL, et al. Combinatorial therapy with neurotrophins and cAMP promotes axonal regeneration beyond sites of spinal cord injury. *J Neurosci*. 2004;24(28): 6402–6409.

54. He Z, Koprivica V. The Nogo signaling pathway for regeneration block. *Annu Rev Neurosci*. 2004;27:341–368.

55. Dergham P, Ellezam B, Essagian C, et al. Rho signaling pathway targeted to promote spinal cord repair. *J Neurosci*. 2002;22(15):6570–6577.

56. Fournier AE, Takizawa BT, Strittmatter SM. Rho kinase inhibition enhances axonal regeneration in the injured CNS. *J Neurosci*. 2003;23(4):1416–1423.

57. David S, Aguayo AJ. Axonal elongation into peripheral nervous system "bridges" after central nervous system injury in adult rats. *Science*. 1981;214(4523):931–933.

58. Menei P, Montero-Menei C, Whittemore SR, et al. Schwann cells genetically modified to secrete human BDNF promote enhanced axonal regrowth across transected adult rat spinal cord. *Eur J Neurosci*. 1998;10(2):607–621.

59. Jones LL, Oudega M, Bunge MB, et al. Neurotrophic factors, cellular bridges and gene therapy for spinal cord injury. *J Physiol*. 2001;533(pt 1):83–89.

60. Houle JD, Tessler A. Repair of chronic spinal cord injury. *Exp Neurol*. 2003;182(2):247–260.

61. Tobias CA, Shumsky JS, Shibata M, et al. Delayed grafting of BDNF and NT-3 producing fibroblasts into the injured spinal cord stimulates sprouting, partially rescues axotomized red nucleus neurons from loss and atrophy, and provides limited regeneration. *Exp Neurol*. 2003;184(1):97–113.

62. Von Meyenburg J, Brosamle C, Metz GA, et al. Regeneration and sprouting of chronically injured corticospinal tract fibers in adult rats promoted by NT-3 and the mAb IN-1, which neutralizes myelin-associated neurite growth inhibitors. *Exp Neurol*. 1998;154(2):583–594.

63. Kwon BK, Liu J, Oschipok L, et al. Rubrospinal neurons fail to respond to brain-derived neurotrophic factor applied to the spinal cord injury site 2 months after cervical axotomy. *Exp Neurol*. 2004;189(1):45–57.

64. Ye JH, Houle JD. Treatment of the chronically injured spinal cord with neurotrophic factors can promote axonal regeneration from supraspinal neurons. *Exp Neurol*. 1997; 143(1):70–81.

65. Storer PD, Dolbeare D, Houle JD. Treatment of chronically injured spinal cord with neurotrophic factors stimulates betaII-tubulin and GAP-43 expression in rubrospinal tract neurons. *J Neurosci Res*. 2003;74(4):502–511.

66. Storer PD, Houle JD. betaII-tubulin and GAP 43 mRNA expression in chronically injured neurons of the red nucleus after a second spinal cord injury. *Exp Neurol*. 2003;183(2):537–547.

67. Edgerton VR, Tillakaratne NJ, Bigbee AJ, et al. Plasticity of the spinal neural circuitry after injury. *Annu Rev Neurosci*. 2004;27:145–167.

68. Krenz NR, Weaver LC. Sprouting of primary afferent fibers after spinal cord transection in the rat. *Neuroscience*. 1998;85(2):443–458.

69. Murray M, Tobias CA. Regeneration and sprouting in the injured spinal cord: a decade of growth. *Top Spinal Cord Inj Rehab*. 2003;8:37–51.

70. Valero-Cabre A, Fores J, Navarro X. Reorganization of reflex responses mediated by different afferent sensory fibers after spinal cord transection. *J Neurophysiol*. 2004; 91(6):2838–2848.

71. Kim D, Adipudi V, Shibayama M, et al. Direct agonists for serotonin receptors enhance locomotor function in rats that received neural transplants after neonatal spinal transection. *J Neurosci*. 1999;19(14):6213–6224.

72. Hayashi Y, Jacob S, Nothias J-M, et al. 5HT Precursor loading enhances motor function after spinal cord contusion in adult rats. *Exp Neurol*. 2005;51:17849–17854.

73. Edgerton VR, Roy RR. Paralysis recovery in humans and model systems. *Curr Opin Neurobiol*. 2002;12(6):658–667.

74. Gazula VR, Roberts M, Luzzio C, et al. Effects of limb exercise after spinal cord injury on motor neuron dendrite structure. *J Comp Neurol*. 2004;476(2):130–145.

75. Bareyre FM, Kerschensteiner M, Raineteau O, et al. The injured spinal cord spontaneously forms a new intraspinal circuit in adult rats. *Nat Neurosci*. 2004;7(3):269–277.

76. Raineteau O, Fouad K, Noth P, et al. Functional switch between motor tracts in the presence of the mAb IN-1 in the adult rat. *Proc Natl Acad Sci USA*. 2001;98(12):6929–6934.

77. Weidner N, Ner A, Salimi N, et al. Spontaneous corticospinal axonal plasticity and functional recovery after adult central nervous system injury. *Proc Natl Acad Sci USA*. 2001;98(6):3513–3518.

78. Murray A, Tobias C. 2003 Regeneration and sprouting in the injured spinal cord. *Top Spinal Cord Inj Rehab*. 2003;8:37–51.

79. Mitsui T, Shumsky JS, Lepore A, et al. Transplantation of neural and glial restricted precursors into contused spinal cord improves bladder and motor functions, decreases allodynia and modified intraspinal circuitry. *J. Neurosci*. 2005;25:9624–9636.

80. Mitsui T, Fischer I, Shumsky JS, et al. Transplants of fibroblasts expressing BDNF and NT-3 promote recovery of bladder and hindlimb function following spinal contusion in rats. *Exp. Neurol*. 2005;194:410–431.

81. Wolpaw JR, Tennissen AM. Activity-dependent spinal cord plasticity in health and disease. *Annu Rev Neurosci*. 2001;24:807–843.

82. Lankhorst AJ, ter Laak MP, van Laar TJ, et al. Effects of enriched housing on functional recovery after spinal contusive injury in the adult rat. *J Neurotrauma*. 2001; 18(2):203–215.

83. Schallert T, Jones TA. "Exuberant" neuronal growth after brain damage in adult rats: the essential role of behavioral experience. *J Neural Transplant Plast*. 1993;4(3):193–198.

84. Biernaskie J, Chernenko G, Corbett D. Efficacy of rehabilitative experience declines with time after focal ischemic brain injury. *J Neurosci*. 2004;24(5):1245–1254.

85. Brown AW, Bjelke B, Fuxe K. Motor response to amphetamine treatment, task-specific training, and limited motor experience in a postacute animal stroke model. *Exp Neurol*. 2004;190(1):102–108.

86. Griesbach GS, Gomez-Pinilla F, Hovda DA. The upregulation of plasticity-related proteins following TBI is disrupted with acute voluntary exercise. *Brain Res*. 2004;1016(2):154–162.

87. Wernig A, Nanassy A, Muller S. Maintenance of locomotor abilities following Laufband (treadmill) therapy in para- and tetraplegic persons: follow-up studies. *Spinal Cord*. 1998;36(11):744–749.

88. Barbeau H, Fung J. The role of rehabilitation in the recovery of walking in the neurological population. *Curr Opin Neurol*. 2001;14(6):735–740.

89. Gomez-Pinilla F, Ying Z, Roy RR, et al. Afferent input modulates neurotrophins and synaptic plasticity in the spinal cord. *J Neurophysiol*. 2004;92(6):3423–3432.

90. De Leon RD, Reinkensmeyer DJ, Timoszyk WK, et al. Use of robotics in assessing the adaptive capacity of the rat lumbar spinal cord. *Prog Brain Res*. 2002;137:141–149.

91. Hutchinson KJ, Gomez-Pinilla F, Crowe MJ, et al. Three exercise paradigms differentially improve sensory recovery after spinal cord contusion in rats. *Brain*. 2004;127(pt 6):1403–1414.

92. Feraboli-Lohnherr D, Barthe JY, Orsal D. Serotonin-induced activation of the network for locomotion in adult spinal rats. *J Neurosci Res*. 1999;55(1):87–98.

93. Antri M, Orsal D, Barthe JY. Locomotor recovery in the chronic spinal rat: effects of long-term treatment with a 5-HT2 agonist. *Eur J Neurosci*. 2002;16(3):467–476.

94. Kim D, Murray M, Simansky KJ. The serotonergic 5-HT(2C) agonist m-chlorophenylpiperazine increases weight-supported locomotion without development of tolerance in rats with spinal transections. *Exp Neurol*. 2001;169(2):496–500.

95. Guertin PA. Synergistic activation of the central pattern generator for locomotion by l-beta-3,4-dihydroxyphenylalanine and quipazine in adult paraplegic mice. *Neurosci Lett*. 2004;358(2):71–74.

96. Giroux N, Rossignol S, Reader TA. Autoradiographic study of alpha1- and alpha2-noradrenergic and serotonin1A receptors in the spinal cord of normal and chronically transected cats. *J Comp Neurol*. 1999;406(3):402–414.

97. Roudet C, Gimenez Ribotta M, Privat A, et al. Regional study of spinal alpha 2-adrenoceptor densities after intraspinal noradrenergic-rich implants on adult rats bearing complete spinal cord transection or selective chemical noradrenergic denervation. *Neurosci Lett*. 1996;208(2):89–92.

98. Barbeau H, Rossignol S. The effects of serotonergic drugs on the locomotor pattern and on cutaneous reflexes of the adult chronic spinal cat. *Brain Res*. 1990;514(1):55–67.

99. Chau C, Barbeau H, Rossignol S. Early locomotor training with clonidine in spinal cats. *J Neurophysiol*. 1998;79(1): 392–409.

100. Nothias J-M, Mitsui T, Shumsky JS, et al. Combined effects of neurotrophin secreting transplants, exercise and serotonergic drug challenge improve function in spinal rats. *Neurorehab Neural Repair*. 2005;19:296–312.

101. Cote MP, Gossard JP. Step training-dependent plasticity in spinal cutaneous pathways. *J Neurosci*. 2004;24(50): 11317–11327.

102. Campos L, Meng Z, Hu G, et al. Engineering novel spinal circuits to promote recovery after spinal injury. *J Neurosci*. 2004;24(9):2090–2101.

103. Grill WM, Kirsch RF. Neuroprosthetic applications of electrical stimulation. *Assist Technol*. 2000;12(1):6–20.

104. Prochazka A, Mushahwar VK, McCreery DB. Neural prostheses. *J Physiol.* 2001;533(pt 1):99–109.

105. Nicolelis MA. Brain-machine interfaces to restore motor function and probe neural circuits. *Nat Rev Neurosci.* 2003;4(5):417–422.

106. Wolpaw JR, McFarland DJ. Control of a two-dimensional movement signal by a noninvasive brain-computer interface in humans. *Proc Natl Acad Sci USA.* 2004;101(51):17849–17854.

107. Mushahwar VK, Collins DF, Prochazka A. Spinal cord microstimulation generates functional limb movements in chronically implanted cats. *Exp Neurol.* 2000;163(2):422–429.

108. Lemay MA, Grill WM. Modularity of motor output evoked by intraspinal microstimulation in cats. *J Neurophysiol.* 2004;91(1):502–514.

109. Saigal R, Renzi C, Mushahwar VK. Intraspinal microstimulation generates functional movements after spinal-cord injury. *IEEE Trans Neural Syst Rehabil Eng.* 2004;12(4):430–440.

110. Shumsky JS, Tobias CA, Tumolo M, et al. Delayed transplantation of fibroblasts genetically modified to secrete BDNF and NT-3 into a spinal cord injury site is associated with limited recovery of function. *Exp Neurol.* 2003;184(1):114–130.

111. Barbeau H, Rossignol S. Recovery of locomotion after chronic spinalization in the adult cat. *Brain Res.* 1987;412(1):84–95.

112. Dietz V, Wirz M, Colombo G, et al. Locomotor capacity and recovery of spinal cord function in paraplegic patients: a clinical and electrophysiological evaluation. *Electroencephalogr Clin Neurophysiol.* 1998;109(2):140–153.

113. Hoyte L, Kaur J, Buchan AM. Lost in translation: taking neuroprotection from animal models to clinical trials. *Exp Neurol.* 2004;188(2):200–204.

114. Thoenen H, Sendtner M. Neurotrophins: from enthusiastic expectations through sobering experiences to rational therapeutic approaches. *Nat Neurosci.* 2002;5(suppl):1046–1050.

115. Fouad K, Schnell L, Bunge MB, et al. Combining Schwann cell bridges and olfactory-ensheathing glia grafts with chondroitinase promotes locomotor recovery after complete transection of the spinal cord. *J Neurosci.* 2005;25(5):1169–1178.

116. Murray M. Therapies to promote CNS repair. In: Ingolia N, Murray, M, eds. *Axonal Regeneration in the Central Nervous System.* New York: Marcel Dekker; 2001:649–674.

Chapter 13

Experimental Techniques of Spinal Imaging

Eric D. Schwartz

INTRODUCTION

Epidemiology and Current Clinical Treatments

Every year, approximately 12,000 people in the United States become victims of spinal cord injury, and there are currently almost 250,000 who are paraplegic or quadriplegic (1,2). Because this disease affects the young more than the old and because better postinjury care has resulted in increased survival, the impact on society is huge and annual medical costs in the United States are close to $9 billion (2). Treatment options for these spinally injured patients are limited. The usefulness of immediate application of methylprednisolone, the only treatment shown to be effective in ameliorating spinal cord injury

(3,4), has been aggressively questioned over the past few years (5). According to the Canadian Neurosurgical Society and the National Association of Emergency Medical Services Physicians (NAEMSP), treatment with methylprednisolone is no longer the "standard of care" (6,7).

Despite this setback in the clinical arena, basic science research has identified many promising treatment options, including both transplantation and pharmacologic therapy (8–14); however, as noted by Naomi Kleitman (15) of the National Institute of Neurological Disorders and Stroke, "the promise (of these basic science advances) has not been fulfilled by improving clinical treatment." The question that arises is what is needed to translate these advances from the lab to the bedside?

One answer is that improved outcome measures are needed for translating basic science advances (16). The evaluation of treatment efficacy in clinical trials faces obstacles that slow the pace of research. The improvement of patient care has reduced the mortality and morbidity of spinally injured patients, and the life expectancy of non-ventilator dependent spinal cord injured patients is close to normal (2,17); thus histologic data may not be forthcoming. Unlike experimental models, behavioral improvement in humans following therapy may take years (18) and is difficult to assess (19), thus slowing the pace of evaluating treatment efficacy. A noninvasive imaging modality that could objectively identify histologic changes to axons would therefore be an important component to a battery of tests designed to evaluate treatment efficacy.

Limitations of Conventional Magnetic Resonance Imaging in the Evaluation of Spinal Cord Injury

Conventional magnetic resonance imaging (MRI) techniques for evaluation of acute spinal cord injury generally include the following pulse sequences: T1-weighted images, T2-weighted images, T2* susceptibility images, and short tau inversion recovery (STIR) images. For these pulse sequences, contrast is based on intrinsic properties of the tissue, referred to as T1 and T2 values. Although these intrinsic properties of tissue may be altered with injury, the effect on contrast differs among the pulse sequences. Increases in water content, such as that seen with spinal cord edema, usually result in longer T1 and longer T2 values. The overall effect is lower signal on T1-weighted images and higher signal on T2-weighted images. Although T1-weighted images provide good evaluation of vertebral alignment and help assess spinal cord size, this pulse sequence is not ideal for evaluation of spinal cord parenchymal injury. The T2-weighted image is usually more sensitive than the T1 weighted images for detecting alterations caused by trauma. The high intensity of cerebrospinal fluid on a T2-weighted image also helps to evaluate for effacement of surrounding cerebrospinal fluid

and spinal cord compression. T2* images are more sensitive for identifying spinal cord hemorrhage, with areas of hemorrhage appearing dark. STIR images are usually T2-weighted with suppression of signal from fat, allowing visualization of edema/injury within the vertebral bodies, soft tissues, and ligaments that surround the spinal canal. Contrast on T1- and T2-weighted images varies with the strength of the main magnetic field, but successful imaging strategies have been implemented across the range of field strengths used for clinical and experimental studies.

These conventional MRI pulse sequences can indicate the presence of hemorrhage, length of contusion-induced edema, level of injury, spinal cord swelling, and cord compression. This information has proven valuable in early diagnosis and treatment planning. These techniques are limited, however, in that their contrast primarily reflects changes in water content or presence of hemorrhage. This limitation is demonstrated in experimental research that attempts to correlate edema and hemorrhage with neurologic and histologic severity. One study using a rat spinal cord contusion model showed that the degree of neurologic recovery following contusion injury did not correlate either with volumetric lesion size as evaluated by T2-weighted abnormal signal (edema) or T2 hypointensity (hemorrhage) (20). Another study with the rat contusion model demonstrated that the water content and average T2 may not change significantly in areas of acute injury (21); therefore, conventional MRI techniques may underestimate the degree of injury. Additionally, some areas of hemorrhage may be too small to be visible on T2* images.

Although MRI is the best imaging modality for the evaluation of spinal cord parenchyma at this time, conventional MRI techniques do not appear to differentiate edema from axonal injury are therefore limited to providing anatomic information about the spinal cord parenchyma, including the degree of spinal cord compression, amount of hemorrhage, and injury localization. The water content or hemorrhagic content does not necessarily reflect the status of the white matter tracts, and, consequently, the functional status of the spinal cord is not well assessed. This reliance on water content and blood products explains why the use of MRI for prognostication of future neurologic status following human spinal cord injury has been minimally or no more successful than neurologic examination alone. Although there has been limited success in correlating these conventional MRI findings with neurologic outcome (22–27), a review of the prognostic ability of MRI in the National Acute Spinal Cord Injury Study 3 (NASCIS) noted that "the present analyses find that MR imaging does not add much to the diagnosis of neurologic function at the time of injury when compared with assessment by more traditional measures of neurologic function" (28). Follow-up imaging of chronic spinal cord injury has also been limited to assessment of spinal cord morphology, and the development of posttraumatic syringomyelia and myelomalacia (29–34). Another methodology is needed for identifying appropriate patient populations for treatment delivery; optimal therapy may need to be delivered in the first few hours or days, yet neurologic examination may require a week's delay before providing an accurate prognosis.

Conventional MRI, therefore, appears restricted to assessing macroscopic changes in the injured spinal cord and does not adequately address integrity of the white matter. This limitation may explain the limited success of MRI as a prognostic tool because it is the degree and location of injured and spared white matter that primarily determine subsequent function. More advanced MRI techniques, however, show great promise in providing structural information concerning the integrity of axons. In this chapter we will review the MRI techniques that have the most potential for impacting the diagnosis and treatment of spinal cord injury, with the greatest emphasis on diffusion-weighted and diffusion-tensor MRI (DWI and DTI). Other promising techniques will be introduced as well, including MR spectroscopy (MRS), magnetization transfer imaging (MTI), blood oxygen level dependent MRI (BOLD), and newer techniques for tracking cells following neurotransplantation.

DIFFUSION-BASED MAGNETIC RESONANCE IMAGING TECHNIQUES

Diffusion-weighted Magnetic Resonance Imaging: Background and Principles

DWI is designed to measure the movement rate of water molecules that results from random (Brownian) motion. Most diffusion-based studies use a pulse sequence derived from the work of Stejskal and Tanner (35). A paired set of diffusion sensitizing gradients is used to encode signal intensity on the resulting images. In this scheme, stationary water molecules retain high-signal and water molecules that move between the first and second gradient pulses and lose signal as a function of the magnitude of displacement. The obtained images are referred to as diffusion weighted because the dominant contrast mechanism is differences in local water diffusion. The degree of diffusion weighting is described by the *b*-value, which is determined by

$$b = \gamma^2 G^2 \delta^2 (\Delta \text{-} \delta/3),$$

with γ = gyromagnetic ratio, G = magnitude of diffusion sensitizing gradients, δ = duration of individual diffusion sensitizing lobe, and Δ = time period between leading edges of the diffusion sensitizing lobes. The gyromagnetic ratio is a constant for protons in a particular magnetic field strength; all of the other factors are under operator control, subject to technical limitations.

In addition to one image with *b* = 0, which is essentially a T2-weighted image, at least one images with *b* >0 is required to quantify water diffusion. Using the signal intensities in the DWI images, we can quantify water diffusion in each voxel with the monoexponential equation:

$$S/So = \exp(\text{-}bD),$$

where S = signal from a DWI image, So = signal without diffusion sensitizing gradients (*b* = 0), D = measured diffusion coefficient, usually referred to as the apparent diffusion coefficient (ADC), and *b* = b-value. Each measured voxel in an ADC map image is therefore an average measurement of water diffusion.

A strength of this technique is that diffusion-sensitizing gradients can be oriented to measure water diffusion in a specific direction. The measured diffusion coefficient D is referred to as an "apparent" diffusion coefficient. The rate of water diffusion is "apparent" because we are not measuring the actual speed of water molecules, but how far the molecules are permitted to move in a specified period of time, taking into account biologic diffusion barriers. DWI can probe the structure of biologic materials and identify these barriers to water diffusion. By measuring water diffusion rates in multiple directions, we can classify water diffusion in biologic tissues as *isotropic* (water diffuses at equal rates in all directions) or *anisotropic* (water diffuses preferentially in one particular direction) (Fig. 13-1). DWI has shown that intact white matter tracts of the central nervous system display anisotropy (36–38). This anisotropic water diffusion has been hypothesized to be due to the axon membrane and myelin sheaths acting as diffusion barriers perpendicular, or transverse, to the axons, whereas few of these barriers are encountered parallel, or longitudinal, to the axons (39–42).

Diffusion-tensor Magnetic Resonance Imaging: Background and Principles

Water diffusion in an anisotropic sample is best described as a tensor, as opposed to a scalar quantity, due to barriers resulting in variations of water diffusion coefficients depending on which direction the diffusivity is measured. Diffusion-tensor MRI (DTI) is a technique that allows us to measure principal diffusivities in a sample without worrying about sample orientations. Diffusion tensors are typically measured by obtaining ADC values in multiple different directions (generally six or greater). From the DTI data, multiple measurements can be obtained:

1. Three diffusivity measures can be derived from the DTI data, the first of which describes the largest direction of diffusivity, and the second and third of which are orthogonal to the first measure, thus delineating a three-dimensional ellipsoid (43). The largest diffusion value is the first eigenvalue ($\lambda 1$), and the

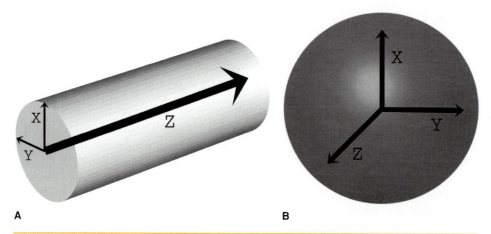

A   **B**

FIGURE 13-1. Schematic representation of anisotropic water diffusion in a cylinder, in which diffusion is preferential in a particular direction, which happens to be the Z-direction in this example **(A)**. Axons in the spinal cord can be conceived as packed cylinders with preferential water diffusion longitudinal (parallel) to their long axis. When no preferential direction of water diffusion exists, this property is referred to as isotropic water diffusion. Schematic representation of isotropic water diffusion in a sphere, in which water diffusion is equal in all measured X-, Y- and Z-directions **(B)**. (Adapted from Schwartz ED, Hackney DB. Diffusion weighted MRI and the evaluation of spinal cord axonal integrity following injury and treatment. *Exp Neurol.* 2003;184(2):570–589, with permission.)

second and third diffusion values are the second ($\lambda2$) and third ($\lambda3$) eigenvalues, respectively (Fig. 13-2). This rotationally invariant measure of water diffusion and orientation can be determined on a voxel-by-voxel basis.

2. Quantitative measures of diffusional anisotropy can then be calculated based on formulas that incorporate the tensor elements (44). Two common measures include:
   a. Fractional anisotropy (FA) is a dimensionless, but quantitative, measure that will acquire a value of 0

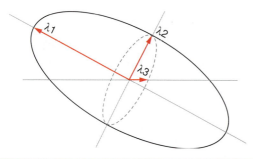

FIGURE 13-2. Schematic of the ellipsoid defined by diffusion tensor imaging. The eigenvalues are the diffusion values in the three orthogonal directions that define the ellipsoid, with the first eigenvalue ($\lambda1$) representing the largest diffusion value (major axis), and the second ($\lambda2$) and third ($\lambda3$) eigenvalues representing the minor axes. The third eigenvalue ($\lambda3$) represents the smallest diffusion value. In white matter, $\lambda1$ is equivalent to "longitudinal diffusion" with $\lambda2$ and $\lambda3$ equivalent to "transverse diffusion."

when tissue is purely isotropic and will tend toward 1 for highly anisotropic, cylindrically symmetric, diffusion (45).
   b. The lattice index (LI) anisotropy also provides a robust, dimensionless measure of diffusion tensor anisotropy (with values tending toward 0 for isotropic diffusion); however, this measure also incorporates local averaging to reduce effects of noise (46).
3. Trace diffusion is an overall measure of diffusion within the voxel (average diffusivity of the tissue) and can be defined by the equation ($\lambda1 + \lambda2 + \lambda3$)/3.
4. The directionality of $\lambda1$ can also be determined, which has been shown in normal white matter to be parallel to the long axis of axons, thus indicating the direction of white matter fiber tracts. There are numerous methods of visualizing this directionality. A color map, similar to proposed schemes (47–49), can be created in which the x, y, and z components of the principal direction of diffusion are assigned respectively to the red, green, and blue pixel channel values. This color map may be displayed as a color sphere in order to indicate direction of principal diffusivity, and the intensity of the voxel can be weighted by the degree of anisotropy.

Using either DWI or DTI techniques, the preferred direction of water diffusion in spinal cord white matter tracts has been shown in numerous ex vivo (21,50–57) and in vivo (58–66) experimental studies, as well as in vivo human studies (67–73), to be parallel, or longitudinal, to the long axis of the axons (Fig. 13-3).

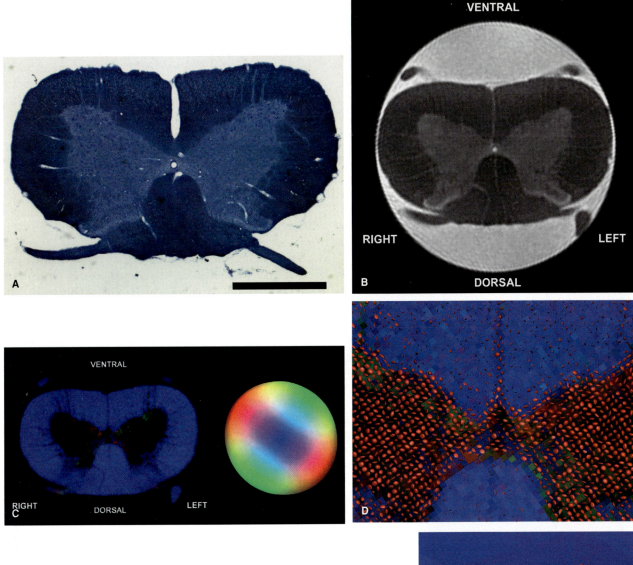

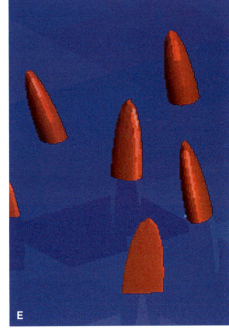

FIGURE 13-3. Normal cervical spinal cord section stained with Nissl-Myelin staining **(A)** (black bar = 1 mm) with corresponding T2 weighted axial image **(B)**, and color-coded diffusion tensor image **(C)** of ex vivo normal rat cervical spinal cord. A color sphere is provided adjacent to the diffusion tensor image in order to indicate the preferential direction of water diffusion seen in the spinal cord. The diffusion tensor image shows white matter to be blue, indicating, as shown with the color sphere, preferential water diffusion to be perpendicular to the plane of the image, in the expected rostral-caudal direction. Another method of presenting anisotropic and directional information is to create a three-dimensional ellipsoid for each pixel in the DTI image. The central portion of the spinal cord with representative ellipsoids for each pixel **(D)** shows how the ellipsoids in the gray matter are more rounded and larger than those in the white matter, indicating less anisotropy and increased trace diffusion. An enlarged image of the ventral white matter **(E)** demonstrates the expected cigar-shape ellipsoids for white matter, indicating strong rostral-caudal anisotropy. (Adapted and reproduced from Schwartz ED, et al. Spinal cord diffusion tensor imaging and fiber tracking can identify white matter tract disruption and glial scar orientation following lateral funiculotomy. *J Neurotrauma*. December 2005;22(12):1388–1398, with permission.)

DIFFUSION-WEIGHTED AND DIFFUSION-TENSOR MAGNETIC RESONANCE IMAGING OF THE EX VIVO SPINAL CORD

Regarding DWI and DTI, the spinal cord has been less studied than the brain. One reason is the small size of the spinal cord, which therefore requires higher field strength magnets and longer imaging times to achieve images comparable to brain research. In vivo imaging of the spinal cord is also hindered by technical factors, including motion artifacts arising from respiratory and cardiac activity, as well as cerebral spinal fluid (CSF) pulsations resulting in movement of the spinal cord itself. Experimental animal studies, however, have permitted the imaging of ex vivo spinal cord specimens, which avoids these problems.

As with white matter tracts in the brain, anisotropy in the spinal cord appears to be due to diffusion barriers encountered as water moves in the direction perpendicular to the fibers. These barriers are believed to be cellular membranes and myelin sheaths, which result in a low tADC (transverse ADC). As water diffuses longitudinally in the spinal cord, these diffusion barriers are not encountered, and lADC (longitudinal ADC) is therefore large in comparison to tADC.

Ex vivo studies of the spinal cord have confirmed its anisotropic properties. Pattany et al. (50) studied both fresh and fixed cat spinal cords and demonstrated anisotropic diffusion in the spinal cord white matter tracts with tADC values ranging from approximately $0.1 - 0.3 \times 10^{-3}$ mm²/s and lADC values ranging from approximately $0.6 - 1.0 \times 10^{-3}$ mm²/s. Measurements of white matter in formaldehyde fixed rat spinal cords from two different studies showed similar ADC values (21,53). These studies of fixed rat and cat spinal cord demonstrated that the lADC was significantly greater than the tADC, as would be expected in white matter. In these three studies, the tADC was measured in only one direction, which may be either anterior-posterior or left-right.

Other ex vivo studies have utilized DTI, which again confirm the anisotropic properties of the spinal cord. Additionally, the longitudinal orientation of the axons has also been shown to result in cylindrical symmetry (74), so that the anterior-posterior tADC is equivalent to the left-right tADC if the spinal cord is properly aligned without curvature. Therefore, a full diffusion tensor may not be necessary in the spinal cord, as the principal diffusivities derived from the tensor can be derived from one lADC and one tADC measurement. Inglis et al. (59) compared diffusion tensor imaging with ADC mapping, however, and found that ADC measurements tended to underestimate high diffusivities and overestimate low diffusivities in white matter, thereby underestimating the degree of anisotropy. These findings would suggest that obtaining ADC values without tensors might not be sufficient to evaluate principal diffusivities in the spinal cord. Gulani et al. (74) demonstrated cylindrical symmetry by obtaining four of the six elements of the diffusion tensor with resulting principal diffusivities similar to those obtained with all six tensor elements. They also noted that differences in anterior-posterior and left-right diffusion values with measured diffusion coefficients were within experimental error. Interestingly, the measured ADC values in the left-right, anterior-posterior, and longitudinal directions were within experimental error of principal diffusivities obtained with tensor imaging. This finding is different from that reported by Inglis et al. (59), and suggests that if spinal cords are carefully oriented in the magnetic field frame of reference, ADC values will provide an accurate assessment of principal diffusivities of the spinal cord white matter. Recent reports, however, indicate that obtaining a full diffusion tensor may provide more information concerning white matter fiber architecture. The directionality of the second eigenvalue (second eigenvector) appears to correlate with collateral nerve fibers (75). High-resolution DTI has also shown that white matter fibers running transversely toward the exiting nerve roots can be identified (76) (Fig. 13-4).

All these studies have demonstrated anisotropic diffusion within the white matter. The situation in gray matter is not as clear. In general, the tADC values and lADC matters of gray matter are similar, with tADC values greater than white matter, and lADC values less than white matter. Two studies of fixed rat spinal cord have shown slight anisotropy, with a larger lADC than tADC (21,77), while fixed cat spinal cords showed a slightly elevated tADC as compared to lADC (50). The direction of the tADC measurement (left-right or anterior-posterior) may be important, as high-resolution diffusion tensor imaging showed variability within the gray matter that appeared to correspond to anatomic fiber orientation (59,76). More rapid longitudinal diffusion was seen in the substantia gelatinosa where small fibers from the tract of Lissauer are ascending and descending, whereas there was left-right anisotropy in the gray commissure where these axons cross (Fig. 13-4).

The confirmation of anisotropy within spinal cord white matter tracts helps substantiate the hypotheses that tADC measures water diffusion in the presence of barriers, such as the cell membrane and myelin sheath, and that lADC measures water diffusion without significant restrictive effects from cell membranes. These theories received further support by Gulani et al. (56) in which diffusion tensor measurements were obtained from fixed ex vivo specimens of myelin deficient rats. Anisotropic diffusion was demonstrated in these myelin deficient rats, but there was a greater degree of anisotropy in their normal controls. Analysis of principal diffusivities derived from the diffusion tensor showed that there was a greater proportional increase of transverse diffusivity compared to

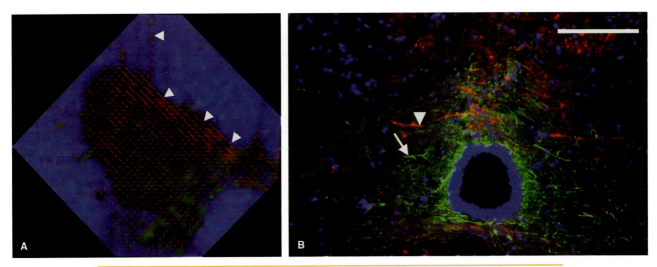

FIGURE 13-4. An enlarged view of the central and lateral gray matter of the normal spinal cord **(A)** from Figure 13-3, with lines for each pixel indicating the direction of primary ($\lambda 1$) diffusivity. The central gray matter surrounding the central canal, which is black, appearing to be a combination of red and green; this finding indicates left-right diffusional anisotropy that is seen with the left-right orientation of the primary diffusivity and may be expected due to left-right orientation of crossing axons and glial processes. Histologic image **(B)** shows the glial processes (*white arrowhead*—stained green for GFAP, a glial marker), and axonal fibers (*white arrow*—stained red for RT-97, an axonal marker), confirm their left-right orientation in the midline. Also note that the lines of principal diffusivity also appear to track axons that exit ventrally through the white matter (*A, arrowheads*). (Adapted and reproduced from Schwartz ED, Duda J, Shumsky JS, et al. Spinal cord diffusion tensor imaging and fiber tracking can identify white matter tract disruption and glial scar orientation following lateral funiculotomy. *J Neurotrauma*. December 2005;22(12):1388–1398, with permission.)

longitudinal diffusivity in myelin deficient rats than in normal controls. Although myelination is not solely responsible for diffusion anisotropy, it nevertheless does play an important role in generating diffusion anisotropy in white matter. The fact that longitudinal diffusivity also increased suggests that myelin may restrict diffusion in any direction. Therefore, as expected, the overall trace diffusion (average of three principal diffusivities) was greater in myelin deficient rats, suggesting that the lack of myelination resulted in an overall decrease in diffusion barriers. Gray matter was also studied and there were only minimal changes between the myelin deficient and normal rats, likely due to the relatively small number of myelinated axon fibers present in normal gray matter.

Observed differences in diffusion measurements between experimental settings may be due to a number of factors. Differences in fixation methods and fixative may affect diffusion values. In order to evaluate fixative effect, we obtained ADC values in normal spinal cords perfusion fixed with formaldehyde alone or with a combination of glutaraldehyde/formaldehyde. A glutaraldehyde/formaldehyde solution has been shown to preserve the myelin sheath and ultrastructural proteins such as intra-axonal cytoskeletal proteins better than buffered formaldehyde alone (78). We found there was a significant decrease in anisotropy (as measured with the ratio tADC/lADC) in the white matter of

glutaraldehyde/formaldehyde fixed specimens compared to formaldehyde only fixed specimens, mostly due to lower lADC values in the glutaraldehyde/formaldehyde fixed specimens (53). This finding may be due to better preservation of the cytoskeletal proteins, as research has shown that breakdown of the cytoskeletal proteins will decrease intra-axonal water diffusion (79). Interestingly, there were no differences between the two fixatives with respect to tADC; a smaller tADC may have been expected with glutaraldehyde/formaldehyde as it better preserves the myelin sheath than formaldehyde alone, and it may be that actual loss of myelin is required to affect tADC values.

Another factor to consider when comparing and reviewing ADC values is the temperature of acquisition, as measured water diffusion increases with temperature. Differing MRI equipment and pulse sequences may also affect ADC measurements. It is clear that normal controls for each research model are necessary.

MATHEMATICAL MODELS AND COMPUTER SIMULATIONS OF WATER DIFFUSION

The correlation between observed diffusion behavior and underlying physiological mechanism is not fully understood. Therefore, in order to facilitate interpretations of experimental observations and to delineate pathology of the spinal cord injury, numerical methods have been developed to simulate water diffusion behavior in spinal cord for both normal and injured models (80–84). By making certain assumptions, such as intracellular and extracellular diffusion rates and axonal shape, this approach allows for adjustments in both imaging parameters and possible histologic parameters in the simulations. Subsequent comparisons of simulations to actual data can help determine the effect of histologic factors (i.e., axonal size, axonal spacing, myelin sheath integrity/permeability, and myelin sheath thickness) on diffusion data, both with normal and injured spinal cords.

More realistic computer models have been recently developed (80,85–87) that are based on histologic images, as opposed to geometric approximations of axons, such as square prisms (84), cylinders (82,83), and ellipsoids (81). Myelin comprises a significant proportion of white matter cross-sectional area and can undergo morphologic changes during injury and repair (88,89). Therefore, instead of modeling myelin sheaths as infinitesimally thin membranes, myelin is more accurately modeled as multiple concentric bilipid layers, which result in anisotropic diffusion. The model thus provides flexibility in modeling various pathologic changes. To validate this model, Chin et al. (87) looked at the effects of time dependency and permeability on diffusion simulations with a digitized histologic section of the spinal cord. Their findings suggest that factors other than volume fractions of intracellular (intra-axonal) space (ICS), extracellular space (ECS) may be important in deriving ADC values in white matter. Histologic factors include the permeability of the axonal membrane and geometric spacing/orientation of the axons. Water exchange among cellular components is another important factor in determining ADC values, which suggests that proximity of water to the myelin sheath may be important and that differences in ADC will be seen in white matter with differing average axon diameters, even if overall volume fraction does not change.

Direct Correlation of Axon Morphometry with Diffusion Values

A critical goal of spinal cord imaging research is a noninvasive quantifiable predictor of axon loss. Although the mathematical models and computer simulations of water diffusion discussed above have been useful in determining the histologic factors that affect the changes in diffusion parameters seen following injury, we have taken a more straightforward approach by directly correlating axon morphometric parameters with transverse and longitudinal water diffusion. In order to obtain quantifiable histology, we developed an automated computer program that

segments axons and quantifies their morphometric parameters from a digitized histologic image (Fig. 13-5). Using these data, we have shown that the natural variation of differing axon morphometric parameters (including axon density, axon spacing, axon diameter) between normal spinal cord tracts significantly correlates with different directional water diffusion values (54). Using regression analysis, we also showed that these quantitative measures of transverse and longitudinal diffusion could predict axon density with $R^2 = 64$. Thus it is possible to create predictive mathematic equations that can translate diffusion data into precise measures of axon density and morphometry. We found that transverse water diffusion was related to the tortuosity of the extracellular space, with decreased transverse water diffusion in those white matter tracts with densely packed axons. Longitudinal diffusion appeared to be related to axon diameter, with larger axons having increased diffusion; this may reflect decreased overall density of cytoskeletal proteins in larger axons, resulting in fewer barriers to water diffusion. These findings seem to suggest that measurements of anisotropy based on different directional ADC values may not be solely an appropriate measure of axonal damage. If the ADC in each direction is based on different histologic parameters, then solely obtaining a ratio provides no more information than evaluating each of the ADC values separately and may actually provide less information.

DIFFUSION-WEIGHTED AND DIFFUSION-TENSOR MAGNETIC RESONANCE IMAGING OF THE IN VIVO RODENT SPINAL CORD

In vivo imaging of the rat spinal cord is difficult due to the small size of the spinal cord, motion, and time limitations. Nevertheless, there have been a number of publications confirming the anisotropic properties of spinal cord white matter in vivo. Nakada et al. (66) used a 7-T magnet to obtain in vivo diffusion encoding information in three directions in a rat. From this data, the authors constructed a color-coded image that displayed anisotropic directional information. Differentiation of gray and white matter was possible, and anisotropic water diffusion was seen in the white matter. These studies were limited by long acquisition times, as a single spin-echo sequence took almost 52 minutes. The data presented were qualitative, however, and no diffusion coefficients were provided.

Fenyes and Narayana (62,90,91) have published a series of papers that discuss and provide possible solutions to the difficulties arising from in vivo diffusion imaging of the rat spinal cord. The spinal cord in vivo is located further from the MRI receiver coil than an ex vivo specimen, resulting in decreased signal-to-noise ratio (SNR) with resultant poorer quality images. Fenyes and

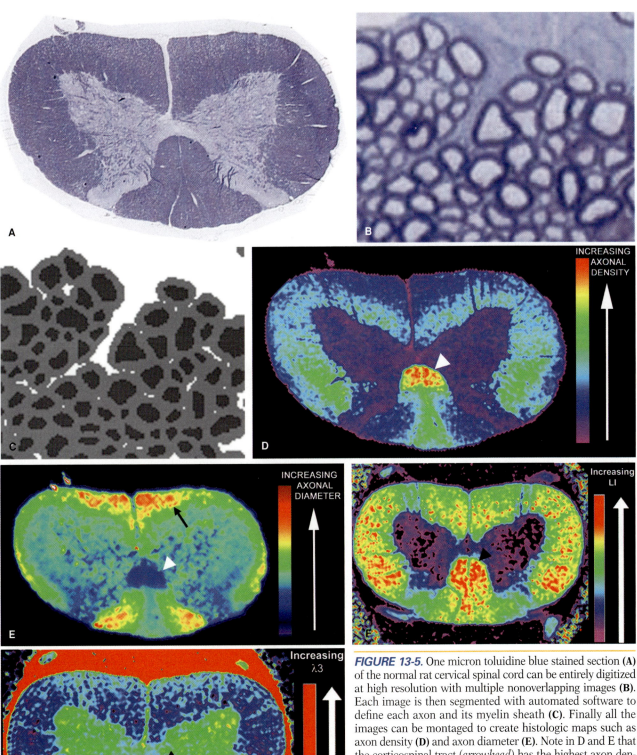

FIGURE 13-5. One micron toluidine blue stained section **(A)** of the normal rat cervical spinal cord can be entirely digitized at high resolution with multiple nonoverlapping images **(B)**. Each image is then segmented with automated software to define each axon and its myelin sheath **(C)**. Finally all the images can be montaged to create histologic maps such as axon density **(D)** and axon diameter **(E)**. Note in D and E that the corticospinal tract (*arrowhead*) has the highest axon density and smallest axon diameter, as expected. Also as expected, the vestibular spinal tract has the largest axons (*arrow, E*). These histologic maps can potentially be registered with DTI maps, such as lattice index anisotropy **(F)** and λ3 **(G)**. Note that the corticospinal tract (*arrowhead, F and G*) has the greatest anisotropy and smallest λ3, also consistent with previous studies that suggest that tightly packed axons have the smallest transverse diffusion and greatest anisotropy.

Narayana alleviate this problem by using surgically placed inductively coupled implantable coils over the dorsal aspect of the thoracic spine to increase SNR, a strategy used by other researchers as well (92,93). Motion artifacts from breathing were minimized by respiratory gating the MRI sequence. This required intubating the rats and using ventilators to ensure that MRI data acquisition was performed at the same point in the respiratory cycle. Other methods that decrease artifact include shimming the magnetic field, and postprocessing the data with reference scans. Fenyes and Narayana then could obtain a diffusion tensor of the spinal cord in vivo using a standard spin echo technique in 43 minutes, and multishot echoplanar imaging (EPI) sequence that decreased imaging time to 9 minutes. Although the spatial resolution was not as fine as in the ex vivo studies, anisotropy was seen in the white matter with longitudinal diffusion coefficient values in the white matter ranging from 2.22×10^{-3} mm^2/s (spin echo) to 2.11×10^{-3} mm^2/s (EPI) and transverse diffusion coefficients ranging from $0.36 - 0.56 \times 10^{-3}$ mm^2/s (higher values obtained with EPI). Gray matter was also noted to be anisotropic with longitudinal values ranging from $1.36 - 1.46 \times 10^{-3}$ mm^2/s and transverse values ranging from $0.41 - 0.59 \times 10^{-3}$ mm^2/s. Silver et al. (60) described similar in vivo anisotropic findings with an implantable coil, and, although no diffusion values were presented, they did provide a color-coded map of diffusion anisotropy. Much of this in vivo research with implantable coils has been performed in the thoracic spine, as the cervical spine is technically more difficult due to the necessity of maintaining coil configuration in a more mobile portion of the spinal column.

In vivo diffusion imaging of the spinal cord has also been performed without implantable coils as well (58,94). Although anisotropic water diffusion was seen in both gray and white matter, the values in these reports differed from those reported by Fenyes and Narayana. While these findings raise issues of reproducibility, it should be noted that measurements were taken in different parts of the spinal cord (cervical versus thoracic) and full diffusion tensor measurements were not obtained. Therefore, ADC values could be less accurate due to inadvertent misalignment of the experimental (spinal cord) and laboratory (MRI gradient) frame of reference.

Applicability of Ex Vivo Findings to the In Vivo Setting

Although the use of fixed tissue allows for higher resolution imaging, the question of whether findings from ex vivo studies are applicable in the in vivo setting is often raised. A DTI study comparing in vivo mouse brain with fixed mouse brain showed that while overall trace diffusions decreases in fixed tissue, the directional ADC values decrease proportionally, resulting in identical anisotropy

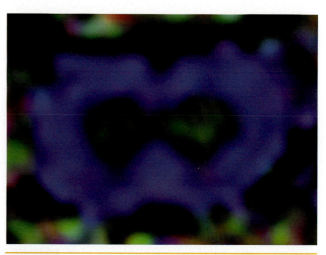

FIGURE 13-6. In vivo axial color-coded diffusion tensor image of the normal rat spinal cord at the thoracic-lumbar junction. As with ex vivo imaging, there is strong rostral-caudal anisotropic diffusion in the white matter, again seen as blue.

data (95). Recently, Madi et al. (63) also looked at this issue in a study that compared in vivo and ex vivo DTI data of the rat spinal cord. As with Sun et al. (95), they found decreased average diffusivity in the fixed, excised spinal cord; however, they also found increased anisotropy (measured with FA) in the in vivo setting. They did see a linear relationship between the in vivo and ex vivo values ($r = 0.99$ for FA), however, they noted that care needs to be taken in interpreting in vivo pathology from ex vivo data.

We performed in vivo DTI of the rat thoracic spinal cord using a 4.7-T magnet with a standard spin echo diffusion tensor sequence for both cardiac gating and respiratory gating to minimize spinal cord motion (Fig. 13-6). In addition to evaluating measures of anisotropy, we also looked at eigenvalues between different spinal cord tracts. Our diffusion values for white matter appeared similar to those of Madi et al. (63). By looking at specific spinal cord tracts, we found significant differences that correlated with our previous ex vivo studies (53), in that spinal cord tracts with the larger axons, such as the vestibulospinal tract in the ventral white matter, had larger longitudinal and transverse diffusivities. Therefore, the same histologic factors that were related to ex vivo diffusion data (see above, "Direct Correlation of Axon Morphometry with Diffusion Values") appear to be important in determining in vivo diffusion data as well.

Biexponential Diffusion in Neural Tissue

Prior publications have discussed the presence of two diffusion fractions (fast and slow) in neural tissue based on biexponential DWI models using high b-values (96–98) and have argued that these diffusion fractions correlate with volume fractions of the extracellular and intracellular spaces, respectively (99). Computer simulations, however, do not support the notion that the fast and slow components obtained with biexponential fits correspond solely to the intracellular and extracellular volume fractions (87).

In general, biexponential diffusion is seen using *b*-values ranging from 4,000 to 10,000 s/mm^2 (96,98–100). Elshafiey et al. (61), however, reported biexponential diffusion in the rat spinal cord in vivo, and suggested that biexponential diffusion may be seen with *b*-values as low as 1,600 s/mm^2. If not taken into account, this property could result in artifactually low ADC values. In our ex vivo studies with *b*-values ranging up to 3,100 s/mm^2, we performed linear regression analysis and demonstrated robust linear fit to our data, both in the transverse and longitudinal directions, with R^2 >0.99 (53). Although a slow diffusing component may be identified with much larger *b*-values, we have used a monoexponential fit for our data as the diffusion values appear to primarily arise from the fast diffusing component.

DIFFUSION-WEIGHTED AND DIFFUSION-TENSOR MAGNETIC RESONANCE IMAGING IN EXPERIMENTAL SPINAL CORD INJURY

Evaluation of Axonal Integrity

Axonal transection is only partly responsible for the functional deficits resulting from spinal cord injury. Much of the damage is due to secondary injury that expands the size of the lesion with additional degeneration of axonal fiber tracts (101,102,103). Within 15 minutes, intact myelinated axons swell and there is a reduction in intact neurofilaments (104). Myelin sheaths then begin to split, and vesicles may form in larger axons (105). It may be postulated that damage to the myelin sheath should increase membrane permeability, which would subsequently increase the tADC. The effect of myelin on lADC values is not as strong, and therefore the cellular swelling seen in damaged axons, as well as loss of energy dependent systems in transected axons, may be expected to lower the lADC. Treatments for spinal cord injury, however, may attenuate these diffusion changes, and perhaps correct diffusion values over time. Early experimental research has supported these hypotheses.

Ford et al. (21) showed that alterations in ADC values were more sensitive than conventional MRI techniques in detecting spinal cord injury. They measured tADC and lADC values in fixed rat spinal cords that had been subjected to thoracic spinal cord weight drop injury and then sacrificed seven days later. T2 maps were created with a spin echo sequence utilizing identical slice thickness and positioning. Conventional MRI was used to subjectively evaluate the spinal cord, and in areas where gray matter

and white matter could be differentiated, the gray matter, dorsal white matter, and lateral white matter were described as normal appearing versus abnormal appearing. At the lesion center, large portions of the spinal cord were so severely damaged that gray matter could not be distinguished from white matter. As expected, the axial slices farthest from the lesion center appeared more normal. At all sites, whether appearing abnormal or normal, the T2 values did not differ significantly from normal controls. Following injury, tADC values increased and lADC values decreased in both normal and abnormal appearing white matter. These changes resulted in decreased anisotropy. These results imply that there are consequences of spinal cord injury that dramatically alter axon structure without changing water content or T2, and, therefore, would not be detected by conventional MRI. If we assume that the myelin sheaths and cell membranes restrict water diffusion in the transverse direction, then the loss of diffusion anisotropy at the lesion epicenter may be due to mechanical disruption of the axons and their myelin sheaths. Farther from the lesion center, axonal swelling may have decreased the lADC, while the increased tADC may be attributed to increased permeability of damaged and degenerating myelin sheaths or cell membranes.

Nevo et al. (55) has recently shown that measurement of ADC values and anisotropy can be used to quantify spinal cord injury and neuroprotection. Rats were subjected to a weight drop contusion injury. Untreated rats were then compared with rats treated with T cells specific to the central nervous system self-antigen myelin basic protein, an intervention that has been shown to be neuroprotective (106). Rats were sacrificed after more than 3 months and ex vivo MRI was performed. Anisotropy maps were created and visual inspection of these maps suggested that there was lower anisotropy in both treated and untreated rats compared to control animals, possibly reflecting spinal cord injury and disruption of anisotropic axon fibers. There also appeared to be less anisotropic tissue at the lesion site and surrounding tissue in untreated rats compared to treated rats, perhaps due to neuroprotection in treated rats. Histograms were constructed from portions of the spinal cord near the injury center, revealing greater loss of anisotropy in untreated rats compared to treated rats. Locomotor scores were obtained for these animals and improved scores were seen in the treated animals, and decreased anisotropy appeared to correspond with poorer locomotor performance. Although detailed histologic analysis was not performed, the authors attribute the improved anisotropy in the treated rats to enhanced survival of myelinated fibers and decreased formation of cysts. This study suggests that measures of anisotropy in the injured spinal cord may be used to evaluate injury severity and possibly evaluate treatment effects.

Changes in apparent diffusion coefficients in spinal cord white matter have been correlated with behavioral recovery following cervical lateral funiculus lesion and transplantation of fibroblasts genetically modified to express brain-derived neurotrophic factor (BDNF) (51). BDNF acts on the TrkB receptors located on rubrospinal tract (RST) axons and red nucleus neurons, and BDNF secreting fibroblasts placed into spinal cord lesions have been shown to promote neuroprotection of red nucleus neurons, regeneration of RST axons, and growth of other axons, as well as improving behavioral recovery, when compared with transplants of unmodified fibroblasts (Fb-UM) (107–112). After 12 weeks of behavioral testing, rats, with either Fb-BDNF or Fb-UM transplants, were sacrificed and fixed spinal cords were imaged in a 9.4-T magnet. ADCs perpendicular (tADC) and parallel (lADC) to the long axis of the cord were measured in the dorsal lateral white matter up to 2.5 mm rostral and caudal to the transplant, and an anisotropy index (AI = tADC/lADC) was also derived. Within the white matter rostral and caudal to the transplant, the tADC values and AI were elevated, and the lADC values were decreased, in both transplant types, however, rats with Fb-BDNF transplants had values were significantly closer to normal controls (Fig. 13-7). Histological and immunocytochemical examinations showed comparable lesion sizes and transplant survival in the two groups, with substantial growth of axons into Fb-BDNF grafts but little growth into Fb-UM grafts. Therefore, DWI may be able to provide noninvasive

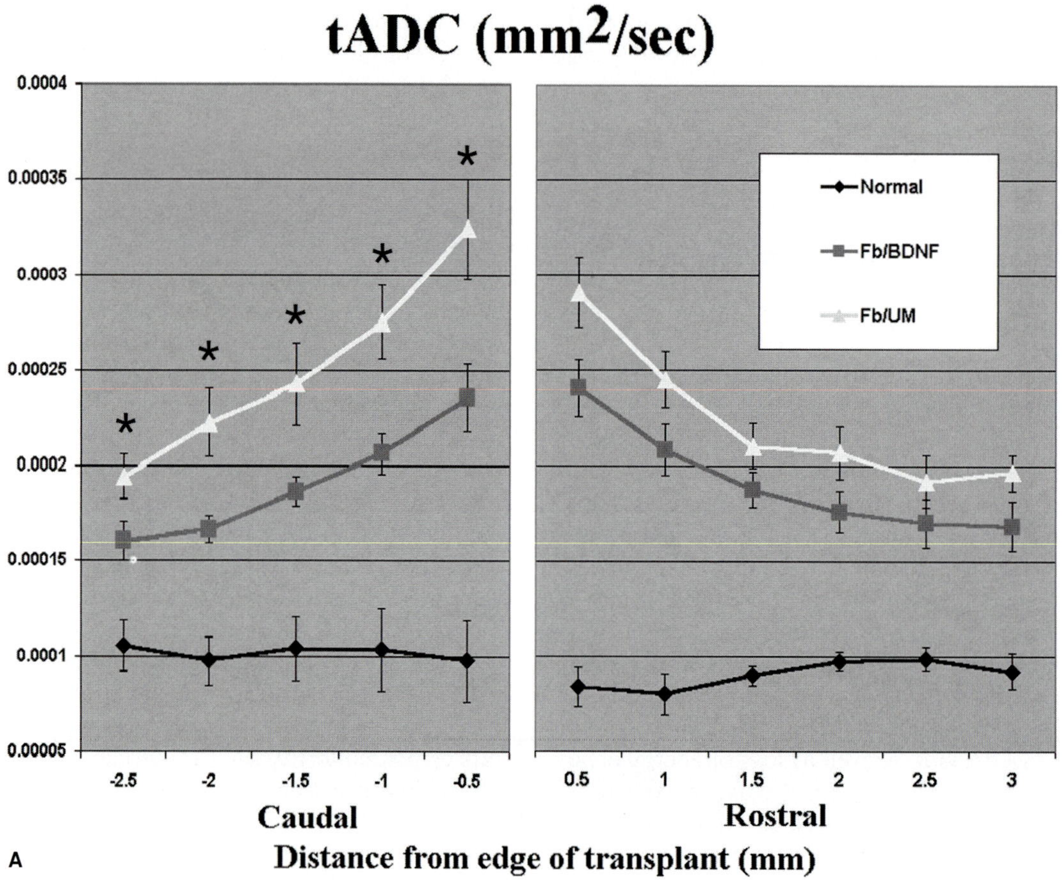

FIGURE 13-7. Graphs show tADC **(A)**, lADC **(B)**, and AI **(C)** values of the right dorsal lateral white matter versus distance from the rostral or caudal edge of the transplant. All values of operated animals with functioning transplants (Fb-BDNF) and nonfunctioning transplants (Fb-UM) were significantly different ($p < 0.05$) from normal values at each distance point. Asterisks indicate statistically significant ($p < 0.05$) differences between Fb-UM and Fb-BDNF animals at a specific distance point; note that those animals with functioning transplants had DWI values closer to normal. Note that values become closer to normal farther from the site of injury, which is expected as the amount of indirect injury should decrease with increasing distance from direct lesion center. (Reproduced from Schwartz ED, Shumsky JS, Wehrli S, et al. MR determined apparent diffusion coefficients correlate with motor recovery mediated by intraspinal transplants of fibroblasts genetically modified to express BDNF. *Exp Neurol.* 2003;82(1):49–63, with permission.)

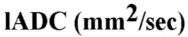

lADC (mm²/sec)

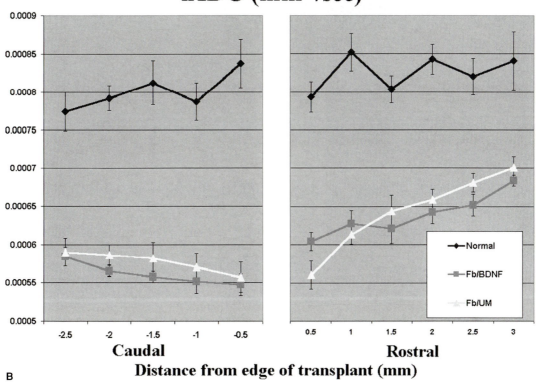

B

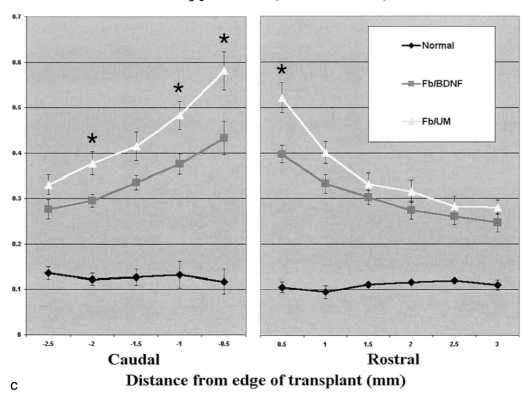

C

FIGURE 13-7. (CONTINUED).

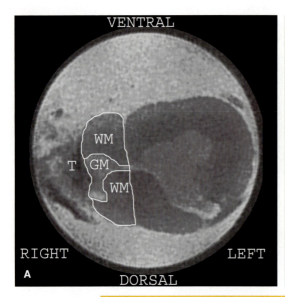
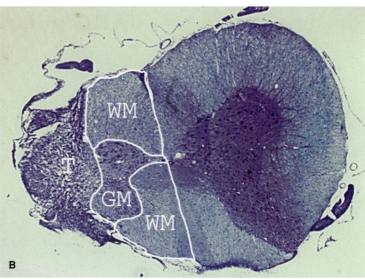

FIGURE 13-8. T2 weighted axial image of an ex vivo rat spinal cord following partial hemisection and transplantation **(A)** clearly delineates white matter (*WM*) and gray matter (*GM*) from the transplant (*T*). Corresponding histologic image **(B)** stained with nissl-myelin confirms the MRI findings. (Reproduced and adapted from Schwartz ED, Shumsky JS, Wehrli S, et al. MR determined apparent diffusion coefficients correlate with motor recovery mediated by intraspinal transplants of fibroblasts genetically modified to express BDNF. *Exp Neurol*. 2003;182(1):49–63, with permission.)

measurements that reflect axon regrowth and neuroprotection. Over 12 weeks, rats with Fb-BDNF transplants showed significantly greater behavioral recovery than did Fb-UM animals as measured by tests of forelimb exploration and open field locomotor activity. The tADC and AI values 0.5 mm caudal to the transplant were correlated with the extent of behavioral recovery. The correlation of DWI measures with behavior also suggests that these measures are functionally significant.

In a follow-up study, we used the tract tracer biotinylated dextran amine (BDA) to provide a quantitative measure of axon survival and dieback, also following partial cervical hemisection and fibroblast transplantation (52). Prior to sacrifice, BDA was injected into the left red nucleus, predominantly labeling the contralateral and descending right rubrospinal tract. Following ex vivo imaging of the spinal cord in a 9.4-T magnet, axons of the rubrospinal tract rostral to the site of injury could be counted on transverse histologic sections. As expected, there was retraction, or dieback, of the rubrospinal axons, with fewer axons seen closer to the site of injury. ADC values were also significantly more abnormal as measurements were obtained closer to the site of injury. There was also a linear correlation between the degree of axonal loss and the diffusion values (tADC:$r = 0.72$, lADC:$r = -0.69$, and anisotropy index tADC/lADC:$r = 0.77$), providing the first evidence that ADC values can quantitate the degree of axonal pathology following injury. As seen in the prior study, the ADC values in functioning BDNF producing transplants were lower than in unmodified transplants. In

this study, it was seen that these lower ADC values also correlated with decreased axonal dieback, suggesting that functioning grafts, which stimulate axonal sprouting or regrowth, can be identified by their lower ADC values.

In the two prior studies, it was seen that the T2 weighted images could be used to accurately segment the graft from the remaining white and gray matter (51,52) (Fig. 13-8). This finding supports two previous studies by Wirth et al. (113,114) that used in vivo MRI to evaluate fetal graft survival in the injured feline spinal cord. Other studies suggest that the temporal evolution of diffusion values may reflect changes in graft composition that are not seen with conventional MRI, with such diffusion values decreasing as cellularity increases (40).

Fraidakis et al. (58) used a standard diffusion weighted spin echo sequence in a 4.7-T magnet with a surface coil to obtain in vivo images 2 to 6 months following transection of rat spinal cords. In this study, diffusion anisotropy was seen to progressively decline toward the cut ends of the spinal cord. Abnormalities in the surrounding intact spinal cord, both rostral and caudal, were seen up to 6.6 mm from the transection site, suggesting that degenerative changes can be seen in the spinal cord away from the actual site of injury. However, histologic evaluation was unable to determine whether these changes were due entirely to axonal degeneration or partially due to the development of microcysts.

Banasik et al. (115) performed in vivo DWI in three orthogonal directions following a weight drop injury to the rat spinal cord, with some animals receiving treatment with a glutamate receptor antagonist (2-methyl-6-(pheny-lethynyl)pyridine; MPEP) that is thought to decrease excitatory amino acid toxicity following spinal cord injury (SCI). At 48 hours postinjury, they found that transverse ADC values in white matter at the injury level were elevated only in the surgical control animals, while the MPEP-treated animals had values similar to normal controls. In gray matter, the ADC values of the injured animals are elevated; however, the values of the MPEP-treated animals are closer to those of normal controls. Although there was no difference in locomotor recovery between the two sets of injured animals, the authors conclude that DWI can detect the neuroprotective effects of treatment for SCI.

Deo et al. (116) used implantable coils and a 7-T magnet to perform serial in vivo DTI up to 56 days postcontusion SCI. They found that FA values, as well as individual directional diffusivities, could evaluate endogenous tissue recovery and remyelination.

We have seen that at 24 hours posthemisection injury, transverse diffusion decreases in the white matter rostral and caudal to the injury. This finding may be related to the axonal swelling that occurs prior to breakdown of the myelin sheath. This swelling results in a more tortuous extracellular space, which, as noted above (see "Direct Correlation of Axon Morphometry with Diffusion Values"), correlates with transverse diffusion. Longitudinal diffusion decreases, and this may be related to breakdown of cytoskeletal components acutely, which may decrease intra-axonal water diffusion (79) prior to subsequent clearing of these breakdown products.

Evaluation of Gray Matter and Transplants

Late changes in SCI also include liquefaction and necrosis of tissue resulting in cystic lesions. ADC values were measured in a rat model of syringomyelia, in which an excitatory amino acid is injected into gray matter, resulting in cavities within the spinal cord parenchyma that have histologic properties similar to posttraumatic syringes (77). Ex vivo MRI and DWI was performed at 1, 4, and 8 weeks following injections. By 1 week after injection, tADC and lADC maps at the level of injection could detect regions of cavitation; however, conventional T1 and T2 weighted images showed cystic changes only at 4 and 8 weeks (Fig. 13-9). ADC values also were seen to

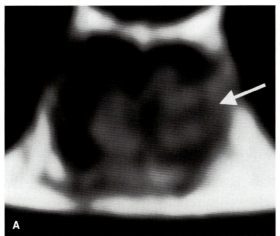
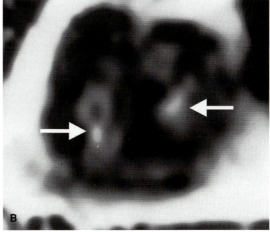
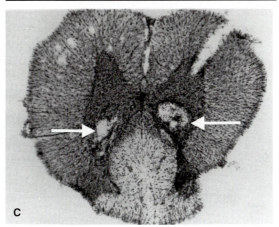

FIGURE 13-9. DWI syringomyelia. T2-weighted image **(A)** of rat spinal cord 1-week postquisqualic acid injection shows abnormal heterogeneous signal in the gray matter, worse on the left, with associated loss of normal gray/white differentiation (*white arrow*). Corresponding ADC map **(B)** shows two areas of increased signal (*arrows*), corresponding to the two cavities partially filled with cellular debris on the histopathologic specimen (*white arrows*) **(C)**. (Reproduced from Schwartz ED, Yezierski RP, Pattany PM, et al. MR and diffusion weighted imaging in a rat model of syringomyelia following excitotoxic spinal cord injury. *AJNR Am J Neurorad.* 1999;20:1422–1428, with permission.)

increase in the cystic areas as time progressed, possibly represent subsequent clearing of necrotic debris that otherwise would restrict water diffusion. These findings imply that diffusion imaging can reveal structural changes before conventional MRI, perhaps because alterations in water content only became apparent with conventional MRI after necrotic debris was replaced by fluid, while DWI could detect the early breakdown of diffusion barriers such as cell membranes.

DWI imaging has also been shown to differentiate between functioning and nonfunctioning transplants (51). In an ex vivo study, we saw that by 12 weeks spinal cord transplants that had functioning BDNF grafts had lower ADC values than nonfunctioning grafts. This finding appeared to correspond to greater ingrowth of axons into the graft, perhaps resulting in more diffusion barriers. It should be noted that diffusion was isotropic in both functioning and nonfunctioning grafts, again suggesting that evaluation of individual ADC values may be more important than calculated measures of anisotropy.

DTI may also be able to determine the degree of glial scarring in the gray matter following injury, which may go undetected with conventional MRI (76). We saw significantly increased left-right fractional anisotropy in the gray matter adjacent to a partial hemisection; this area appeared normal on T2 weighted images (Fig. 13-10). Histologic analysis indicated that the directionality and degree of glial scarring appeared to correlate with the DTI findings. As some current therapies are focused on decreasing the degree of glial scarring following injury, DTI may provide an important noninvasive outcome measure.

Traumatic Brain Injury

Diffusion imaging and evaluation of white matter following traumatic axonal injury to the brain has produced similar findings. Clinical studies have shown decreased anisotropy in areas of the brain that appeared normal with conventional MRI techniques (117,118), although diffusion tensor imaging was less sensitive than T2* sequences for identifying hemorrhagic lesions (119). Huisman et al. (120) have also shown that FA measurements in white matter correlated better with outcome than mean diffusivity in patients imaged within 1 week of injury. Diffusion tensor imaging of white matter following acute diffuse axonal injury in humans has shown that the principal diffusivity (equivalent to spinal cord lADC) decreased, and the second and third diffusivities (equivalent to spinal cord tADC) increased, subsequently decreasing anisotropy (121). These findings are similar to those seen in experimental spinal cord research. The authors suggest that the decreased anisotropy within 24 hours of injury is due initially to misalignment of the cytoskeletal network and axonal

membranes, which would increase the perpendicular diffusion measurements and decrease longitudinal diffusion, thus decreasing anisotropy. They note that axon swelling as well as impairment of axoplasmic transport may decrease diffusion along the axon long axis, while degeneration of axonal membranes would increase diffusion perpendicular to the axon long axis. At 1 month following injury, the diffusion tensor values appeared to partially correct or, in some cases, completely correct to normal values. Interestingly, as seen with spinal cord research, diffusion longitudinal to the white matter tracts did not significantly increase at 1 month following injury (121), despite Wallerian degeneration, which may be expected to remove barriers to water diffusion. Vorisek et al. (122) provide a possible explanation; they evaluated experimental traumatic brain injury with both DWI and real-time iontophoretic tetramethylammonium method to measure changes in the extracellular space. Initially there was significant increase in extracellular volume fraction (ECS volume/total tissue volume), however, by 1 month, the extracellular volume fraction had returned to control levels. They attribute these findings to the proliferation of astrocytes. There was also decreased water diffusion in areas without changes in extracellular volume, which they attribute to modifications in the extracellular matrix, and such increased expression of chondroitin sulfate proteoglycan may have increased diffusion barriers. These findings may help explain why lADC values decrease following experimental spinal cord injury despite axon loss (21,51).

Which Parameters Should Be Evaluated?

There is no consensus as yet on how to image (apparent diffusion coefficients only versus diffusion tensor imaging), and, similarly, there is no consensus on how to interpret the data. Some have looked at each separate diffusion coefficient, while others have focused on measurements of anisotropy. There are several ways of measuring anisotropy. Fractional anisotropy (FA) and LI anisotropy index derived from DTI tensor imaging yields values between 0 (isotropic diffusion as in a sphere) and 1 (perfectly anisotropic), representing the magnitude of the anisotropic component of the tensor as a percentage of the magnitude of the total diffusion tensor. Nevo et al. (55) defined other ratios to describe anisotropy. Others have used a simple ratio of tADC and lADC. Some authors prefer a more qualitative approach and have developed color traces designed to visually present anisotropic data. One of the difficulties with using anisotropy measures, however, is that they are derived from diffusion coefficient values. Since the diffusion coefficient may change in each orientation, reviewing only the ratios, and not the underlying diffusion values,

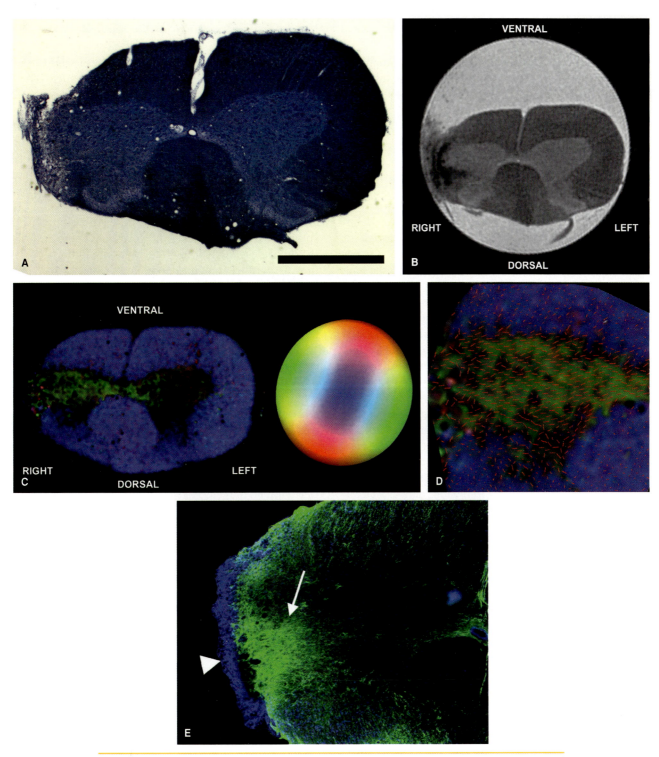

FIGURE 13-10. Nissl myelin stained section of cervical rat spinal cord section following partial hemisection **(A)** with corresponding ex vivo T2 weighted image **(B)** and color coded diffusion tensor image **(C)**. Although the right-sided white matter adjacent to the injury site appears to have normal signal on the T2 weighted image, the diffusion tensor image shows increased left-right diffusional anisotropy (indicated by green, refer to color coded sphere in C) as compared to normal animals (Fig. 13-3C). This finding is confirmed in the enlarged image **(D)** with lines indicating the principal direction of diffusivity in each pixel. **E:** Histologic image shows a left-right orientation of reactive glial processes in the gray matter adjacent to the transplant and extending to the midline (*arrow*, glial processes are stained green for GFAP, a glial marker). Arrowhead indicates blue-stained nuclei of a fibroblast transplant that was placed in the partial hemisection cavity. (Adapted and reproduced from Schwartz ED, Dude J, Shumsky JS, et al. Spinal cord diffusion tensor imaging and fiber tracking can identify white matter tract disruption and glial scar orientation following lateral funiculotomy. *J Neurotrauma*. December 2005;22(12):1388–1398, with permission.)

may be misleading. Therefore, it may be more valuable to look at individual diffusion coefficients, because differing histologic factors may be important for each directional ADC that is obtained.

DIFFUSION-TENSOR MAGNETIC RESONANCE IMAGING AND WHITE MATTER FIBER TRACTOGRAPHY

Recently, there has been an interest in using DTI to delineate axonal tracts based on intrinsic properties of anisotropy within white matter. As discussed above, water has been observed to diffuse preferentially along the long axis of the axon in white matter tracts. The primary explanation for this property has been that myelin sheaths and axon cellular membranes are barriers to water diffusion. Consequently, the direction of greatest water diffusion is felt to be oriented parallel to the axon or axon tract, while there is restricted diffusion in the transverse direction (perpendicular to the axon long axis). The direction of axon tracts in the brain can then be tracked by looking for anisotropic voxels that are adjacent to one another and that delineate known axon bundles. As axons may not run directly orthogonal to the magnetic field of the MRI scanner, axon-tracking methods generally rely on DTI (44). By assuming that the direction of greatest diffusion (longest axis of the ellipsoid) is parallel to the long axis of an axon bundle, an axon tract may be inferred by tracking the principal (largest) direction of diffusivity along many voxels. Although much of the research in axon tracking relies on known neuroanatomy, recent experimental studies have validated this method in the optic tracts by directly correlating diffusion tensor findings with an MRI detectable axon tracer (122).

In the spinal cord, fiber tractography may be used to evaluate integrity and continuity of white matter following injury. This fast method of graphically presenting DTI data may be important in the clinical setting when rapid decisions need to be made. In a study with ex vivo spinal cords following partial hemisection and transplantation, fiber tractography could accurately demonstrate disruption (and sparing) of the axons on the affected side (76) (Fig. 13-11). In vivo DTI of experimental hemisection spinal cord injury also showed similar findings (Fig. 13-12).

DIFFUSION-WEIGHTED AND DIFFUSION-TENSOR MAGNETIC RESONANCE IMAGING OF THE HUMAN SPINAL CORD

Perhaps what makes DWI and DTI of the spinal cord a relevant methodology is that new research has already

shown promise for the application of these sequences to human subjects (37,69,70,73,124–133). Although DWI is routinely applied to clinical brain MRI, there are technical difficulties associated with in vivo imaging of the spinal cord that are not as problematic in brain imaging. These difficulties include susceptibility artifacts from surrounding bony structures, motion from CSF pulsations, pulsation from carotid/vertebral arteries, respiratory motion, and the intrinsic small size of the spinal cord resulting in signal contamination from surrounding CSF (133). These challenges have limited development of spinal cord DWI and DTI; however, advances in pulse sequence development and hardware, including application of parallel imaging technology (Fig. 13-13), have improved image quality. Many of these initial studies have confirmed what was learned with experimental data, suggesting that this technique is valid and applicable to human spinal cord disease.

As with the animal studies, there appears to be evidence of cylindrical symmetry in human spinal cord white matter. Clark et al. (69,124) have used a sagittal spin echo sequence on a 1.5-T magnet to obtain tADC (both left-right and anterior-posterior) and lADC values. Their resolution was less than 1 mm, however gray-white differentiation was not possible. The tADC values they obtained were ~0.6 × 10-3 mm²/s for both directions and the lADC value was ~1.5 to 2.0 × 10-3 mm²/s. As the transverse values were similar, they suggested that the spinal cord had cylindrical symmetry and that the determination of the diffusion tensor can be achieved with ADC values in two directions. Ries et al. (133) performed diffusion tensor imaging of the spinal cord and also noted that differences between the anterior-posterior and right-left tADC values were not statistically significant.

In addition to normal studies, there have been reports of applying DWI and DTI to diseases of the spinal cord. Spinal cord ischemia has been studied mostly with nondirectional DWI, and it appears the findings are similar to those in the brain; following spinal cord infarction, there is early restriction of diffusion, followed by pseudonormalization and then increase of ADC values (134–142). In patients with demyelination, significant increases in mean diffusivities are seen in spinal cord white matter (69), and there have been reports of increased FA in normal appearing spinal cord white matter (143). In patients with spondylosis and spinal cord compression, it has been seen that diffusion MRI improves sensitivity to cervical myelopathy (144); however, there have been conflicting reports of both increased and decreased ADC values, and it may be that the age and clinical severity of a lesion may be important in relating the imaging finding to pathophysiology (123,131,145). White matter tractography also appears to be feasible in the clinical setting (67,68). Ducreux et al. (146) have shown that DTI and white matter tractography can be used to evaluate the effects of

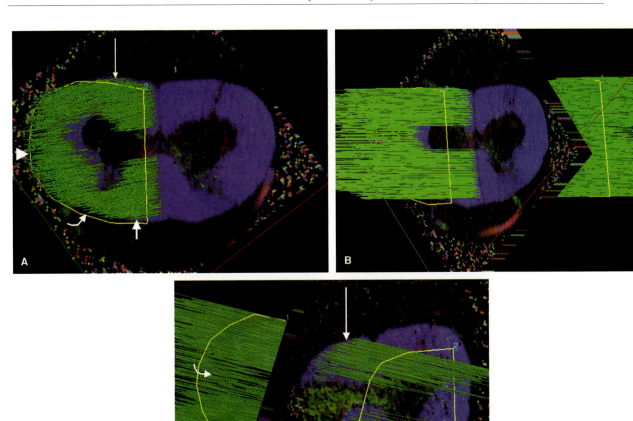

FIGURE 13-11. Ex vivo fiber tractography. For fiber tracking in an ex vivo specimen, we defined the entire right side of the spinal cord (white and gray matter) 2 mm rostral to the center of the injury as the source and the entire right side of the spinal cord 2 mm caudal to the center of the injury as the target. Fiber tracking would then look for continuity of presumed white matter tracts starting rostral to the injury site and extending caudal to the injury site. Although fiber tractography does not distinguish between ascending and descending tracts, we decided to start rostral to the center of the injury because the dorsal lateral white matter contains the rubrospinal tract, a descending white matter tract. In a normal spinal cord specimen **(A,B)** fiber tractography shows no disruption of right-sided white matter tracts, including the ventral (*long arrow, A*), lateral (*arrowhead, A*), and dorsal white matter (*short arrow, A*). White matter tracking is also seen in the region of the Lissauer tract (*curved arrow, A*) at the periphery of the dorsal horn. The yellow lines outline the source and target regions of interest (ROIs), which incorporate the entire right side of the spinal cord. Intact white matter tracts are seen as uninterrupted green lines extending through both the source and target ROIs. In a spinal cord specimen with right-sided partial hemisection **(C)**, white matter fiber tractography indicates preservation of the ventral (*long arrow, C*) and dorsal (*short arrow, C*) white matter, with disruption of the majority of the dorsal lateral white matter caudal to the injury; the dorsal lateral white matter tracts rostral to the injury are indicated with a curved arrow and do not extend to the target ROI. Note how fiber tractography appears to indicate preservation of some axons in the dorsal lateral white matter (*arrowhead indicating green lines extending through both the source and target ROIs, C*); this finding was confirmed on histologic analysis. (Adapted and reproduced from Schwartz ED, Duda J, Shumsky, JS, et al. Spinal cord diffusion tensor imaging and fiber tracking can identify white matter tract disruption and glial scar orientation following lateral funiculotomy. *J Neurotrauma.* December 2005;22(12):1388–1398, with permission.)

astrocytoma infiltration in the spinal cord. There has only been one report of DWI in acute spinal cord injury, and it was noted that diffusion values decreased acutely at the site of injury, potentially due to cellular and axonal swelling (147). In a case report of a patient with syringomyelia, DTI was able to identify spared white matter around the periphery of the syrinx, underscoring the potential for visualizing spared white matter following trauma (148).

All the human imaging discussed above has utilized a 1.5-T magnet. It may be that the next generation of 3-T magnets, as well as continually improving hardware, may be necessary before the resolution and image quality is sufficient to routinely implement spinal cord DWI (149). Nakada et al. (129) have performed diffusion imaging of the brainstem with a 3-T magnet, and they obtained

detailed images of pontine and midbrain fiber tracts, and the effects of mass lesions and Wallerian degeneration on specific fiber tracts were visualized.

MAGNETIC RESONANCE MICROSCOPY OF SEA LAMPREY AXONS

Recent work with the sea lamprey (*Petromyzon marinus*), and its giant unmyelinated axons, has increased our understanding of diffusion coefficients. The sea lamprey have unmyelinated axons in their spinal cords, including the giant reticular neurons, Mauthner and Müller axons, with axon diameters up to 30 to 40 μm. Unlike mammals,

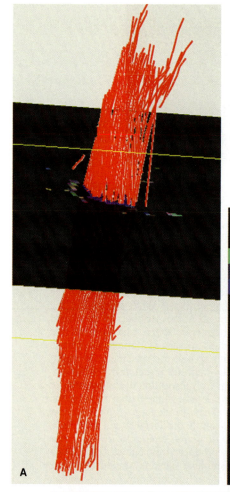
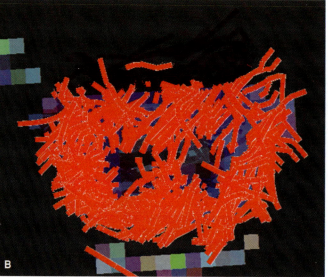

FIGURE 13-12. In vivo spinal cord fiber tractography at 4.7T shows intact white matter in a normal rat **(A)**. An end-on view of the fiber tracking **(B)** shows how the fibers are confined to the white matter. In a rat with a complete hemisection, fiber tractography clearly indicates disruption of the white at the site of injury (*arrow*) **(C)**.

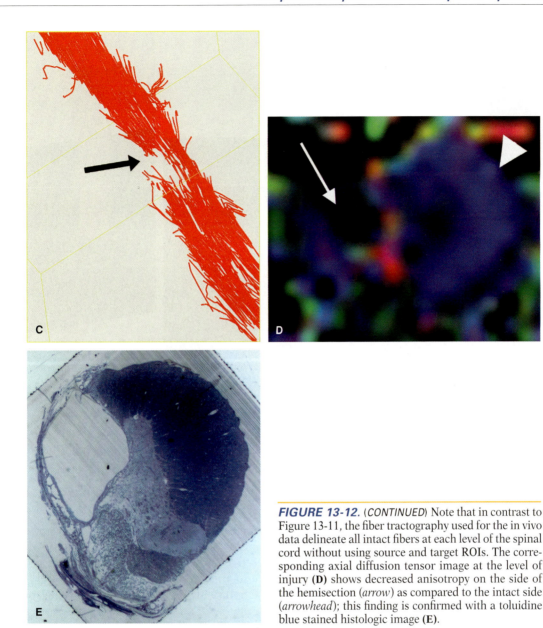

FIGURE 13-12. (*CONTINUED*) Note that in contrast to Figure 13-11, the fiber tractography used for the in vivo data delineate all intact fibers at each level of the spinal cord without using source and target ROIs. The corresponding axial diffusion tensor image at the level of injury (**D**) shows decreased anisotropy on the side of the hemisection (*arrow*) as compared to the intact side (*arrowhead*); this finding is confirmed with a toluidine blue stained histologic image (**E**).

these species have robust spontaneous regeneration of axons following injury, and axonal dieback, degeneration, and regeneration following traumatic injury in a spinal cord have been well documented for over a decade (101,150,151).

Larval sea lampreys were subjected to complete spinal cord transactions and diffusion imaging was performed in a 9.4-T magnet (150). The tADC and lADC diffusion coefficients were calculated in regions of interest encompassing the entire spinal cord. Anisotropy was simply defined as the ratio lADC/tADC. The tADC values rostral and caudal to the injury site increased at 1 week posttransection, subsequently decreasing to below normal controls at 5 weeks and then returning to normal control

values by 10 weeks. Histologically, there was early regeneration of small diameter fibers at 5 weeks, with enlargement of these axons at 10 weeks. These histologic findings may explain tADC decreasing to below normal control at 5 weeks and then increasing to normal levels by 10 weeks, as intracellular water may encounter diffusion barriers sooner in smaller diameter axons than in larger axons. The lADC values rostral to the transection site decreased up to 2 or 5 weeks, then increased at 10 weeks; however, lADC values caudal to the transaction gradually decreased throughout the time points studied. Diffusional anisotropy decreased at 1 and 2 weeks after transection while increasing from weeks 5 to 10, relative to earlier time points, which may be related to initial loss of axons

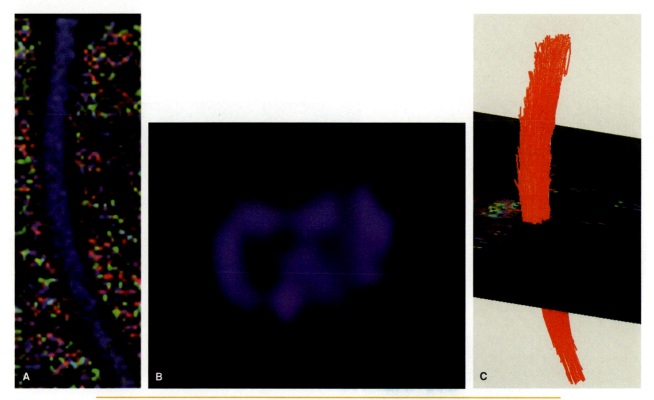

FIGURE 13-13. Sagittal color-coded diffusion tensor image of the normal human cervical spinal cord in vivo at 1.5T using parallel imaging technology **(A)** demonstrates expected rostral-caudal anisotropy, indicated by blue. Axial color-coded diffusion tensor image in the upper cervical human spinal cord **(B)** shows greater diffusional anisotropy in the white matter as compared to the gray matter. Fiber tractography **(C)** shows expected continuity of fibers.

followed by regeneration. In summary, the ADC values were sensitive to the initial loss of axons following injury and the axonal regeneration was reflected in return of diffusion measures toward normal values.

Recent developments in magnetic resonance microscopy and MRI coil development allow for diffusion MRI to be performed within the intracellular space of giant Mauthner and Müller axons, as well as in small subregions in the white matter (153,154) (Fig. 13-14). This assessment will allow for determining the effect of fiber tract anatomy on ADCs. These anatomic factors include mean axonal diameter, axonal density, regional volume fraction, and longitudinal orientation. As the lamprey axons are unmyelinated, the effects of the cell membrane alone could be evaluated.

Live excised lamprey spinal cords were maintained in cold buffer and diffusion weighed imaging was performed at 9.4-T (153). Extensive experience has documented that the tissue remains viable for many hours under these conditions (155). The tADC values in the giant Mauthner axon was the largest measured, and it progressively decreased as subregions included smaller axons. It may be inferred that subregions with smaller

axons have increased numbers of membrane barriers, resulting in decreased diffusion coefficients. Anisotropy increased as axons decreased in size, which may mostly be due to variations of the tADC values. Additionally, when regions of interest (ROIs) were placed entirely within the Mauthner axon, diffusion was isotropic, as in

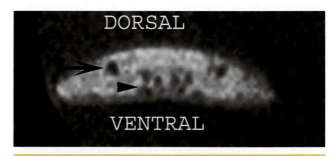

FIGURE 13-14. MR image of individual axons in the fixed excised sea lamprey spinal cord obtained in a 9.4-T magnet. Arrow points to Mauthner axon and arrowhead points to a cluster of Müller axons. These giant axons can reach diameters of 30 to 40 μm. (Reproduced from Schwartz ED, Chin CH, Takahashi M, et al. Diffusion weighted imaging of the spinal cord. *Neuroimaging Clin N Am*. 2002;12(1):125–146, figure 5, with permission.)

gray matter; this finding again supports the theory that barriers, such as cell membranes, are a determinant of anisotropy in the white matter.

Q-SPACE MAGNETIC RESONANCE IMAGING OF THE SPINAL CORD

Q-space imaging is a diffusion-based MRI technique that is analogous to observing the diffraction of light waves traveling through an aperture. Instead of observing light waves, however, the diffraction pattern of water molecular spins provides morphologic information based on water displacement profiles that can detect diffusion to a few microns. The water displacement profiles obtained from q-space data are thought to reflect average diffusion barrier spacing, which should correlate to the structural integrity of spinal cords. The concept of q-space imaging has proven useful for obtaining information on heterogeneous systems that exhibit structural regularity on the scale of the diffusion distance (156,157). The potential importance of the q-space imaging technique is that this approach provides indirect measurement to assess the structural integrity of spinal cord at the cellular level resolution, which is beyond any other available MRI method.

Assaf et al. (158) have employed q-space imaging to assess the maturation of spinal cords and demonstrated that as spinal cord white matter became more myelinated, the water displacement profile narrowed, suggesting that water diffusion was limited by myelin barriers and perhaps increased axonal tortuosity. Barrier permeability and water exchange is also thought to be important in q-space imaging. Nossin-Manor et al. (159) used q-space imaging to evaluate injury in the rat spinal cord; the mean displacement of water molecules perpendicular to the long axis of the spinal cord increased with injury and the probability for zero displacement of water molecules decreased. The probability for zero displacement represents the probability of water molecules to stay close to their point of origin; this probability is high with restricted diffusion. Their findings, therefore, were felt to reflect decreased restriction to water diffusion secondary to structural damage. They point out that these findings were more sensitive to injury than conventional T1 and T2 weighted images. Similar findings have been seen in the spinal cord with experimental models of ischemia/axonal degeneration (160) and experimental allergic encephalomyelitis (161).

Using a combination of computer simulations and high-resolution ex vivo imaging in a 9.4-T magnet, Chin et al. (162) showed that q-space imaging could provide quantitative morphometric data such as mean axonal diameter. In the evaluation of three spinal cord tracts in the rat spinal cord, it was noted that the displacement profiles corresponded to axonal size; the least displacement was seen in the spinal cord tract with smallest axons and higher density, which was expected based on the simulations (Fig. 13-15).

Although this technique has been applied to the brain in patients with multiple sclerosis (MS) (163,164), the need for long *b*-values makes imaging in a small, motion prone structure like the spinal cord challenging. Fast acquisition techniques such as echo-planar imaging will likely be necessary (160).

CONTRAST ENHANCED MAGNETIC RESONANCE IMAGING: EVALUATION OF THE BLOOD-SPINAL CORD BARRIER

Disruption of the blood-spinal cord barrier (BSCB) following traumatic spinal cord injury may be an important cause of propagating injury following spinal cord trauma and is therefore a potential target for therapy (165). Loss of BSCB integrity appears to be biphasic. There is primary mechanical disruption of the spinal vasculature at the time of traumatic injury, resulting in hemorrhage and ischemia. There is then a cascade of secondary events that expand the injury, including toxicity from blood products, as well as excitatory amino acids. The secondary injury, however, is not just due to the sequelae of mechanical disruption; there is a second phase of BSCB permeability that begins 3 to 4 days following initial injury (166) and may last up to 28 days. This second phase of BSCB disruption may result in more injury to the spinal cord, allowing entry of inflammatory cells and small toxic molecules into the extracellular space. Subsequently, there is increased tissue damage, including areas of intact spinal cord adjacent to the central hemorrhagic core. As protection of less than 10% of axons in spinal cord white matter may result in significant functional recovery (167), this penumbra of tissue surrounding the central hemorrhagic core may be a promising target for therapy. One line of research has involved matrix metalloproteinases (MMPs), which are excessively expressed by inflammatory cells following spinal cord injury. MMPs are thought to increase BSCB permeability, resulting in an influx of inflammatory cells and excitatory amino acids that are toxic to the spinal cord. Mice that do not express these proteinases, as well as mice administered an MMP inhibitor, show improved recovery to spinal cord injury (168,169). These papers utilized histologic techniques for evaluating the BSCB, such as staining for IgG leakage, or measuring leakage of intravenous-injected macromolecules through the BSCB. All these methods, however, are performed postmortem and thus at only one time point. MRI may provide a method for serial and in vivo analysis of the BSCB disruption and subsequent restoration (170), and there have been a few papers that explore this issue.

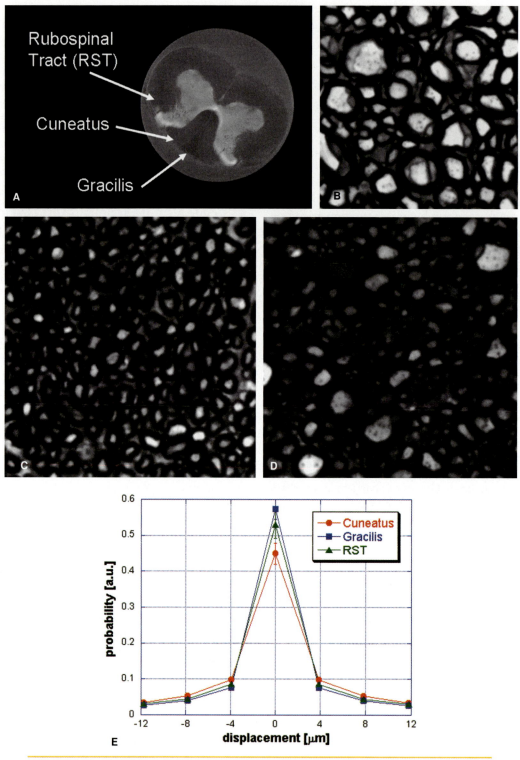

FIGURE 13-15. MRI q-space imaging. T2-weighted spin-echo image of the ex vivo rat spinal cord **(A)**, showing the fiber tract locations where histologic images and the localized q-space data were acquired. Histologic images of cuneatus **(B)**, gracilis **(C)**, and rubrospinal tracts **(D)**. As would be expected, the displacement profile graph **(E)** shows the narrowest profile was for the tract with the highest axonal density and smallest axons (gracilis). Water molecules in the gracilis tract appear to stay closer to their point of origin during the pulse sequence than in other tracts, presumably due to barriers (such as myelin sheath/cell membranes) that are more closely spaced. (Reproduced from Chin CL, Wehrli FW, Fan Y, et al. Assessment of axonal fiber tract architecture in excised rat spinal cord by localized NMR q-space imaging: simulations and experimental studies. *Magn Reson Med*. 2004;52:733–740, figures 1 and 5, with permission.)

In a model of contusive injury, Runge et al. (171) used contrast enhancement to demonstrate early breakdown of the BSCB. As they followed the animals over time, no significant enhancement could be seen by 28 days. Berens et al. (172) also saw no evidence of BSCB disruption in a contrast enhanced MRI at 17 to 24 days postinjury in a rodent model of posttraumatic cavity formation. The lack of enhancement 4 weeks postinjury would appear to correspond to the expected timing of the BSCB postinjury. In a series of papers, Bilgen et al. (173–175) has looked at dynamic contrast enhanced MRI in experimental spinal cord injury. Proposing a multicompartmental pharmacokinetic model, they used this MRI technique to quantify the integrity of the BSCB; they saw early disruption of the BSCB with subsequent restoration corresponding to behavioral recovery over the next few weeks.

MAGNETIC RESONANCE SPECTROSCOPY

Magnetic resonance spectroscopy (MRS) is a noninvasive technique used to assess the biochemistry in the human body. The most common application in the central nervous system is proton (1H) spectroscopy, which looks at the resonance frequencies of protons on specific metabolites. As the most abundant proton is attached to water, sufficient water suppression is required in order to visualize these other resonance frequencies. In the evaluation of central nervous system injury, a few metabolites have proven to be most helpful. For example, N-acetyl aspartate (NAA) is thought to be exclusively localized within neurons and is therefore a putative neuronal marker. A decrease in NAA has been correlated with neuronal and axonal loss following brain trauma, ischemia, demyelination, or with neurodegenerative diseases. Choline (Cho) is a marker of membrane turnover, and increases may be seen with rapid cell turnover, such as that associated with tumors. MRS can also identify an increase in lactate (lac), which is associated with anaerobic metabolism and will be increased with cell ischemia or death.

Although MRS has been successfully applied to the brain, applications to the spinal cord have been limited, with only a few published manuscripts describing the technique in the human cervical spinal cord. This lack of research is likely due to technical challenges in performing MRS in the spinal cord. First, the small size of the spinal cord is limiting because of the generally large voxels that are required to obtain sufficient MRI signal. Additionally, the surrounding bone of the vertebral bodies results in susceptibility artifact that degrades spectra. The spinal cord also moves with the cardiac cycle, posing further problems as the tissue may move in and out of voxel, resulting in inaccurate spectra. Cooke et al. (176) detail their methods for overcoming these difficulties using

magnetic susceptibility maps, accurate voxel placement, and cardiac gating, and they show that MRS in the spinal cord is feasible. A recent study by Kendi et al. (177) has shown that patients with multiple sclerosis have decreased NAA in their spinal cords, indicative of axonal loss and damage; these findings are similar to those seen in the brain.

Other researchers have used MRS to evaluate changes in the brain following spinal cord injury. Pattany et al. (178) evaluated patients with SCI and paraplegia and found that patients with chronic neuropathic pain had decreased NAA and increased myoinositol in their thalami (Fig. 13-16). They hypothesize that the decreased NAA may be due to dysfunction of inhibitory neurons due to deafferentation. The increased myoinositol, a glial marker, may be due to gliosis in the thalami. The authors suggest that MRS may be used to predict and to evaluate effectiveness of treatments for managing pain in SCI patients. Puri et al. (179) reported increases in NAA within the motor cortex following incomplete SCI. The authors suggest that the increased NAA may be due to neuronal adaptation and point out that MRS could be used noninvasively to monitor recovery following SCI.

Experimentally, there have also been only a few publications that utilize MRS to evaluate spinal cord injury. Falconer et al. (180) used non-MRI ex vivo techniques, UV spectroscopy, and gas chromatography mass spectrometry, to identify changes in lactate and NAA respectively. They showed that following experimental spinal cord injury there were decreases in NAA and increases in lactate that appeared to reflect both abnormal NAA metabolism and neuronal death. The authors noted that the changes in metabolites should be significant enough to be detected with MRS. Although application to an animal model is technically difficult, two studies have shown the feasibility of in vivo MRS within the rat spinal cord by utilizing implantable radiofrequency coils (60,64).

Vink et al. (181,182) also used a slightly different technique, phosphorus (31P) MRS, which is used to evaluate energy metabolites, such as ATP. They performed 1H and 31P MRS in vivo following experimental spinal cord injury in the rabbit and showed that there were early elevations in lactic acid and loss of high-energy metabolites in regions that progressed to necrosis and cavitation, suggesting that MRS could evaluate changes in metabolism and predict irreversible tissue damage. Durozard et al. (183) applied in vivo 31P MRS to the question of metabolism in rat gastrocnemius muscle following spinal cord transection. Following electrical stimulation of the muscle, anaerobic metabolism increased and mitochondrial oxidative metabolism decreased; these findings suggest that 31P MRS could be used to evaluate therapies designed to improve muscle function in SCI patients.

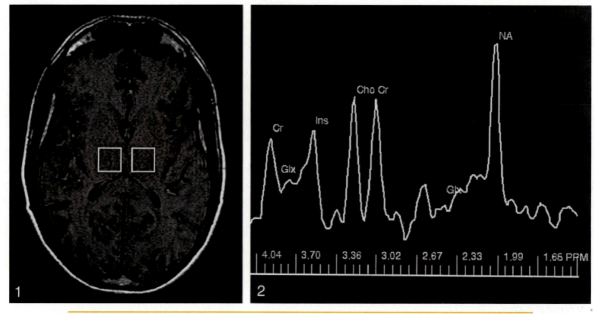

FIGURE 13-16. Axial T1-weighted image (*left*) shows the location of the 2 by 2 by 2-cm voxel in the region of the left thalamus and the corresponding location of the right thalamus. MRS data were separately acquired from each voxel for the three groups: SCI patients with pain, SCI patients without pain, and healthy control subjects. Typical MRS spectrum (*right*) from a healthy control subject with peaks representing cerebral metabolites: N-acetyl, NA; total creatine, Cr; choline compounds, Cho; glutamate, Glu; glutamine, Gln; Glu and Gln, Glx; and myo-inositol, Ins. In spinal cord injured patients with neuropathic pain, the NA is decreased and the Ins is increased. (Reproduced from Pattany PM, Yezierski RP, Widerstrom-Noga EG, et al. Proton magnetic resonance spectroscopy of the thalamus in patients with chronic neuropathic pain after spinal cord injury. *AJNR Am J Neuroradiol.* 2002;23(6):901–905, with permission.)

MAGNETIZATION TRANSFER MAGNETIC RESONANCE IMAGING

Magnetization transfer MRI (MTI) is a technique that takes advantage of differences in resonance frequencies between water protons that are free and water protons that are bound to large macromolecules.

MRI signal is derived from mobile, or free, water protons; however, this pool of mobile protons can exchange or "transfer" magnetization with a pool of bound protons that exist on macromolecules. The application of an off-resonance radiofrequency (RF) pulse can "saturate" the pool of bound protons, however, as there is "saturation transfer or magnetization transfer" in which some of the bound protons exchange magnetization with the pool of free protons (184,185). A saturated proton does not contribute an MRI signal. Therefore, when this transfer occurs, there are now "saturated" free protons that decrease the overall signal intensity from the free proton pool. The degree of magnetization transfer in a particular region will be dependent on factors including the concentration of macromolecular structures, the number of sites that bound protons can interact with free protons, and surface chemistry. Although qualitative information can be obtained from viewing the MT images, quantitative evaluation can be obtained with the magnetization transfer ratio (MTR) histogram (186). MTR is calculated with the following equation:

$$MTR = (1 - Ms/Mo) * 100\%$$

where Ms = signal intensity of pixels in a region of interest with application of a saturating off-resonance RF pulse and Mo = signal intensity of pixels in the same region of interest without a saturation pulse.

In addition to looking at average MTR in a particular region of interest, histograms can be generated that plot MTR values versus the number of pixels for each MTR value.

Myelin is thought to have a surface structure that is ideal for magnetization transfer (187), and MTI has been applied to white matter diseases, such as multiple sclerosis. Whole brain MTR histograms of the brain in patients with MS show a leftward shift and decrease of the peak MTR value as compared to normal controls; this finding is felt to reflect the MTR reduction seen in both plaques and normal appearing white matter in patients with MS (188). The MTR reduction is felt to be related to the structural compromise and loss of myelin within the white matter of patients with MS (189). In an ex vivo study of spinal cords from patients with MS, Mottershead et al. (190) showed strong correlations between the MTR and axonal density and myelin content, with reduced MTR values being seen in areas with fewer axons and less myelin. Interestingly, the correlation of MTR values with axon density/myelin content was stronger than with mean diffusivity; measures of anisotropy and directional diffusion, however, were not evaluated. Another ex vivo study with human spinal cords by Bot et al. (191) also compared MTR findings with histopathologic findings and they found a good correlation of decreased MTR with myelin loss; however, they did not find as strong a relationship between MTR and axonal density, and they suggest that MRI findings are dominated by demyelination rather than axonal density.

Experimental studies in animal models of MS (experimental allergic encephalitis or EAE) have continued to determine the histopathologic correlations of reduced MTR, and findings have suggested that the degree of myelin loss does not solely affect MTR. Gareau et al. (192) have shown that decreased MTR values in the brain may not necessarily indicate myelin loss, but may reflect pathophysiologic changes due to inflammation. Cook et al. (193) used a 4.0-T magnet to evaluate demyelination in the lumbar spinal cord of guinea pigs and found that MTR, as well as conventional imaging, was sensitive to the presence of demyelination as well as cellular infiltrates; however, there was no difference to degree of MTR decrease and was therefore nonspecific as to the underlying pathology. In an MRI microscopy study with the unmyelinated lamprey spinal cord at 9.4-T, Uemtsu et al. (194) found regional differences in the spinal cord that appeared to correlate with the density of cell membranes (axonal and glial), and suggest that MTR may be useful measure of axonal density.

Two papers have been published that utilize MTI for the evaluation of experimental spinal cord injury in the rat. The degree of MTR reductions theoretically should correlate with injury severity, as the degree of MTR reduction is thought to be related to the extent of macromolecular breakdown that occurs with both injury to myelin and axons. In addition, MTR may be reduced by increases in water content that accompany spinal cord edema, and this edema would be expected to increase with the severity of spinal cord injury. In a weight drop model of experimental spinal cord injury, McGowan et al. (195) imaged ex vivo spinal cords 4 weeks postinjury in a 1.9-T magnet. As the severity of injury increased MTR histograms showed decreasing peak heights and further leftward shifts. Additionally, the range of normal white matter values decreased with increasing spinal cord damage. The authors found that the degree of MTR alterations correlated with histologic measures of myelin and neurofilament damage; however, not as well with edema, suggesting that edema did not contribute as much to the MTR reduction. This distinction is important as edema contributes strongly to conventional MRI findings, such as T2

weighted images, and may indicate that MTR provides more specific information concerning spinal cord pathology. Gareau et al. (196) studied MTI in vivo following clip compression injury in rats utilizing a 4.0-T magnet. They found that the average MTR in white matter could discriminate between mild and severe spinal cord injury at 1 day following injury, with lowest MTRs seen in severe spinal cord injury, as opposed to proton density imaging, which did not allow for discrimination of injury severity. They also found some recovery in MTR values 1 week following severe injury, which they suggested was due to a decrease in edema and hemorrhage, as well as an increase in inflammatory cells and gliosis. These two studies suggest that MTI may visualize changes in myelin and neurofilament structure that may go unseen with conventional MRI.

FUNCTIONAL MAGNETIC RESONANCE IMAGING

Functional MRI (fMRI) is an imaging technique that has been used extensively as a tool for mapping brain activity in vivo. The most utilized fMRI technique is the blood oxygen level–dependent (BOLD) pulse sequence. The underlying mechanism is based on the differences in signal obtained from oxyhemoglobin (Hb) and deoxyhemoglobin (dHb). Deoxyhemoglobin, as opposed to Hb, causes a magnetic susceptibility effect, resulting in decreased signal intensity due to shorter T2* relaxation rate. When using the BOLD pulse sequence, which is sensitive to changes in T2* relaxation rate, signal intensity increases when relative dHb is decreased, and signal intensity decreases when relative dHb is increased. In the central nervous system, changes in hemodynamics that would affect the relative amount of dHb can be exploited to localize neuronal activation. A few seconds following neuronal activation there is actually an increase in BOLD signal in the activated CNS region because of an increase in cerebral blood flow that overcompensates for the increase in oxygen demand, resulting in an oversupply of Hb and a relative decrease in dHb (197,198). Although the vast majority of fMRI is brain related, there has been interest in applying this technique to the spinal cord. Unfortunately, BOLD imaging of the spinal cord is limited by the small size of the spinal cord, by spinal cord motion, and by nearby location of large pial vessels; all of these factors can result in poor localization of the BOLD signal. Additionally, the magnetic susceptibility of the surrounding vertebral bodies and ligaments can also result in distortions to the MRI signal. Consequently, there have been relatively few articles published with BOLD fMRI applied to the spinal cord.

Following a unilateral hand-closing task, Yoshizawa et al. (199) noted a 4.8% change in BOLD signal intensity in the ipsilateral cervical spinal cord utilizing a 1.5-T magnet and Backes et al. (200) noted localized spinal cord activation (8% to 15% BOLD signal increase) following median nerve stimulation and hand clenching, although lateralization was not visualized. Stroman et al. (201) used a 3-T magnet to evaluate the lower cervical spinal cord following hand exercises and found a 7.0% increase in BOLD signal that corresponded to the expected location of both motor and sensory activation. Madi et al. (202) used a series of different exercised to determine if they could demonstrate a task-dependent change in the spinal cord BOLD signal at 1.5-T (Fig. 13-17). They found that BOLD signal increased at the expected spinal cord level; elbow flexion showed activation at C5 and C6, wrist extension at C6 and C7, and finger abduction at T1 and T2. They also reported a linear dependence of the fMRI signal with the force applied by the muscle group. Stroman et al. (203) also showed that following sensory stimulation, the distribution of spinal cord activity with fMRI matched the expected location of neuronal activation; however, a separate report by Stracke et al. (204) using BOLD imaging also showed consistent activation at higher cervical levels as well, which they attribute to synaptic transmissions at interneurons.

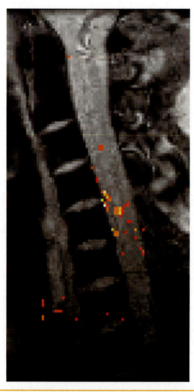

FIGURE 13-17. BOLD fMRI of the human spinal cord. In a subject performing isometric exercises with the arm, sagittal BOLD fMRI image shows first order activation in the expected C5-6 region of the spinal cord; this finding suggests a linear relationship between BOLD signal and applied force. (Image courtesy of Adam Flanders, MD, Thomas Jefferson University.)

It has been suggested, however, that the changes seen in fMRI of the spinal cord may not be due to the BOLD effect. Changes in proton density may actually predominate, which can then be imaged with a proton-density spin echo sequence, eliminating much of the susceptibility artifacts that limited spinal fMRI (205,206). The mechanism for the signal changes on proton density imaging appears to be due to water protons in the extravascular space, and not due to water protons in the blood where the BOLD effect takes place; this effect has been termed by Stroman et al. (207) as signal enhancement by extravascular water protons (SEEP). It has been proposed that the underlying mechanism for the SEEP effect is that hemodynamic changes in regions of activated neurons result in increased perfusion and movement of water molecules from the vascular to the extravascular spaces. Additionally, the swelling of glial cells following neurotransmitter release may also contribute to the SEEP effect. This technique has been optimized to perform spinal fMRI, both in the cervical (208) and lumbar spine (209). One advantage of this technique is that it can be performed on low field strength magnets, such as 0.2-T, whereas the BOLD technique relies on susceptibility changes, which are best seen with higher strength magnetic fields (210,211). Two articles by Stroman et al. (212,213) have applied this technique to patients with SCI. Graded thermal stimuli were applied to normal controls and SCI patients below the level of injury. Lumbar spinal cord activity is seen in both controls and patients; however, the pattern of activation is altered in the injured patients. Also preserved in SCI patients is a stimulus response pattern similar to uninjured subjects, as the signal changes increased with more noxious (colder) stimuli.

There have been a few papers that have also looked at fMRI in the spinal cords of animals. These studies have shown activation in the cervical (214) and lumbar (215,216) spinal cord of rats following noxious stimuli. Confirming the robustness of fMRI, Lawrence et al. (217) demonstrated agreement between the areas of activation seen with fMRI and C-*fos* (upregulated in neurons following repeated stimuli) expression seen on immunochemistry.

BOLD fMRI of brain activation following spinal and peripheral nerve injury has shown that there is reorganization, expansion, and shifting of motor cortical representations in nonaffected limbs (218–220). Interestingly, Sabbah et al. (221) demonstrated that in patients with complete SCI, activation could be seen in the motor regions with both an attempts to move as well as mental imagery of movement in affected limbs. These findings suggest that the cortical networks involved with motion and sensation remain intact despite complete injury. Komisaruk et al. (222) used fMRI to demonstrate that women with complete spinal cord injury could use the vagus nerve to provide a spinal-cord bypass pathway for vaginal-cervical sensation, and that the degree of sensation was sufficient to achieve orgasm. In a rodent model of spinal cord injury, fMRI showed the expected expansion of cortical representation of nonaffected limbs as well as loss of sensory cortical representation in the affected limb; in mild SCI, there was recovery of sensory function detectable with fMRI, as opposed to moderate SCI (223). Two recent experimental studies have shown that fMRI may be used as a noninvasive test of recovery following experimental treatment. Hofstetter et al. (224) showed fMRI could detect sensory recovery in rats treated with modified neural stem cells following contusion injury and Liebscher et al. (225) demonstrated that fMRI could detect the recovery of sensory function in rats that were treated with Nogo-A antibody following a surgically induced lesion to the dorsal columns. In both studies, no recovery was seen in untreated surgical controls. These findings, both clinical and experimental, suggest that fMRI may be a noninvasive technique of evaluating the effects of SCI and treatment, both within the spinal cord and the brain.

MAGNETIC RESONANCE IMAGING TRACKING OF MAGNETICALLY LABELED NEUROTRANSPLANTS

Recently, there has been interest in using noninvasive methods for the tracking of engrafted cells into the injured spinal cord. One technique utilizing MRI is performed by magnetically labeling the cells, prior to transplantation, with super paramagnetic iron nanoparticles. MRI will then show the labeled cells to be hypointense as compared to the remainder of the spinal cord (Fig. 13-18). Bulte et al. (226) have shown the feasibility of this technique in the spinal cord by labeling oligodendrocyte precursors and injecting these cells into the spinal cord of myelin deficient rats; there was a close correlation between the hypointense regions seen with ex vivo MRI and histologic confirmation of cell location and myelination. This technique can be used for tracking the migration of cells following neurotransplantation (Fig. 13-18). More recent studies have shown that this technique is feasible in vivo, with Lee et al. (227) demonstrating that labeled olfactory ensheathing cells could not cross an experimental spinal cord transection site following neurotransplantation. This technique has also demonstrated that labeled bone marrow stromal cells and embryonic stem cells will migrate to a site of injury in the brain or spinal cord following either direct implantation into the CNS or intravenous injection (228,229). One of the disadvantages of this technique, however, in that the labeled cells cannot be reliably differentiated from blood products (which also appear hypointense), thus adding a confounding factor when imaging an injury that also contains hemorrhage; however, recent reports suggest that

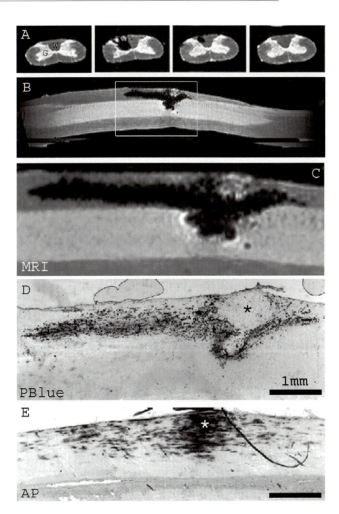

FIGURE 13-18. Neural-restricted precursor stem cells (NRPs) and glial-restricted precursor stem cells have been labeled with iron oxide (Ferridex; Berlex Laboratories, Wayne, NJ), and then grafted into the intact rat spinal cord. Ex vivo axial **(A)** and sagittal **(B,C)** MR images obtained 5 weeks posttransplantation show the grafted cells as dark areas. Histologic image stained with the iron stain Prussian blue **(D)** shows a correspondence between the MR and iron containing cells. The grafted cells were from a transgenic alkaline phosphatase (AP) rat, and a histologic image stained for AP **(E)** shows that the dark areas in the MRI correspond to grafted cells. Note that this technique is able to detect grafted cells that have migrated rostral and caudal to the implantation site. There is less MRI-histology correspondence at the central portion of the graft site *(asterisk)* due to high degree of cell proliferation that dilutes the iron oxide label. (Figure courtesy of Angelo Lepore, PhD, Johns Hopkins University.)

newer pulse sequences and labeling techniques have potential to overcome this limitation (230,231).

SUMMARY

Prior research has shown that small amounts of fiber sparing may contribute to substantial recovery of function.

Based on results from a study evaluating a transaction injury and a contusion injury in rats, Basso et al. (232) suggest that sparing of as little as 5% to 10% of axon fibers may be enough to recover basic locomotion. They also note that animals with 45% to 90% white matter preservation all recovered equally well. Kakulas (167) counted spared axons in injured human spinal cords and noted that less than 10% residual fibers, if in the appropriate location, could subserve voluntary motor function. Subsequently, the detection of the location and amount of preserved white matter, especially in severely injured patients, would help with prognosis and possibly selection of treatment. Although it remains to be seen whether these advanced imaging techniques will be sensitive enough to detect the small amounts of preserved axon fibers that may be important in determining function following injury, it is clear that the potential exists.

REFERENCES

1. Sekhon LH and Fehlings MG. Epidemiology, demographics, and pathophysiology of acute spinal cord injury. *Spine*. 2001;26(24 Suppl):S2–12.
2. DeVivo MJ. Epidemiology of traumatic spinal cord injury. In: Kirshblum S, Campagnolo DI, Delisa, JA, eds. Spinal Cord Medicine. Philadelphia: Lippincott, Williams & Wilkins, 2002;69–81.
3. Bracken MB, Shepard MJ, Collins WF, et al. A randomized, controlled trial of methylprednisolone or naloxone in the treatment of acute spinal-cord injury. Results of the Second National Acute Spinal Cord Injury Study. *N Engl J Med*. 1990;322(20):1405–1411.
4. Bracken MB. Methylprednisolone and acute spinal cord injury: an update of the randomized evidence. *Spine*. 2001;26(24 Suppl):S47–54.
5. Hurlbert RJ. The role of steroids in acute spinal cord injury: an evidence-based analysis. *Spine*. 2001;26(24 Suppl):S39–46.
6. Bledsoe BE, Wesley AK, Salomone JP. High-dose steroids for acute spinal cord injury in emergency medical services. *Prehosp Emerg Care*. 2004;8(3):313–316.
7. Hugenholtz H, Cass DE, Dvorak MF, et al. High-dose methylprednisolone for acute closed spinal cord injury—only a treatment option. *Can J Neurol Sci*. 2002;29(3):227–235.
8. Murray M. Therapies to promote CNS repair. In: Ingoli NA, Murray M, eds. Axonal Regeneration in the Central Nervous System. New York: Marcel Dekker; 2001:649–656.
9. Bregman BS, Coumans JV, Dai HN, et al. Transplants and neurotrophic factors increase regeneration and recovery of function after spinal cord injury. *Prog Brain Res*. 2002;137: 257–273.
10. McDonald JW, Becker D, Holekamp TF, et al. Repair of the injured spinal cord and the potential of embryonic stem cell transplantation. *J Neurotrauma*. 2004;21(4):383–393.
11. Qu Y, Vadivelu S, Choi L, et al. Neurons derived from embryonic stem (ES) cells resemble normal neurons in their vulnerability to excitotoxic death. *Exp Neurol*. 2003;184(1):326–336.
12. Kwon BK, Tetzlaff W, Grauer JN, et al. Pathophysiology and pharmacologic treatment of acute spinal cord injury. *Spine J*. 2004;4(4):451–464.
13. Dobkin BH, Havton LA. Basic advances and new avenues in therapy of spinal cord injury. *Annu Rev Med*. 2004;55: 255–282.
14. Reier PJ. Cellular Transplantation Strategies for Spinal Cord Injury and Translational Neurobiology. *Neurorx*. 2004;1(4):424–451.
15. Kleitman N. Keeping promises: translating basic research into new spinal cord injury therapies. *J Spinal Cord Med*. 2004;27(4):311–318.
16. NIH. Translating promising strategies for spinal cord injury therapy. Paper presented at NINDS Workshop, 2003; http://www.ninds.nih.gov/news_and_events/proceedings/ sci_translation_workshop.htm.
17. Houle JD and Tessler A. Repair of chronic spinal cord injury. *Exp Neurol*. 2003;182(2):247–260.
18. Raineteau O, Schwab ME. Plasticity of motor systems after incomplete spinal cord injury. *Nat Rev Neurosci*. 2001;2(4): 263–273.
19. Ellaway PH, Anand P, Bergstrom EM, et al. Towards improved clinical and physiological assessments of recovery in spinal cord injury: a clinical initiative. *Spinal Cord*. 2004;42(6):325–337.
20. Falconer JC, Narayana PA, Bhattacharjee MB, et al. Quantitative MRI of spinal cord injury in a rat model. *MRM Magn Reson Med*. 1994;32:484–491.
21. Ford JC, Hackney DB, Alsop DC, et al. MRI characterization of diffusion coefficients in a rat spinal cord injury model. *Magn Reson Med*. 1994;31(5):488–494.
22. Ramon S, Dominguez R, Ramirez L, et al. Clinical and magnetic resonance imaging correlation in acute spinal cord injury. *Spinal Cord*. 1997;35:664–673.
23. Takhtani D, Melhem ER. MR imaging in cervical spine trauma. Magn Reson Imaging Clin N Am. 2000;8(3):615–634.
24. Ditunno JF, Flanders AE, Kirshblum S, et al. Predicting outcome in traumatic spinal cord injury. In: Kirshblum S, Campagnolo DI, Delisa JA, eds. *Spinal Cord Medicine*. Philadelphia: Lippincott, Williams & Wilkins; 2002:108–122.
25. Flanders AE, Spettell CM, Friedman DP, et al. The relationship between the functional abilities of patients with cervical spinal cord injury and the severity of damage revealed by MR imaging. *Am. J. Neuroradiol*. 1999;20:926–934.
26. Kulkarni MV, McArdle CB, Kopanicky D, et al. Acute spinal cord injury: MR imaging at 1.5 T. *Radiology*. 1987;164(3): 837–843.
27. Bondurant FJ, Cotler HB, Kulkarni MV, et al. Acute spinal cord injury. A study using physical examination and magnetic resonance imaging. *Spine*. 1990;15(3):161–168.
28. Shepard MJ and Bracken MB. Magnetic resonance imaging and neurological recovery in acute spinal cord injury: observations from the National Acute Spinal Cord Injury Study 3. *Spinal Cord*. 1999;37(12):833–837.
29. Milhorat TH, Johnson RW, Milhorat RH, et al. Clinicopathologic correlations in syringomyelia using axial magnetic resonance imaging. *Neurosurgery*. 1995;37:206–213.
30. Jinkins JR, Reddy S, Leite CC, et al. MR of parenchymal spinal cord signal change as a sign of active advancement in clinically progressive posttraumatic syringomyelia. *AJNR Am J Neuroradiol*. 1998;19:177–182.
31. Quencer RM, Sheldon JJ, Post MJ, et al. MRI of the chronically injured cervical spinal cord. *AJR Am J Roentgenol*. 1986;147:125–132.
32. Schurch B, Wichmann W, Rossier AB. Post-traumatic syringomyelia (cystic myelopathy): a prospective study of 449 patients with spinal cord injury. *J Neurol Neurosurg Psychiatry*. 1996;60:61–67.
33. Schwartz ED, Falcone SF, Quencer RM, et al. Posttraumatic syringomyelia: pathogenesis, imaging, and treatment. *AJR Am J Roentgenol*. 1999;173:487–492.
34. Bodley R. Imaging in chronic spinal cord injury—indications and benefits. *Eur J Radiol*. 2002;42(2):135–153.
35. Stejskal EO and Tanner JE. Spin diffusion measurements: Spin echoes in the presence of a time-dependent field gradient. *J Chem Phys*. 1965;42:288–292.
36. Barkovich AJ. Concepts of myelin and myelination in neuroradiology. *AJNR Am J Neuroradiol*. 2000;21(6):1099–1109.
37. Hajnal JV, Doran M, Hall AS, et al. MR imaging of anisotropically restricted diffusion of water in the nervous system: technical, anatomic, and pathologic considerations. *J Comput Assist Tomogr*. 1991;15(1):1–18.

38. Doran M and Bydder GM. Magnetic resonance: perfusion and diffusion imaging. *Neuroradiology*. 1990;32(5):392–398.

39. Schwartz ED and Hackney DB. Diffusion-weighted MRI and the evaluation of spinal cord axonal integrity following injury and treatment. *Exp Neurol*. 2003;184(2):570–589.

40. Schwartz ED, Chin CL, Takahashi M, et al. Diffusion-weighted imaging of the spinal cord. *Neuroimaging Clin N Am*. 2002;12(1):125–146.

41. Beaulieu C. The basis of anisotropic water diffusion in the nervous system—a technical review. *NMR Biomed*. 2002; 15(7-8):435–455.

42. Clark CA, Werring DJ. Diffusion tensor imaging in spinal cord: methods and applications—a review. *NMR Biomed*. 2002;15(7-8):578–586.

43. Basser PJ, Mattiello J, LeBihan D. MR diffusion tensor spectroscopy and imaging. *Biophys J*. 1994;66(1):259–267.

44. Melhem ER, Mori S, Mukundan G, et al. Diffusion tensor MR imaging of the brain and white matter tractography. *AJR Am J Roentgenol*. 2002;178(1):3–16.

45. Dong Q, Welsh RC, Chenevert TL, et al. Clinical applications of diffusion tensor imaging. *J Magn Reson Imaging*. 2004;19(1):6–18.

46. Pierpaoli C, Basser PJ. Toward a quantitative assessment of diffusion anisotropy. *Magn Reson Med*. 1996;36(6):893–906.

47. Pierpaoli C. *Oh no! One more method for color mapping of fiber tract direction using diffusion MR imaging data*. in *ISMRM Proceedings*. 1997. Vancouver, Canada.

48. Jones DK, Williams SC, Horsfield MA. *Full representation of white-matter fibre direction on one map via diffusion tensor analysis*. in *ISMRM Proceedings*. 1997. Vancouver, Canada.

49. Pajevic S, Pierpaoli C. Color schemes to represent the orientation of anisotropic tissues from diffusion tensor data: application to white matter fiber tract mapping in the human brain. *Magn Reson Med*. 1999;42(3):526–540.

50. Pattany PM, Puckett WR, Klose KJ, et al. High-resolution diffusion-weighted MR of fresh and fixed cat spinal cords: evaluation of diffusion coefficients and anisotropy. *AJNR Am J Neuroradiol*. 1997;18(6):1049–1056.

51. Schwartz ED, Shumsky JS, Wehrli S, et al. Ex vivo MR determined apparent diffusion coefficients correlate with motor recovery mediated by intraspinal transplants of fibroblasts genetically modified to express BDNF. *Exp Neurol*. 2003;182(1):49–63.

52. Schwartz ED, Chin CL, Shumsky JS, et al. Apparent diffusion coefficients in spinal cord transplants and surrounding white matter correlate with degree of axonal dieback after injury in rats. *AJNR Am J Neuroradiol*. 2005;26(1):7–18.

53. Schwartz ED, Cooper ET, Chin CL, et al. Ex vivo evaluation of ADC values within spinal cord white matter tracts. *AJNR Am J Neuroradiol*. 2005;26(2):390–397.

54. Schwartz ED, Cooper ET, Fan Y, et al. MRI diffusion coefficients in spinal cord correlate with axon morphometry. *Neuroreport*. 2005;16(1):73–76.

55. Nevo U, Hauben E, Yoles E, et al. Diffusion anisotropy MRI for quantitative assessment of recovery in injured rat spinal cord. *Magn Reson Med*. 2001;45(1):1–9.

56. Gulani V, Webb AG, Duncan ID, et al. Apparent diffusion tensor measurements in myelin-deficient rat spinal cords. *Magn Reson Med*. 2001;45(2):191–195.

57. Weglarz WP, Adamek D, Markiewicz J, et al. Analysis of the diffusion weighted MR microscopy data of excised spinal cord of a rat on the basis of the model of restricted diffusion. *Solid State Nucl Magn Reson*. 2004;25(1-3):88–93.

58. Fraidakis M, Klason T, Cheng H, et al. High-resolution MRI of intact and transected rat spinal cord. *Exp Neurol*. 1998; 153(2):299–312.

59. Inglis BA, Yang L, Wirth ED, 3rd, et al. Diffusion anisotropy in excised normal rat spinal cord measured by NMR microscopy. *Magn Reson Imaging*. 1997;15(4):441–450.

60. Silver X, Ni WX, Mercer EV, et al. In vivo 1H magnetic resonance imaging and spectroscopy of the rat spinal cord using an inductively-coupled chronically implanted RF coil. *Magn Reson Med*. 2001;46(6):1216–1222.

61. Elshafiey I, Bilgen M, He R, et al. In vivo diffusion tensor imaging of rat spinal cord at 7 T. *Magn Reson Imaging*. 2002;20(3):243–247.

62. Fenyes DA and Narayana PA. In vivo diffusion characteristics of rat spinal cord. *Magn Reson Imaging*. 1999;17(5):717–722.

63. Madi S, Hasan KM, and Narayana PA. Diffusion tensor imaging of in vivo and excised rat spinal cord at 7 T with an icosahedral encoding scheme. *Magn Reson Med*. 2005;53(1): 118–125.

64. Bilgen M, Elshafiey I, and Narayana PA. In vivo magnetic resonance microscopy of rat spinal cord at 7 T using implantable RF coils. *Magn Reson Med*. 2001;46(6):1250–1253.

65. Bobek J and Wilk L. [Cervical pain as the only complaint in a patient with metastatic advanced lung carcinoma (case report)]. *Neurol Neurochir Pol*. 1999;33(5):1187–1193.

66. Nakada T, Matsuzawa H, and Kwee IL. Magnetic resonance axonography of the rat spinal cord. *Neuroreport*. 1994;5(16): 2053–2056.

67. Wheeler-Kingshott CA, Hickman SJ, Parker GJ, et al. Investigating cervical spinal cord structure using axial diffusion tensor imaging. *Neuroimage*. 2002;16(1):93–102.

68. Tsuchiya K, Fujikawa A, and Suzuki Y. Diffusion tractography of the cervical spinal cord by using parallel imaging. *AJNR Am J Neuroradiol*. 2005;26(2):398–400.

69. Clark CA, Werring DJ, and Miller DH. Diffusion imaging of the spinal cord in vivo: estimation of the principal diffusivities and application to multiple sclerosis. *Magn Reson Med*. 2000;43(1):133–138.

70. Holder CA, Muthupillai R, Mukundan S, Jr., et al. Diffusion-weighted MR imaging of the normal human spinal cord in vivo. *AJNR Am J Neuroradiol*. 2000;21(10):1799–1806.

71. Bammer R, Augustin M, Prokesch RW, et al. Diffusion-weighted imaging of the spinal cord: interleaved echo-planar imaging is superior to fast spin-echo. *J Magn Reson Imaging*. 2002;15(4):364–373.

72. Dietrich O, Herlihy A, Dannels WR, et al. Diffusion-weighted imaging of the spine using radial k-space trajectories. *Magma*. 2001;12(1):23–31.

73. Murphy BP, Zientara GP, Huppi PS, et al. Line scan diffusion tensor MRI of the cervical spinal cord in preterm infants. *J Magn Reson Imaging*. 2001;13(6):949–953.

74. Gulani V, Iwamoto GA, Jiang H, et al. A multiple echo pulse sequence for diffusion tensor imaging and its application in excised rat spinal cords. *Magn Reson Med*. 1997;38(6): 868–873.

75. Mamata H, De Girolami U, Hoge WS, et al. Collateral nerve fibers in human spinal cord: Visualization with magnetic resonance diffusion tensor imaging. *Neuroimage*. 2006; 31(1):24–30.

76. Schwartz ED, Duda J, Shumsky JS, et al. Spinal cord diffusion tensor imaging and fiber tracking can identify white matter tract disruption and glial scar orientation following lateral funiculotomy. *J Neurotrauma*. 2005;22(12):1388–1398.

77. Schwartz ED, Yezierski RP, Pattany PM, et al. Diffusion-weighted MR imaging in a rat model of syringomyelia after excitotoxic spinal cord injury. *AJNR Am J Neuroradiol*. 1999;20(8):1422–1428.

78. Baccarini I and Powell EW. A comparison of fixation by formaldehyde and glutaraldehyde-formaldehyde for combined light and electron microscopy of axonal degeneration in the mamillary body. *Stain Technol*. 1973;48(2):77–83.

79. Beaulieu C and Allen PS. Determinants of anisotropic water diffusion in nerves. *Magn Reson Med*. 1994;31(4):394–400.

80. Hwang SN, Chin CL, Wehrli FW, et al. An image-based finite difference model for simulating restricted diffusion. *Magn Reson Med*. 2003;50(2):373–382.

81. Stanisz GJ, Szafer A, Wright GA, et al. An analytical model of restricted diffusion in bovine optic nerve. *Magn Reson Med*. 1997;37(1):103–111.

82. Ford JC, Hackney DB, Lavi E, et al. Dependence of apparent diffusion coefficients on axonal spacing, membrane permeability, and diffusion time in spinal cord white matter. *J Magn Reson Imaging*. 1998;8(4):775–782.

83. Ford JC and Hackney DB. Numerical model for calculation of apparent diffusion coefficients (ADC) in permeable cylinders—comparison with measured ADC in spinal cord white matter. *Magn Reson Med*. 1997;37(3):387–394.

84. Sfazer A, Zhong J, and Gore JC. Theoretical model for water diffusion in tissues. *MRM Magn Reson Med*. 1995;33:697–712.

85. Hwang S, Hackney DB, and Wehrli F. The effect of myelin loss on the diffusion-sensitized MRsignal in the spinal cord: application of a new finite difference method. *Radiology*. 2000;217(P):390.

86. Hwang S, Wehrli F, and Hackney DB. *A finite difference method for simulating restricted diffusion in the spinal cord*. in *ISMRM Scientific Meeting and Exhibition*. 2000. Denver.

87. Chin CL, Wehrli FW, Hwang SN, et al. Biexponential diffusion attenuation in the rat spinal cord: Computer simulations based on anatomic images of axonal architecture. *Magn Reson Med*. 2002;47(3):455–460.

88. Balentine JD. Pathology of experimental spinal cord trauma II. Ultratructure of axons and myelin. *Lab Invest*. 1978;39:254–266.

89. Salgado-Ceballos H, Guizar-Sahagun G, Feria-Velasco A, et al. Spontaneous long-term remyelination after traumatic spinal cord injury in rats. *Brain Res*. 1998;782:126–135.

90. Fenyes DA and Narayana PA. In vivo echo-planar imaging of rat spinal cord. *Magn Reson Imaging*. 1998;16(10):1249–1255.

91. Fenyes DA and Narayana PA. In vivo diffusion tensor imaging of rat spinal cord with echo planar imaging. *Magn Reson Med*. 1999;42(2):300–306.

92. Wirth ED, Mareci TH, Beck BL, et al. A comparison of an inductively coupled implanted coil with optimized surface coils for in vivo NMR imaging of the spinal cord. *Magnetic Resonance in Medicine*. 1993;30(5):626–633.

93. Ford JC, Hackney DB, Joseph PM, et al. A method for in vivo high resolution MRI of rat spinal cord injury. *Magn Reson Med*. 1994;31:218–223.

94. Franconi F, Lemaire L, Marescaux L, et al. In vivo quantitative microimaging of rat spinal cord at 7T. *Magn Reson Med*. 2000;44(6):893–898.

95. Sun SW, Neil JJ, and Song SK. Relative indices of water diffusion anisotropy are equivalent in live and formalin-fixed mouse brains. *Magn Reson Med*. 2003;50(4):743–748.

96. Buckley DL, Bui JD, Phillips MI, et al. The effect of ouabain on water diffusion in the rat hippocampal slice measured by high resolution NMR imaging. *Magn Reson Med*. 1999;41(1):137–142.

97. Bui JD, Buckley DL, Phillips MI, et al. Nuclear magnetic resonance imaging measurements of water diffusion in the perfused hippocampal slice during N-methyl-D-aspartate-induced excitotoxicity. *Neuroscience*. 1999;93(2):487–490.

98. Grant SC, Buckley DL, Gibbs S, et al. MR microscopy of multicomponent diffusion in single neurons. *Magn Reson Med*. 2001;46(6):1107–1112.

99. Inglis BA, Bossart EL, Buckley DL, et al. Visualization of neural tissue water compartments using biexponential diffusion tensor MRI. *Magn Reson Med*. 2001;45(4):580–587.

100. Shepherd TM, Thelwall PE, Blackband SJ, et al. Diffusion magnetic resonance imaging study of a rat hippocampal slice model for acute brain injury. *J Cereb Blood Flow Metab*. 2003;23(12):1461–1470.

101. Schwab ME and Bartholdi D. Degeneration and regeneration of axons in the lesioned spinal cord. *Physiol Rev*. 1996;76(2):319–369.

102. Liu XZ, Xu SM, Hu R, et al. Neuronal and glial apoptosis after traumatic spinal cord injury. *J Neurosci*. 1997;17(14):5395–5406.

103. Shuman S, Bresnehan J, Beattie M. Apoptosis of microglia and oligodendrocytes after spinal cord contusion in rats. *J Neurosci Res*. 1997;50:798–808.

104. Banik NL, Hogan EL, Powers JM, et al. Degradation of cytoskeletal proteins in experimental spinal cord injury. *Neurochem Res*. 1982;7:1465–1475.

105. Banik NL, Powers JM, and Hogan EL. The effects of spinal cord trauma on myelin. *J Neuropath Exper Neurol*. 1980;39:232–244.

106. Hauben E, Nevo U, Yoles E, et al. Autoimmune T cells as potential neuroprotective therapy for spinal cord injury. *Lancet*. 2000;355(9200):286–287.

107. Kim D, Liu Y, Browarek T, et al. Transplants of fibroblasts genetically modified to express BDNF promote recovery of forelimb and hindlimb funtions in the adult rat. *Soc. Neurosci. Abstr*. 1999;25:492.

108. Liu Y, Kim D, Himes BT, et al. Transplants of fibroblasts genetically modified to express BDNF promote regeneration of adult rat rubrospinal axons and recovery of forelimb function. *J Neurosci*. 1999;19(11):4370–4387.

109. Himes BT and Tessler A, *Neuroprotection from cell death following axotomy*, in *Axonal Regeneration in the Central Nervous System*, NA Ingoglia and M Murray, Editors. 2001, Marcel Dekker: New York. 477–503.

110. Kim D, Schallert T, Liu Y, et al. Transplantation of genetically modified fibroblasts expressing BDNF in adult rats with a subtotal hemisection improves specific motor and sensory functions. *Neurorehabil Neural Repair*. 2001;15(2):141–150.

111. Liu Y, Himes BT, Murray M, et al. Grafts of BDNF-producing fibroblasts rescue axotomized rubrospinal neurons and prevent their atrophy. *Exp Neurol*. 2002;178(2):150–164.

112. Murray M, Kim D, Liu Y, et al. Transplantation of genetically modified cells contributes to repair and recovery from spinal injury. *Brain Res Rev*. 2002;40(1-3):292–300.

113. Wirth ED, Theele DP, Mareci TH, et al. Dynamic assessment of intraspinal neural graft survival using magnetic resonance imaging. *Exp. Neurol*. 1995;136:64–72.

114. Wirth ED, Theele DP, Mareci TH, et al. In vivo magnetic resonance imaging of fetal cat neural tissue transplants in the adult cat spinal cord. *J Neurosurg*. 1992;76:261–274.

115. Banasik T, Jasinski A, Pilc A, et al. Application of magnetic resonance diffusion anisotropy imaging for the assessment neuroprotecting effects of MPEP, a selective mGluR5 antagonist, on the rat spinal cord injury in vivo. *Pharmacol Rep*. 2005;57(6):861–866.

116. Deo AA, Grill RJ, Hasan KM, et al. In vivo serial diffusion tensor imaging of experimental spinal cord injury. *J Neurosci Res*. 2006;83(5):801–810.

117. Rugg-Gunn FJ, Symms MR, Barker GJ, et al. Diffusion imaging shows abnormalities after blunt head trauma when conventional magnetic resonance imaging is normal. *J Neurol Neurosurg Psychiatry*. 2001;70(4):530–533.

118. Chan JH, Tsui EY, Peh WC, et al. Diffuse axonal injury: detection of changes in anisotropy of water diffusion by diffusion-weighted imaging. *Neuroradiology*. 2003;45(1):34–38.

119. Huisman TA. Diffusion-weighted imaging: basic concepts and application in cerebral stroke and head trauma. *Eur Radiol*. 2003;13(10):2283–2297.

120. Huisman TA, Schwamm LH, Schaefer PW, et al. Diffusion tensor imaging as potential biomarker of white matter injury in diffuse axonal injury. *AJNR Am J Neuroradiol*. 2004;25(3):370–376.

121. Arfanakis K, Haughton VM, Carew JD, et al. Diffusion tensor MR imaging in diffuse axonal injury. *AJNR Am J Neuroradiol*. 2002;23(5):794–802.

122. Vorisek I, Hajek M, Tintera J, et al. Water ADC, extracellular space volume, and tortuosity in the rat cortex after traumatic injury. *Magn Reson Med*. 2002;48(6):994–1003.

123. Lin CP, Tseng WY, Cheng HC, et al. Validation of diffusion tensor magnetic resonance axonal fiber imaging with registered manganese-enhanced optic tracts. *Neuroimage*. 2001;14(5):1035–1047.

124. Clark CA, Barker GJ, and Tofts PS. Magnetic resonance diffusion imaging of the human cervical spinal cord in vivo. *Magn Reson Med*. 1999;41(6):1269–1273.

125. Bammer R, Fazekas F, Augustin M, et al. Diffusion-weighted MR imaging of the spinal cord. *AJNR Am J Neuroradiol*. 2000;21(3):587–591.

126. Bammer R, Augustin M, Prokesch RW, et al. Diffusion-weighted imaging of the spinal cord: interleaved echo-planar imaging is superior to fast spin-echo. *J Magn Reson Imaging*. 2002;15(4):364–373.

127. Holder CA. MR diffusion imaging of the cervical spine. *Magn Reson Imaging Clin N Am*. 2000;8(3):675–686.

128. Robertson RL, Maier SE, Mulkern RV, et al. MR line-scan diffusion imaging of the spinal cord in children. *AJNR Am J Neuroradiol*. 2000;21(7):1344–1348.

129. Nakada T, Nakayama N, Fujii Y, et al. Clinical application of three-dimensional anisotropy contrast magnetic resonance axonography. *J Neurosurg*. 1999;90:791–795.

130. Barker GJ. Diffusion-weighted imaging of the spinal cord and optic nerve. *J Neurol Sci*. 2001;186 Suppl 1:S45–49.

131. Alsop DC, Schwartz ED, and Hackney DB. *The effects of spinal cord motion on imaging of diffusion and anisotropy in the human spinal cord. in Proceedings of the International Society for Magnetic Resonance in Medicine 8th Scientific Meeting and Exhibition*. 2000. Denver.

132. Nagayoshi K, Kimura S, Ochi M, et al. Diffusion-weighted echo planar imaging of the normal human cervical spinal cord. *J Comput Assist Tomogr*. 2000;24(3):482–485.

133. Ries M, Jones RA, Dousset V, et al. Diffusion tensor MRI of the spinal cord. *Magn Reson Med*. 2000;44(6):884–892.

134. Gass A, Back T, Behrens S, et al. MRI of spinal cord infarction. *Neurology*. 2000;54(11):2195.

135. Stepper F and Lovblad KO. Anterior spinal artery stroke demonstrated by echo-planar DWI. *Eur Radiol*. 2001;11(12):2607–2610.

136. Weidauer S, Nichtweiss M, Lanfermann H, et al. Spinal cord infarction: MR imaging and clinical features in 16 cases. *Neuroradiology*. 2002;44(10):851–857.

137. Fujikawa A, Tsuchiya K, Koppera P, et al. Case report: spinal cord infarction demonstrated on diffusion-weighted MR imaging with a single-shot fast spin-echo sequence. *J Comput Assist Tomogr*. 2003;27(3):415–419.

138. Fujikawa A, Tsuchiya K, Takeuchi S, et al. Diffusion-weighted MR imaging in acute spinal cord ischemia. *Eur Radiol*. 2004;14(11):2076–2078.

139. Loher TJ, Bassetti CL, Lovblad KO, et al. Diffusion-weighted MRI in acute spinal cord ischaemia. *Neuroradiology*. 2003;45(8):557–561.

140. Sagiuchi T, Iida H, Tachibana S, et al. Case report: diffusion-weighted MRI in anterior spinal artery stroke of the cervical spinal cord. *J Comput Assist Tomogr*. 2003;27(3):410–414.

141. Sibon I, Menegon P, Moonen CT, et al. Early diagnosis of spinal cord infarct using magnetic resonance diffusion imaging. *Neurology*. 2003;61(11):1622.

142. Kuker W, Weller M, Klose U, et al. Diffusion-weighted MRI of spinal cord infarction—high resolution imaging and time course of diffusion abnormality. *J Neurol*. 2004;251(7):818–824.

143. Hesseltine S, Law M, Rad M, et al. *Changes in cervical spinal cord anisotropy in multiple sclerosis measured by diffusion tensor imaging. in 43rd Annual Meeting of the American Society of Neuroradiology*. 2005. Toronto, Canada.

144. Demir A, Ries M, Moonen CT, et al. Diffusion-weighted MR imaging with apparent diffusion coefficient and apparent diffusion tensor maps in cervical spondylotic myelopathy. *Radiology*. 2003;229(1):37–43.

145. Mamata H, Jolesz FA, and Maier SE. Apparent diffusion coefficient and fractional anisotropy in spinal cord: age and cervical spondylosis-related changes. *J Magn Reson Imaging*. 2005;22(1):38–43.

146. Ducreux D, Lepeintre JF, Fillard P, et al. MR diffusion tensor imaging and fiber tracking in 5 spinal cord astrocytomas. *AJNR Am J Neuroradiol*. 2006;27(1):214–216.

147. Sagiuchi T, Tachibana S, Endo M, et al. Diffusion-weighted MRI of the cervical cord in acute spinal cord injury with type II odontoid fracture. *J Comput Assist Tomogr*. 2002; 26(4):654–656.

148. Agosta F, Rovaris M, Benedetti B, et al. Diffusion tensor MRI of the cervical cord in a patient with syringomyelia and multiple sclerosis. *J Neurol Neurosurg Psychiatry*. 2004; 75(11):1647.

149. Quencer RM and Pattany PM. Diffusion-weighted imaging of the spinal cord: is there a future? *AJNR Am J Neuroradiol*. 2000;21(7):1181–1182.

150. Selzer ME. Mechanisms of functional recovery and regeneration after spinal cord transection in larval sea lamprey. *J Physiol*. 1978;227:395–408.

151. Cohen AH, Mackler SA, and Selzer ME. Behavioral recovery following spinal transection: functional regeneration in the lamprey CNS. *Trends Neurosci*. 1988;11(5):227–231.

152. Takahahsi M, Zhang G, Selzer ME, et al. *Diffusion MR studies characterize axonal degeneration and dieback in the injured larval sea lamprey spinal cord. in Proc Int Soc Magn Res Medicine*. 2001. Glasgow.

153. Takahashi M, Hackney DB, Zhang G, et al. Magnetic resonance microimaging of intraaxonal water diffusion in live excised lamprey spinal cord. *Proc Natl Acad Sci U S A*. 2002;99(25):16192–16196.

154. Wright AC, Wehrli SL, Zhang G, et al. Visualization of individual axons in excised lamprey spinal cord by magnetic resonance microscopy. *J Neurosci Methods*. 2002;114(1):9–15.

155. Mathews G and Wickelgreen WO. Evoked depolarizing and hyperpolarizing potentials in reticulospinal axons of the lamprey. *J Physiol*. 1978;279:551–567.

156. Callaghan PT, Principle of Nulcear Magnetic Resonance Microscopy. 1991, New York: Oxford University Press.

157. Callaghan PT. NMR imaging, NMR diffraction and applications of pulsed gradient spin echoes in porous media. *MRM Magn Reson Med*. 1996;14:701–709.

158. Assaf Y, Mayk A, and Cohen Y. Displacement imaging of spinal cord using q-space diffusion-weighted MRI. *Magn Reson Med*. 2000;44(5):713–722.

159. Nossin-Manor R, Duvdevani R, and Cohen Y. q-Space high b-value diffusion MRI of hemi-crush in rat spinal cord: evidence for spontaneous regeneration. *Magn Reson Imaging*. 2002;20(3):231–241.

160. Assaf Y, Mayk A, Eliash S, et al. Hypertension and neuronal degeneration in excised rat spinal cord studied by high b-value q-space diffusion magnetic resonance imaging. *Exp Neurol*. 2003;184(2):726–736.

161. Biton IE, Mayk A, Kidron D, et al. Improved detectability of experimental allergic encephalomyelitis in excised swine spinal cords by high b-value q-space DWI. *Exp Neurol*. 2005;195(2):437–446.

162. Chin CL, Wehrli FW, Fan Y, et al. Assessment of axonal fiber tract architecture in excised rat spinal cord by localized NMR q-space imaging: simulations and experimental studies. *Magn Reson Med*. 2004;52(4):733–740.

163. Assaf Y, Chapman J, Ben-Bashat D, et al. White matter changes in multiple sclerosis: correlation of q-space diffusion MRI and (1)H MRS. *Magn Reson Imaging*. 2005;23(6):703–710.

164. Assaf Y, Ben-Bashat D, Chapman J, et al. High b-value q-space analyzed diffusion-weighted MRI: application to multiple sclerosis. *Magn Reson Med*. 2002;47(1):115–126.

165. Mautes AE, Weinzierl MR, Donovan F, et al. Vascular events after spinal cord injury: contribution to secondary pathogenesis. *Phys Ther*. 2000;80(7):673–687.

166. Pan W, Kastin AJ, Gera L, et al. Bradykinin antagonist decreases early disruption of the blood-spinal cord barrier after spinal cord injury in mice. *Neurosci Lett*. 2001;307(1):25–28.

167. Kakulas BA. A review of the neuropathology of human spinal cord injury with emphasis on special features. *J Spinal Cord Med*. 1999;22(2):119–124.

168. Noble LJ, Donovan F, Igarashi T, et al. Matrix metalloproteinases limit functional recovery after spinal cord injury by modulation of early vascular events. *J Neurosci*. 2002; 22(17):7526–7535.

169. Wells JE, Rice TK, Nuttall RK, et al. An adverse role for matrix metalloproteinase 12 after spinal cord injury in mice. *J Neurosci*. 2003;23(31):10107–10115.

170. Schwartz ED. MRI and the evaluation of the blood-spinal cord barrier following injury. *AJNR Am J Neuroradiol.* 2005; 26(7):1609–1610.

171. Runge VM, Wells JW, Baldwin SA, et al. Evaluation of the temporal evolution of acute spinal cord injury. *Invest Radiol.* 1997;32(2):105–110.

172. Berens SA, Colvin DC, Yu CG, et al. Evaluation of the pathologic characteristics of excitotoxic spinal cord injury with MR imaging. *AJNR Am J Neuroradiol.* 2005;26(7):1612–1622.

173. Bilgen M and Narayana PA. A pharmacokinetic model for quantitative evaluation of spinal cord injury with dynamic contrast-enhanced magnetic resonance imaging. *Magn Reson Med.* 2001;46(6):1099–1106.

174. Bilgen M, Dogan B, and Narayana PA. In vivo assessment of blood-spinal cord barrier permeability: serial dynamic contrast enhanced MRI of spinal cord injury. *Magn Reson Imaging.* 2002;20(4):337–341.

175. Bilgen M, Abbe R, and Narayana PA. Dynamic contrast-enhanced MRI of experimental spinal cord injury: in vivo serial studies. *Magn Reson Med.* 2001;45(4):614–622.

176. Cooke FJ, Blamire AM, Manners DN, et al. Quantitative proton magnetic resonance spectroscopy of the cervical spinal cord. *Magn Reson Med.* 2004;51(6):1122–1128.

177. Kendi AT, Tan FU, Kendi M, et al. MR spectroscopy of cervical spinal cord in patients with multiple sclerosis. *Neuroradiology.* 2004;46(9):764–769.

178. Pattany PM, Yezierski RP, Widerstrom-Noga EG, et al. Proton magnetic resonance spectroscopy of the thalamus in patients with chronic neuropathic pain after spinal cord injury. *AJNR Am J Neuroradiol.* 2002;23(6):901–905.

179. Puri BK, Smith HC, Cox IJ, et al. The human motor cortex after incomplete spinal cord injury: an investigation using proton magnetic resonance spectroscopy. *J Neurol Neurosurg Psychiatry.* 1998;65(5):748–754.

180. Falconer JC, Liu SJ, Abbe RA, et al. Time dependence of N-acetyl-aspartate, lactate, and pyruvate concentrations following spinal cord injury. *J Neurochem.* 1996;66(2):717–722.

181. Vink R, Knoblach SM, and Faden AI. 31P magnetic resonance spectroscopy of traumatic spinal cord injury. *Magn Reson Med.* 1987;5(4):390–394.

182. Vink R, Noble LJ, Knoblach SM, et al. Metabolic changes in rabbit spinal cord after trauma: magnetic resonance spectroscopy studies. *Ann Neurol.* 1989;25(1):26–31.

183. Durozard D, Gabrielle C, and Baverel G. Metabolism of rat skeletal muscle after spinal cord transection. *Muscle Nerve.* 2000;23(10):1561–1568.

184. Balaban RS and Ceckler TL. Magnetization transfer contrast in magnetic resonance imaging. *Magn Reson Q.* 1992;8(2):116–137.

185. McGowan JC, Filippi M, Campi A, et al. Magnetisation transfer imaging: theory and application to multiple sclerosis. *J Neurol Neurosurg Psychiatry.* 1998;64 Suppl 1:S66–69.

186. van Buchem MA, McGowan JC, and Grossman RI. Magnetization transfer histogram methodology: its clinical and neuropsychological correlates. *Neurology.* 1999;53(5): S23–28.

187. Petrella JR, Grossman RI, McGowan JC, et al. Multiple sclerosis lesions: relationship between MR enhancement pattern and magnetization transfer effect. *AJNR Am J Neuroradiol.* 1996;17(6):1041–1049.

188. Grossman RI and McGowan JC. Perspectives on multiple sclerosis. *AJNR Am J Neuroradiol.* 1998;19(7):1251–1265.

189. Grossman RI, Gomori JM, Ramer KN, et al. Magnetization transfer: theory and clinical applications in neuroradiology. *Radiographics.* 1994;14(2):279–290.

190. Mottershead JP, Schmierer K, Clemence M, et al. High field MRI correlates of myelin content and axonal density in multiple sclerosis—a post-mortem study of the spinal cord. *J Neurol.* 2003;250(11):1293–1301.

191. Bot JC, Blezer EL, Kamphorst W, et al. The spinal cord in multiple sclerosis: relationship of high-spatial-resolution quantitative MR imaging findings to histopathologic results. *Radiology.* 2004;233(2):531–540.

192. Gareau PJ, Rutt BK, Karlik SJ, et al. Magnetization transfer and multicomponent T2 relaxation measurements with histopathologic correlation in an experimental model of MS. *J Magn Reson Imaging.* 2000;11(6):586–595.

193. Cook LL, Foster PJ, Mitchell JR, et al. In vivo 4.0-T magnetic resonance investigation of spinal cord inflammation, demyelination, and axonal damage in chronic-progressive experimental allergic encephalomyelitis. *J Magn Reson Imaging.* 2004;20(4):563–571.

194. Uematsu H, Popescu A, Zhang G, et al. Magnetization transfer micro-MR imaging of live excised lamprey spinal cord: characterization and immunohistochemical correlation. *AJNR Am J Neuroradiol.* 2004;25(10):1816–1820.

195. McGowan JC, Berman JI, Ford JC, et al. Characterization of experimental spinal cord injury with magnetization transfer ratio histograms. *J Magn Reson Imaging.* 2000;12(2):247–254.

196. Gareau PJ, Weaver LC, and Dekaban GA. In vivo magnetization transfer measurements of experimental spinal cord injury in the rat. *Magn Reson Med.* 2001;45(1):159–163.

197. Logothetis NK and Pfeuffer J. On the nature of the BOLD fMRI contrast mechanism. *Magn Reson Imaging.* 2004; 22(10):1517–1531.

198. Logothetis NK and Wandell BA. Interpreting the BOLD signal. *Annu Rev Physiol.* 2004;66:735–769.

199. Yoshizawa T, Nose T, Moore GJ, et al. Functional magnetic resonance imaging of motor activation in the human cervical spinal cord. *Neuroimage.* 1996;4(3 Pt 1):174–182.

200. Backes WH, Mess WH, and Wilmink JT. Functional MR imaging of the cervical spinal cord by use of median nerve stimulation and fist clenching. *AJNR Am J Neuroradiol.* 2001;22(10):1854–1859.

201. Stroman PW, Nance PW, and Ryner LN. BOLD MRI of the human cervical spinal cord at 3 tesla. *Magn Reson Med.* 1999;42(3):571–576.

202. Madi S, Flanders AE, Vinitski S, et al. Functional MR imaging of the human cervical spinal cord. *AJNR Am J Neuroradiol.* 2001;22(9):1768–1774.

203. Stroman PW, Krause V, Malisza KL, et al. Functional magnetic resonance imaging of the human cervical spinal cord with stimulation of different sensory dermatomes. *Magn Reson Imaging.* 2002;20(1):1–6.

204. Stracke CP, Pettersson LG, Schoth F, et al. Interneuronal systems of the cervical spinal cord assessed with BOLD imaging at 1.5 T. *Neuroradiology.* 2005;47(2):127–133.

205. Stroman PW. Magnetic resonance imaging of neuronal function in the spinal cord: spinal FMRI. *Clin Med Res.* 2005;3(3):146–156.

206. Stroman PW, Krause V, Malisza KL, et al. Characterization of contrast changes in functional MRI of the human spinal cord at 1.5 T. *Magn Reson Imaging.* 2001;19(6):833–838.

207. Stroman PW, Krause V, Malisza KL, et al. Extravascular proton-density changes as a non-BOLD component of contrast in fMRI of the human spinal cord. *Magn Reson Med.* 2002;48(1):122–127.

208. Stroman PW, Kornelsen J, and Lawrence J. An improved method for spinal functional MRI with large volume coverage of the spinal cord. *J Magn Reson Imaging.* 2005;21(5):520–526.

209. Kornelsen J and Stroman PW. fMRI of the lumbar spinal cord during a lower limb motor task. *Magn Reson Med.* 2004;52(2):411–414.

210. Ng MC, Wong KK, Li G, et al. Proton-density-weighted spinal fMRI with sensorimotor stimulation at 0.2 T. *Neuroimage.* 2006;29(3):995–999.

211. Stroman PW, Malisza KL, and Onu M. Functional magnetic resonance imaging at 0.2 Tesla. *Neuroimage.* 2003;20(2): 1210–1214.

212. Stroman PW, Kornelsen J, Bergman A, et al. Noninvasive assessment of the injured human spinal cord by means of functional magnetic resonance imaging. *Spinal Cord.* 2004;42(2):59–66.

213. Stroman PW, Tomanek B, Krause V, et al. Mapping of neuronal function in the healthy and injured human spinal cord with spinal fMRI. *Neuroimage.* 2002;17(4):1854–1860.

214. Malisza KL and Stroman PW. Functional imaging of the rat cervical spinal cord. *J Magn Reson Imaging*. 2002;16(5): 553–558.

215. Malisza KL, Gregorash L, Turner A, et al. Functional MRI involving painful stimulation of the ankle and the effect of physiotherapy joint mobilization. *Magn Reson Imaging*. 2003;21(5):489–496.

216. Porszasz R, Beckmann N, Bruttel K, et al. Signal changes in the spinal cord of the rat after injection of formalin into the hind-paw: characterization using functional magnetic resonance imaging. *Proc Natl Acad Sci USA*. 1997;94(10): 5034–5039.

217. Lawrence J, Stroman PW, Bascaramurty S, et al. Correlation of functional activation in the rat spinal cord with neuronal activation detected by immunohistochemistry. *Neuroimage*. 2004;22(4):1802–1807.

218. Turner JA, Lee JS, Schandler SL, et al. An fMRI investigation of hand representation in paraplegic humans. *Neurorehabil Neural Repair*. 2003;17(1):37–47.

219. Foltys H, Kemeny S, Krings T, et al. The representation of the plegic hand in the motor cortex: a combined fMRI and TMS study. *Neuroreport*. 2000;11(1):147–150.

220. Mikulis DJ, Jurkiewicz MT, McIlroy WE, et al. Adaptation in the motor cortex following cervical spinal cord injury. *Neurology*. 2002;58(5):794–801.

221. Sabbah P, de SS, Leveque C, et al. Sensorimotor cortical activity in patients with complete spinal cord injury: a functional magnetic resonance imaging study. *J Neurotrauma*. 2002;19(1):53–60.

222. Komisaruk BR, Whipple B, Crawford A, et al. Brain activation during vaginocervical self-stimulation and orgasm in women with complete spinal cord injury: fMRI evidence of mediation by the vagus nerves. *Brain Res*. 2004;1024(1-2):77–88.

223. Hofstetter CP, Schweinhardt P, Klason T, et al. Numb rats walk - a behavioural and fMRI comparison of mild and moderate spinal cord injury. *Eur J Neurosci*. 2003;18(11): 3061–3068.

224. Hofstetter CP, Holmstrom NA, Lilja JA, et al. Allodynia limits the usefulness of intraspinal neural stem cell grafts; directed differentiation improves outcome. *Nat Neurosci*. 2005;8(3):346–353.

225. Liebscher T, Schnell L, Schnell D, et al. Nogo-A antibody improves regeneration and locomotion of spinal cord-injured rats. *Ann Neurol*. 2005;58(5):706–719.

226. Bulte JW, Zhang S, van Gelderen P, et al. Neurotransplantation of magnetically labeled oligodendrocyte progenitors: magnetic resonance tracking of cell migration and myelination. *Proc Natl Acad Sci U S A*. 1999;96(26):15256–15261.

227. Lee IH, Bulte JW, Schweinhardt P, et al. In vivo magnetic resonance tracking of olfactory ensheathing glia grafted into the rat spinal cord. *Exp Neurol*. 2004;187(2):509–516.

228. Jendelova P, Herynek V, Urdzikova L, et al. Magnetic resonance tracking of transplanted bone marrow and embryonic stem cells labeled by iron oxide nanoparticles in rat brain and spinal cord. *J Neurosci Res*. 2004;76(2):232–243.

229. Sykova E and Jendelova P. Magnetic resonance tracking of implanted adult and embryonic stem cells in injured brain and spinal cord. *Ann N Y Acad Sci*. 2005;1049:146–160.

230. Dunn EA, Weaver LC, Dekaban GA, et al. Cellular imaging of inflammation after experimental spinal cord injury. *Mol Imaging*. 2005;4(1):53–62.

231. Dunning MD, Kettunen MI, Ffrench Constant C, et al. Magnetic resonance imaging of functional Schwann cell transplants labelled with magnetic microspheres. *Neuroimage*. 2006;31(1):172–180.

232. Basso DM, Beattie MS, and Bresnahan JC. Graded histological and locomotor outcomes after spinal cord contusion using the NYU weight-drop device versus transection. *Exp. Neurol*. 1996;139:244–256.